American Academy of Orthopaedic Surgeons
American Academy of Pediatrics

Essentials
of
Musculoskeletal
Care
4

John F. Sarwark, MD
Editor

AAOS
AMERICAN ACADEMY OF ORTHOPAEDIC SURGEONS

Published 2010 by the
American Academy of Orthopaedic Surgeons
6300 North River Road
Rosemont, IL 60018

Fourth Edition
Copyright 2010
by the American Academy of Orthopaedic Surgeons

The material presented in *Essentials of Musculoskeletal Care,* Fourth Edition, has been made available by the American Academy of Orthopaedic Surgeons for educational purposes only. This material is not intended to present the only, or necessarily best, methods or procedures for the medical situations discussed, but rather is intended to represent an approach, view, statement, or opinion of the author(s) or producer(s), which may be helpful to others who face similar situations. The recommendations in this publication do not indicate an exclusive course of treatment or serve as a standard of medical care. Variations, taking into account individual circumstances, may be appropriate.

Some drugs or medical devices demonstrated in Academy courses or described in Academy print or electronic publications have not been cleared by the Food and Drug Administration (FDA) or have been cleared for specific uses only. The FDA has stated that it is the responsibility of the physician to determine the FDA clearance status of each drug or device he or she wishes to use in clinical practice.

Furthermore, any statements about commercial products are solely the opinion(s) of the author(s) and do not represent an Academy endorsement or evaluation of these products. These statements may not be used in advertising or for any commercial purpose.

CPT® is copyright 2010 American Medical Association. All rights reserved. No fee schedules, basic units, relative values, or related listings are included in CPT. The AMA assumes no liability for the data contained herein.

ISBN 978-0-89203-579-3

Printed in the USA

Cover art
Robert Liberace

Anatomic Illustrations
Scott Thorn Barrows, MA, CMI, FAMI

Editorial Board Disclosures

Contributors

Albert J. Aboulafia, MD, MBA
Co-Director of Sarcoma Services
Department of Orthopaedic Surgery
The Alvin & Lois Lapidus
Cancer Institute
Baltimore, Maryland

Lindsay Andras, MD
Orthopaedic Resident
Emory Orthopaedics
Emory University
Atlanta, Georgia

Sigurd H. Berven, MD

Rebecca Carl, MD
Professor of Pediatrics
Department of Orthopaedic Surgery
Northwestern University
Feinberg School of Medicine
Chicago, Illinois

Brian D. Dierckman, MD
Resident
Department of Orthopaedic Surgery
Emory University
Atlanta, Georgia

Julie A. Dodds, MD
Associate Clinical Professor
College of Human Medicine
Michigan State University
East Lansing, Michigan

Robert T. Floyd, EdD, ATC
Director of Athletic Training
and Sports Medicine
Chair and Professor of Physical
Education and Athletic Training
Department of Athletic Training
The University of West Alabama
Livingston, Alabama

Jordyn Griffin, BA
Medical Student
Medical College of Georgia
Augusta, Georgia

George N. Guild III, MD
Orthopaedic Surgeon
Department of Orthopaedic Surgery
Emory University
Atlanta, Georgia

Stephen C. Hamilton, MD
Resident
Department of Orthopaedic Surgery
Emory University
Atlanta, Georgia

Kyle E. Hammond, MD
Resident Physician
Department of Orthopaedic Surgery
Emory University
Atlanta, Georgia

James S. Kercher, MD
Department of Orthopaedic Surgery
Emory University
Atlanta, Georgia

Yukiko Kimura, MD
Chief of Pediatric Rheumatology
Joseph M. Sanzari Children's Hospital
Hackensack University Medical Center
Hackensack, New Jersey

L. Andrew Koman, MD
Chair and Professor
Department of Orthopaedic Surgery
Wake Forest University
School of Medicine
Winston-Salem, North Carolina

Lindsey Snyder
Knowles, DPT, STC
Department of Outpatient
Orthopaedics and Sports
Physical Therapy
Atlanta Sport & Spine Physical
Therapy
Atlanta, Georgia

Joseph M. Lane, MD
Chief
Metabolic Bone Service
Department of Orthopaedics
Hospital for Special Surgery
New York, New York

Thomas J. Moore, MD
Associate Professor
Department of Orthopaedic Surgery
Emory University
Atlanta, Georgia

Robert Murphy, MS, ATC
Assistant Athletic Director
for Sports Medicine
Department of Intercollegiate Athletics
Georgia State University
Atlanta, Georgia

Shane J. Nho, MD, MS
Assistant Professor
Section of Sports Medicine
Department of Orthopaedic Surgery
Rush University Medical Center
Chicago, Illinois

Michael S. Pinzur, MD
Professor of Orthopaedic Surgery
Department of Orthopaedic Surgery
Loyola University Health System
Maywood, Illinois

Michael S. Sridhar, MD
Resident
Department of Orthopaedic Surgery
Emory University
Atlanta, Georgia

Harlan M. Starr, MD
Resident Physician
Department of Orthopaedic Surgery
Emory University School of Medicine
Atlanta, Georgia

Brian L. Thomas, MD
Chairman
Department of Anesthesiology
Piedmont Hospital
Atlanta, Georgia

Lawrence Wells, MD
Attending Orthopaedic Surgeon
Department of Orthopaedic Surgery
The Children's Hospital
of Philadelphia
Assistant Professor
of Orthopaedic Surgery
University of Pennsylvania School
of Medicine
Philadelphia, Pennsylvania

Contributors' Disclosures

Neither Dr. Aboulafia nor any immediate family member has received anything of value from or owns stock in a commercial company or institution related directly or indirectly to the content of this publication.

Dr. Andras or an immediate family member has received research or institutional support from Osteotech and owns stock or stock options in Eli Lilly.

Dr. Berven or an immediate family member serves as a board member, owner, officer, or committee member of the Bone and Joint Decade, USA, the North American Spine Society, and the Scoliosis Research Society; serves as a paid consultant to or is an employee of Alphatec Spine, Biomet, DePuy, Medtronic Sofamor Danek, Osteotech, Stryker: Pioneer; and US Spine; has received research or institutional support from OREF and the AO Foundation; and owns stock or stock options in Baxano, Simpirica, Providence, Axis, and AccuLif.

Neither Dr. Carl nor any immediate family member has received anything of value from or owns stock in a commercial company or institution related directly or indirectly to the content of this publication.

Dr. Dierckman or an immediate family member has received research or institutional support from Surgical Monitoring Associates and Stryker and has received nonincome support (such as equipment or services), commercially derived honoraria, or other non–research-related funding (such as paid travel) from Synthes.

Dr. Dodds or an immediate family member serves as a board member, owner, officer, or committee member of the Arthroscopy Association of North America and the Saint Lawrence Outpatient Surgery Center.

Mr. Floyd or an immediate family member serves as a board member, owner, officer, or committee member of the National Athletic Trainers Association and the National Athletic Trainers Association Research and Education Foundation.

Ms. Griffin or an immediate family member serves as a board member, owner, officer, or committee member of the Piedmont Hospital.

Neither Dr. Guild nor any immediate family member has received anything of value from or owns stock in a commercial company or institution related directly or indirectly to the content of this publication.

Neither Dr. Hamilton nor any immediate family member has received anything of value from or owns stock in a commercial company or institution related directly or indirectly to the content of this publication.

Neither Dr. Hammond nor any immediate family member has received anything of value from or owns stock in a commercial company or institution related directly or indirectly to the content of this publication.

Neither Dr. Kercher nor any immediate family member has received anything of value from or owns stock in a commercial company or institution related directly or indirectly to the content of this publication.

Dr. Kimura or an immediate family member serves as a board member, owner, officer, or committee member of the Arthritis Foundation; has received royalties from Oxford University Press and UpToDate; and has received research or institutional support from Roche.

Dr. Koman or an immediate family member serves as a board member, owner, officer, or committee member of DT Scimed and Keranetics; serves as a paid consultant to or is an employee of DT Scimed and QRxPharma; has received research or institutional support from Datatrace, Allergan, Biomet, DT Scimed, Johnson & Johnson, Keranetics, Smith & Nephew, Synthes, Wright Medical Technology, and Zimmer; owns stock or stock options in Wright Medical Technology; and has received nonincome support (such as equipment or services), commercially derived honoraria, or other non–research-related funding (such as paid travel) from Datatrace, DT Scimed, and Keranetics.

Neither Dr. Knowles nor any immediate family member has received anything of value from or owns stock in a commercial company or institution related directly or indirectly to the content of this publication.

Dr. Lane or an immediate family member is a member of a speakers' bureau or has made paid presentations on behalf of GlaxoSmithKline, Eli Lilly, Procter & Gamble, Sanofi-Aventis, Novartis, and Roche; serves as a paid consultant to or is an employee of Biomimetic, Orthovita, Osteotech, Zimmer, Innovative Clinical Solutions, D'Fine, Biomimetics, Soteria, Zelos Thearpeutics, and Kuros; and has received nonincome support (such as equipment or services), commercially derived honoraria, or other non–research-related funding (such as paid travel) from Amgen.

Dr. Moore or an immediate family member is a member of a speakers' bureau or has made paid presentations on behalf of Osteotech and Synthes, serves as an unpaid consultant to Osteotech, and has received research or institutional support from Synthes.

Dr. Murphy or an immediate family member serves as a board member, owner, officer, or committee member of College Athletic Trainers' Society and owns stock or stock options in Stryker.

Dr. Nho or an immediate family member has received research or institutional support from Arthrex, DJ Orthopaedics, Linvatec, Ossur, Smith & Nephew, Athletico, and Miomed.

Dr. Pinzur or an immediate family member is a member of a speakers' bureau or has made paid presentations on behalf of SBI, Smith & Nephew, and Ascension; serves as a paid consultant to or is an employee of SBI and Smith & Nephew; and has received research or institutional support from Synthes and Biomimetic.

Neither Dr. Sridhar nor any immediate family member has received anything of value from or owns stock in a commercial company or institution related directly or indirectly to the content of his chapter.

Neither Dr. Starr nor any immediate family member has received anything of value from or owns stock in a commercial company or institution related directly or indirectly to the content of this publication

Neither Dr. Thomas nor any immediate family member has received anything of value from or owns stock in a commercial company or institution related directly or indirectly to the content of this publication.

Neither Dr. Wells nor any immediate family member has received anything of value from or owns stock in a commercial company or institution related directly or indirectly to the content of this publication.

Dedication

To health care providers everywhere—who devote their careers to the health and well-being of individual patients and families, both young and old.

Preface

Essentials of Musculoskeletal Care bridges the gap between what primary care physicians were taught in medical school and what they need to know to evaluate and manage common musculoskeletal conditions. This text is used for immediate, point-of-care guidance in decision making and intervention. Physicians and allied health care providers also often use the images in this text to educate their patients regarding conditions and treatments. *Essentials* also helps physicians decide which cases to treat themselves and which to refer. Since the first edition of *Essentials of Musculoskeletal Care* was published in 1997, more than 120,000 copies have been sold.

Essentials of Musculoskeletal Care is used by physicians in family practice, internists, specialists in physical medicine and rehabilitation, pediatricians, physicians in the armed forces, physicians in occupational medicine, physicians in sports medicine, athletic trainers, physical therapists, emergency medicine physicians, nurse practitioners, physician assistants, residents in family practice and orthopaedic surgery, orthopaedic surgeons, osteopathic physicians, and many others. In addition, although not designed as a textbook, *Essentials* has been adopted as a required or recommended text by numerous teaching programs, both for clinical rotations and for courses such as Concepts in Primary Care, Orthopaedic Injuries, Primary Care of Adults, and Musculoskeletal Clinical Medicine.

This fourth edition of *Essentials of Musculoskeletal Care* has been improved and enhanced with additional illustrations, tables, and video for even greater clarity and ease of reading. All sections and chapters have been reviewed and updated, some completely, and several new topics have been added. In addition, rehabilitation prescriptions with home exercise programs and general musculoskeletal conditioning programs are available in the text and as patient handouts that can be printed from the DVD that accompanies this book. Enhancements to the DVD are extensive, including the inclusion of adult and pediatric musculoskeletal physical examinations and tests. Also new to this edition is the availability of online access to the contents of the book.

I am indebted to the Board of Directors of the American Academy of Orthopaedic Surgeons (AAOS) and to the executive staff of AAOS for their commitment to excellence in education. My thanks also go to the Editorial Board for this fourth edition for their commitment to this project: section editors Letha Yurko Griffin (General Orthopaedics); Leesa M. Galatz (Shoulder); April D. Armstrong (Elbow and Forearm); John G. Seiler III (Hand and Wrist); Craig J. Della Valle and Kathleen Weber (Hip and Thigh); Jason L. Koh (Knee and Lower Leg); Jerome M. Benavides and Thomas O. Clanton (Foot and Ankle); Dan M. Spengler (Spine); David Andrew Spiegel (Pediatric Orthopaedics); and Michael Huxford, who oversaw the rehabilitation content. I also am indebted to the following AAOS staff: Laurie Braun, Managing Editor, and Steven Kellert, Senior Editor, who worked diligently to ensure an updated and accurate professional publication according to a strict production schedule; Marilyn Fox, PhD, Director of Publications, whose leadership and long-term guidance is "essential"; and Mary Steermann Bishop, Courtney Astle, Suzanne O'Reilly, and everyone in the Publications Department who contributed to the design and production of this book.

Once again, we are grateful for the support of the American Academy of Pediatrics (AAP) and thank them for serving as a valuable professional Academy partner in the Essentials project. The comments from the AAP as well as from the internists, physiatrists, family practitioners, orthopaedic residents, medical students, and others who use this book have helped us continuously improve this publication.

John F. Sarwark, MD
Editor

How to Use

Essentials of Musculoskeletal Care 4th Edition

Essentials of Musculoskeletal Care provides concise content in an easy-to-use format. The book chapters are also available online. To access the online content, follow the instructions provided on the inside cover of this book.

Pain diagram opens each section. Shows areas of pain and identifies conditions typically associated with each pain location. Names chapter where condition is discussed.

Table of contents lists conditions in alphabetic order and indicates topics with an accompanying video on the DVD.

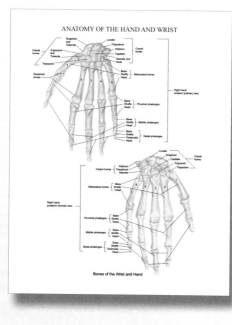

Anatomic art at beginning of section for handy reference.

Physical examination shows photographs and step-by-step descriptions of physical examination maneuvers: inspection and palpation, range of motion, muscle testing, and special tests. Symbol indicates that videos are available on the DVD.

Conditions chapters include:

a. ICD-9 codes
b. Synonyms
c. Clinical symptoms
d. Physical examination pearls
e. Diagnostic tests
f. Differential diagnosis
g. Adverse outcomes of the disease
h. Treatment
i. Rehabilitation prescription
j. Adverse outcomes of treatment
k. Referral decisions/Red flags

Home exercise program includes:

a. Symbol indicating customizable pdf of the home exercise program is available on the DVD and can be printed from your computer
b. Handy table of exercises
c. Step-by-step instructions and illustrations

Procedures include:

a. CPT code(s)
b Symbol indicating video is available on the DVD
c. List of materials
d. Step-by-step instructions

Table of Contents

SECTION ONE

General Orthopaedics

SECTION TWO

Shoulder

SECTION FIVE

Hip and Thigh

SECTION SIX

Knee and Lower Leg

SECTION EIGHT

Spine

SECTION NINE

Pediatric Orthopaedics

PAIN DIAGRAM
General Orthopaedics

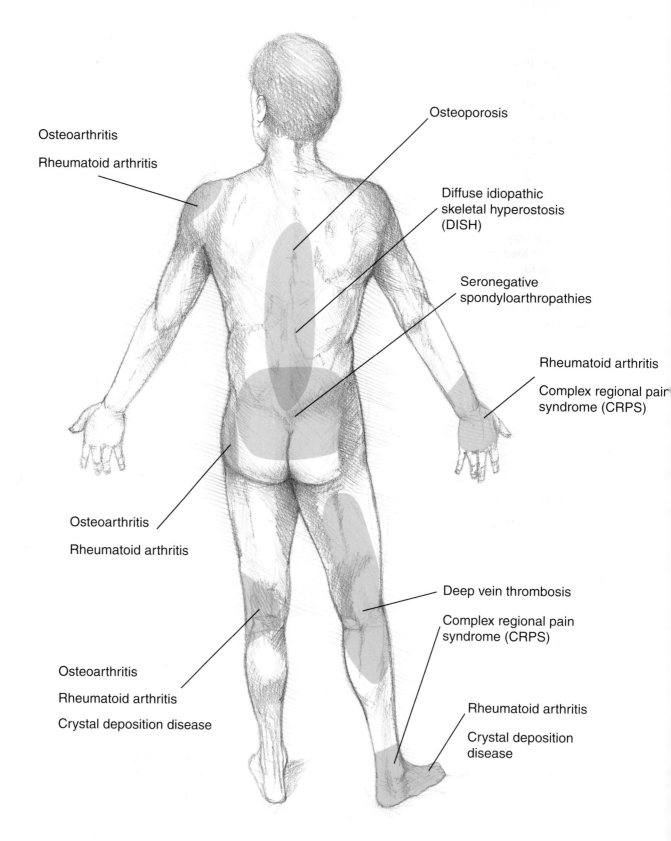

Osteoporosis

Osteoarthritis

Rheumatoid arthritis

Diffuse idiopathic skeletal hyperostosis (DISH)

Seronegative spondyloarthropathies

Rheumatoid arthritis

Complex regional pain syndrome (CRPS)

Osteoarthritis

Rheumatoid arthritis

Deep vein thrombosis

Complex regional pain syndrome (CRPS)

Osteoarthritis

Rheumatoid arthritis

Crystal deposition disease

Rheumatoid arthritis

Crystal deposition disease

General Orthopaedics

Section Editor

Letha Y. Griffin, MD, PhD
Team Physician
Georgia State University
Department of Sports Medicine
Peachtree Orthopaedic Clinic
Atlanta, GA

Contributors

...ert J. Alboulafia, MD, MBA
...-Director of Sarcoma Services
Department of
Orthopaedic Surgery
The Alvin & Lois Lapidus
Cancer Institute
Baltimore, MD

Lindsay Andras, MD
Orthopaedic Resident
Emory Orthopaedics
Emory University
Atlanta, GA

Brian D. Dierckman, MD
Resident
Department of
Orthopaedic Surgery
Emory University
Atlanta, GA

Julie A. Dodds, MD
Associate Clinical Professor
College of Human Medicine
Michigan State University
East Lansing, MI

Jordyn Griffin, BA
Medical Student
Medical College of Georgia
Augusta, GA

George N. Guild III, MD
Orthopaedic Surgeon
Department of
Orthopaedic Surgery
Emory University
Atlanta, GA

Stephen C. Hamilton, MD
Resident
Department of
Orthopaedic Surgery
Emory University
Atlanta, GA

Kyle E. Hammond, MD
Resident Physician
Department of
Orthopedic Surgery
Emory University
Atlanta, GA

Michael Huxford, MEd, ATC, CSCS
Sports Medicine Coordinator
Rehabilitative Services
Institute for Sports Medicine
Children's Memorial Hospital
Chicago, IL

James S. Kercher, MD
Department of
Orthopaedic Surgery
Emory Univesrity
Atlanta, GA

L. Andrew Koman, MD
Chair and Professor
Department of
Orthopaedic Surgery
Wake Forest University
School of Medicine
Winston-Salem, NC

Lindsey Snyder Knowles, DPT, STC
Department of Outpatient
Orthopaedics and Sports
Physical Therapy
Atlanta Sport & Spine Physical
Therapy
Atlanta, GA

Joseph M. Lane, MD
Chief
Metabolic Bone Service
Department of Orthopaedics
Hospital for Special Surgery
New York, NY

Thomas J. Moore, MD
Associate Professor
Department of
Orthopaedic Surgery
Emory University
Atlanta, GA

Robert Murphy, MS, ATC
Assistant Athletic Director for
Sports Medicine
Department of
Intercollegiate Athletics
Georgia State University
Atlanta, GA

Michael S. Pinzur, MD
Professor of Orthopaedic Surgery
Department of
Orthopaedic Surgery
Loyola University Health System
Maywood, IL

Michael S. Sridhar, MD
Resident
Department of
Orthopaedic Surgery
Emory University
Atlanta, GA

Harlan M. Starr, MD
Resident Physician
Department of
Orthopaedic Surgery
Emory University School
of Medicine
Atlanta, GA

Brian L. Thomas, MD
Chairman
Department of Anesthesiology
Piedmont Hospital
Atlanta, GA

ANATOMY—MAJOR BONES OF THE BODY

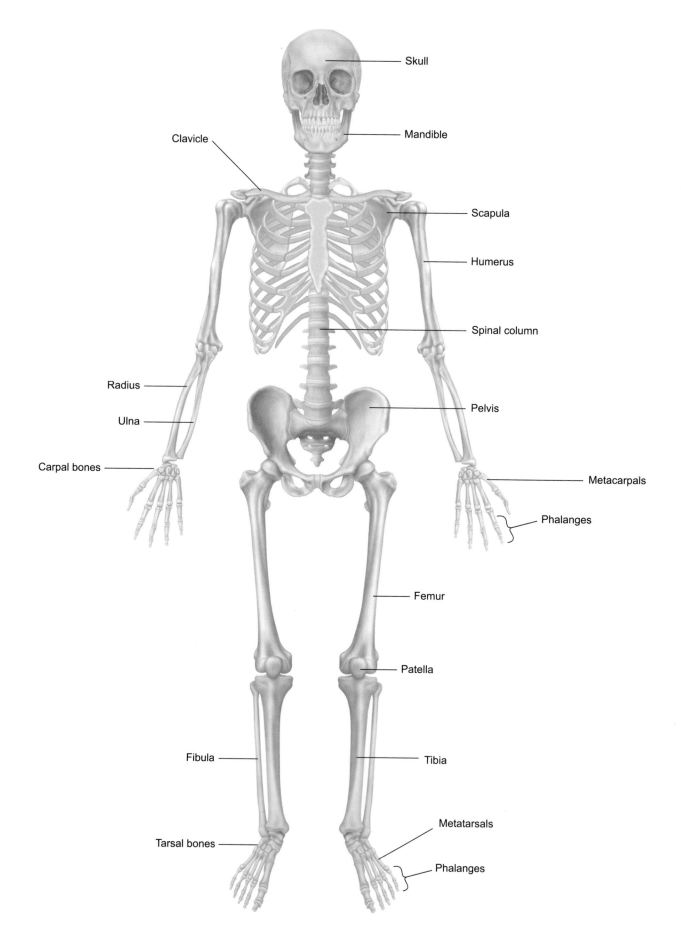

Skull

Clavicle

Mandible

Scapula

Humerus

Spinal column

Radius

Pelvis

Ulna

Carpal bones

Metacarpals

Phalanges

Femur

Patella

Fibula

Tibia

Metatarsals

Tarsal bones

Phalanges

Overview of General Orthopaedics

Bone, cartilage, muscle, tendon, ligament, and their supporting nerve and vascular supplies are the specialized structures that make up the musculoskeletal system. In combination, these structures provide remarkable strength, movement, durability, and efficiency. Disease or injury to any of these tissues may adversely affect function and the ability to perform daily activities. This General Orthopaedics section of *Essentials of Musculoskeletal Care* describes conditions that affect multiple joints, bones, or regions; conditions that have systemic effects; and therapeutic modalities commonly used in the nonsurgical treatment of musculoskeletal conditions. An anatomic drawing showing the major bones of the human body is on page 2; detailed anatomic drawing showing the bones and muscles of the various anatomic areas appear at the beginning of each anatomic section. A glossary of commonly used orthopaedic terms is provided on page 1202.

Arthritis

The etiologies of arthritis range from degenerative processes associated with aging (osteoarthritis) to acute infectious processes (septic arthritis). Likewise, disability from arthritis ranges from inconsequential stiffness to severe pain and crippling dysfunction. Two of the most common forms of adult arthritis encountered in clinical practice are osteoarthritis and rheumatoid arthritis (**Figure 1**). Distinguishing characteristics are listed in **Table 1**.

Other types of inflammatory arthritis include the seronegative spondyloarthropathies, crystal deposition diseases, and septic arthritis. Of these conditions, septic arthritis is the most urgent, as it demands immediate diagnosis and efficacious treatment to prevent joint destruction. Diagnosis typically involves joint fluid analysis and culture, followed by appropriately tailored antibiotics, and in most cases, surgical drainage and lavage. The crystal arthropathies present as acute monoarticular arthritis with an abrupt onset of intense pain and swelling. The seronegative spondyloarthropathies are a group of disorders characterized by oligoarticular peripheral joint arthritis, enthesitis, inflammatory changes in axial skeletal joints (sacroiliitis and spondylitis), extra-articular sites of inflammation, association with human leukocyte antigen B27 (HLA-B27), and negative rheumatoid factor.

SECTION 1   GENERAL ORTHOPAEDICS

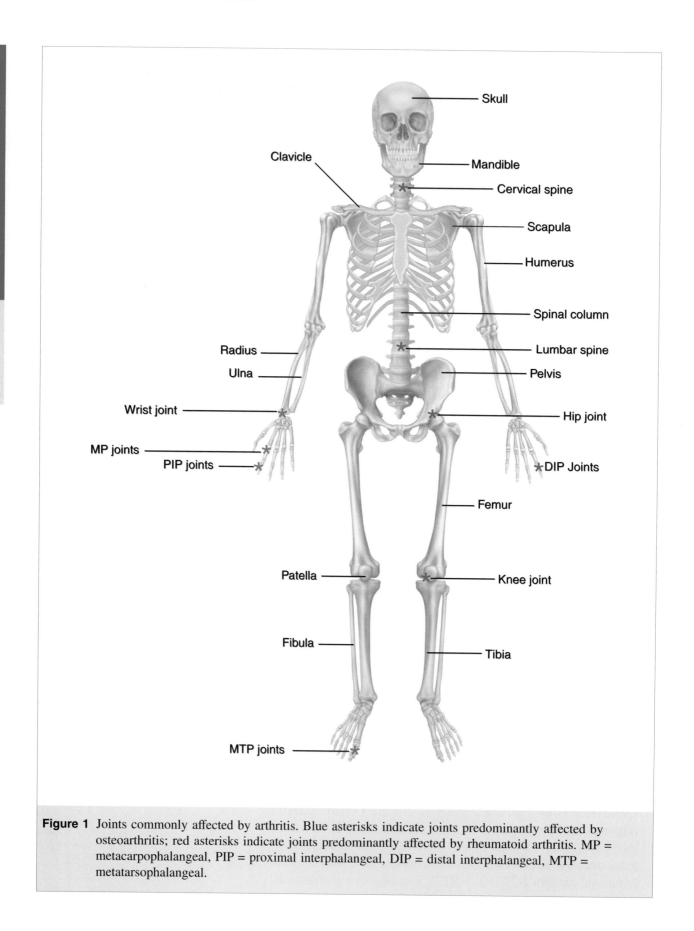

Figure 1 Joints commonly affected by arthritis. Blue asterisks indicate joints predominantly affected by osteoarthritis; red asterisks indicate joints predominantly affected by rheumatoid arthritis. MP = metacarpophalangeal, PIP = proximal interphalangeal, DIP = distal interphalangeal, MTP = metatarsophalangeal.

Table 1   Characteristics of Osteoarthritis Versus Rheumatoid Arthritis

	Osteoarthritis	Rheumatoid Arthritis
Pathophysiology	Noninflammatory, asymmetric, articular cartilage deterioration "Wear and tear"	Autoimmune, inflammatory Cytokines target synovial membranes
Demographics	Most common arthritis Incidence increases with age Obesity History of joint trauma or other joint disease (secondary to OA)	Affects 1% of population 3:1 female-to-male Peak onset in the fourth and fifth decades
Clinical	Increased pain with use, fast-resolving stiffness Classically affects knees, hips, spine, DIP joints Decreased crepitus, joint ROM	Morning stiffness Classically affects MP, PIP, wrists, MTP joints Symmetric and deforming joint erosion Synovial thickening and joint tenderness to palpation
Work-up	Radiographs: joint space narrowing, subchondral sclerosis, osteophytes	Laboratory tests: RF (high sensitivity), anti-CCP (high specificity) Radiographs: bony erosions
Treatment	Exercise and weight loss, NSAIDs, corticosteroid injections, glucosamine and chondroitin sulfate, hyaluronic acid, total joint arthroplasty	NSAIDs, DMARDs, TNF-α antagonists, glucocorticoids Goal of treatment is to prevent irreversible joint erosion and deformity

OA = osteoarthritis, MP = metacarpophalangeal, PIP = proximal interphalangeal, MTP = metatarsophalangeal, DIP = distal interphalangeal, ROM = range of motion, RF = rheumatoid factor, CCP = cyclic citrullinated peptide, DMARDs = disease-modifying antirheumatic drugs, TNF-α = tumor necrosis factor-α.

Bursitis and Tenosynovitis

Sterile inflammation of bursae (bursitis) and tendon sheaths (tendinitis) occurs frequently in adults, particularly following an injury or repetitive motion. Characteristic symptoms include localized pain that is exacerbated by specific movements and is frequently relieved with rest. Classic bursitis locations include the olecranon, greater trochanter, and prepatellar bursae, whereas tenosynovitis frequently affects tendon sheaths of the wrist and hand flexor tendons and tendons about the ankle (peroneal, posterior tibial, and Achilles). Common treatments for bursitis and tenosynovitis include activity modification, NSAIDs, splinting, and the judicious use of corticosteroid injections. Infectious tenosynovitis or infectious bursitis can follow minor trauma, especially if the skin is violated. The cardinal signs of Kanavel (Table 2) signal infection in pyogenic flexor tenosynovitis. Infectious bursitis or tenosynovitis requires prompt recognition with culture (if feasible) of the area and initial treatment with broad-spectrum antibiotics until culture results are known. Prompt referral for consideration of surgical drainage is essential.

Table 2 Cardinal Signs of Kanavel for Hand Flexor Tendon Sheath Infection

Fusiform swelling of digit

Tenderness along tendon sheath

Digit held in flexed position

Severe pain with passive digit extension

Table 3   Major Risk Factors for Osteoporotic Fractures

Not Modifiable	Possibly Modifiable
Advanced age	Low bone mineral density
Female sex	Oral glucocorticoid use
History of fracture as an adult	Recurrent falls
History of fracture in first-degree relative	Current tobacco use
Dementia	Alcoholism
Poor health/frailty	Estrogen deficiency, including menopause onset before age 45 years
Caucasian or Asian race	Lifelong low calcium intake
	Low body weight
	Little or no physical activity

Osteoporosis

Osteoporosis is a common skeletal disorder with significant health cost. Associated fragility (low-energy) fractures seen primarily in the hip, distal radius, proximal humerus, and vertebrae total 1.5 million per year in the United States alone and are a significant source of morbidity and mortality in an increasingly aging population. Dual-energy x-ray absorptiometry (DEXA) is used to screen for osteoporosis, defined as a bone density 2.5 SDs below the healthy young adult mean. Treatment osteoporosis includes modifying risk factors (Table 3), vitamin D and calcium supplementation, and pharmacologic therapy. All physicians should encourage patients to include calcium-rich foods in their diet, obtain appropriate "sunshine" vitamin D, and exercise regularly to avoid the development of osteoporosis.

Trauma

Trauma to the musculoskeletal system may involve bones, ligaments, or tendons. Initial management should include a thorough history; physical examination, including assessment of neurovascular status; imaging; and appropriate immobilization via splinting or bracing. Inspect the skin for wounds that extend into fractures or joints. Open injuries necessitate urgent irrigation and débridement to minimize the chance of infection. Injured patients should be monitored for traumatic compartment syndrome, especially in leg and forearm fractures, as immediate surgical fasciotomy is required to prevent catastrophic sequelae. Following trauma, immobilization of the injured body part provides pain relief, limits further bone and soft-tissue damage, and may aid in the definitive treatment. Injury type and severity, along with patient-specific considerations, factor into the decision of nonsurgical versus surgical management in musculoskeletal trauma.

Musculoskeletal Oncology

Primary bone malignancy is uncommon. Evaluation involves clinical, radiographic, and pathologic correlation. Metastatic bone disease in adults is significantly more prevalent than primary bone cancer. Malignancies frequently associated with bone metastasis include breast, prostate, lung, kidney, and thyroid tumors.

Abuse

Abuse involving children, spouses, or the elderly is a complex social and medical problem. Recognizing abuse can prevent catastrophic consequences; therefore, it is essential that the appropriate social service agencies be notified when a patient's injuries are recognized as potentially from abuse. Child abuse is discussed in the Pediatric Orthopaedics section. Spouse or elder abuse may be identified by recognizing the signs listed in **Table 4**. The complexity of these problems and the seriousness of the consequences demand familiarity with them and with available community resources.

Table 4 Signs of Elder Abuse

Signs of Physical Abuse
Abrasions
Bruises
Fractures

Signs of Emotional Abuse
Overbearing caregiver
New-onset depression
Dementia-like behavior

Signs of Sexual Abuse
Signs of minor trauma to anogenital area
Sexually transmitted disease (STD)

Signs of Neglect
Malnutrition
Failure to take medications
Poor grooming
Bedsores

Signs of Financial Exploitation
Abrupt changes in finances
Failure to pay bills
Suspicious changes in legal documents

SECTION 1 GENERAL ORTHOPAEDICS

Principles of Musculoskeletal Evaluation

Patients presenting with musculoskeletal problems may report pain, deformity, or weakness. General principles for evaluating these patients are described here.

History

The history of the presenting condition should include onset, location, duration, aggravators/relievers, character, and temporal factors tailored to the specific symptom(s) (Table 1). Additional questions about the patient's medical history and family history and a review of systems may reveal clues that suggest the correct diagnosis. For example, weight loss may suggest that low back pain is secondary to metastatic disease, whereas back pain in a postmenopausal woman may relate to a vertebral compression fracture. When dealing with musculoskeletal disorders, it is important to understand the patient's level of function before the injury or illness.

Physical Examination

The general principles of examining the musculoskeletal system, including inspection, palpation, range of motion, muscle testing, motor and sensory evaluation, and special tests, are described later in this section. The specific techniques are detailed in subsequent anatomic sections. When examining the extremities, comparison with the opposite, asymptomatic extremity is often helpful in defining the specific abnormalities in the symptomatic extremity.

Table 1 History Questions Pertinent to Musculoskeletal Conditions

Pain	Joints	Back
Nature: sharp, dull, achy, radiating, associated with fatigue or weakness? *Timing*: increasing, decreasing, intermittent, related to time of day, related to activity, related to injury?	Decreased range of motion? Swelling? Warmth/erythema? Morning or activity-related pain/stiffness? Catching or giving way? Instability? Loss of function? Unilateral or bilateral? Crepitus? Related to deformity?	Radiation to buttocks or legs? Midline versus paravertebral? Sharp or aching? Postural or height change? Paresthesias? Night pain? Bowel or bladder incontinence?

Inspection/Palpation

Inspect the patient's standing posture. Compare the affected extremity with the opposite extremity for any difference in symmetry or length. Note if the patient has any abnormal spine curvature or axial asymmetry.

Watch the patient walk. Analyze the stance and swing phases of gait. Look for an antalgic gait, which is characterized by limited stance phase on the affected extremity. Weakness of the swing-phase muscles—for example, weakness of the ankle dorsiflexors (peroneal nerve dysfunction)—is manifested by a drop foot gait.

Ask the patient to place one finger on the one spot that hurts the most to localize the problem and narrow the differential diagnosis (**Figure 1**). After exposing the area, look for swelling, erythema, ecchymosis, and muscular atrophy.

The affected area should be palpated for tenderness, abnormal masses, fluctuance, crepitus, or temperature changes.

Figure 1 Localizing the point of maximal tenderness (PMT). Patients can best localize a problem by identifying the one spot that hurts the most.

Range of Motion

Measure the motion of the joints in the affected extremity or spine and compare with normal or the unaffected side. Restricted joint motion may herald trauma, infection, arthritis, or another inflammatory process. Measure both passive and active range of motion. A discrepancy between active and passive range of motion may indicate joint injury or may represent an underlying muscle weakness.

Basic Principles

Joint range of motion is an objective measurement. The parameters for rating musculoskeletal disability, whether for government or other agencies, are based on the degree to which joint motion is impaired. Joint motion can be estimated visually, but a goniometer enhances accuracy and is preferred for evaluating motion of the elbow, wrist, digits, knee, ankle, and great toe. A goniometer is less useful in measuring hip and shoulder motion because the overlying soft tissues do not allow the same degree of precision.

Zero Starting Position

Describing joint motion with reference to the accepted Zero Starting Position for each joint is necessary to provide consistent communication between observers. The Zero Starting Position for each joint is described in the examination chapter of each section and in **Figure 2** and **3**. For most joints, the Zero Starting Position is the anatomic position of the extremity in extension.

SECTION 1 GENERAL ORTHOPAEDICS

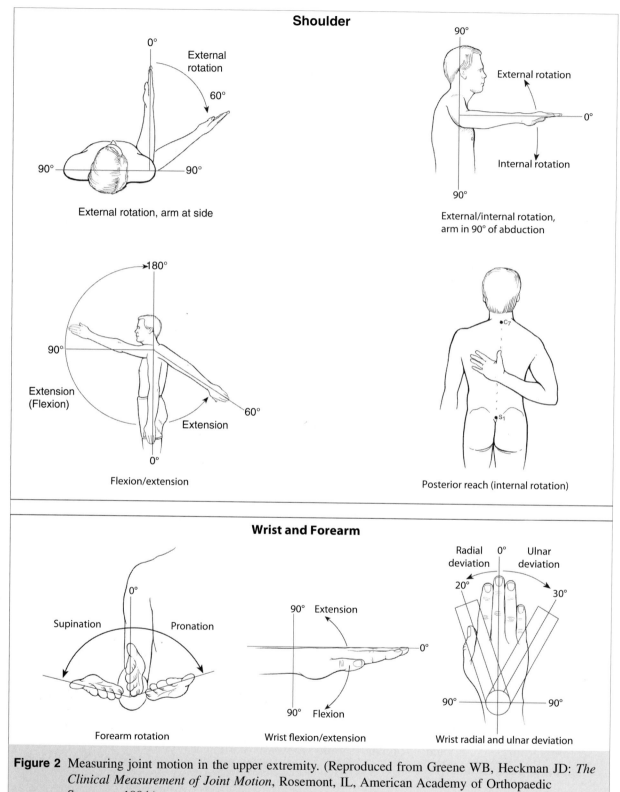

Figure 2 Measuring joint motion in the upper extremity. (Reproduced from Greene WB, Heckman JD: *The Clinical Measurement of Joint Motion*, Rosemont, IL, American Academy of Orthopaedic Surgeons, 1994.)

Figure 3 Measuring joint motion in the lower extremity. (Reproduced from Greene WB, Heckman JD: *The Clinical Measurement of Joint Motion*, Rosemont, IL, American Academy of Orthopaedic Surgeons, 1994.)

To measure joint motion, start by placing the joint in the Zero Starting Position. Place the center of the goniometer at the center of the joint. Align one arm of the goniometer with the bony axis of the proximal segment and the other end of the goniometer with the bony axis of the distal segment (**Figure 4**). The examiner holds the upper end of the goniometer in place while the joint is moved through its arc of motion. At the farthest extent of the arc of motion, the distal arm of the goniometer is then realigned with the axis of the distal segment, and the degree of joint motion is read off the goniometer.

Definitions of Limited Motion

The terminology for describing limited motion is illustrated in **Figure 5**. The knee joint depicted in this photograph can be neither fully extended nor fully flexed. The restricted motion is recorded as either "The knee flexes from 30° to 90° (30° → 90°)," or "The knee has a 30° flexion contracture with further flexion to 90° (30° FC → 90° or 30° FC W/FF 90°)."

Range of motion is slightly greater in children, particularly those younger than 10 years. Decreased motion occurs as adults age, but the loss of motion is relatively minimal in most joints.

Figure 4 Using a goniometer to measure joint motion.

Figure 5 Photographs illustrate the terminology for describing restricted range of motion in a joint. This patient has both restricted extension (**A**) and flexion (**B**) of the knee.

SECTION 1 GENERAL ORTHOPAEDICS

Except for motion at the distal finger joints, it is safe to say that any substantial loss of mobility should be viewed as abnormal and not attributable to aging.

Motion of an injured or diseased joint may be painful. In such a situation, it is better to observe active motion first. The examiner will then know how much support to provide the limb when the passive arc of motion is analyzed.

Muscle Testing

Examination techniques used in muscle testing include placing the muscle in a shortened position and asking the patient to perform an activity that lengthens the muscle while the examiner resists the movement. For example, when testing the biceps muscle, the patient should position the elbow in flexion and supination; the examiner then tests the strength of the biceps by attempting to pull the elbow into extension as the patient resists (**Figure 6**).

Manual muscle testing provides a semiquantitative measurement of muscle strength (**Table 2**). For example, if the patient can actively extend or lift the knee to only 20° of flexion, then, by definition, the quadriceps strength is less than grade 3. A muscle of this strength cannot function against gravity and thus creates a disability for the patient.

Motor and Sensory Evaluation

Nerve root function should be tested if the patient's presenting symptoms suggest a neck or back problem. Peripheral nerve function should be tested if the disorder is localized to the extremities. This is most efficiently accomplished by evaluating one muscle and one area of sensation for each nerve root or peripheral nerve in question. The guidelines for assessing nerve root function are presented on page 901. A guide to the evaluation of the peripheral nerves is outlined in **Table 3**.

Figure 6 Testing biceps strength.

Table 2 Grading of Manual Muscle Testing

Numeric Grade	Descriptive Grade	Description
5	Normal	Complete range of motion against gravity with full or normal resistance
4	Good	Complete range of motion against gravity with some resistance
3	Fair	Complete range of motion against gravity
2	Poor	Complete range of motion with gravity eliminated
1	Trace	Muscle contraction but no or very limited joint motion
0	Zero	No evidence of muscle function

SECTION 1 GENERAL ORTHOPAEDICS

Table 3 Evaluation of Peripheral Nerves

Nerve	Muscle	Sensory
Upper extremity		
Axillary	Deltoid—shoulder abduction	Lateral aspect arm
Musculocutaneous	Biceps—elbow flexion	Lateral proximal forearm
Median	Flexor pollicis longus—thumb flexion	Tip of thumb, volar aspect
Ulnar	First dorsal interosseous—abduction	Tip of little finger, volar aspect
Radial	Extensor pollicis longus—thumb extension	Dorsum thumb web space
Lower extremity		
Obturator	Adductors—hip adduction	Medial aspect, midthigh
Femoral	Quadriceps—knee extension	Proximal to medial malleolus
Peroneal		
Deep branch	Extensor hallucis longus—great toe extension	Dorsum first web space
Superficial branch	Peroneus brevis—foot eversion	Dorsum lateral foot
Tibial	Flexor hallucis longus—great toe flexion	Plantar aspect foot

Other Considerations

Stretch exacerbates pain or contracture of an injured or deformed structure. If a muscle/tendon crosses two joints, then both joints must be positioned to stretch the injured part. For example, if the hamstrings are injured, their involvement is elucidated by placing these structures on stretch (eg, flexing the hip to 90° and then extending the knee). Pain and/or limited knee extension typically occurs with this maneuver when a patient has an injury or contracture of the hamstring muscles.

Tests specific to individual anatomic injuries are described in the appropriate sections.

Amputations of the Lower Extremity

Definition

Limb amputation is the removal of all or part of an extremity through the level of a bone. Disarticulation is the removal of all or part of an extremity through the level of a joint.

Indications

Certain disease states, particularly diabetes mellitus, severe infections, and peripheral vascular disease, are the cause of approximately 70% of all lower extremity amputations. In fact, these conditions account for more than 100,000 lower extremity amputations performed yearly in the United States. Each year, trauma accounts for approximately 20% of lower extremity amputations and tumors for another 5%, with another approximately 5% of amputations related to congenital limb deficiency. Prevalence data, obtained through surveys of all individuals living with limb loss, show that approximately 55% of lower limb amputees and 85% of upper limb amputees experienced limb loss as a result of trauma. The differences between the incidence and prevalence data can be explained by understanding that traumatic amputations more often occur in younger individuals, who typically live with the amputation for many more years than do individuals who undergo amputation because of chronic disease.

Amputations frequently are performed after the patient has undergone extensive medical or surgical intervention to salvage the limb. In these situations, the patient and even the medical team may have a negative attitude concerning the amputation and subsequent rehabilitation, regarding it as a sign of failure. This attitude is inappropriate, however, because most lower extremity amputees regain functional ambulation. Almost 90% of transtibial (below-knee) amputees achieve a functional ambulatory capacity that approaches their preamputation level. Therefore, the physician should maintain a positive attitude and aggressively pursue early rehabilitation, including prosthesis fitting, to allow patients to resume their normal daily activities.

The energy requirements of walking generally increase with more proximal levels of amputation. Therefore, amputations should usually be performed at the most distal level possible; residual limb ("stump") length is sometimes sacrificed, however, to create a soft-tissue envelope that will optimize prosthetic limb fitting and comfortable ambulation for the prospective amputee.

ICD-9 Codes	
997.60	Amputation stump complication, unspecified
997.61	Amputation of stump complication, neuroma of amputation stump
997.62	Amputation of stump complication, infection (chronic)
997.69	Amputation of stump complication, other

For example, an amputation performed at the hindfoot often compromises prosthetic function. In this case, an amputation at the next higher level (ankle disarticulation) may provide better function.

Levels of Amputation and Prosthetic Considerations

Toe Amputation

Dysvascular amputees note no significant loss of function after toe amputation because of their low baseline activity level. Young, active adults with traumatic hallux (great toe) amputations lose some propulsive power and walking stability but are able to walk reasonably well. Little disability is associated with the loss of the lesser toes. Isolated amputation of the second toe should retain the base of the proximal phalanx whenever possible to prevent hallux valgus. In elderly patients, toe amputations often indicate a foot at high risk for ulceration or pressure problems from standard shoes because of poor vascular perfusion and difficulty healing minor injuries and wounds. Therefore, shoes for these individuals should include extra depth and extra width and, often, custom-molded insoles to accommodate and protect a high-risk foot. Following trauma, patients are typically most comfortable in shoes with a more rigid sole and wide toe box to minimize pressure on the amputation site.

Ray Resection

A ray resection includes a toe and all or part of the corresponding metatarsal. A foot with a single-ray resection of ray 2, 3, 4, or 5 will function well in either standard shoes or diabetic footwear, depending on the shape and size of the remaining foot. Amputation of the first ray or resection of more than one ray leads to a residual foot that is more difficult to manage. A custom-molded, multidurometer orthosis is required to load the remaining metatarsal shafts and to unload the amputation site and the remaining metatarsal heads, and it can improve comfort and lessen the chance of re-ulceration. This type of orthosis almost always requires footwear with extra depth and extra width.

Midfoot Amputation

Midfoot amputation is performed at either the transmetatarsal or tarsometatarsal level. Muscle rebalancing at the time of surgery and postoperative rehabilitation can help prevent the two most common postoperative contractures of the foot, equinus and varus. Prosthetic requirements vary tremendously at this level. A widened foot at the amputation site is almost universal, and tenderness at the end of the amputation is very common.

Because of the increased width of the foot, accommodative footwear and prosthetic or orthotic management are usually needed. A low-profile prosthetic device that cups the heel and provides a long footplate will prevent the shoe from folding and putting pressure on the amputation site. If the foot is hypersensitive, or if balance and weakness are major symptoms, a prosthetic device that encloses the calf may improve function.

Hindfoot Amputation

Poor function and difficult prosthetic management are common after amputations in the hindfoot. The retained talus and calcaneus frequently are pulled into equinus, and attempts at weight bearing put excessive pressure directly on the amputation site. Surgical muscle rebalancing consists of reattachment of the anterior tendons and a complete release of the Achilles tendon. Advances in prostheses have improved function, especially for elderly individuals, and household ambulation and transfer skills can be very successful. Even with state-of-the-art prostheses, however, aggressive walking and impact activities are still very compromised with a hindfoot amputation (**Figure 1**).

Ankle Disarticulation

Disarticulation of the entire foot at the ankle and using the heel pad to cover the amputation site is known as a Syme ankle disarticulation. Surgical revision of the bony malleoli flush with the articular cartilage creates a very smooth weight-bearing surface. When combined with durable heel pad coverage, the resulting residual limb usually can tolerate direct pressure and end weight bearing. A prosthesis is required for routine walking, but the amputation site usually can tolerate transfer pressure and the pressure required for a limited number of steps for bathroom activities without a prosthesis, a benefit to many amputees. The prosthesis socket extends up to the proximal tibia region, very similar to a transtibial prosthesis. The foot component must be very low profile because the amputated limb is almost as long as the nonamputated limb. The gait pattern is stable and requires minimal training (**Figure 2**).

Transtibial Amputation

A transtibial amputation is also referred to as a below-knee, or BK, amputation. Various surgical methods are used, but a long posterior flap usually results in more durable padding over the distal end of the tibia and a cylindrical shape, which tolerates prosthetic fitting better than a dramatically tapered residual limb. This durable padding can be very important for minimizing residual limb ulcerations, particularly in patients with diabetes mellitus or peripheral vascular disease. The optimal functional length of the remaining tibia is 12 to 15 cm below the knee joint. Some experts recommend longer transtibial amputations

SECTION 1 GENERAL ORTHOPAEDICS

Figure 1   Hindfoot amputation. **A,** Hindfoot amputation performed at the level of the talonavicular joint. Even a successful hindfoot amputation, as shown here, provides a very small surface area for weight bearing and requires custom footwear to prevent the shoe from falling off. The patient also will have an apropulsive gait because of the loss of the forefoot lever arm, which, in the normal foot, is used during the terminal stance phase of gait. **B,** AP radiograph obtained following a hindfoot amputation shows a too-common result, hindfoot equinus. Bearing weight on the plantar surface of the residual foot is painful and is likely to be associated with skin breakdown.

when the vascular status and skin condition are adequate. Amputation in the lower third of the tibia is not recommended because the padding is simply not adequate below the level of the calf muscle.

Even if walking is expected to be minimal, providing a simple prosthesis and a wheelchair can enhance a transtibial amputee's functional independence if safe transfer skills can be achieved. New developments in flexible sockets are providing a more comfortable fit and better proprioception through improved suspension. The springlike design of dynamic elastic-response feet both absorbs the shock and rotation of impact and actually returns energy at the end of each stride.

Knee Disarticulation

A knee disarticulation extends through the knee joint itself. Like the Syme disarticulation at the ankle joint, the goal of knee

Figure 2 The Syme ankle disarticulation creates an excellent weight-bearing platform. By removing the talus and calcaneus, room is created to place a dynamic elastic-response ("energy-storing") prosthetic foot. **A,** Appearance of the lower limb after a Syme disarticulation. **B,** Canadian Syme prosthesis.

disarticulation is to create a smooth surface that can directly tolerate end weight bearing, improving function. Early knee disarticulation prostheses had two major drawbacks: they were bulky around the knee area, and the prosthetic knee joint attached below the socket at a level lower than that of the contralateral, unaffected knee. Newer prosthetic knee joints minimize these disadvantages and have greatly improved the walking function of patients with knee disarticulations. For individuals who are nonambulatory because of paraplegia, neurologic conditions, or other chronic diseases, knee disarticulation is preferable to a more proximal amputation because it maintains a full-length thigh to maximize sitting support and can improve function. It also minimizes the risk of skin problems associated with more distal amputations.

Transfemoral Amputation
A transfemoral (through the thigh) amputation is commonly referred to as an above-knee, or AK, amputation. Contractures are common following this surgery because the muscle attachments at the hip pull the residual thigh into flexion and abduction. Rebalancing the muscles surgically by attaching the adductor muscle and hamstrings can minimize postoperative problems associated with severe hip joint contractures.

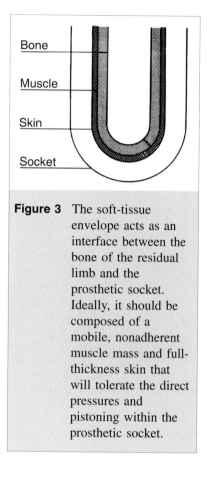

Figure 3 The soft-tissue envelope acts as an interface between the bone of the residual limb and the prosthetic socket. Ideally, it should be composed of a mobile, nonadherent muscle mass and full-thickness skin that will tolerate the direct pressures and pistoning within the prosthetic socket.

Aggressive rehabilitation also is helpful. The energy requirements of walking are significantly higher with this level of amputation than with more distal amputations, and many dysvascular transfemoral amputees do not have adequate cardiac function for functional ambulation using a prosthesis. Also, the transfemoral amputation loses the power of the knee joint, which the prosthesis cannot replace. Therefore, many transfemoral amputees never become very proficient with a prosthesis or may find wheelchair ambulation more efficient.

The weight of a transfemoral prosthesis acts as an anchor and makes transfer more difficult. Therefore, to be a candidate for a prosthetic limb, a high-level amputee should have three skills: (1) the ability to independently transfer from bed to chair; (2) the ability to independently rise from sitting to standing; and (3) the ability to ambulate up and down parallel bars with a one-legged gait. Many transfemoral amputees master these skills within days or weeks of surgery, but others simply cannot. Being able to go a short distance without a prosthesis on the parallel bars or with a walker is an excellent indication that the transfemoral amputee will have the energy to use a prosthesis safely.

Hip Disarticulation

Amputations and disarticulations at the hip and pelvic level lead to significant loss of function. For many individuals, sitting balance and sitting support to prevent decubitus ulcers are the first priority, followed by learning independent transfer and safe toilet skills. The patient should be educated about the importance of mastering the three vital independence skills listed above under transfemoral amputation before the decision is made to proceed with a prosthesis. Even young adults with this level of amputation find use of a prosthesis very challenging because of the high energy requirements and the need to control three joints (hip, knee, and ankle). Many individuals with amputations at this level therefore prefer walking with crutches rather than using a prosthesis.

Principles of Prosthetic Fitting

The soft-tissue envelope over the end of the amputation site is the interface, or cushion, between the bone of the residual limb and the prosthetic socket (**Figure 3**). Disarticulations at the ankle and knee levels can allow weight bearing directly through the end of the residual limb because the bone surface is broad and smooth (**Figure 4**). The soft-tissue envelope acts as a cushion, and the function of the prosthetic socket is simply to prevent the prosthesis from falling off.

In amputations at the transtibial and transfemoral levels, the bone is transected through the diaphysis and cannot accept much

Figure 4 Load transfer in knee disarticulation and Syme ankle disarticulations. Weight bearing is accomplished directly through the end of the residual limb in knee disarticulations (**A**) and Syme ankle disarticulations (**B**).

Figure 5 Load transfer in transfemoral and transtibial amputations. Indirect load transfer is required in transfemoral amputations. This is accomplished with either a standard quadrilateral socket (**A**) or an adducted, narrow, medial-lateral socket (**B**). The transtibial amputation socket (**C**) transfers weight indirectly with the knee flexed approximately 10°.

direct force at the end. With these amputations, the socket distributes the load over the entire surface of the residual limb. With transtibial amputations, much more load is directly proximal to the amputation site over the sides of the amputated limb and the contours of the knee; with transfemoral amputation, the load is placed on the hip area (**Figure 5**). Intimate fit of the prosthetic socket is crucial. If the patient loses weight or the residual limb atrophies, the limb will "bottom out," or drop down in the socket, resulting in the development of a pressure ulcer caused by increased end-bearing pressure. In many cases, a prosthetist can add pads inside the socket to improve the fit of a socket that is too big. Conversely, if the patient gains weight, the residual limb will not fit down into the socket and the end of the limb will swell into the void and create tender, weeping skin lesions from lack of any distal contact. A socket that is too small cannot be modified easily and needs to be replaced.

Perfect, intimate prosthetic fit is impossible; therefore, all amputees experience pistoning within the prosthetic socket, which produces shear forces. Good surgical technique produces a residual limb composed of mobile muscle and durable skin; however, if the soft-tissue envelope is thin (eg, composed of split-thickness skin graft, or adherent to bone), blisters and

SECTION 1 GENERAL ORTHOPAEDICS

shearing ulcers will develop. In this situation, the prosthetist attempts to compensate by using pressure- and shear-dissipating materials and by maximizing the suspension of the prosthesis to the residual limb.

A prosthetic socket can be expected to last 18 months to 3 years, but it should be modified or replaced sooner if the fit is poor. Socket liners should be replaced when torn or worn out, and they do not last as long as the socket itself. Liners made of foam may last 6 to 24 months, but the new elastomeric and silicon liners often tear within 3 to 4 months of normal use. Prosthetic components such as feet, ankle units, and knee units should be replaced when they are broken or show signs of fatigue failure. Typically, the components should last 3 to 5 years, and many have warranties for this time span.

Adverse Outcomes

If pressure problems or pain develops, referral to an amputee clinic, a certified prosthetist, or a rehabilitation physician should be considered. The initial approach for most pain- and pressure-related problems is to adjust the residual limb/prosthesis interface by modifying the socket. If problems persist, the cause may be heterotopic bone, bone spurs, increased pressure or bruising of the residual nerve ending, or the formation of symptomatic neuromas.

Residual Limb Ulcers or Infection

Most blisters, ulcers, and infections are caused by an inadequate soft-tissue envelope on the residual limb or poor prosthetic fit. If these problems develop, the patient should stop wearing the prosthesis until it can be adjusted. Often, simply modifying the socket will relieve pressure points, and this modification, combined with simple, nonbulky dressings, will allow the wounds to heal. Antibiotics are necessary only if the patient has signs of local or systemic infection. Surgical revision of the amputation is indicated when (1) superficial wounds fail to heal within 4 to 8 weeks following prosthetic modification, (2) infection fails to resolve with appropriate antibiotics, or (3) wounds become deep, exposing muscle, tendon, or bone.

Skin Conditions

The prosthetic socket is a closed environment, so excessive sweating or poor hygiene will lead to dermatologic eruption on the residual limb. To prevent this, the prosthetic socket and residual limb should be kept clean and dry. Absorbent powders (other than talcum powder) or creams should be used for this purpose.

Folliculitis, which typically develops in the groin of a transfemoral amputee or in the popliteal area of a transtibial amputee, may be just a nuisance or it may be painful, and it can compromise prosthetic fit. Good hygiene, including keeping the prosthesis clean, can help minimize folliculitis. Treatment with warm soaks and topical agents resolves many mild cases. If cellulitis is present, oral antibiotics may be required. When folliculitis becomes chronic or when cystic lesions develop, surgical excision of the involved skin may be required.

Extreme swelling of the residual limb, similar in appearance to severe venous insufficiency disease, may develop if the socket fit is not intimate. The hyperemic, weeping skin may become very painful and develop superficial infection. Treatment includes topical agents and antibiotics as well as improving the fit of the socket.

Amputation-Related Sensation

Various types of sensation are experienced by individuals with limb loss, including nonpainful phantom limb sensations, phantom limb pain, residual limb pain, and back and neck pain.

Nonpainful phantom limb sensations may include a feeling that the missing foot is wrapped in cotton or that the missing limb is actually present. These sensations can take a variety of forms such as touch, pressure, temperature, itch, posture, or location in space. They also can involve feelings of movement in the phantom limb. "Telescoping," the sensation that the distal part of the phantom limb is moving progressively closer to the residual limb, sometimes occurs. Phantom limb sensations may initially be frightening or annoying, but most individuals adjust to these sensations, and they rarely require treatment.

Phantom limb pain refers to painful sensations in the phantom, or missing, portion of the amputated limb. Early reports in the literature suggested that the incidence of chronic phantom limb pain was low, but it is now thought that as many as 55% to 85% of limb amputees continue to experience phantom limb pain from time to time. Fortunately, however, severe, persistent phantom limb pain is unusual. Phantom limb pain tends to be more episodic and more intense than nonpainful phantom limb sensations. Persistent symptoms are best controlled with antiseizure membrane-stabilizing drugs, such as pregabalin and gabapentin. Modalities such as transcutaneous electrical nerve stimulation (TENS) have been reported as helpful for some individuals, especially for short-term flare-ups, but surgery has not been successful. As in many chronic pain syndromes, treatment often requires multiple modalities. Unrelenting phantom limb pain is best managed as a major causalgia with guidance from a specialist in pain management.

Residual limb pain is pain in the portion of the amputated limb that is still physically present. Existing studies disagree regarding the prevalence of chronic residual limb pain after wound healing. Localized residual limb pain may be caused by poor prosthetic socket fit or alignment, and evaluation and adjustment by a prosthetist often resolves the problem. When persistent residual limb pain is caused by bone spurs, which can be visualized on radiographs, surgical excision is indicated. Painful nodules or masses that cause an electrical sensation when palpated or tapped may indicate symptomatic nerve endings or neuromas. Prosthetic modification to relieve local pressure should be tried initially, but if it is not successful, surgical excision with repositioning of the end of the nerve can help.

Back and neck pain are common following amputation of an extremity. Likely contributing factors are asymmetric pelvic motion, weight shifts, and shoulder motion during gait; asymmetric standing posture; and overuse of the remaining extremities. Such back and neck pain is often more functionally limiting than is phantom limb pain or residual limb pain. A careful examination for spine-related causes of pain is necessary. Treatment typically consists of rehabilitation, stretching, and other physical modalities.

Referral Decisions/Red Flags

Referral for amputation may be required for vascular disease, trauma, diabetes-related ulceration or infection, or amputation site complications. Orthopaedic surgeons, vascular surgeons, general surgeons, and plastic surgeons all may have training in amputation-related care. Orthopaedic surgeons and rehabilitation medicine specialists typically have the most experience with prosthetic rehabilitation and complications. The choice between these two specialists will depend on the individual specialists' particular interests in the care and management of limb loss.

Anesthesia for Orthopaedic Surgery

Anesthesia Techniques

General Anesthesia

The safety of general anesthesia has increased over time thanks to improvements in patient preparation and monitoring and the introduction of modern, short-acting anesthetic agents such as propofol, sevoflurane, and desflurane. Laryngeal mask airways, widely adopted in the 1990s, allow for rapid induction and speedy recovery, especially in the outpatient setting. Expanded use of peripheral nerve blocks and infiltration of local anesthetic agents into the surgical incision reduces the need for potent opioids, decreasing the incidence of respiratory depression, postoperative nausea and vomiting, and prolonged sedation and recovery.

Epidural and Spinal Anesthesia

Epidural and spinal anesthesia techniques for procedures involving the lower extremities decrease postoperative sedation in the elderly and provide excellent perioperative pain control. Despite the advantages of spinal and epidural anesthesia, no prospective studies have shown improved outcomes compared with general anesthesia. Reports of epidural hematoma following neuraxial anesthesia have become more common because of the use of low-molecular-weight heparins such as enoxaparin for thromboembolic prophylaxis, even when practitioners have followed appropriate safety guidelines. Often, patients presenting for orthopaedic surgery are on antiplatelet medication after cardiovascular intervention. The anesthesiologist and surgeon should discuss the plan for management of anticoagulation during the perioperative period. Given the potential for devastating complications, the use of epidural anesthesia has decreased in many practices over the last several years.

Peripheral Nerve Blocks

Peripheral nerve blocks of the upper and lower extremity are effective and may be used alone or in combination with general anesthesia or monitored anesthesia care (MAC). Potential complications of peripheral blockade are less severe than those seen with epidural or spinal techniques. The use of a peripheral nerve stimulator or ultrasound targeting of the nerves minimizes patient discomfort and allows for successful nerve blocks under minimal sedation. Nerve blocks of the brachial plexus at the level of the interscalene groove, the infraclavicular area, or in

Table 1 ASA Physical Status Classification System

P1	A normal healthy patient
P2	A patient with mild systemic disease
P3	A patient with severe systemic disease
P4	A patient with severe systemic disease that is a constant threat to life
P5	A moribund patient who is not expected to survive without the operation
P6	A declared brain-dead patient whose organs are being removed for donor purposes

(Reprinted from the ASA website, www.asahq.org/clinical/physicalstatus.htm. Accessed May 14, 2010.)

the axilla are commonly used for surgery of the upper extremity. Postoperative pain from lower extremity surgery may be managed with femoral and/or sciatic nerve blocks in the groin or popliteal fossa or at the ankle.

Intravenous Regional Anesthesia

Intravenous regional anesthesia is safe, easy to perform, and effective for short procedures on the forearm, wrist, and hand.

Preoperative Evaluation

Medical centers and outpatient facilities have developed their own preoperative testing and screening protocols based on the characteristics of their particular patient populations. Information from the patient's history, physical examination, and other diagnostic tests can identify the patient's risk factors and guide the anesthesiologist to either a routine or high-risk care plan, taking into account:

- The patient's preference and understanding of the proposed procedures
- Procedure-appropriate anesthesia techniques: regional versus general anesthesia, peripheral nerve block
- Need for enhanced intravenous access or invasive monitoring
- Strategies for postoperative pain management
- Perioperative pharmacologic interventions: antacids/H2 antagonists, beta-blockers, inhalers, anticoagulants

The American Society of Anesthesiologists (ASA) Physical Status Classification System (Table 1) is widely used to stratify risk prior to surgical procedures. In general, healthy patients (ASA class P1 or P2) undergoing routine inpatient or outpatient surgery are unlikely to benefit from extensive preoperative testing. Routine laboratory tests are obtained much less frequently in this group. A hematocrit may be indicated for

Table 2 Preoperative Screening Tests for Orthopaedic Patients

Procedure	Indication	Advantages/Disadvantages
Electrocardiogram	Indicated for men >50 years and women >60 years (younger if diabetes, hypertension, or history of coronary disease is present) If normal, valid for 1 year	Inexpensive Many false-positives and false-negatives Most useful if prior tracing available
Exercise (treadmill) stress testing	Patient exercises to PMHR; evaluate for ST segment changes, ectopy	Least expensive of "advanced" screening procedures Orthopaedic patients often unable to attain PMHR due to pain or limited mobility
Nuclear stress testing	Imaging obtained with radioactive tracer at rest and under pharmacologic stress; may show areas at risk for ischemia	Expensive Not always predictive of adverse outcome Requires several hours to complete
Dobutamine stress echo	Beta-agonist dobutamine infused during echocardiography; evaluate for appropriate increase in contractility Wall motion abnormalities suggest ischemia	Relatively expensive Risk of dysrhythmia during infusion Gives information about valve and ventricular function Requires experienced physician to interpret study

PMHR = predicted maximal heart rate.

women beyond menarche and for men older than 65 years. If extensive blood loss is expected, a baseline complete blood count may be helpful. Electrolyte levels may be obtained in elderly patients and in those taking diuretics if renal dysfunction is present. Perioperative glucose testing should be performed on all patients with diabetes. A growing number of studies have shown improved postoperative outcome "in patients in whom blood sugar was strictly controlled perioperatively."

Patients in ASA class P3 or P4 may benefit from preoperative screening for a severe underlying medical condition such as coronary artery disease, particularly if their musculoskeletal condition limits their exercise tolerance. A listing of these tests is included in Table 2. Screening tests have limitations, with occasional false-negatives and frequent false-positives, which may lead to more invasive and costly diagnostic procedures.

Outpatient Surgery Centers

A growing number of orthopaedic procedures are routinely performed outside the hospital setting in specialty surgery centers. Many orthopaedic procedures, short of joint replacement, complex spine surgery, and surgery for severe fractures, may be performed in a day surgery setting. Patients and families often prefer the convenience of these centers to a hospital experience. A single specialty focus allows for

Table 3 Patient Selection Criteria for Outpatient Orthopaedic Surgery Centers

Condition	Criteria
Cardiac disease	Patients with stable angina should have undergone recent (within 6 months) evaluation by cardiologist. Patients with unstable angina, MI, or CHF within last 6 months should be cared for in hospital. AICD patients should be treated in hospital setting. Pacemaker depends on procedure considered
Pulmonary disease	If unable to walk up one flight of steps or on home O_2, consider hospital setting. Severe COPD may lead to need for postoperative ventilation.
Morbid obesity	BMI criteria vary among centers; BMI > 40 may lead to difficult airway, which can be hard for one anesthesiologist to manage. High risk of postoperative respiratory complications
Sleep apnea/airway	Patient with history of difficult airway best done in hospital setting Patient with rheumatoid arthritis on gold, methotrexate, or other immunosuppressants may require cervical spine clearance. Patient with sleep apnea may be safe for outpatient surgery if normal body habitus, but require longer postoperative observation period. Sleep apnea with morbid obesity should be treated in hospital.
Diabetes	Most often OK for outpatient unless in combination with other diseases. Young or "brittle" diabetics may do best in hospital setting.
Pregnancy	Fetal monitoring difficult in freestanding outpatient setting
Chronic pain	Implanted device or chronic narcotic therapy may make postoperative pain control in outpatient setting impossible.
Latex allergy	True allergy best treated in hospital Latex sensitivity usually OK
Malignant hyperthermia	If history of disease or susceptible, should be treated in hospital

MI = myocardial infarction, CHF = congestive heart failure, AICD = automated implantable cardiovascular defibrillator, COPD = chronic obstructive pulmonary disease, BMI = body mass index.

operational efficiencies. Appropriate patient selection, however, is critical to patient safety in these centers, where backup personnel and services for high-risk patients are unavailable. In general, patients who have significant cardiac or pulmonary disease may be better served in a hospital setting. A list of selection criteria is found in **Table 3**.

Surgical Procedures

The various anesthesia considerations for selected orthopaedic surgical procedures are summarized in **Table 4**. Specific procedures are discussed below.

Hip Fracture

The patient who undergoes surgery for hip fracture is typically an elderly individual, often from a chronic care facility, who sustained the fracture as a result of a fall. Induction of general anesthesia must take into consideration the mental and

Table 4 Anesthesia Considerations for Selected Orthopaedic Surgical Procedures

Procedure	Typical Patient/ Procedure Characteristics	Common Anesthesia Technique
Repair of hip fracture	Older patient, often >80 years Impaired mental, nutritional status Analgesia required for positioning At risk for thromboembolism, hypothermia, postoperative cognitive dysfunction	General (spinal in some circumstances)
Hip or knee arthroplasty	Predominantly older patients Congenital, rheumatic, or traumatic joint changes; reduced mobility Obesity, often morbid Concurrent health issues, including coronary disease and diabetes At risk for thromboembolism, intraoperative reaction to acrylic bone cement Disabling pain, history of chronic pain therapy	Knee arthroplasty: general with femoral nerve block Hip arthoplasty: general, spinal in some circumstances Postoperative pain therapy directed by consultant
Knee arthroscopy/ ACL reconstruction	Younger patients Outpatient setting Short procedure Minimal blood loss Significant postoperative pain	General plus local anesthesia and/or nerve block
Shoulder procedures	Arthroscopic or open procedures Beach chair or lateral position Severe postoperative pain	General plus brachial plexus block
Spine surgery	Chronic pain Potential for difficult airway (cervical) Potential for blood loss Need for specialized monitoring	General
General trauma surgery	Nonorthopaedic injuries, such as cardiac contusion, lung trauma, head injury, blood loss Unstable cervical spine Intoxication	General

ACL = anterior cruciate ligament.

nutritional status of the patient and may need to be performed before the patient can be moved onto the operating table. The choice of airway management, anesthetic drugs, and extent of intraoperative monitoring is determined by the preoperative assessment. Some practitioners prefer spinal anesthesia; however, this can present challenges with patient positioning.

Hip or Knee Replacement Surgery

In the past, patients undergoing hip or knee replacement surgery received regional anesthesia. The rare but devastating risk of epidural hematoma with common current anticoagulation regimens now outweighs the potential benefits of regional anesthesia (improved postoperative analgesia and cognitive function in the elderly). Postoperative spinal opioids, given as a "single shot" technique without placement of an epidural catheter, may be appropriate, although effective monitoring by a dedicated pain management team and properly trained nursing staff is mandatory. Patient preference and certain conditions such as an abnormal coagulation profile, previous spine surgery, or morbid obesity (leading to technical difficulty with block placement) may favor the use of general anesthesia in many patients. Intravenous patient-controlled analgesia (PCA) in combination with peripheral nerve block usually provides satisfactory postoperative pain management for these patients.

Knee Arthroscopy/ACL Reconstruction

General anesthesia is ideal for the typically young, healthy patient undergoing a knee arthroscopy or anterior cruciate ligament (ACL) reconstruction. This type of anesthesia allows for fast recovery and discharge from the outpatient center. Intra-articular injection of local anesthetics by the surgeon or the administration of a suitable nerve block often provides excellent postoperative analgesia. Preoperative administration of the popular "three-in-one" block (femoral, lateral femoral cutaneous, and obturator nerves) significantly reduces the amount of general anesthesia needed and provides excellent analgesia during and after ACL reconstruction. The reduced need for postoperative narcotics may contribute to less nausea and vomiting and allow for faster discharge from an outpatient center.

Shoulder Procedures

General anesthesia is the technique of choice for most procedures involving the shoulder. The addition of an interscalene brachial plexus block provides excellent, long-lasting perioperative pain relief and should be considered for rotator cuff operations. The beach chair and lateral decubitus positions require careful positioning of the head and neck as well as meticulous protection of the face and the eyes. Extreme head-up positions may warrant maintenance of higher blood pressure as measured on the arm to maintain adequate cerebral perfusion, especially in older patients. Intraoperative surges in heart rate or blood pressure may be the result of epinephrine-containing irrigation fluid being absorbed systemically.

Shoulder replacement surgery is a complex surgical procedure that is often performed in elderly patients. Because of the length of the surgery and the potential for significant blood loss, close monitoring and adequate intravenous access are required. Postoperative pain control is best achieved with a brachial plexus block.

Surgical Procedures Involving the Extremities

Patients requiring surgical procedures involving the extremities cannot be characterized by a consistent set of features because their age and health status varies widely. Depending on the particular surgical procedure and the particular patient, any of a wide variety of anesthesia techniques and agents may be appropriate.

Most patients presenting for surgery of the upper extremity, the foot, or the ankle will do well with modern agents used for general anesthesia. Also, short and minimally invasive procedures can be accomplished by using a peripheral/field block and MAC. Intravenous regional anesthesia (Bier block) may be an excellent choice for short procedures for the hand, wrist, or forearm. Brachial plexus blocks (interscalene, infraclavicular, axillary) provide excellent, long-lasting anesthesia of the upper extremity. A popliteal or ankle block alone or in combination with general anesthesia or MAC creates excellent surgical conditions for most interventions on the ankle or foot, at the same time reducing postoperative pain, nausea, and vomiting.

Spine Surgery

The most common spine surgery procedures are related to instability and herniation of intervertebral disks. Patients may have a long-standing history of back or neck pain that requires chronic administration of narcotic analgesics, which will most likely need to be continued in the immediate postoperative period. After induction of general anesthesia, control of the airway may require fiberoptic intubation if cervical instability or malformation is present. In addition, the competing needs for surgical exposure and for controlling and maintaining of ventilation and circulation make positioning of the patient challenging. Somatosensory-evoked potentials (SSEPs) are useful in assessing spinal cord function during major corrective surgeries of the spine. Potential problems for the anesthesiologist include major blood loss, air embolism, pneumothorax, ventilation perfusion mismatch, and injury to face and eyes when the patient is in the prone position. Postoperative bleeding with formation of a hematoma in the neck requires immediate decompression, as would any bleeding in or around the spinal canal that compromises cord function. Postoperative pain can be significant and is best treated with PCA; help from a pain consultant is often required.

Arthritis: Osteoarthritis

Synonyms

Degenerative joint disease
Osteoarthrosis
Wear-and-tear arthritis

Definition

Osteoarthritis (OA), or osteoarthrosis, is a progressive, irreversible condition involving loss of articular cartilage that leads to pain and sometimes deformity, principally in the weight-bearing joints of the lower extremities and spine. It is the most common type of arthritis and is associated with genetics, age, obesity, and previous trauma or other disorders that change the mechanics of the joint.

Clinical Symptoms

The common symptoms of OA are stiffness, pain, and deformity. Even when a joint effusion is present, the patient will commonly report stiffness rather than swelling. Swelling in the back of the knee (a Baker cyst) is a common cause of posterior knee pain. OA occurs frequently in the fingers, knees, hips, and spine and is relatively rare in the elbow, wrist, and ankle. The most common reason patients seek medical attention for OA is joint pain. The pain is deep, poorly localized, and aching and is exacerbated by activity and relieved by rest. Initial signs include decrease in range of motion that may be caused by a loss of cartilage, muscle spasm, and joint capsule contraction. Osteophytes (bone spurs) and articular cartilage fragments also may decrease motion, and the patient may report grating, catching, and grinding (crepitus). With disease progression, pain is noted with less activity and may eventually occur at rest and at night. Joints may enlarge as the disease progresses secondary to adaptive changes in the bone such as sclerosis (increased density of bone) or osteophyte formation. Adaptive changes occur as the articular cartilage pad becomes thinned and the stress to the bone beneath increases. Osteophytes may block motion in advanced disease. The patient may report that changes in symptoms correlate with changes in weather, but the results of studies on the effects of barometric pressure, temperature, and precipitation on OA have been conflicting.

Figure 1 **A,** Photograph of the hands of a patient with osteoarthritis (OA). Note the prominences at the distal interphalangeal joint caused by osteophytes (arrow). These are called Heberden nodes and are characteristic of OA of the hands. **B,** Close-up of little finger with Heberden nodes (arrows).

Tests

Physical Examination

On physical examination, a joint with OA may be tender to palpation and have bone spurs and limited range of motion. An effusion may be present that, on analysis, demonstrates mild pleocytosis, normal viscosity, and slightly elevated protein. Range of motion of the joint may be decreased. The loss of motion typically is mild unless the disease is severe. Joint crepitus (grinding) is a common finding; it results from softening of the articular cartilage.

In the hand, limited range of motion with distal interphalangeal (DIP) and proximal interphalangeal (PIP) joint enlargement is common (Heberden and Bouchard nodes, respectively) (**Figure 1**). OA of the first carpometacarpal joint is common and presents with swelling, bony enlargement of the joint, and restricted motion; the typical deformity is illustrated in **Figure 2**.

Common sites of OA in the foot are the first metatarsophalangeal joint (hallux valgus and rigidus) (**Figures 3A and 3B**), the subtalar joints, and the articulations between the talus, calcaneus, and navicular bones.

In the knee, genu varum (bowleg) or genu valgum (knock-knee) can result from loss of articular cartilage in the medial (genu varum) or lateral (genu valgum) knee compartment. The varus knee is much more common than the valgus knee. Patellofemoral disease also is common, and joint crepitus often can be felt when palpating the patella while taking the knee through range of motion. A Baker cyst can occur with a knee effusion. This fluid-filled cavity communicates with the joint between the interval of the gastrocnemius and semimembranosus muscles.

SECTION 1 GENERAL ORTHOPAEDICS

Figure 2 Carpometacarpal arthritis of the thumb. **A,** Clinical photograph. Note the typical deformity of adduction of the metacarpal and compensatory hyperextension of the metacarpophalangeal joint. **B,** Radiograph of the hand demonstrates sclerosis (dense bone, arrows), joint space narrowing, osteophytic spur, and cystic changes of the carpometacarpal joint of the thumb.

Figure 3 **A,** AP radiograph of foot with hallux valgus and OA. **B,** Weight-bearing AP view of the forefoot shows hallux rigidus (or OA) of the metatarsophalangeal joint of the great toe. Note the joint space narrowing (black arrow), subchondral sclerosis, and medial and lateral osteophytes (white arrows).

With OA of the hip, the patient often walks "toes out," with the limb externally rotated, and tilts or lurches to the affected side with each step. Patients often have pain that radiates to the groin or to the anterior knee as well as pain on internal rotation. Internal rotation also may be limited.

Figure 4 Radiographs of a knee with OA. **A,** AP view shows joint space narrowing in the medial compartment (black arrows) and osteophyte formation (white arrows), characteristic of OA. **B,** Lateral view shows joint space narrowing (black arrows) and osteophyte formation in the posterior femur and off the superior aspect of the patella (white arrows). (Reproduced from Johnson TR, Steinbach LS, eds: *Essentials of Musculoskeletal Imaging.* Rosemont, IL, American Academy of Orthopaedic Surgeons, 2004, p 531.)

Figure 5 Coronal MRI of a knee with OA. Note the decreased joint space (white arrow), flattening of the joint surface (asterisk), osteophyte formation at the joint margin (black arrow), subchondral cyst (black arrowhead), and marrow edema (white arrowhead).

GENERAL ORTHOPAEDICS

SECTION 1

Diagnostic Tests

Radiographs of the affected joint demonstrate loss of joint space, sclerosis, subchondral cysts, and/or osteophytes (bone spurs) at the joint margin (**Figures 4A** and **4B**). Radiographs confirm the disease, but the correlation between the patient's symptoms and findings on radiographs varies. Radiographs are not sensitive in detecting early OA, but they are quite specific when osteoarthritic changes are present. Advanced imaging (MRI, CT, etc) is usually not required if classic signs of OA are present on radiographs. MRI obtained in a patient with moderate to severe OA typically reveals decreased articular cartilage space, subchondral cysts, osteochondral defects, and marrow edema (**Figure 5**).

Differential Diagnosis

- Charcot joint (primarily foot and ankle, diabetic neuropathy)
- Chondrocalcinosis (crystals in joint aspirate)
- Degenerative changes secondary to inflammatory arthritis (positive rheumatoid factor)
- Epiphyseal dysplasia (short stature)
- Hemochromatosis (abnormal liver function studies)
- Hemophilia (bleeding tendency)

- Ochronosis (dark urine and pigmentation of cartilage, skin, and/or sclera)
- Osteonecrosis (areas of bone infarcts seen on routine radiographs and/or MRIs)

Adverse Outcomes of the Disease

Pain, deformity, loss of joint motion, loss of limb function, and joint instability are possible. The natural history of OA is classically described as relentless with progressive degeneration of articular cartilage; however, longitudinal studies in patients with OA of the hip and knee report that over a 10-year period, one third to two thirds of patients do not have radiographic progression. Radiographic findings and patient presentation do not always correlate. Over time, OA may remain stable, have periods of symptomatic improvement, or have periods of rapid progression of symptoms and radiographic appearance.

Treatment

Nonpharmacologic treatment includes continued reassurance, patient education, and avoiding activities that cause intense torsional and impact loading of joints. Weight reduction is an essential part of the treatment of lower extremity arthritis in the obese patient. Weight reduction is critical in arthritis prevention programs. A 10-pound weight loss over 10 years may decrease the risk for OA development by 50%. Joint protection is an important concept that includes exercises that do not cyclically load the joint. Gentle, regular joint exercises help maintain function as strong muscle can protect the joint. Water exercise, bicycling, tai chi, and use of an elliptical machine provide nonimpact exercise that can help to reduce symptoms and preserve muscle support in the affected joints without causing increased stress to the joint. Isometric exercises improve strength if patients are unable to tolerate exercises involving joint motion. Data on outcomes regarding rehabilitation show that a standardized knee exercise program can improve pain, function, and stiffness.

Resting the joint is reasonable for acute pain but should not exceed 12 to 24 hours to prevent muscle atrophy and loss of range of motion. Shock-absorbing heel inserts can help decrease weight-bearing stress to the joints of the lower extremities. Braces also may help decrease forces to the joint in some patients; however, the brace should not be too tight, because this will decrease circulation and can increase the risk of deep vein thrombosis (DVT).

Pharmacologic treatment is indicated for patients who do not respond to nonpharmacologic treatment (**Table 1**). NSAIDs are indicated for inflammatory OA and should be given prior to

Table 1 Pharmacologic Treatment for Osteoarthritis

Drug	Administration	Indications	Comments
NSAIDs (aspirin, ibuprofen, naproxen)	Oral	Inflammatory OA	Contraindications include stomach ulcers, reflux, and liver or kidney disease. Mechanism: NSAIDs block prostaglandin production.
Acetaminophen	Oral; up to 4 g/d	Hip and knee OA	Hepatotoxicity can occur, especially with alcohol use.
COX-2 selective NSAIDs (celecoxib)	Oral	Pain not controlled with acetaminophen	Contraindications include cardiac risk factors.
Tramadol	Oral or intramuscular injection	Pain not controlled by NSAIDs or pain not controlled by acetaminophen in a person with GI sensitivity to NSAIDs	Nonaddictive
Corticosteroids	Intra-articular injection	OA or inflammatory arthritis with symptoms not controlled by acetaminophen or NSAIDs	Relief duration is variable, as little as 1 to 2 weeks
Viscosupplementation	Intra-articular injection	Knee OA	Anti-inflammatory benefit, but cartilage regeneration is not documented.
Glucosamine-chondroitin sulfate	Oral	OA	Benefit not scientifically documented.
Opioids (propoxyphene, codeine, oxycodone)	Oral	Short-term relief	Addictive Synergistic with NSAIDs Contraindicated in elderly Not for chronic pain

OA = osteoarthritis, COX-2 = cyclooxygenase-2, GI = gastrointestinal.

narcotic medications if the patient has no contraindications. Acetaminophen is an over-the-counter analgesic that is superior to placebo but less efficacious than NSAIDs in relieving hip and knee OA.

Opioid analgesics such propoxyphene, codeine, or oxycodone are beneficial for short-term relief of symptoms and are synergistic with NSAIDs. These analgesics should be avoided in the elderly because they may cause increased confusion, sedation, and delirium. Moreover, for chronic arthritis pain, opioids should be avoided because of their addictive potential. Tramadol, a nonaddictive pain reliever, is useful especially when used in combination with acetaminophen or NSAIDs and has been shown in meta-analysis to be more efficacious than placebo in improving pain scores.

Cyclooxygenase-2 (COX-2)–selective NSAIDs such as celecoxib have gastrointestinal side effects similar to acetaminophen. The COX-2–selective inhibitors rofecoxib and valdecoxib have been withdrawn because of increased risk of cardiovascular events. Celecoxib remains on the market and is acceptable for patients with no cardiac risk factors and pain not controlled by acetaminophen. Adverse side effects of NSAIDs include hypersensitivity reaction, platelet inhibition, nephrotoxicity, hypersensitivity, and central nervous system disturbances in the elderly. Glucosamine and chondroitin sulfate are other popular options for pain management. (See page 39.)

Intra-articular corticosteroids often relieve symptoms, but the duration of relief is variable and can be as short as 1 to 2 weeks. Viscosupplementation injections may be useful for OA of the knee (see page 39).

Joint replacement or arthrodesis (joint fusion) is appropriate when patients with unacceptable loss of joint function or those who have pain at rest or at night that is unresponsive to nonsurgical management. Hip, knee, ankle, and shoulder replacement surgery is especially effective in reducing pain and increasing function. Arthrodesis may relieve the joint pain, but the fusion will result in increased stress above and below the fused level.

Adverse Outcomes of Treatment

Salicylates and NSAIDs often help but are associated with renal, hepatic, or gastric problems.

Removal of prosthetic implants because of infection or loosening may be required in rare circumstances. Patients who have undergone an earlier, preemptive procedure, such as an arthroscopic joint débridement or osteotomy, may ultimately require a second operation (ie, joint replacement).

Referral Decisions/Red Flags

Consider referral for patients who have pain at rest, pain at night, a rapid onset of disabling pain, pain unrelieved by nonsurgical methods, or unacceptable loss of joint function.

Complementary and Alternative Medicine Therapies for Osteoarthritis

Osteoarthritis (OA) is the most common form of arthritis and is a leading cause of disability. NSAIDs are commonly used to alleviate the symptoms of OA, but these medications have significant side effects. For this and other reasons, the field of complementary and alternative medicine (CAM) has grown, especially as it relates to OA. A telephone survey in 1997 found that more than 40% of Americans used some form of CAM, accounting for 629 million visits to CAM providers and far exceeding the 386 million visits to primary care physicians that same year. This chapter reviews just a few of the complementary and alternative practices sought out by patients for the treatment of OA.

CAM Providers

Certification and/or licensing are available in specific CAM specialties (Table 1). The amount of training required for licensing or certification varies from hundreds of hours to several years.

Chiropractic Care

Chiropractic care is the most widely used CAM modality in the United States today, used by more than 50 million Americans per year. The most common applications of chiropractic care are for back pain and arthritis, but chiropractors often also treat extremity pain, including pain from OA. The main focus of chiropractic treatment is manipulation, or "adjustment," aimed at realigning spinal segments. Chiropractic treatment may be beneficial in shortening the duration of acute back pain, but caution must be exercised in applying manipulative therapy to patients with OA and osteoporosis because of the risk of fracture. Although no evidence exists that chiropractic care can reverse the joint degeneration associated with OA, some clinical studies suggest that spinal manipulation may increase range of motion, relax the muscles, improve joint coordination, and reduce pain.

SECTION 1 GENERAL ORTHOPAEDICS

Table 1 Complementary and Alternative Medicine Providers

Type of Provider	Complementary or Alternative Medicine Therapeutic Principles/Techniques
Acupuncturist	The acupuncturist inserts fine needles at points along the body's meridians to correct the flow of life energy, or "chi," to restore health and relieve pain.
Ayurvedic practitioner	Ayurveda focuses on wellness and healthy living through diet, exercise, moderation, and meditation; practitioners advise patients on practices to restore mental, physical, and spiritual well-being.
Chinese herbalist	Herbalists prepare various formulations of herbs in an attempt to restore balance to the body.
Chiropractor	Chiropractic is based on the theory that misalignment of vertebrae is the cause of most neuromuscular and related functional diseases and disorders. Chiropractors use spinal manipulation to restore proper vertebral alignment.
Homeopath	Homeopathy is based on the theory that "like cures like." Homeopaths administer minuscule amounts of natural substances such as herbs, minerals, and animal products in serially diluted preparations in an attempt to induce the patient's body to heal itself.
Massage therapist	Massage uses manual touch to improve health and well-being.
Naturopath	Naturopathy encourages healthy living habits, especially proper nutrition, and allowing the body to heal itself. Naturopaths often work closely with physicians and other health providers.

Acupuncture

Acupuncture is an ancient Chinese practice consisting of the placement of needles in specific acupuncture points on the body to promote the flow of "chi," or body energy, throughout the body in pathways called meridians. Acupuncture has been used for a variety of purposes, including weight loss and smoking cessation, as well as for decreasing pain and swelling such as is associated with OA. Several studies have shown that acupuncture can ease the pain of arthritis, back pain, and fibromyalgia. Several controlled clinical trials suggest that acupuncture is an effective treatment for pain associated with OA, as well as for other aspects of the condition, including diminished joint function and reduced waking ability. In fact, a few clinical studies have shown that people with OA experience better pain relief and improvement in function from acupuncture than from certain NSAIDs.

Qi Xiong and Tai Chi

Qi xiong and tai chi have recently gained popularity for increasing the activity level and enhancing the feeling of well-being of elderly individuals. These ancient Chinese practices, which are based on meditation and gentle movements based on the movements of animals in nature, have been credited with decreasing the rate of falls and hip fractures, increasing circulation, and improving mobility in the elderly.

Magnet Therapy

Relatively inexpensive and easy to use, magnets have become a $1.5 billion-per-year business. Magnets have been used to reduce pain and swelling associated with OA. It is said that Cleopatra slept with a magnet to prevent aging. Magnets often come with wraps or bandages to hold them in place. Little scientific evidence supports the claims that magnets alleviate arthritis symptoms, although anecdotal evidence abounds.

Nutritional Supplements

In the United States, more than one third of the population uses nutritional supplements for health purposes, spending more than $3.5 billion annually. The content of these supplements is poorly regulated, and potential interactions of these supplements with prescribed medications are not well publicized. Also, many supplements are contraindicated in the presence of certain medical conditions. Some studies have shown nutritional supplements to be beneficial, but the physician should exercise caution when recommending any supplement. **Table 2** lists commonly used herbal supplements and the potential hazards they pose.

Glucosamine and Chondroitin

Articular cartilage is composed of chondrocytes, water, collagen, and proteoglycans. OA is associated with a breakdown of the proteoglycans, resulting in increased water permeability and deterioration of cartilage. Glycosaminoglycans are an important component of proteoglycans.

Glucosamine is hexosamine sugar and a building block for glycosaminoglycans. The nutritional supplement is extracted from cow tracheas and is sold in either a sulfate or hydrochoride form. Chondroitin sulfate is a glycosaminoglycan that is found in proteoglycans. The nutritional supplement is usually derived from shellfish. Glucosamine and chondroitin are often sold in combination as over-the-counter supplements, with recommended dosages of 1,500 mg/day and 1,200 mg/day, respectively. Only mild side effects such as dyspepsia have been reported in humans, but glucosamine has been shown to increase blood glucose levels in laboratory animals, and some concern exists that chondroitin may increase clotting times in patients taking anticoagulants. A recent large study by the National Institutes of Health has shown that in patients with moderate to severe pain, relief was noted with the combination of glucosamine and chondroitin; no difference was shown in patients with mild pain. In this study, the supplements showed no slowing of progression of OA as compared with control patients, although other studies have suggested this benefit.

Table 2 Herbal Supplement/Drug Interactions

Herbal Supplement	Common Uses	Potential Problems	Potential Interactions
Dong Quai (*Angelica*)	To treat menopausal symptoms, PMS, dysmenorrhea	Enhances bleeding	Anticoagulants
Echinacea	To treat colds, flu, and mild infections, especially upper respiratory infections	Hepatotoxicity; intestinal upset	Other hepatotoxic drugs; anabolic steroids; methotrexate
Ephedra (*Ma Huang, Ephedrine, Pseudoephedrine*)	To treat asthma and cough, and to induce weight loss	Seizures; adverse cardiovascular events, hypertension	Cardiac glycosides; general anesthesia; MAO inhibitors; decongestants, stimulants
Garlic	To decrease cholesterol and blood clot formation	Enhances bleeding	Anticoagulants
Ginger	To relieve nausea, decrease inflammation	Enhances bleeding; CNS depression; hypotension; cardiac arrhythmia; hypoglycemia	Anticoagulants; enhances the effects of barbiturates; antihypertensives; cardiac drugs; hypoglycemic drugs
Ginkgo Biloba	To improve circulation, especially to brain; for memory loss, dizziness, and headache	Enhances bleeding; cramps, muscle spasms	Anticoagulants
Ginseng	To increase energy and reduce stress, and decrease inflammation	Enhances bleeding; tachycardia and hypertension; mania	Anticoagulants; stimulants; antihypertensives; antidepressants/phenelzine; digoxin; potentiates the effects of corticosteroids and estrogens
Goldenseal	To treat sore throats and upper respiratory infections (as a mild antibiotic)	Increases fluid retention; hypertension; nausea; nervousness	Diuretics; antihypertensives
Kava Kava	To treat anxiety, nervousness, and insomnia	Upset stomach; allergic skin reaction, yellow discoloration of skin; CNS depression, liver toxicity	Potentiates the effects of antidepressants, barbiturates, and benzodiazepines; skeletal muscle relaxants; anesthetics
Licorice	To treat hepatitis and peptic ulcers	Hypertension; hypokalemia; edema	Antihypertensives; potentiates the effects of corticosteroids
SAM-e (*S-adenosyl-L-methionine*)	To treat depression or osteoarthritis	Mimics serotonin; nausea, upset stomach	Drugs that can increase or mimic serotonin, such as antidepressants
St. John's Wort	To treat mild depression, anxiety, and seasonal affective disorder	Enhances bleeding; hastens metabolic breakdown of drugs; contraindicated for organ transplant recipients	Anticoagulants; antidepressants; decreases the effectiveness of cyclosporine, antiviral drugs; digoxin; dextrometorphan; prolongs the effects of general anesthetics; MAO inhibitors
Valerian	To treat insomnia, anxiety	Sedation; digestion problems	Potentiates the effects of barbiturates

This table was compiled by the AAOS Committee on Complementary and Alternative Medicine. The information contained here is based on literature searches conducted in July and August of 2001 and was updated in 2003, and it may not be exhaustive. Physicians should rely on their own judgment concerning the care of specific patients and use this table for general guidance only. Common medical practice is that patients cease using most of these preparations at least 2 weeks prior to surgical interventions. PMS = premenstrual syndrome, CNS = central nervous system, MAO = monoamine oxidase.

S-Adenosyl-ʟ-Methionine

S-adenosyl-ʟ-methionine (SAMe) is available as an over-the-counter dietary supplement used to treat OA and depression. The usual dosage is 200 to 400 mg three times a day. SAMe is synthesized in the body from the essential amino acid methionine. SAMe is theorized to augment cartilage formation by forming sulfur compounds. Some clinical studies have shown SAMe to be as effective as NSAIDs in relieving pain and to have fewer side effects, but more evidence is needed to prove whether it promotes cartilage repair.

Methylsulfonylmethane

Methylsulfonylmethane (MSM) is a sulfur compound formed in the breakdown of dimethyl sulfoxide (DMSO). It is sold as an over-the-counter nutritional supplement and lotion that has been touted as a "cure" for arthritis. DMSO has been widely used in veterinary medicine for musculoskeletal problems, including arthritis. Both DMSO and MSM are proposed to act as potent anti-inflammatories. Results of a few clinical studies have shown that MSM modestly reduced pain and swelling associated with OA.

Omega-3 Fatty Acids

Omega-3 fatty acids are essential for human health but cannot be manufactured by the human body; therefore, they must be obtained through food or supplements. Certain fish, such as salmon and tuna, are especially high in this nutrient. Extensive research indicates that omega-3 fatty acids reduce inflammation and help prevent risk factors associated with chronic diseases such as heart disease, some cancers, and arthritis. Omega-3 fatty acids have been more extensively studied for the control of symptoms associated with rheumatoid arthritis than for OA, but it has been suggested that they have similar beneficial effects on decreasing stiffness and pain associated with OA. Omega-3 fatty acids should be used with caution, as they may increase the effect of prescription blood thinners (warfarin [Coumadin] or clopidogrel bisulfate [Plavix]), and taking more than 3 g/day of this supplement has been associated with increased risk of bleeding and severe disorders such as hemorrhagic stroke.

Viscosupplementation

A relatively recent development in the treatment of OA is viscosupplementation. This involves injecting hyaluronic acid (HA) into a joint to improve joint function and decrease pain. HA is a large glycosaminoglycan usually produced by chondrocytes and type B synoviocytes. HA is essential for synovial viscoelasticity, joint lubrication, and joint motion. Patients with OA have a diminished concentration of HA within

SECTION 1 · GENERAL ORTHOPAEDICS

Table 3 Comparative Prescribing Information for Viscosupplements

	Hyalgan (Sodium Hyaluronate)*	Orthovisc (High-Molecular-Weight Hyaluronan)*	Supartz (Sodium Hyaluronate)*	Synvisc (Hylan G-F 20)*	Euflexxa (Sodium Hyaluronate)	Synvisc One (HylanG-F20)
FDA-Approved Course of Therapy	5 injections	3 or 4 injections	3 or 5 injections	1 or 3 injections	3 injections	1 injection
Dose per injection	20 mg	30 mg	25 mg	16 mg	20 mg	48 mg
Description	High-molecular-weight fraction of purified natural sodium hyaluronate derived from rooster combs	High-molecular-weight, ultra-pure natural hyaluronan derived from bacterial cells	Solution of purified, high-molecular-weight sodium hyaluronate derived from rooster combs	Hylan polymers produced from chicken combs by cross-linking of hyaluronan molecules (hylan A + B)	High-molecular-weight hyaluronan extracted from bacterial cells	Hylan polymers produced from chicken combs by crosslinking of hyaluronan molecules (hylan A + B)
Molecular Weight ($\times 10^6$)	0.5 to 0.73	1.0 to 2.9	0.62 to 1.17	6 (hylan A only)	2.4 to 3.6	6 (hylan A only)
HA Concentration (mg/mL)	10	15	10	8	10	8

HA = hyaluronic acid.

*Refer to Hyalgan, Orthovisc, Supartz, and Synvisc, prescribing information. The information given here is not intended to imply a comparison of efficacy or safety.

the affected joint(s). Because it is poorly absorbed in the gastrointestinal tract, HA must be injected into the joint rather than taken orally. Possible mechanisms by which HA may be therapeutic include (1) providing additional lubrication of the synovial membrane; (2) controlling permeability of the synovial membrane, thus diminishing joint effusions; and (3) directly blocking inflammation by scavenging free radicals. Several clinical trials have shown decreased pain and improved function, especially at 5 to 12 weeks after injection.

Currently, the U.S. Food and Drug Administration (FDA) approves viscosupplementation for OA of the knee only, although it has also been used in hip, ankle, and shoulder arthritis. Several preparations produced either from rooster combs or from bacterial cultures are available, with varying molecular weights (Table 3). Intra-articular injections are administered weekly for 3 or 5 weeks, or as a one-time injection of a larger volume of HA. Local reactions of increased joint pain, swelling, erythema, and itching have been reported. Viscosupplementation has been most effective in less severe OA (ie, OA without bone-on-bone changes).

Arthritis: Rheumatoid Arthritis

Definition

Rheumatoid arthritis (RA) is a systemic autoimmune disorder characterized by acute and chronic inflammation in the synovium causing proliferative and erosive joint changes. The etiology is unknown, but it is theorized that an unknown agent activates an immune response in synovial tissue. Genetic predisposition, hormonal changes, infectious agents, and immunologic cytokines all have been postulated to trigger the abnormal immune response seen in RA.

RA affects women more often than men (ratio, 3:1). The prevalence increases with age, with peak onset in the late 40s and early 50s. The arthritis typically is symmetric and most often involves the joints of the hands, wrist, knees, feet, and ankles (**Figure 1**).

ICD-9 Codes
714.0 Rheumatoid arthritis
714.1 Rheumatoid arthritis with splenoadenomegaly and leukopenia

Clinical Symptoms

Pain, morning stiffness, swelling, and systemic symptoms are common. According to the 1987 revised criteria of the American College of Rheumatology, at least four of the following seven criteria must be satisfied for a diagnosis of RA to be established.

- Morning stiffness lasting at least 1 hour and present for at least 6 weeks
- Arthritis (synovitis with periarticular soft-tissue swelling) of three or more joints for at least 6 weeks
- Swelling of hand joints (wrist, metacarpophalangeal, or proximal interphalangeal) for at least 6 weeks
- Symmetric joint swelling for at least 6 weeks
- Rheumatoid nodules (subcutaneous nodules over extensor surfaces or bony prominences)
- Positive serum rheumatoid factor
- Radiographic changes in the hand including erosions or bony decalcification

The onset of RA is typically insidious. The patient reports pain, stiffness, and swelling in many joints. Joints of the hands and feet are usually affected first; proximal joint involvement occurs later in the disease course. The distal interphalangeal joints of the hands are spared from rheumatic changes.

The hypertrophic synovium stretches the ligaments and joint capsules. As a result, these supporting structures become less effective. Erosion of the articular cartilage in combination with

Figure 1   PA view of the left hand of a 42-year-old woman with advanced rheumatoid arthritis (RA). Note the ulnar translocation of the carpus (black arrow); the pencil shape of the ulna (white arrow); the dislocation of the metacarpophalangeal (MCP) joints of the index and middle fingers (black arrowheads); the destruction of the interphalangeal joint of the thumb and the proximal interphalangeal joints of the long, ring, and little fingers (gray arrows); and the arthritic changes in the distal interphalangeal joints (gray arrowheads). (Reproduced from Johnson TR, Steinbach LS, eds: *Essentials of Musculoskeletal Imaging*. Rosemont, IL, American Academy of Orthopaedic Surgeons, 2004, p 394.)

the ligamentous changes results in deformity and contractures such as ulnar drifting and subluxation of the metacarpophalangeal joints in the hand (**Figure 2**) and hallux valgus and claw toe deformities in the foot. Although involvement of the joints is symmetric in RA, the severity of joint disease and deformity is commonly asymmetric. This asymmetry is attributed to increased use of a dominant extremity or protection of a painful extremity. Peripheral joint involvement is almost universal in RA, and 20% to 50% of patients have involvement of central and axial joints. Neck pain and stiffness occur, and with atlantoaxial subluxation, cervical myelopathy develop rarely.

Figure 2 Clinical photographs of the left hand of a patient with RA. Note the characteristic volar subluxation (**A**) and ulnar drift of the digits at the MCP joints (**B**). (Reproduced from Abboud JA, Beredjiklian PK, Bozentka DJ: Metacarpophalangeal joint arthroplasty in rheumatoid arthritis. *J Am Acad Ortho Surg* 2003;11:184-191.)

Table 1 Extra-articular Manifestations of Rheumatoid Arthritis

System	Manifestation	Symptoms
Pulmonary	Nodules, fibrosis	Pleurisy, effusion
Cardiovascular	Vasculitis, pericarditis	Digital infarcts, ischemic mononeuropathy
Musculoskeletal	Nodules, tenosynovitis	Carpal/tarsal tunnel syndrome, trigger finger
Ocular	Keratoconjunctivitis, scleritis	Dry eyes, corneal ulcer, scleral injection

Extra-articular symptoms are more common in patients who are seropositive for rheumatoic factor (RF) and rarely occur in the absence of clinical arthritis. In patients with extra-articular symptoms, anemia, generalized malaise, fatigue, vasculitis, scleritis, rheumatoid nodules, pleuropericarditis, and renal disease may develop (Table 1). Tenosynovitis causes carpal tunnel syndrome in 1% to 5% of patients with RA. Nodules along the tendon sheath may cause trigger finger or tendon ruptures, most commonly in the extensor pollicis longus, resulting in lack of thumb extension.

Both the course of disease activity and speed of joint destruction vary markedly in patients with RA. In most patients, disease activity fluctuates over periods lasting from weeks to months throughout the disease course. In 10% to 20% of patients, however, disease activity does not subside. Remission is rare without disease-modifying antirheumatic drugs (DMARDs). Studies have demonstrated remission rates up to 20% after 3 years of DMARD therapy. Even though disease activity is variable, joint structural damage is cumulative and irreversible.

Tests

Physical Examination

Pain and swelling of the affected joints, along with diminished range of motion and pain elicited by pressure, are the predominant physical findings in early RA. Erythema and marked warmth are not predominant physical examination findings. Synovial hypertrophy causes a boggy feeling in swollen joints. Joint aspirations often produce less fluid than expected because much of the enlargement comes from synovial hypertrophy, not effusions. The characteristic joint deformities seen in RA are late manifestations of the disease.

Swelling of the proximal interphalangeal joints and stiffness in the hands usually occur early. Distal interphalangeal joints are typically spared. Reduced grip strength is common, as is carpal tunnel syndrome as noted by symptoms of numbness and tingling in the median nerve distribution of the hand and as tested by the Phalen test (see page 413). The elbow is the most common site of subcutaneous rheumatoid nodules. Lateral drift of the toes and plantar subluxation of the metatarsal heads are common foot deformities in patients with RA (**Figure 3**). Heel pain can be caused by retrocalcaneal bursitis or tarsal tunnel syndrome, which is caused by impingement of the posterior tibial nerve. In the knee, ligamentous laxity, effusion, and genu valgum deformity (knock-knee) are common.

Diagnostic Tests

Laboratory tests are used for diagnostic purposes and to assess disease activity in RA. RF, an immunoglobulin M (IgM) antibody against the Fc portion of immunoglobulin G (IgG), is elevated in 75% to 90% of patients. Higher titers are seen in patients with more severe disease, but this test is not specific for RA. Anti-CCP antibodies are as sensitive as RF and are more specific. When both RF and anti-CCP are tested in patients with early stage arthritis, the tests are 55% sensitive and 97% specific in identifying patients in whom clinical RA would develop. The C-reactive protein level and erythrocyte sedimentation rate are acute phase reactants that correlate with the degree of joint inflammation. Patients with RA are commonly anemic, but the hemoglobin level is usually above 9.0 g/dL. Platelet counts are

Figure 3 Clinical photograph of the plantar aspect of the feet of a patient with RA. The left foot demonstrates forefoot deformities typical of RA, including hallux valgus, claw toes, and plantar keratoses beneath the second and third metatarsal heads. The right forefoot has been surgically reconstructed. (Reproduced from Abdo RV, Iorio LJ: Rheumatoid arthritis of the foot and ankle. *J Am Acad Orthop Surg* 1994;2:326-333.)

elevated in patients with an acute flare, but serial platelet counts are not useful. Serum albumin has been shown to be decreased in active disease and to correlate with disease activity.

Radiographic changes vary according to disease activity. Common signs are periarticular osteopenia and bony erosion at the joint margin, which correlates with the insertion site of the synovium. Lateral flexion and extension views of the neck may demonstrate C1-C2 instability secondary to erosion of the ligaments that hold the odontoid in place. These findings are important if the patient is anticipating any surgery that involves intubation or manipulation of the neck, as it could lead to quadriparesis or death (Figure 4). Regional anesthesia should be considered in all patients with RA. If general anesthesia is necessary, an awake, fiberoptic intubation may be warranted if significant instability exists at C1-C2.

Differential Diagnosis

- Hepatitis (abnormal liver function tests)
- Lyme disease (serology, rash, anemia)
- Seronegative arthropathies (human leukocyte antigen [HLA] tests, abnormal radiographs, urethritis)
- Systemic lupus erythematosus (antinuclear antibodies, peripheral blood smear)

Figure 4   Images of a patient with RA. **A**, Lateral cervical spine radiograph demonstrates atlantoaxial subluxation. Sagittal (**B**) and axial (**C**) T2-weighted MRIs of the cervical spine show decreased space available for the spinal cord and a soft-tissue pannus posterior to the odontoid. The line on the inset indicates the level at which the image was obtained. (Reproduced from Kim DH, Hilibrand AS: Rheumatoid arthritis in the cervical spine. *J Am Acad Ortho Surg* 2005;13:463-474.)

Adverse Outcomes of the Disease

Joint contractures, pain, loss of function, loss of ambulation, and multisystem disorders leading to death are possible. Osteoporosis is common, in part related to the disease, inactivity, and steroids that are commonly used in treating the disease. Patients can have impaired immune function when using DMARDs.

Treatment

Drug therapy is the main treatment for patients with RA to prevent complications and reduce morbidity. Analgesics are available in both topical (capsaicin) and oral forms. Oral agents such as acetaminophen, tramadol, and opioids are used in RA, but opioids should be used with great discretion in treating the chronic pain of this disease. NSAIDs are the first-line treatment, providing both analgesic and anti-inflammatory benefits. Glucocorticoids have anti-inflammatory properties and are administered by various routes in the treatment of RA, including orally, intravenously, and intra-articularly. Corticosteroid injections into selected joints and the carpal tunnel may relieve acute synovitis and thereby decrease pain and improve function.

DMARDs alter the inflammatory cascade on a molecular level. Two classes of DMARDs have been developed: nonbiologic and biologic. These drugs reduce or prevent articular damage and the development of joint deformities. The nonbiologic agents include hydroxychloroquine, sulfasalazine, minocycline, and the two most commonly used nonbiologic agents, methotrexate and leflunomide. The biologic agents are produced with recombinant DNA technology and target cytokines or their receptors in the inflammatory cascade. Biologic agents include tumor necrosis factor–α (TNF-α) inhibitors (etanercept, infliximab, adalimumab), interleukin-1 (IL-1) antagonists (anakinra), and anti-CD20 B-cell depleting monoclonal antibodies (rituximab).

Splints and orthoses may help manage acute episodes of pain associated with synovitis as well as position joints to minimize progressive deformity and improve function. Custom shoes are helpful for severe foot deformities. Physical and occupational therapy for modalities to decrease swelling and pain as well as for information on range-of-motion and strengthening exercises should be part of a multidisciplinary treatment program. Selective surgical intervention by synovectomy or tenosynovectomy may prevent tendon rupture and progression of joint deformity. End-stage arthritis requires total joint arthroplasty or arthrodesis.

Adverse Outcomes of Treatment

Infection secondary to injections or surgery; gastric, hepatic, or renal complications associated with NSAID use; and osteonecrosis of bone or osteoporosis associated with steroid use are possible. Skin rash and other side effects of various medications also can develop. DMARDs weaken the immune system, so patients should be monitored for serious infections.

Referral Decisions/Red Flags

Patients whose symptoms persist for more than 3 months or who have uncontrollable joint pain at rest despite nonsurgical care as well as those who have significant deformity or extra-articular manifestations of the disease are appropriate for referral for consideration of surgical options.

Arthritis: Seronegative Spondyloarthropathies

Synonyms

Ankylosing spondylitis
Psoriatic arthritis
Psoriatic arthropathy
Reactive arthritis
Reiter syndrome

Definition

The seronegative spondyloarthropathies—including ankylosing spondylitis, reactive arthritis (Reiter syndrome), psoriatic arthritis, and arthritis associated with inflammatory bowel disease—are a group of arthritides that have common clinical and genetic features (**Table 1**). They are called seronegative because laboratory results are negative for rheumatoid factor and antinuclear antibodies. The axial skeleton is commonly involved, and patients report back pain. Ocular, dermatologic, and gastrointestinal manifestations are frequent. Patients develop enthesitis, an inflammation at the site of ligament and tendon insertions onto bone. These arthropathies share a common genetic factor, human leukocyte antigen B27 (HLA-B27), so a strong familial association exists. However, not all patients with seronegative spondyloarthropathies are positive for the

Table 1 Seronegative Spondyloarthropathies

Disorder	Arthritis Characteristics	Commonly Affected Areas	Associated Conditions	Treatment
Ankylosing spondylitis	Sacroiliitis	Sacroiliac joint; rarely peripheral joints	Uveitis, carditis, enthesitis	NSAIDs, exercise
Arthritis associated with inflammatory bowel disease	Asymmetric, oligoarticular	Sacroiliac joint, knee, ankle	Crohn disease, ulcerative colitis, enthesitis	NSAIDs
Psoriatic arthritis	5 clinical patterns, erosive	Hands, wrist, ankle, sacroiliac joint	Skin lesions, nail involvement, dactylitis, iritis, enthesitis	NSAIDs, methotrexate, biologics
Reiter syndrome	Asymmetric, oligoarticular	Knee, ankle, sacroiliac joint	Iritis, urethritis, dactylitis, enthesitis	Treatment of precipitating infection, NSAIDs

Figure 1   AP view of the pelvis shows iliac sclerosis at the middle aspect of the right sacroiliac joint (arrow). The left sacroiliac joint appears normal (arrowhead). Lack of involvement of the inferior sacroiliac joint excludes sacroiliitis.

HLA-B27 antigen. The strongest association is found in ankylosing spondylitis, with an 88% positive rate for HLA-B27.

Ankylosing Spondylitis

Ankylosing spondylitis is a systemic inflammatory disorder that primarily affects the axial skeleton. Sacroiliitis (**Figure 1**) and kyphosis are seen on radiographic imaging. Ankylosing spondylitis typically begins in the second or third decade of life and is three times more common in men. Peripheral joint involvement correlates with the severity of the disease but is typically less severe than is observed in the other seronegative spondyloarthropathies. The shoulders and hips are the peripheral joints most commonly affected by arthritic changes. Association with the HLA-B27 antigen is high, particularly in white patients, who have an HLA-B27–positive rate of approximately 95%. Systemic manifestations, including uveitis, iritis, aortitis, and cardiac conduction abnormalities, occur in 33% of patients.

Reactive Arthritis

Reactive arthritis is an acute spondyloarthropathy precipitated by gastrointestinal or genitourinary infection. The HLA-B27 antigen has been documented in 63% to 96% of these patients. Reiter syndrome is a type of reactive arthritis that causes arthritis, urethritis, conjunctivitis, and mucocutaneous lesions. Sexually transmitted and dysenteric diseases are common 2 to 8 weeks prior to the onset of joint pain. *Chlamydia trachomatis*, *Shigella*, *Salmonella*, *Yersinia*, and *Campylobacter* are common inciting pathogens.

Table 2 Patterns of Psoriatic Arthritis

Type	Diagnostic Pattern	Commonly Affected Areas
DIP joint	Nail involvement common (5%-10% of patients)	DIP joint
Asymmetric oligoarthritis	Fewer than 5 joints affected, dactylitis	Hands, feet
Symmetric polyarthritis	Similar to rheumatoid arthritis, but DIP joint involvement and negative rheumatoid factor	Hands, wrist, ankles, feet
Arthritic mutilans	Osteolysis at joint	DIP joint
Sacroiliitis	Asymmetric vertebral involvement	Sacroiliac

DIP = distal interphalangeal.

Psoriatic Arthritis

Psoriatic arthritis affects approximately 5% to 10% of patients with psoriasis. The sex ratio is approximately equal, and age of onset is typically in the late 30s. Five patterns of psoriatic arthritis have been described: distal interphalangeal (DIP) joint arthritis, asymmetric oligoarthritis, symmetric polyarthritis, arthritic mutilans, and sacroiliitis (**Table 2**). DIP joint involvement and absence of rheumatoid nodules differentiates symmetric polyarthritis from rheumatoid arthritis.

Arthritis Associated with Inflammatory Bowel Disease

Arthritis associated with inflammatory bowel disease occurs in patients with ulcerative colitis or Crohn disease. The incidence is 10% to 20% and is more common in patients with Crohn disease. The HLA-B27 antigen is present in 50% to 70% of these patients.

Clinical Symptoms

Back pain may be the presenting symptom in all seronegative spondyloarthropathies, particularly in young men with ankylosing spondylitis. With ankylosing spondylitis, patients report nocturnal back pain and morning stiffness that is relieved by activity and leaning forward.

Patients with reactive arthritis report pain in the large joints of the lower extremity. Joint involvement is typically an asymmetric oligoarthritis involving the large joints of the lower extremity. Other musculoskeletal manifestations include enthesitis of the Achilles tendon or plantar fascia, dactylitis ("sausage digit"; swelling of an entire toe or finger), and sacroiliitis. Conjunctivitis and nongonococcal urethritis commonly develop. Other associated lesions include iritis and cutaneous ulcerations. Reactive arthritis commonly resolves in 3 to 4 months, but up to 50% of patients experience recurrent symptoms lasting years.

DIP joint pain associated with scaly, cutaneous lesions is the usual clinical presentation of psoriatic arthritis. Skin disease usually, but not always, precedes joint symptoms. Patients with joint problems commonly have nail disorders, including pitting, ridging, and oncolysis (**Figure 2**).

Sacroiliitis, spondylitis, and arthritis of the knee and ankle are common in patients with arthritis associated with inflammatory bowel disease. Peripheral arthritis symptoms usually worsen during gastrointenstinal flares, but the spondylitis symptoms typically do not.

Enthesitis, particularly at the Achilles tendon insertion, and extraskeletal manifestations, such as iritis, conjunctivitis, and urethritis, are common manifestations in patients with seronegative spondyloarthropathies.

Figure 2 Finger of patient with psoriatic arthritis. Note the pitting, ridging, and oncolysis of the nail.

Tests

Physical Examination

With ankylosing spondylitis, limited spinal motion is common. Measure a 15-cm span in the midline distally from the posterior iliac spine (dimples of Venus) to the upper lumbar region. Then have the patient flex (lean forward) as much as possible. The distance between the two points should increase by 5 to 7 cm (see page 901). With ankylosing spondylitis, spinal motion is limited, and the skin distraction on forward flexion is decreased. The FABER maneuver (flexion, abduction, and external rotation of the hip) places stress across the sacroiliac joint; patients with sacroiliitis have increased pain with this maneuver. Examine the patient's hands carefully for swelling, inflammation, and nail abnormalities. Also examine the patient for enthesitis, particularly of the lower extremity.

Diagnostic Tests

Laboratory Tests

Although many of these patients are positive for the HLA-B27 antigen, the test for this antigen is relatively expensive and usually is not needed to make the diagnosis. The erythrocyte sedimentation rate and C-reactive protein level are inconsistently elevated during acute episodes. Rheumatoid factor and antinuclear antibody tests are negative. A detailed history and examination are more important than laboratory testing.

Radiographs

Resorption of terminal phalanges and proliferative bone reaction are common radiographic findings in the DIP joints of patients with psoriatic arthritis. In diagnosing sacroiliitis, radiographs demonstrating narrowing of the sacroiliac joints can be helpful. With ankylosing spondylitis, early radiographic findings in the spine include squaring of the superior and anterior margins of the vertebral bodies, thought to be caused by enthesitis at the attachment of the anulus fibrosus onto the vertebral body. Later findings include ossification of the anterior longitudinal ligament of the spine and autofusion of the facet joints leading to the classic "poker spine." The spine may be fused along its the entire length.

Differential Diagnosis

- Achilles tendinitis or plantar fasciitis (no associated symptoms)
- Degenerative disk disease (no associated symptoms, normal skin distraction on flexion of the spine)
- Rheumatoid arthritis (positive rheumatoid factor, peripheral joint involvement)

Adverse Outcomes of the Disease

Severe spinal deformity may occur in ankylosing spondylitis. End-stage arthritis may affect the peripheral joints. Uveitis with visual impairment may occur. Occasionally, carditis may cause aortic insufficiency in patients with ankylosing spondylitis.

Treatment

NSAIDs, particularly indomethacin, are effective in controlling symptoms in many patients with seronegative spondyloarthropathies. Tumor necrosis factor–α (TNF-α) inhibitors, such as enteracept and infliximab, are administered to patients with ankylosing spondylitis when symptoms are not controlled by NSAIDs. Regular exercise is important, particularly for patients with ankylosing spondylitis. An occasional patient may require a spinal osteotomy for correction of deformity associated with ankylosing spondylitis. Treatment of the inciting genitourologic or gastrointestinal infection is imperative in treatment of reactive arthritis. Methotrexate may be useful for severe reactive arthritis. Both nonbiologic and biologic disease-modifying antirheumatic drugs (DMARDs) are effective in treating psoriatic arthritis. The dermatologic manifestations of psoriatic arthritis are often treated with phototherapy. Surgery (total joint replacement) can provide relief for end-stage arthritic pain.

Adverse Outcomes of Treatment

NSAIDs can cause gastric, renal, or hepatic complications. Postoperative infection and/or loosening of total joint implants is possible, and heterotopic ossification can complicate total hip arthroplasty.

Referral Decisions/Red Flags

Patients with kyphosis, pain at rest, or pain at night in a weight-bearing joint may benefit from orthopaedic evaluation. Accompanying problems with the eyes, skin, or pulmonary system may require referral to an ophthalmologist, dermatologist, or pulmonologist.

Compartment Syndrome

ICD-9 Codes

355.8
Mononeuritis of lower limb, unspecified (Chronic compartment syndrome)

958.8
Other early complications of trauma (Acute compartment syndrome)

Refer to 729 series of ICD-9 for specific body area.

Definition

A muscle compartment is defined as a group of one or more muscles and their associated nerves and vessels surrounded by fascia that is relatively unyielding. Compartment syndrome occurs when intracompartmental pressure exceeds vascular perfusion pressure, leading to ischemia of the muscles, nerves, and vessels in a closed fibro-osseous space.

The leg comprises four compartments (**Figure 1**): anterior, lateral, superficial posterior, and deep posterior. Some authors consider the tibialis posterior muscle as being located in its own compartment.

The forearm comprises three compartments (**Figure 2**): volar (flexors, pronators, supinators), dorsal (extensors), and mobile wad (brachioradialis, extensor carpi radialis longus, extensor carpi radialis brevis). The thigh has three compartments (**Figure 3**): medial, anterior, and posterior.

Acute compartment syndrome is usually the result of trauma. It is most often seen in the leg with tibia fractures but also can occur with long-bone fractures in the thigh, arm, or forearm. Additionally, it can occur in the hand, foot, or gluteal region.

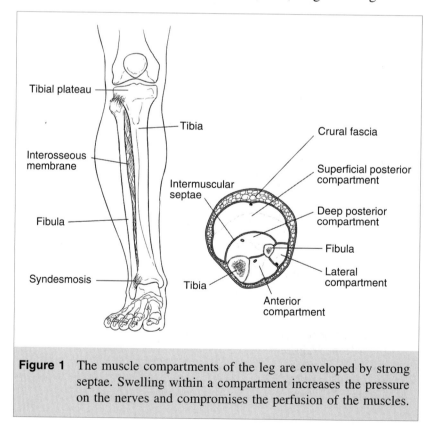

Figure 1 The muscle compartments of the leg are enveloped by strong septae. Swelling within a compartment increases the pressure on the nerves and compromises the perfusion of the muscles.

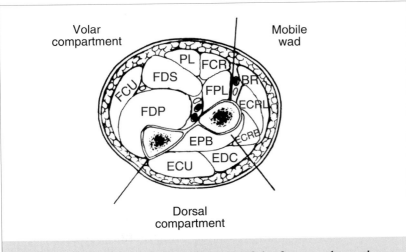

Figure 2   Cross section of the midportion of the forearm shows the location of the various compartments. BR = brachioradialis; ECRB = extensor carpi radialis brevis; ECRL = extensor carpi radialis longus; ECU = extensor carpi ulnaris; EDC = extensor digitorum communis; EPB = extensor pollicis brevis; FCR = flexor carpi ulnaris; FDP = flexor digitorum profundus; FDS = flexor digitorum superficialis; FPL = flexor pollicis longus; PL = palmaris longus.

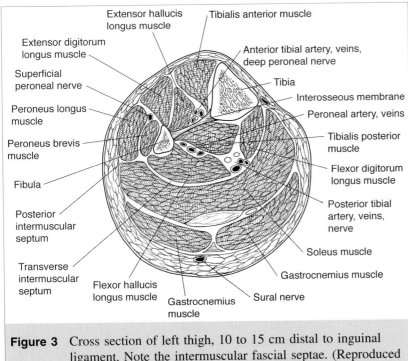

Figure 3   Cross section of left thigh, 10 to 15 cm distal to inguinal ligament. Note the intermuscular fascial septae. (Reproduced from Fraipont MJ, Adamson GJ: Chronic exertional compartment syndrome. *J Am Acad Orthop Surg* 2003;11:268-276.)

Table 1 Acute Compartment Syndrome Versus Chronic Exertional Compartment Syndrome

Parameter	Acute Compartment Syndrome	Chronic Exertional Compartment Syndrome
Mechanism	Usually traumatic	Overuse
Population	Any	Athlete
Areas of body most commonly affected	Leg, forearm, thigh	Leg, forearm, thigh
Symptoms	7 Ps: pain, pallor, paresthesias, paresis poikilothermia, pressure, pulselessness	Cramping, weakness, paresthesias
Diagnosis	Compartment pressures	Rest/exertional compartment pressures
Rest provides relief?	No	Yes
Treatment	Emergent fasciotomies	Elective fasciotomies
Permanent damage	Yes, if untreated	No
Notification	Immediate referral to surgeon	Nonurgent referral to surgeon's clinic

Patients with systemic hypotension are particularly susceptible. Patients with peripheral vascular disease also are at risk, as their poor tissue perfusion leads to mild ischemia and transudation of fluid, which increases the local compartment pressure. Acute compartment syndrome also may develop after direct, crushing blows that cause only muscular injury and hemorrhage without fracture. In these situations, the clinician should also monitor renal function and adequately hydrate the patient to avoid myoglobinuric renal failure secondary to rhabdomyolysis. Other causes include tight external dressings, thermal injury (ie, burn eschar), extravasation of intravenous infusion, reperfusion following prolonged ischemia, and penetrating trauma.

Chronic exertional compartment syndrome (CECS) results when muscles that are metabolically active during exercise swell pathologically, compressing neurovascular structures within the same compartment. Patients have elevated pressures at rest and with exertion. CECS usually occurs in the anterior and lateral compartments of the leg but also may affect all compartments of the leg, shoulder, upper arm, forearm, hand, gluteus, thigh, and foot. Potential causative factors in the leg include fascial defects anterolaterally and arteriolar dysfunction. CECS may develop in long-distance runners, new military recruits, or others involved in a major change in activity level. In these patients, the symptoms are less acute and tend to improve with rest following exercise; long-term sequelae are uncommon. **Table 1** outlines the differences in presentation, diagnosis, and management between acute compartment syndrome and CECS.

As an acute compartment syndrome develops, the intracompartmental tissue pressure becomes elevated, producing a secondary elevation in venous pressure that obstructs venous outflow. This causes an escalating cycle of continued increases in intracompartmental tissue pressure and a resultant decrease in arterial flow. It has been shown that muscles are tolerant of ischemia at 4 hours, damage may occur at 6 hours, and irreversible damage sets in after 8 hours.

Failure to recognize an acute compartment syndrome can lead to a tragic outcome: the muscle first becomes necrotic and then is replaced by fibrotic scar tissue, muscular contracture, and permanent dysfunction of all nerves traveling through the compartment. Avoidance of this outcome requires early recognition and, in most cases, urgent surgical intervention.

Clinical Symptoms

The anterior compartment of the leg and the volar aspect of the forearm are the muscular compartments most commonly affected in acute compartment syndrome. Pain that is disproportionate to the injury and sensory hypoesthesia distal to the involved compartment (deep peroneal nerve distribution in the foot and median nerve distribution in the hand) are characteristic early symptoms. Other symptoms may include paresthesias, weakness, and coolness distally.

In CECS, the patient often experiences a dull ache over the affected compartment that occurs with exertion and progresses to pain severe enough that the activity must be stopped. The symptoms become predictable and reproducible. The patient may report transient numbness, tingling, or weakness in the involved compartments.

Tests

Physical Examination

Acute compartment syndrome is often diagnosed with reference to the "7 Ps": pain, pallor, parasthesias, paresis, poikilothermia (cool extremity distally), pressure, and pulselessness (**Table 1**). The most important symptom is recalcitrant pain, and the most important physical sign is extreme pain on stretching of the long muscles that pass through a compartment. For example, extension of the fingers will stretch the volar forearm muscles, and plantar flexion of the ankle and toes will place the anterior leg muscles on stretch. The inability to actively contract these muscles, as when making a fist or dorsiflexing the toes, is an indication of paresis or paralysis and along with diminishing pulses, is often a late finding possibly indicative of irreversible soft-tissue damage.

Passive or active stretching of muscles around fractured bones is always painful, but it is usually tolerable; intolerable pain may indicate a compartment syndrome. A patient who has an extraordinary amount of pain in the leg or forearm should be examined carefully. Distracting the patient with conversation is sometimes useful when testing for tolerance of passive range of motion as most patients with long-bone fractures will become quite anxious with any attempt to examine the extremity.

Examination of a patient who is wearing a cast or dressing begins with removing the cast, splint, or any compressive bandage to carefully evaluate the muscular compartments. Sometimes, simply loosening a splint and elevating the limb relieves the patient's pain significantly and may prevent an impending compartment syndrome. If compartment syndrome is a concern, the examiner should never hesitate to loosen a dressing because of worry about losing fracture reduction or wound protection. Assessment of increased compartment pressure by palpation is subjective, but a tight or rigid compartment should raise suspicion for compartment syndrome because a normal compartment is soft. Assess motor and sensory function of the peripheral nerves passing through the compartments, as well as passive stretch of the involved muscles.

Pulselessness indicates arterial trauma or a very advanced acute compartment syndrome. It is important to remember that a compartment syndrome may exist in combination with vascular ischemia. Pulses are typically completely normal in early compartment syndrome because at that time, the intracompartmental pressure rarely exceeds systolic pressure levels.

Clinical acumen becomes increasingly vital in the setting of an obtunded patient. With a patient who is intubated or sedated or has sustained head trauma, especially a hypotensive and inadequately resuscitated patient, consultation with a surgeon for evaluation and possible measurement of compartment pressures is indicated, as a physical examination and interview would not be reliable. A high index of suspicion for an evolving compartment syndrome is critical. Serial examinations, interviews, and a knowledgeable nursing staff are essential.

In CECS, the physical examination is more difficult. With the extremity at rest, muscular atrophy, which may be apparent if the disease is unilateral, may be the only clue. With provocation, tenderness and tension of the affected compartment and parasthesias distally may be appreciated.

Diagnostic Tests

When necessary, compartment pressures can be measured directly. One technique is the historic Whitesides infusion technique (**Figure 4**). In recent years, easier techniques have

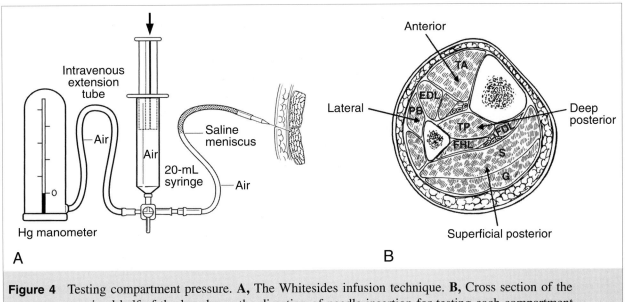

Figure 4 Testing compartment pressure. **A,** The Whitesides infusion technique. **B,** Cross section of the proximal half of the leg shows the direction of needle insertion for testing each compartment. EDL = extensor digitorum longus; FDL = flexor digitorum longus; FHL = flexor hallucis longus; G = gastrocnemius; PB = peroneus brevis; S = soleus; TA = tibialis anterior; TP = tibialis posterior.

been developed, including one involving a basic arterial line setup that is zeroed with normal saline prior to each compartment measurement. Other advances include handheld devices such as the one shown in **Figure 5**. Pressures should be measured in each suspected compartment within 5 cm of the level of injury. Ischemic damage begins when tissue pressure is 10 to 20 mm Hg below diastolic pressure. Therefore, compartment syndrome usually is present when tissue pressure is more than 20 mm Hg less than the diastolic pressure. Many general surgery trauma services use an absolute tissue pressure, usually around 30 mm Hg, as the threshold for diagnosis.

The surgeon should be the one who measures compartment pressures. Many surgeons will have already made up their mind to proceed with surgical intervention when they obtain the compartment pressure measurements. Some general guidelines for when to measure pressures are listed in **Table 2**.

In CECS, pressures are measured a variety of ways. The commonly accepted criteria for diagnosis are (1) a resting pressure measurement of 15 mm Hg or higher; a measurement of 30 mm Hg or higher obtained after 1 minute of exercise; or (3) a measurement of 20 mm Hg or higher obtained after 5 minutes of exercise. **Table 3** lists the differential diagnoses for CECS.

Figure 5 An intracompartmental pressure monitoring system is used to measure the pressure in the deep posterior compartment of the leg.

Table 2 Indications for Compartment Pressure Measurement

One or more symptoms of compartment syndrome with confounding factors (eg, neurologic injury, regional anesthesia, undermedication)

No symptoms other than increased firmness or swelling in the limb in an awake, alert patient receiving postoperative pain control

Unreliable or unobtainable examination with firmness or swelling in the injured extremity

Prolonged hypotension and a swollen extremity with equivocal firmness

Spontaneous increase in pain in the limb after receiving adequate pain control

(Reproduced from Olson SA, Glasgow RR: Acute compartment syndrome in lower extremity musculoskeletal trauma. *J Am Acad Orthop Surg* 2005;13:436-444.)

Table 3 Differential Diagnosis for Chronic Exertional Compartment Syndrome

Diagnosis	Findings	Confirmatory Studies
Stress fracture	Localized tenderness directly over the tibia; pain with torsional or bending stress	Plain radiograph, bone scan, MRI
Medial tibial stress syndrome (periostitis at the muscular attachment site along the posteromedial tibia)	Manual resistance to active plantar flexion and inversion leading to pain along the distal posteromedial aspect of the tibia; localized to diffuse tibial tenderness	Bone scan, MRI
Chronic regional pain syndrome (reflex sympathetic dystrophy)	Allodynia and trophic skin changes	Three-phase bone scan, thermography, sympathetic block
Tenosynovitis of the ankle dorsiflexors or the posterior tibialis tendon	Tenderness along the extent of the tendon aggravated by flexion and extension maneuvers	MRI
Peripheral nerve entrapment syndromes	Tingling or numbness associated with a specific location (Tinel sign)	EMG, nerve conduction study
Venous stasis disease	Trophic skin changes	Duplex ultrasonography
Deep vein thrombosis	Palpable cords or pain with plantar flexion; calf swelling	Duplex ultrasonography, venogram
Radiculopathy	Sensory losses, weakness	EMG, central nervous system evaluation
Arterial vascular disease	Pain, paresthesias, and coolness with activity; claudication	Ankle-brachial index
Popliteal artery entrapment syndrome	Pain and coolness; paradoxical claudication	Arteriogram

EMG = electromyogram.

(Reproduced from Fraipont MJ, Adamson GJ: Chronic exertional compartment syndrome. *J Am Acad Ortho Surg* 2003;11:268-276.)

Differential Diagnosis

- Arterial injury (pulse deficit)
- Muscle contusion (local soft-tissue bleeding)

Adverse Outcomes of the Disease

Without immediate treatment, acute compartment syndrome may result in permanent loss of function. The muscles necrose, fibrose, and shorten; fingers and toes are often clawed and have little motion. The wrist is held in flexion, and sensation is impaired. Late reconstructive surgery, usually involving tendon transfers, has little chance of restoring normal function.

Treatment

Because muscle necrosis may develop within as few as 8 hours of injury, treatment must not be delayed. Suspicion of acute compartment syndrome may indicate treatment, especially if intracompartmental pressure measurements support the diagnosis. Surgical fasciotomy of the compartments is essential. This is accomplished in the leg through either medial and lateral incisions or a single-incision perifibular approach. In the forearm, decompression is achieved either with a volar or combined volar and dorsal approaches. The wounds are left open, supported by vessel loops or a wound vacuum, with delayed closure or skin grafting performed after swelling subsides. Inadequate decompression is possible, so these patients should be closely monitored postoperatively.

In the emergency department and the postanesthesia care unit, strict instructions should be given to return the patient for repeat evaluation immediately if the patient experiences severe, uncontrolled pain or a diminishing ability to move or feel his or her toes. Patients must be able to actively extend their fingers or toes before leaving the emergency department or office so that they or their parents/guardians have a benchmark for acceptable motion and function.

Elevating the affected extremity on a pillow placed under the calf will help reduce edema. (If an upper extremity is affected, the arm can be elevated by placing a pillow beneath it.) The extremity should be elevated only to the level of the heart; excessive elevation should be avoided because this increases hydrostatic pressure and can lower arterial pressure enough to decrease compartment perfusion. Traction is often used in long-bone fracture care, but recent evidence suggests that traction tightens the fascial planes, decreasing the available intracompartmental volume and possibly predisposing a patient to acute compartment syndrome.

Another important consideration is the use of chemical anticoagulants in patients predisposed to an acute compartment syndrome. Compartment syndrome has been reported with ballistic tibial or femoral fractures or nailed long bones after aggressive therapy with anticoagulants. In these patients, the treating surgeon should be consulted before anticoagulant therapy is initiated.

Adverse Outcomes of Treatment

Treating an acute compartment syndrome with fasciotomy carries very little risk, except that the scar may be unsightly. Failure to perform a fasciotomy can be catastrophic for the patient.

Referral Decisions/Red Flags

Even a tentative diagnosis of compartment syndrome requires urgent evaluation so that surgical decompression by emergency fasciotomy can be considered. If a patient with CECS is unwilling to modify or restrict provocative activities, surgical treatment is indicated.

Complex Regional Pain Syndrome

Synonyms

Algodystrophy

Causalgia

Pain dysfunction syndrome

Reflex sympathetic dystrophy (RSD)

Shoulder-hand syndrome

Sudeck atrophy

Sympathetically maintained pain (SMP)

ICD-9 Codes
337.21 Reflex sympathetic dystrophy of the upper limb
337.22 Reflex sympathetic dystrophy of the lower limb
337.9 Unspecified disorder of autonomic nervous system
355.9 Causalgia NOS
733.70 Sudeck's atrophy

Definition

Complex regional pain syndrome (CRPS), also known as reflex sympathetic dystrophy (RSD), algodystrophy, and causalgia, is a clinical diagnosis comprised of pain, autonomic dysfunction, trophic changes, and functional impairment. CRPS is classified as type 1 (RSD, algodystrophy) if there is no identifiable nerve injury or type 2 (causalgia) if an identifiable nerve lesion exists. Part of the spectrum of pain dysfunction syndromes, CRPS is characterized by pain that is generally out of proportion to what would be expected after the original injury and persists despite the absence of ongoing cellular damage or death. CRPS is the abnormal prolongation of normal postinjury physiologic responses and, in part, involves receptor dysfunction. It is a dynamic process that is initiated and manifested in the extremity but is affected by spinal cord and cortical events. The precise etiology of CRPS has not been defined, and no pathognomonic marker has been identified.

The worldwide incidence of CRPS is unknown; however, one report from Minnesota showed an incidence of 5.5 per year and a prevalence of 20.7 per 100,000 residents. In the Netherlands, the prevalence was 26.2 per 100,000. Women are affected at a rate three to four times that of men, and smokers are at increased risk. Individuals between 30 and 50 years of age are most likely to be affected; however, CRPS does occur in children. No identifiable psychologic profile or psychiatric disorder is linked causally to CRPS.

Although CRPS is classically associated with the upper extremity, the lower extremity is affected almost as often. Injuries that commonly precipitate CRPS include fracture of the distal radius and injuries of the infrapatellar branch of the saphenous nerve; the latter occurs after contusion or arthroscopy.

Up to 30% of patients have no apparent injury, indicating the innocuous nature of the events that may precipitate CRPS in some individuals. A persistent and associated nociceptive focus—either neural or mechanical—is identifiable in less than 50% of patients. Early, appropriate treatment is important for the best prognosis. With the exception of CRPS after fracture of the distal radius (in which poor finger function 3 months following the fracture correlates significantly with the presence of components of algodystrophy after 10 years), 80% of patients who are diagnosed and treated within 1 year of the injury improve significantly. After 1 year, however, 50% of patients for whom treatment is initiated have significant long-term morbidity. Some patients deteriorate and manifest long-term disability in spite of early diagnosis and appropriate intervention.

Clinical Symptoms

The clinical presentation of CRPS varies from classic dystrophy to indolent forms. A delay in the onset of dystrophic pain is common. Classic symptoms of CRPS may not be present for 3 to 14 days after the initiating event, with the affected area progressing from localized to diffuse pain that involves the entire extremity. Patients with classic symptoms have difficulty sleeping, and narcotics provide incomplete pain relief. The injured body part and surrounding area are hot/swollen and allodynic and manifest autonomic dysfunction. In addition, temperature changes and abnormal sweat gland function compared with the contralateral extremity is common. Variant presentations are common, and classic staging with time intervals is often unreliable. The hallmark pain of CRPS is described as "burning," "tearing," "searing," and "throbbing"; it is associated with allodynia (pain caused by a normally nonpainful stimulus), hyperpathia (perception of pain that is delayed and extends beyond the normal nerve distribution), and hyperesthesia.

In later or chronic presentations, pain, autonomic dysfunction, and functional impairment persist, and trophic change may be obvious. Contractures are common, and the involved part of the extremity is often cool.

Tests

Physical Examination

Signs of CRPS include swelling, hypersensitivity, abnormal sweating, stiffness, contracture, temperature change, and/or atrophy of hair, skin, and soft tissue. An evaluation to identify underlying nociceptive foci (coexistent carpal tunnel syndrome, etc) is important and should be done both before and after sympatholytic intervention.

Instruments

The use of functional and health-related quality-of-life instruments such as the DASH (Disabilities of the Arm, Shoulder, and Hand) questionnaire, the Rand 36-Item Health Survey, and the McGill Pain Questionnaire may be helpful for documenting symptoms in patients with CRPS.

Diagnostic Tests

Radiographs may show spotty areas of osteopenia or demineralization in the bones of the affected extremity. Three-phase bone scans may show increased uptake in the extremity, especially in the third phase of the scan. Autonomic function may be evaluated with temperature and laser Doppler flowmetric measurements obtained after cold stress testing and QSART (quantitative sudomotor axon reflex testing). Functional impairment may be quantified with endurance testing. Nutritional blood flow may be analyzed with vital capillaroscopy. Response to sympatholytic oral or injectable drugs should be evaluated to assess whether the patient has sympathetically maintained pain (SMP) or sympathetically independent pain (SIP). Pain relief after sympatholysis from intravenous phentolamine defines SMP, which has a more favorable prognosis than SIP. Similarly, a positive response to stellate block, other autonomic blocks, and/or oral agents supports the diagnosis and suggests SMP. It should be remembered, however, that CRPS is a dynamic process, and the pain of CRPS can change from SMP to SIP.

Differential Diagnosis

- Factitious syndromes (SHAFT—sad, hostile, anxious, factitious, tenacious syndrome; Munchausen syndrome; etc); malingering (skin breakdown, unexplainable and massive edema, recurrent and mixed flora infections, abnormal posturing, spread to other areas beyond the affected extremity)
- Other neuropathic pain disorders (localized to the site of nerve damage)

Adverse Outcomes of the Disease

Chronic, possibly debilitating, pain; joint contractures and stiffness; and skin and muscle atrophy may develop. Loss of function in the affected extremity, osteopenia, and delayed healing also may occur.

SECTION 1 GENERAL ORTHOPAEDICS

Table 1 Oral Medications Used to Treat Complex Regional Pain Syndrome

Drug	Usual Dosage	Mechanism	Major Short-term Disadvantages or Side Effects
Vitamin C	500 IU/d	Unknown	None
Amitriptyline hydrochloride (Elavil hydrochloride)	25 mg tid or 50 mg qhs	Inhibits amine pump–decreased (norepinephrine) uptake	Drowsiness; should not be taken with guanethidine sulfate
Pregabalin (Lyrica)	50-200 mg tid	Antinociceptive-binding alpha 2–delta subunit; blocks calcium channels	Dizziness, somnolence, peripheral edema
Gabapentin (Neurontin)	300-600 mg tid	Blocks calcium channels	Dizziness, peripheral edema, asthenia
Fluoxetine (Prozac)	20 mg/d AM	Serotonin inhibitor	Minimal drowsiness
Phenytoin (Dilantin)	100 mg tid	Decreases resting membrane potentials, inhibits amine pump, stabilizes synaptic membrane	Minimal drowsiness
Phenoxybenzamine hydrochloride (Dibenzyline)	40-120 mg/d	Al-receptor blocking agent	Orthostatic hypertension
Nifedipine (Procardia)	10 mg tid, may increase slowly to 30 mg tid	Ca++ channel blocking agent, prevents arteriovenous shunting, increases nutritional flow	Headache, postural hypotension
Amlodipine (Norvasc)	5-10 mg qd	Ca++ channel blocking agent, prevents arteriovenous shunting, increases nutritional flow	Headache, postural hypotension
Corticosteroids	20-80 mg/d, prednisone equivalents × 5-40 days	Stabilizes membranes, increases nutritional flow, decreases inflammatory pain	Adrenal suppression, osteonecrosis (dose-related)

Treatment

Early recognition and prompt treatment are crucial. Treatment includes rehabilitation, oral medications (**Table 1**), biofeedback, therapeutic modalities, parenteral medications, and surgery. Generally, several modalities are used simultaneously, starting with less invasive treatments and progressing to more invasive treatments if the response to the initial interventions is unsatisfactory. Recently, a prophylactic use of vitamin C (550 IU/day orally) was demonstrated in a randomized clinical trial to decrease the incidence of CRPS after fractures of the distal radius.

Initial management frequently includes a combination of oral medications and rehabilitation with physical therapy or occupational therapy. Although analgesics (nonnarcotic and narcotic) and NSAIDs treat pain resulting from underlying nociceptive insults and trauma, pharmacologic management of CRPS is designed to block sympatholytic events and/or improve nutritional blood flow. This treatment is accomplished by the use of multiple drug classes, none of which are FDA-labeled for chronic pain. Commonly used drug classes include antidepressants (tricyclic antidepressants and serotonin-reuptake inhibitors), anticonvulsants, membrane stabilizers, and calcium channel blockers. Effective oral medications include prednisone, amitriptyline, gabapentin, pregabalin, phenytoin, amlodipine besylate, clonidine, and calcitonin. Two or more of these oral agents are commonly prescribed together.

Rehabilitation

Although therapy programs to manage CRPS include passive range of motion, they emphasize active range of motion, including stress loading. Frequently, adaptive modalities such as contrast baths, transcutaneous electrical nerve stimulation (TENS), or iontophoresis are used.

Psychologic counseling may be helpful and often incorporates coping techniques and biofeedback to control the autonomic functions of the body that regulate sweating, skin temperature, and blood flow. Acupuncture and injections of corticosteroid and local anesthetic into trigger points also can provide transient pain relief.

Parenteral medications such as bupivacaine may be used for stellate blocks. Continuous brachial plexus autonomic blocks may be used for diagnosis and/or management of symptoms.

Continuous intrathecal administration of drugs such as clonidine are used as a salvage treatment for refractory symptoms, as are dorsal column stimulators, brainstem stimulators, and other implanted central nervous system devices. Phenol or partial radiofrequency stellate ganglion interruption can provide palliative relief, but nerve transection should be avoided to prevent receptor up-regulation and potential late exacerbation of symptoms.

In acute CRPS, identification and surgical management of associated nerve injury (compression or mechanical injury) is desirable. Perioperative continuous or intermittent autonomic blockade may be used to prevent dystrophic exacerbation if less invasive modalities are ineffective (Figure 1). The sequelae of CRPS, including joint contractures and deformity, can be managed surgically, using appropriate monitoring and pharmacologic management as needed. Patients with CRPS can undergo surgical interventions during all stages of the dystrophic process.

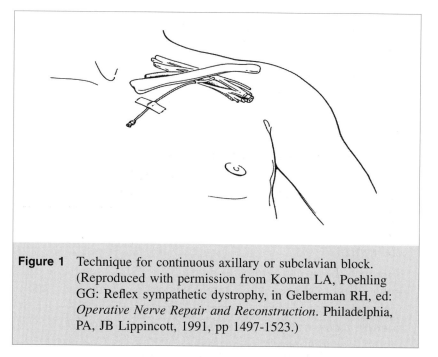

Figure 1   Technique for continuous axillary or subclavian block. (Reproduced with permission from Koman LA, Poehling GG: Reflex sympathetic dystrophy, in Gelberman RH, ed: *Operative Nerve Repair and Reconstruction*. Philadelphia, PA, JB Lippincott, 1991, pp 1497-1523.)

Adverse Outcomes of Treatment

Side effects of treatment are minimal when the therapeutic modalities are used judiciously. Undertreatment is common. Significant side effects of stellate ganglion blocks, which include hoarseness, weakness, numbness in the arm, pneumothorax, and possible seizures from vertebral artery injection, are infrequent. Use of narcotics may lead to addiction, and excessive use of NSAIDs may result in gastric, hepatic, and renal symptoms. Fractures also may occur from too-vigorous manipulations during therapy sessions.

Referral Decisions/Red Flags

If symptoms fail to respond to initial pharmacologic and therapeutic treatments, patients should consider consultation with a pain specialist. Additional evaluations performed at a center where a multidisciplinary team is available to treat this difficult problem should be used as needed.

Crystal Deposition Diseases

Synonyms

Calcium pyrophospate crystal deposition disease
Calcium pyrophospate deposition disease (CPDD)
Calcium pyrophospate dihydrate crystal deposition disease
Gout
Podagra
Pseudogout

Definition

Crystal deposition disease is an arthritis characterized by abrupt episodes of severe joint pain and swelling, typically involving a single joint. The pain and swelling result from the lysis of polymorphonuclear cells triggered when these cells engulf crystals deposited in synovium, cartilage, and other tissues.

Gout

All patients with gout have hyperuricemia (elevated serum levels of uric acid), but not all patients with hyperuricemia develop gout. Uric acid is a by-product of purine metabolism. Urine excretion levels are used to categorize patients as overproducers or underexcretors of uric acid. In certain patients with hyperuricemia, the excess monosodium urate crystals deposit in tissue, causing the inflammatory process of gout. The disease is relatively common, and its prevalence increases with age. The most frequent manifestation of gout is recurrent attacks of acute inflammatory arthritis, but the uric acid crystals may also be deposited in other tissues. Accumulation of urate crystals causes the formation of tophaceous deposits, or tophi (soft-tissue masses from urate crystal deposition noted several years after the onset of gout; (**Figure 1**), and renal manifestations, such as uric acid nephrolithiasis and chronic nephropathy.

Calcium Pyrophosphate Deposition Disease

Calcium pyrophosphate deposition disease (CPDD), which is caused by the precipitation of calcium pyrophosphate dihydrate (CPPD) crystals in connective tissues, has a wide spectrum of clinical manifestations. The clinical spectrum includes asymptomatic disease, pseudogout (**Table 1**), pseudo-rheumatoid arthritis, pseudo-osteoarthritis, and pseudo-neuropathic joint disease. Most patients with radiographic evidence of crystal deposition due to CPDD are asymptomatic.

Figure 1   Dorsal (**A**) and lateral (**B**) photographs of tophi affecting the hand, primarily the metacarpophalangeal joints. (Reproduced from Fitzgerald BT, Setty A, Mudgal CS: Gout affecting the hand and wrist. *J Am Acad Orthop Surg* 2007;15:625-635.)

Table 1 Characteristics of Gout and Pseudogout

Disease	Crystals	Arthritis	Commonly Affected Joints	Treatment
Gout	Monosodium urate monohydrate, negative birefringence	Acute monoarticular	First MTP joint, ankle, knee	Colchicine, indomethacine, NSAIDs, allopurinol
Pseudogout	Calcium pyrophosphate, positive birefringence	Acute monoarticular or oligoarticular	Knee, wrist	Joint aspiration, intra-articular steroids, NSAIDs

MTP = metatarsophalangeal.

Clinical Symptoms

Gout

Acute gouty arthritis, interval gout, and chronic tophaceous gout represent three stages of progressive urate crystal deposition. Acute gouty arthritis occurs after years of asymptomatic hyperuricemia. At least 80% of initial attacks involve a single joint. The metatarsophalangeal joint of the great toe is most commonly affected (podagra), accounting for approximately 50% of the initial episodes of gouty arthritis. Other frequent sites of involvement include the ankle, the tarsal joints, and the knee. Patients report severe pain, redness, and swelling in the affected joint, with maximal severity of symptoms reached over several hours. The overlying erythema may be confused with cellulitis or a septic joint. During the acute event, serum uric acid concentrations are often normal or low. After resolution of the acute attack, patients are often asymptomatic for a variable period of time, with most patients experiencing another attack within 2 years. Tophi develop in only approximately 5% of patients who are compliant with antihyperuricemic therapy. They can develop in many locations, including the olecranon bursa, the extensor surface of the forearm, the Achilles tendon, or the tendon sheaths in the hand. Tophi may be confused with rheumatoid nodules.

Calcium Pyrophosphate Deposition Disease

CPDD commonly affects patients older than 65 years. It is characterized by acute or subacute attacks of arthritis and radiographic evidence of CPPD crystal deposition. Chondrocalcinosis is the calcification of articular cartilage or menisci caused by deposition of CPPD crystals. Most patients with chondrocalcinosis are asymptomatic or have only mild arthritic symptoms. This disorder is more common in women and increases with age, affecting approximately one half of the population older than 80 years.

Patients with pseudogout experience acute or subacute attacks of arthritis, usually in one joint. The knee joint is affected in more than 50% of patients, and CPPD crystals are found on examination of synovial fluid aspirate.

Progressive joint degeneration in a pattern similar to osteoarthritis affects 50% of patients with symptomatic CPDD. The knees are the most commonly affected joints, followed by the wrist, metacarpophalangeal joints, hips, shoulders, elbows, and spine. Evidence of CPPD crystals in synovial fluid and radiographic evidence of CPPD crystal deposition help distinguish this clinical entity from osteoarthritis. Approximately half of the patients experience intermittent acute inflammatory attacks similar to pseudogout.

CPPD arthropathy may be confused with rheumatoid arthritis (RA), but patients do not have bony erosions or other features of RA, such as tenosynovitis. CPDD crystal deposition has been associated with severe neuropathic joint degeneration, but these patients typically suffer from other underlying disorders such as diabetes mellitus or tabes dorsalis.

Tests

Physical Examination

In both gout and pseudogout, examination of the affected joint reveals marked tenderness to palpation, swelling, erythema, and limited motion.

Diagnostic Tests

Laboratory serum analysis for calcium, phosphorous, magnesium, alkaline phosphatase, ferritin, iron, transferrin, and thyroid-stimulating hormone are performed to screen for these disorders.

Figure 2 **A,** Monosodium urate crystals as seen under polarized light. These crystals are characteristic of gout and are found in the fluid of the inflamed joint and in other affected tissues. **B,** Birefringent rhomboid-shaped calcium pyrophosphate crystals, characteristic of pseudogout. (Courtesy Ann Faber, photographer.)

Gout

The clinical picture of acute gouty arthritis is similar to that of acute septic arthritis. Patients are often febrile with a leukocytosis and elevated erythrocyte sedimentation rate. Serum uric acid levels should be checked; however, these levels may be normal during an acute episode. Joint aspiration and analysis of synovial fluid with white blood cell count, Gram stain, and culture are critical in distinguishing gout from septic arthritis. Examination of joint fluid under polarized microscopy reveals the characteristic negatively birefringent urate crystals (**Figure 2**). Early in the disease, radiographs are normal except for soft-tissue swelling. Radiographs of established gout are characterized by subchondral bony erosions and peripheral articular spurs (**Figure 3**).

Calcium Pyrophosphate Deposition Disease

Patients with acute CPDD inflammatory arthritis present with a clinical picture similar to an acute gout attack, hence the name *pseudogout*. Patients are often febrile with a leukocytosis and elevated erythrocyte sedimentation rate. Joint aspiration and synovial fluid analysis with cell count, Gram stain, culture, and polarized microscopy help distinguish this clinical entity from gout or a septic joint. CPPD crystals in synovial fluid appear as weakly positive, birefringent rhomboid-shaped crystals (**Figure 2B**). The deposition of CPPD crystals in soft tissues can cause

Figure 3 **A,** AP view of the foot of a patient with gout. Note the erosions with sharp margins, the overhanging edge in the metatarsophalangeal joint of the great toe (arrow), and a soft-tissue mass around the first metatarsal consistent with a deposit of sodium urate (arrowheads). **B,** AP view of the great toe of a patient with advanced gout. The black arrows indicate large, well-marginated erosions on both sides of the metatarsophalangeal joint, and the white arrowheads indicate a large soft-tissue mass, findings consistent with advanced gout. (Reproduced from Johnson TR, Steinbach LS [eds]: Essentials of Musculoskeletal Imaging. Rosemont, IL, American Academy of Orthopaedic Surgeons, 2004, p 627.)

Figure 4 AP view of the knee of a 48-year-old patient with pseudogout. The crystals in the meniscal cartilage demonstrate the linear calcifications characteristic of chondrocalcinosis (arrows).

chondrocalcinosis, which is visualized on radiographs as punctate or linear calcification of articular cartilage and internal joint structures, such as menisci in the knee or the triangular fibrocartilage in the wrist (**Figure 4**). Some metabolic disorders, such as hyperparathyroidism, hemochromatosis, hypophosphatasia, and hypothyroidism, are associated with CPPD.

Differential Diagnosis

- Cellulitis (joint not involved and motion only mildly affected by overlying skin infection)
- Lyme disease (chronic fatigue, memory loss, history of rash, immunoglobulin M [IgM] or immunoglobulin G [IgG] antibody titer)
- Neuropathic arthropathy (underlying neurologic disorder such as diabetes, insignificant pain)
- Osteoarthritis (less acute, pain proportionate to activity)

SECTION 1 | GENERAL ORTHOPAEDICS

- RA arthritis (younger age, multiple joint involvement, associated tenosynovitis)
- Septic arthritis (severe pain, systemic signs, positive Gram stain and culture)
- Trauma (history, hemarthrosis, or fracture)

Adverse Outcomes of the Disease

Before effective control of hyperuricemia was common, the development of tophi and chronic gouty arthritis was the expected course. Chronic hyperuricemia also leads to nephropathy and renal stones. End-stage arthritis may occur with CPPD, but this is infrequent.

Treatment

Gout

Treatment of acute episodes of gout should focus on relieving pain and inflammation. NSAIDs and oral corticosteroids are first-line agents. Indomethacin is a commonly used NSAID, with an initial oral dose of 75 to 100 mg, followed by 50 mg every 6 hours until symptoms subside. The use of oral NSAIDs is limited in patients with gastrointestinal complications, and oral corticosteroids should be used cautiously in patients with diabetes. Intra-articular corticosteroid injections can be used to treat acute gout in a single joint.

Colchicine is a second-line agent in treating acute gouty arthritis because side effects such as nausea, diarrhea, and bone marrow suppression often limit administration of therapeutic doses. Long-term treatment of gout is aimed at limiting hyperuricemia with drugs such as allopurinol and probenecid. Probenecid increases the urinary excretion of uric acid and should not be administered to patients with renal insufficiency. Allopurinol is a xanthine oxidase inhibitor that decreases production of uric acid in purine metabolism. Allopurinol should not be used in the acute setting because it can exacerbate symptoms.

Calcium Pyrophosphate Deposition Disease

Joint aspiration serves both a diagnostic and therapeutic role in pseduogout. Joint aspiration is commonly followed by intra-articular corticosteroid injections if fewer than three joints are involved. Oral NSAIDs or colchicine are administered during acute attacks if multiple joints are affected. Short-term joint immobilization plays a role in reducing pain and inflammation.

Adverse Outcomes of Treatment

NSAIDs can interfere with drugs used concomitantly to control hypertension and often produce gastrointestinal side effects. Complications of corticosteroid use include osteonecrosis, osteoporosis, glaucoma, and elevated blood glucose levels.

Referral Decisions/Red Flags

Joint deformity or destruction, large tophaceous masses, or drainage of tophaceous material may require surgical attention.

Deep Vein Thrombosis

ICD-9 Code

451.1
Phlebitis and thrombophlebitis, of deep vessels of lower extremities

Synonyms

Deep venous thrombosis

Definition

The Virchow triad—hypercoagulability, venous stasis, and endothelial damage—is the impetus behind venous clot formation. Proximal propagation of clots may lead to pulmonary embolism (PE) and even death. Major musculoskeletal procedures (eg, total hip and knee arthroplasty, hip fracture surgery), polytrauma, and spinal cord injuries increase the likelihood of deep vein thrombosis (DVT) and subsequent PE. Risk factors for DVT are summarized in **Table 1**.

Clinical Symptoms

Many patients with DVT are asymptomatic, but some report fever and pain or swelling in the calf or thigh. Patients with PE often report dyspnea, pleuritic or substernal chest pain, and hemoptysis. Clinicians should be alert for postthrombotic syndrome, which is characterized by leg swelling, dermatitis, ulcers, venous insufficiency, and persistent venous occlusion.

Tests

Physical Examination

Clinical signs of DVT are nonspecific. Edema, either tender or not, is common. Clots may be asymptomatic, and PE can occur without warning. Low-grade fever and palpable cordlike veins may be present. A positive Homans sign (calf pain with forced ankle dorsiflexion) may be present. Patients with superficial saphenous vein thrombophlebitis have a tender, warm, ropy vein, which can extend proximally into the common femoral vein.

The clinical signs of PE include chest pain, dyspnea, hemoptysis, tachycardia, tachypnea, and sometimes circulatory collapse.

Diagnostic Tests

If patients report swelling and pain, duplex ultrasonography is indicated and is highly accurate in diagnosing proximal clot formation. The role of a duplex ultrasonographic scan in screening for asymptomatic thrombi remains controversial. Venography remains the gold standard to confirm DVT, but it is

Table 1 Risk Factors for Deep Vein Thrombosis

Major musculoskeletal operations

Polytrauma

Vertebral column/spinal cord injuries

History of thrombosis or PE

Immobilization

Stroke

Congestive heart failure

Malignancy

Antithrombin-III deficiency

Protein C deficiency

Protein S deficiency

Prothrombin 20210 defect

Factor V Leiden

Myeloproliferative diseases

Estrogen use (including oral contraceptives)

Smoking

Inflammatory bowel disease

Diabetes mellitus

Obesity

Age >40-50 years

PE = pulmonary embolism.

an invasive procedure and may cause pain, allergic reactions to contrast medium, or, rarely, DVT. Pulmonary angiography is the gold standard for detecting a PE, but the PE protocol at most centers is to obtain a CT scan. Other tests that should be ordered include a chest radiograph, an electrocardiogram (to look for tachycardia, new-onset atrial fibrillation, S1QT3, etc), and arterial blood gas (to look for respiratory alkalosis). Auscultation may reveal a pleural rub.

Differential Diagnosis

- Baker cyst (ruptured popliteal cyst) (no history of prior trauma or surgery)
- Cellulitis (erythema, superficial tenderness)
- Contusion of calf muscles (direct blow, subsequent ecchymosis and tenderness)
- Lymphedema (nontender, diffuse swelling)
- Strain of the calf or thigh muscles (history of injury, pain with stretch of the involved muscle)

Adverse Outcomes of the Disease

Both distal and proximal clots can lead to PE and/or death. Symptomatic proximal leg vein thromboses may have silent PEs in as many as 50% of patients. Other possible problems include postthrombotic syndrome.

Treatment

Prophylaxis

Most DVTs and PEs are clinically silent, and it is difficult to know in which patients they will be symptomatic. Trying to identify at-risk individuals with a physical examination and screening modalities has been largely ineffective. The cost of treating the sequelae of venous thromboembolism (VTE) is substantial, and each event carries with it an increased risk of recurrent disease and its sequelae (chronic postthrombotic syndrome). The ultimate goal of prophylaxis is to prevent a symptomatic PE, which is the end point of research in the orthopaedic literature. Most patients who die as a result of a PE do so within 30 minutes of the acute event, which is too soon for therapeutic anticoagulation to be effective or interventional radiologic catheter-based measures to begin. Consequently, prevention of PE depends on prevention of lower extremity thromboses. General agreement exists that patients undergoing total hip or knee arthroplasty and polytrauma patients (including those with spinal injuries) require DVT prophylaxis. Despite extensive research, however, controversy remains regarding the best regimen. The ideal prophylactic regimen would be practical, easy to use, and cost effective, would have no side effects, and would require no monitoring. Unfortunately, this regimen does not exist. Today's anticoagulants require constant balancing of the risk of clots against the risk of bleeding. Most orthopaedic surgeons' practices are based on the literature dealing with arthroplasty procedures. American Academy of Orthopaedic Surgeons' guidelines for prevention of symptomatic PE are available at www.aaos.org/research/guidelines/PEguide.asp.

The mainstays of prophylaxis today include parenteral heparin (including low-molecular-weight heparin [LMWH] formulations), fondaparinux, oral warfarin, and aspirin. Desirudin, a hirudin derivative, has been recently approved by the FDA for VTE prevention. Many more medications are in various stages of development, including oral heparin and direct and indirect inhibitors of factors IIa, IXa, and Xa. **Table 2** lists the characteristics of the most commonly used medications in DVT prevention.

Enoxaparin is the most commonly used LMWH for hip and knee arthroplasty. Enoxaparin and heparin are both frequently used in the setting of polytrauma or long-bone fractures. Enoxaparin is renally cleared, so heparin may be a better choice in patients with underlying renal insufficiency.

Oral warfarin is the agent most commonly used for anticoagulation. Studies indicate that an international normalized ratio (INR) of 2.0 to 2.5 is associated with the lowest bleeding risk while maintaining efficacy. Warfarin alone is not sufficient for clot prevention, and it has been shown to be more effective in preventing proximal clots than distal ones in total hip arthroplasty patients.

Aspirin, although inferior in effectiveness to LMWH and warfarin, may be effective if combined with mechanical prophylaxis.

Mechanical prophylaxis reduces VTE disease secondary to increased fibrinolysis and decreasing stasis with accelerated venous emptying. Foot, calf, and calf/thigh pumps are the three basic devices. They work using pneumatic compression, sequential inflation, or rapid inflation. Elastic stockings are useful as well. They should be applied preoperatively, intraoperatively, and postoperatively. Mechanical devices have very low complication rates. Patient compliance can be a problem, however, so the modality the patient will be most compliant with should be used. These devices should be used as an adjunct to pharmacologic prophylaxis.

Procoagulant medication should be discontinued prior to admission. Autologous blood donation is encouraged because it has been proven to significantly reduce the prevalence of DVT in total hip and knee arthroplasty. Regional anesthesia decreases blood loss and the rate of DVT. A surgical time of less than

Table 2 Characteristics of Pharmacologic Prophylactic Agents

Medication	Mechanism of Action	Advantages	Disadvantages
Heparin (including LMWH)	Activation of antithrombin-III	Can be used in patients with renal insufficiency	Risk of bleeding; can lead to HIT; can cause hyperkalemia; can cause elevation in serum aminotransferase levels
Desirudin (Iprivask)	Direct thrombin inhibitor Effects reversed by protamine sulfate	Can be used in patients with a history of or at risk for HIT; monitoring usually not required	Risk of bleeding; requires renal dosing
Enoxaparin (Lovenox)	Activation of antithrombin-III	Rapid onset; linear pharmacokinetics; little variability among patients; monitoring not required; practical for outpatient use; can be dosed every 12 or 24 hours	High cost; risk of bleeding (intraoperative and postoperative); use prohibited with epidural catheters; renally cleared
Warfarin (Coumadin)	Inhibits Vitamin K–dependent carboxylation of factors II, VII, IX, X, protein C, and protein S	Proved efficacy; oral administration; effects reversed using vitamin K	Requires outpatient monitoring; low but real risk of bleeding; possibly inferior to LMWH for primary thrombosis prevention; warfarin alone not sufficient for clot prevention; multiple drug and dietary interactions
Aspirin (ASA)	Inhibits platelet aggregation via inhibition of COX-1 and thus production of thromboxane-A2	Inexpensive; easy to take; monitoring not required; safe; combats heterotopic ossification	Efficacy inferior to LMWH, warfarin; no rapid reversal, as this is a permanent inhibition of COX-1
Fondaparinux (Arixtra)	Factor Xa inhibitor	Effectively prevents VTE; lower risk of HIT	Risk of major bleeding; risk of thrombocytopenia

LMWH = low-molecular-weight heparin, HIT = heparin-induced thrombocytopenia, COX = cyclooxygenase, VTE = venous thromboembolism.

70 minutes decreases the rate of DVT in total knee arthroplasty patients and a single, intraoperative dose of unfractionated heparin may do so in total hip arthroplasty patients. The effect of early hospital discharge on the duration of prophylaxis and the prevalence of symptomatic thromboembolism following discharge is unclear.

The standard inpatient regimen for arthroplasty patients is intermittent pneumatic compression and pharmacologic prophylaxis (warfarin or aspirin if warfarin is contraindicated). Some have even advocated and achieved excellent results with low-dose oral chemoprophylaxis prior to surgery. Prophylaxis should continue after discharge, and patients should be educated on signs and symptoms of VTE. Studies have shown that even if screening tests are negative, discharging total knee and hip

Table 3 Perioperative Modalities for Optimization of Deep Vein Thrombosis Prophylaxis

Preoperative	Cessation of procoagulant medication
	Rehabilitation
	Weight loss
	Smoking cessation
	Low-dose chemoprophylaxis in select cases
Intraoperative	Pneumatic compression of uninvolved extremity
	Autologous blood for transfusion if required
	Regional anesthesia
	Short surgical time
	Intraoperative dose of heparin in select cases
Postoperative	Pharmacologic prophylaxis (eg, warfarin, enoxaparin)
	Pneumatic compression bilaterally
	Rehabilitation
	Adherence to outpatient pharmacologic regimen for instructed duration
	Patient education with regard to signs/symptoms of DVT/PE

DVT = deep vein thrombosis, PE = pulmonary embolism.

arthroplasty patients without continuing prophylaxis is not cost effective. Other regimens exist and are usually used according to the surgeon's preference. LMWH has a short half-life and therefore should not be administered immediately after surgery. Depending on the drug used, the first dose is started 6 to 24 hours postoperatively, and may be started later at the discretion of the surgeon if intraoperative blood loss was high or a concern exists for compartment syndrome. LMWH has been found to be more effective than warfarin in reducing the overall rates of asymptomatic DVT, but no difference has been noted in reducing the prevalence of death from PEs. Table 3 details inpatient and outpatient care to optimize DVT prevention.

The duration of prophylaxis remains controversial. After total hip arthroplasty, total knee arthroplasty, and hip fracture surgery, 7 to 10 days of prophylaxis has been recommended, although some recommend up to 30 days of prophylaxis. Recent large studies in total hip arthroplasty patients have shown that if a diligent multimodal approach in the form of preoperative and intraoperative measures combined with pneumatic compression, compression stockings, early mobilization, and 4 to 6 weeks of oral warfarin or aspirin is administered, chemoprophylactic agents that carry an increased risk of bleeding (eg, LMWH) may be unnecessary. Chemical anticoagulation is usually withheld for 7 to 10 days to reduce the risk of an epidural hematoma in postoperative spinal surgery patients. Spinal trauma patients may require an inferior vena cava filter when (1) a history of VTE exists despite appropriate prophylaxis, (2) prolonged immobilization is expected, or (3) chemical anticoagulation is contraindicated. Filter placement is not without risk, is invasive, and exposes the patient to contrast dye loads. Newer models are retrievable, but some may be left in place permanently.

In the near future, the number of total knee arthroplasties performed is expected to increase, especially in younger, healthier individuals, whose risk for VTE is decreased. Judicious use of more aggressive chemoprophylactic regimens is warranted, both for cost reasons and to avoid placing patients who are at low risk for DVT at risk for complications such as bleeding and wound infection.

Treatment of Distal Clots

The risk of PE and subsequent death is significantly lower for a distal clot than for a proximal one; therefore, many physicians do not treat distal thromboses. Instead, they follow them with serial duplex ultrasonographic imaging, and, if the clot migrates proximally (as occurs in 20% of patients), they treat the DVT. No consensus exists as to how long to follow patients, although one accepted regime recommends following patients every 7 to 10 days for 3 weeks, discontinuing follow-up if the clot does not progress.

Treatment of Proximal Clots

Anticoagulation is recommended in patients diagnosed with a proximal venous thrombosis. This can be done by hospitalization for an intravenous, therapeutic heparin drip, or as an outpatient with LMWH. The patient is usually bridged to warfarin with a goal INR of 2 to 3. This bridging with parenteral therapy is necessary because it takes a few days to achieve a therapeutic INR and warfarin initially reduces circulating protein C and S levels, making the patient temporarily hypercoagulable. Popliteal clots are considered proximal clots. Warfarin therapy is usually continued for 3 months. Therapeutic heparin can be monitored with serial activated partial thromboplastin time measurements. Therapeutic enoxaparin monitoring, if warranted and available, is best done with anti–factor Xa levels.

Contraindications to long-term warfarin therapy include pregnancy, liver insufficiency, severe liver disease, noncompliance, severe alcoholism, uncontrolled hypertension, active major hemorrhage or recent hemorrhagic stroke, and an inability to return for monitoring.

Treatment of Acute PE

Admission to the hospital for intravenous therapeutic heparin, supplemental oxygen, and close monitoring is advised. Coumadin therapy is then initiated, and when INR levels reach the therapeutic range, the intravenous heparin may be discontinued. Oral anticoagulation is typically continued for 6 months for a first episode of PE, including idiopathic cases. With any PE or DVT, it is important to evaluate for causative factors before declaring the event idiopathic.

Adverse Outcomes of Treatment

Bleeding has been associated with anticoagulants. Rare reports have documented death from postoperative bleeding with aggressive chemoprophylaxis. Immune-mediated heparin–induced thrombocytopenia (HIT) type II ("white clot syndrome") is a prothrombotic adverse effect of unfractionated heparin and, less frequently, LMWH. Venous limb gangrene may complicate the transition from heparin to warfarin in HIT type II. Skin necrosis can develop with warfarin but is uncommon.

Referral Decisions/Red Flags

None

Diffuse Idiopathic Skeletal Hyperostosis

Synonyms

Ankylosing hyperostosis
Vertebral osteophytosis

Definition

Diffuse idiopathic skeletal hyperostosis (DISH) is an idiopathic disease characterized by striking osteophyte formation in the spine. Patients with DISH have confluent ossification spanning three or more intervertebral disks, most commonly in the thoracic and thoracolumbar spine. The bridging osteophytes follow the course of the anterior longitudinal ligaments and the peripheral disk margins. The disease primarily affects white men (the male-to-female ratio is 2:1) who are 60 years or older.

Clinical Symptoms

The principal symptom is stiffness in the spine, especially in the morning and evening. Patients often report that symptoms have been present for several months or even years. Nonradicular back pain, especially in the lumbar and thoracolumbar junction area, is mild (**Figure 1**). Patients with cervical spine involvement may notice dysphagia related to a large anterior cervical osteophyte located behind the esophagus. Other weight-bearing joints can be painful, but spinal pain is the most common.

Tests

Physical Examination

Examination reveals stiffness in the spine on forward flexion and on extension. Reduced hip motion or associated knee arthritis also is possible.

Diagnostic Tests

Radiographs of the thoracic and lumbar spine, especially the lateral view, show confluent ossification spanning the intervertebral disks of at least four contiguous vertebral bodies (three disks) (**Figure 2**). The intervertebral disk height is preserved in the fused segments. The posterior apophyseal joints and sacroiliac joints are normal in contrast to the findings characteristic of ankylosing spondylitis.

Figure 1   Distribution of pain in diffuse idiopathic skeletal hyperostosis.

Figure 2 Lateral radiograph of the thoracic spine shows confluent ossification anteriorly spanning multiple disk levels (arrows).

In the cervical spine, ossification of the posterior longitudinal ligament occurs and is the second most common cause of cervical myelopathy, after cervical spondylosis.

The pelvis often shows "whiskering," or shaggy hyperostotic bone at the pelvic rim. Hyperostotic changes may be seen in the ribs as well.

No human leukocyte antigen (HLA) association exists.

Differential Diagnosis

- Acromegaly (facial and phalangeal changes)
- Ankylosing spondylitis (sacroiliac and apophyseal joint involvement, positive HLA-B27)
- Degenerative disk disease (reduced disk height)
- Paget disease (bowing of legs, enlarging head, hearing loss; 32% of patients also have DISH)
- Polymyalgia rheumatica (muscle and joint pain and stiffness associated with systemic symptoms)

Adverse Outcomes of the Disease

Spinal stiffness is common. With widespread involvement, a single mobile segment can remain, but it may become unstable and painful.

Treatment

Walking and exercise programs are recommended as initial treatment. Intermittent NSAIDs may be useful, but pain usually is mild and tolerable.

Adverse Outcomes of Treatment

Heterotopic ossification following hip replacement surgery occurs five times more often in patients with DISH. Preventive intervention may be indicated. NSAIDs can cause gastric, renal, or hepatic complications.

Referral Decisions/Red Flags

Symptoms of neurogenic claudication, myelopathy, or dysphagia indicate the need for further evaluation.

Drugs: Corticosteroid Injections

Introduction

Corticosteroid injections (**Table 1**) are a mainstay of treatment for various musculoskeletal conditions. Depot formulations remain at the injected site for an extended time and have limited systemic effects. The most common depot corticosteroids used are methylprednisolone actetate, triamcinolone hexacetonide, and triamcinolone acetonide. Injection principles are provided in **Table 2**. The use of a particular depot corticosteroid is based on cost, availability, and pharmacokinetics of the agent.

The mechanism of action in the intra-articular injection of corticosteroids is mediated decrease of inflammation of synovial tissue. A transient mild increase in inflammation may occur after injection of a joint. There is minimal systemic response to injected depot corticosteroids. Improvement in inflammatory markers (erythrocyte sedimentation rate and C-reactive protein level) and clinical improvement of other joints suggest some systemic response, however.

Intra-articular Injections

Depot corticosteroids are indicated for a variety of intra-articular conditions, including rheumatoid arthritis, degenerative arthritis, crystal deposition diseases (eg, gout), systemic lupus erythematosus arthrosis, and posttraumatic arthritis. Although few high-level studies (randomized clinical trials) have investigated the long-term efficacy of intra-articular

Table 1 Characteristics of Common Injectable Corticosteroids

Corticosteroid	Relative Potency	Onset	Duration
Hydrocortisone	1	Fast	Short
Prednisolone terbutate	4	Fast	Intermediate
Methylprednisolone acetate	4	Slow	Intermediate
Triamcinolone acetonide	5	Moderate	Intermediate
Triamcinolone hexacetonide	5	Moderate	Intermediate
Betamethasone	25	Fast	Long

Table 2 Corticosteroid Injection Principles

1. Scrub the intended injection site with a bactericidal solution. Wear sterile gloves and handle the syringes and needles with strict aseptic technique. Observe universal precautions.

2. Cleanse the top of the solution vial with an antiseptic solution.

3. Use an 18- or 20-gauge needle for easy withdrawal of solution. Discard this needle.

4. Consider anesthetizing the injection site with ethyl chloride or a small amount of local anesthetic administered with a 25- or 27-gauge needle.

5. Do not use local anesthetics that contain epinephrine when injecting the hand or foot; these can cause arterial constriction and infarction of a digit.

6. Corticosteroid and local anesthetic solutions can be mixed in the same syringe, usually in a 1:2 ratio. Injection of the site with 2 to 3 mL of a rapid-acting local anesthetic solution, advancing the same needle into the joint or tendon sheath, and injecting additional local anesthetic followed by the steroid through the same needle is less traumatic to the patient. Large joints (knee and shoulder) may need an additional 4 mL of local anesthetic.

7. Short- and long-acting local anesthetics also may be mixed in the same syringe.

8. Inject anesthetic or corticosteroid preparation with a sterile 22- to 25-gauge needle.

9. Do not inject anesthetic or corticosteroid into a nerve, a tendon, a ligament, or subcutaneous fat.

10. Use multiple injections only if clear improvement has occurred. Limit the number of injections to three.

11. Following the injection, have the patient rest the extremity for 24 hours and avoid the precipitating cause of the problem.

corticosteroid injections, the therapeutic benefits have been demonstrated. The duration of pain relief with intra-articular injections of corticosteroids ranges from 1 to 13 weeks. Pain relief is longer and more effective in patients with rheumatoid arthritis than in patients with osteoarthritis. Pain relief is enhanced with preliminary aspiration of synovial effusions.

Clinical experience suggests that "resting the injected joint" for a brief period after an intra-articular corticosteroid injection may have a beneficial effect, as contrasted with unrestricted weight bearing.

Little evidence exists on which to base the time sequence of serial intra-articular injections. Animal studies have shown hyaline cartilage damage with serial corticosteroid injections, but in patients with osteoarthritis who underwent intra-articular knee injections every 3 months for up to 2 years, no significant joint space narrowing was seen on weight-bearing radiographs. In patients with rheumatoid arthritis, serial corticosteroid joint injections did not increase the frequency of joint arthoplasty surgery in comparison to patients who did not receive injections. It is generally accepted that the same joint should not be injected with corticosteroids more often than every 3 months. Table 3 lists the suggested dose of methylprednisolone or equivalent by site.

Table 3 Usual Doses of Methylprednisolone or Equivalent by Site

Dose Range (mg)	Anatomic Site
5 to 10	Phalangeal joints
20 to 30	Wrist
20 to 30	Elbow and ankle
40 to 80	Shoulder, hip, or knee

Extra-articular Injections

Corticosteroid injections also are used for several nonarticular conditions, including overuse syndromes, athletic injuries, selected neuropathies, bursitis, and tendinitis. The most common nonarticular injection sites are the subacromial shoulder for rotator cuff tendinitis, the lateral elbow for lateral epicondylitis (tennis elbow), the lateral wrist for de Quervain tenosynovitis and trigger finger, the lateral knee for iliotibial band tendinitis, the lateral hip for trochanteric bursitis, and the lateral heel for plantar fasciitis. A corticosteroid injection into the carpal canal is frequently helpful in alleviating the pain and numbness associated with carpal tunnel syndrome. In the spine, epidural injections can be used for diskogenic pain, and facet injections can be used for axial spine pain. These spinal injections may require radiographic guidance.

Contraindications to Injections and Adverse Outcomes

Intra-articular injection of corticosteroids is contraindicated in the presence of a pyarthrosis. The clinical presentation of a pyarthrosis and nonseptic inflammation of a joint is often similar. If clinical signs of infection are present (fever, leukocytosis, elevated inflammatory markers, or cellulitis), a preliminary aspiration of the joint should be done to obtain a joint fluid leukocyte count and culture. Intra-articular fractures and the presence of prosthetic joint components (eg, total knee replacement) are contraindications to intra-articular corticosteroid injections.

The complication rate for corticosteroid injections is very low, with transient injection pain the most common complication. Postinjection joint pain occurs in 1% to 10% of patients, and may be related to crystal inflammation caused by the injected steroid. Facial flushing, focal skin discoloration, or subcutaneous lipodystrophy (fat atrophy) rarely occurs. Tendon rupture has been associated with corticosteroid injection into the tendon itself or from masking of pain by the corticosteroid. A significant complication of intra-articular injection of corticosteroids is iatrogenic joint infection, which is reported to occur in 1 in 3,000 to 5,000 injections.

Drugs: Nonsteroidal Anti-Inflammatory Drugs

Definition

NSAIDs are a group of drugs used to treat inflammatory conditions such as arthritis, bursitis, and tendinitis (Table 1). Aspirin is an NSAID, but the term usually is reserved for the newer aspirin-like agents that were developed to decrease the severity of gastritis associated with long-term use of aspirin.

Inflammation is an essential, normal protective mechanism associated with injury to the musculoskeletal system, but in addition to trauma, inflammation may also be triggered by infection, allergy, or an autoimmune response, as in rheumatoid arthritis. The inflammatory response is mediated by chemicals, such as prostaglandins, which are released from mast cells, granulocytes, and basophils. NSAIDs block prostaglandin by interfering with the action of the cyclooxygenase (COX) enzyme. Corticosteroids also block the formation of prostaglandins but at a different step in the production chain.

In addition to their anti-inflammatory properties, NSAIDs exhibit analgesic and antipyretic activity. These drugs also decrease platelet adhesiveness and may inhibit the production of prothrombin.

NSAIDs vary in chemical structure, cost, frequency of side effects, and duration of action. Effective use of these drugs often requires some trialing because a patient may respond to one NSAID but not another, and an initial good response may wane with time. Switching to another class of NSAIDs as opposed to switching within the class is likely to be more effective. Table 1 lists NSAIDs by class.

Two forms of COX have been identified. COX-1 is expressed in many tissues, but COX-2 primarily mediates the inflammatory response. Most NSAIDs inhibit COX-1 and COX-2 production, thereby affecting gastric mucosa, renal blood flow, and platelet aggregation as well as inflammation. COX-2 inhibitors selectively affect COX-2 enzymes and are therefore less likely to cause gastric ulcers and bleeding. Renal and hepatic complications have been reported in patients taking COX-2 inhibitors. COX-2 inhibitors also have been associated with an increased risk of stroke and myocardial infarction and should be used with great caution in a susceptible patient population.

Table 1 Types of NSAIDs

Drug	Strength (mg)	Trade Name	Typical Dosage
Salicylates			
Aspirin	300, 325, 600, 650	Several	325 mb qid
Choline magnesium trisalicylate	500, 750, 1,000	Trilisate	1,500 mg bid
Salsalate	500, 700	Disalcid	1,000 mg tid, 1,500 mg bid
Diflunisal	500	Dolobid	250 mg bid or tid, 500 mg bid
Propionic Acids			
Naproxen sodium	220 375, 500 275, DS 550	Aleve Naprelan 375, 500 Anaprox	220 mg bid 750-1,000 mg/day 275 mg bid or tid, 500 mg bid
Naproxen	250, 375, 500	Naprosyn	250, 375, or 500 mg bid
Naproxen EC	375, 500	EC Naprosyn	375 or 500 mg/day
Flurbiprofen	50, 100	Ansaid	100 mg bid
Oxaprozin	600	Daypro	600-1,200 mg/day
Ibuprofen	400, 600, 800	Motrin	400-800 mg bid or tid
Ibuprofen (over the counter)	200	Motrin IB, Advil, Rufin, Nuprin	200-400 mg bid or tid
Ketoprofen	25, 50, 75	Orudis	50 mg qid, 75 mg tid
Ketoprofen extended release	100, 150, 200	Oruvail	200 mg/day
Ketorolac tromethamine	10	Toradol Oral	10 mg qid; 5 days maximum of oral and IM combined
Indolacetic Acids and Related Compounds			
Sulindac	150, 200	Clinoril	150-200 mg bid
Indomethacin	25, 50	Indocin	25-50 mg tid
Indomethacin sustained release	75	Indocin SR	75 mg/day
Etodolac	200-500	Lodine	200-400 mg tid, 500 mg bid

DS = double strength, IM = intramuscular

Side Effects

NSAIDs cause similar side effects, but in varying degrees. Minor dyspepsia is common, even with COX-2 drugs. Gastric ulcers and bleeding are less common but more serious. In patients older than 65 years, approximately 30% of hospitalizations and deaths from gastrointestinal hemorrhage are secondary to NSAID treatment.

Reversible hepatotoxicity is observed with long-term use of some NSAIDs in 10% to 15% of patients. Nephrotoxicity is less common but can develop early in treatment; it results from losing the vasodilatory effects of renal prostaglandins. Fluid retention can increase blood pressure in susceptible patients. The inhibition of prostaglandin synthesis also can be responsible for hives and acute episodes of asthma in some patients.

Choice of Therapeutic Agents

When choosing an NSAID, cost, side effects, dosage schedule, and physician familiarity should be considered. Once- or twice-daily dosage schedules are optimal for patients with poor compliance. Although long-term use is standard practice in patients with rheumatoid arthritis or osteoarthritis, short-term use is encouraged for most other conditions. For osteoarthritis that has a minimal inflammatory component, acetaminophen can be taken for primary management and supplemented with the intermittent use of NSAIDs for breakthrough pain. This dual therapy helps reduce gastric complications caused by NSAIDs.

In general, NSAIDs should be taken with food to decrease gastric irritation. Oral hypoglycemic agents or warfarin sodium may be unfavorably potentiated by some NSAIDs in some patients. Full-dose aspirin or other NSAIDs should not be taken at the same time as another NSAID; however, low-dose aspirin often is used with other NSAIDs in patients with cardiac disease. NSAIDs should be used with caution in patients with hypertension; indomethacin is particularly hazardous in elderly patients.

Patients who are at risk for gastric complications can choose from the following alternatives, in addition to those described previously:

- Nonacetylated NSAIDs such as salsalate (These drugs appear to cause less mucosal injury.)
- NSAIDs that are nonacidic, such as nabumetone
- Prodrugs (drugs that must undergo biotransformation to an active metabolite). These drugs are reported to cause less gastric injury.
- NSAIDs of the pyranocarboxylic acid class, such as etodolac. These drugs are appropriate in high-risk patients.

■ COX-2 inhibitors. These drugs cause the lowest incidence of gastritis; however, they are more expensive than generic NSAIDs that inhibit both COX-1 and COX-2. In light of recent findings of increased risk of cardiovascular events and stroke associated with COX-2 inhibitors, caution must be exercised when prescribing these anti-inflammatories.

SECTION 1 GENERAL ORTHOPAEDICS

Falls and Traumatic Injuries in the Elderly Patient

Definition

Demographics

The elderly are the fastest growing segment of the population, due in part to the aging of the baby boomers. The growth rate of the older adult population greatly exceeds that of the population as a whole. It has been estimated that by 2030, 1 of every 5 people in the United States (nearly 20%) will be older than 65 years. Although older adults today benefit from healthier lifestyles, better nutrition, and advancements in medical care, many still require acute care for traumatic injuries.

For adults 65 years and older, falls are the leading cause of both fatal and nonfatal injuries. Nearly one third of elderly people fall each year, and of these patients, about 50% will fall repeatedly. Both the number of falls and the severity of the injury resulting from the fall increase as people age. The most common serious injuries are head injuries, wrist fractures, spine fractures, and hip fractures. Of these injuries, hip fractures result in the highest health care costs (nearly $35,000 per patient); even more staggering is the total annual cost of nearly $20.2 billion that is spent treating the elderly after falls. Thus, the prevention of falls and management of elderly patients after fall injuries is an important health economics issue, and it will increase in importance as the population of adults older than 65 years continues to grow. (see **Sidebar: Quick Facts About Falls in the Elderly**.)

Risk Factors

Several factors increase the elderly person's risk of falling. These may be categorized as medical risk factors, personal risk factors, and environmental risk factors (**Table 1**).

Medical risk factors are known medical conditions that increase one's risk of falling. Personal risk factors are unique to the individual patient. Age contributes significantly. The rate of hip fractures increases in patients older than 50 years and nearly doubles at 5-year increments. A lack of weight-bearing activity contributes to decreased bone strength and, thus, increased risk of falling. Decreased bone strength due to decreasing estrogen levels puts women at a greater risk than men, with women having two to three times as many hip fractures as men. Habits that increase risk include smoking and heavy alcohol use.

Quick Facts About Falls in the Elderly

The elderly are the fastest growing population segment.

By 2030, 1 in 5 Americans will be older than 65 years.

Falls are the leading cause of death for adults older than 65 years.

Cost of falls in the elderly is $20.2 billion annually.

Falls in the elderly often result in decreased mobility.
Many elderly never return to preinjury activity level.

40% of hip fracture patients require nursing home admission.

Heredity also plays a role in the rate of injury after a fall. Caucasians and Asians with slender bone structures are at higher risk than African Americans and those with larger body structures. Poor nutrition, low calcium intake or absorption, and inadequate vitamin D intake can all lead to osteoporosis, which is known to drastically increase a patient's risk for fall and traumatic injury.

Environmental risk factors may be considered extrinsic factors. Roughly 60% of falls occur at home, 30% occur in the community, and 10% occur in nursing homes/institutions. One quarter of all falls are the result of hazards such as slippery or wet surfaces, poor lighting, and cluttered pathways. Although nearly 4.5 million elderly adults need assistance with activities of daily living, most do not receive the supervision or support that they require. Therefore, they are often forced to engage in activities that put them at risk for a fall and serious injury, including climbing to reach objects high in closets or cabinets, bathing alone, or ambulating through difficult terrain without assistance.

Clinical Symptoms

Symptoms depend on the specific injury sustained as a result of the fall or trauma. For details, see the chapters describing these injuries.

Wrist fractures most often follow a fall on an outstretched hand. Presenting symptoms include pain, swelling, and usually an obvious deformity.

Spine fractures in the elderly are often compression fractures, which are the result of osteoporosis and usually occur in the low thoracic and upper lumbar region. The patient reports pain and occasionally deformity; neurologic complaints are rare.

An elderly patient presenting with a hip fracture is usually nonambulatory. The patient may report pain in the groin, and the leg is shortened and externally rotated.

Tests

Radiographs are indicated to evaluate bone integrity. CT and MRI may be necessary to evaluate soft-tissue injury and may reveal bony injury when radiographs are inconclusive. A dual-energy x-ray absorptiometric (DEXA) scan may be appropriate to diagnose osteoporosis.

Adverse Outcomes of the Disease

Falls and the serious injuries that result can be catastrophic for the older adult. Prolonged immobility can result in a permanent decrease in mobility, leading to a loss of independence. Many

Table 1 Risk Factors for Falls in the Elderly

Medical Risk Factors

Cardiac arrhythmias

Fluctuant blood pressure

Cancer

Arthritis, joint weakness

Pre-existing orthopaedic conditions

Alzheimer/Parkinson disease

Stroke

Multiple sclerosis

Urinary/bladder dysfunction

Vision loss

Hearing loss

Medication side effects

Personal Risk Factors

Age

Activity (lack of weight-bearing activity)

Sex (women at greater risk than men)

Habits (eg, smoking, heavy alcohol use)

Heredity

Nutrition

Environmental Risk Factors

Wet/slippery surfaces

Poor lighting

Cluttered pathways

Poor home layout/design

Inadequate footwear/clothing

Poor supervision

SECTION 1 GENERAL ORTHOPAEDICS

elderly patients with fractures as a result of a fall will not return to their functional baseline, with hip fractures being responsible for the greatest morbidity and mortality in the older adult population. Although approximately 25% of hip fracture patients make a full recovery, 40% require nursing home admission, 50% are dependent on a cane or a walker, and 20% die within 1 year.

Prevention and Treatment

Prevention

Given the high morbidity and mortality associated with falls and traumatic injury in the elderly, it is imperative to consider how to prevent them from occurring. This can best be accomplished by examining each risk factor category and devising a plan to diminish or eliminate that which places one in a high risk stratification.

It may be impossible to eliminate a pre-existing medical condition; however, the older adult may be able to reduce his or her medical risk of a fall caused by a medical condition by seeing a physician regularly to ensure that medical conditions and medications are well managed.

Personal risk factors, such as age, sex, and heredity, are nonmodifiable, but activity level, habits, and diet can be modified. Weight-bearing exercise helps to strengthen bone and improve coordination, resulting in a decreased risk of fall and a decreased risk of fracture after a fall. Consuming adequate calcium and vitamin D strengthens bone. Avoiding smoking and alcohol also lowers risk.

As 60% of falls occur in the home, this is most obvious place to make environmental modifications. For example, stairwells and hallways should be clutter free and well lit, handrails and nonskid rubber mats should be placed in the shower, and throw rugs and loose cords should be removed (Table 2).

Treatment

The goal of treatment is to restore the patient to his or her preinjury level of function. The intervention must be tailored to the specific injury and to the patient, including the patient's ability to participate in and comply with rehabilitation. The presence of comorbid, complex medical conditions in the elderly patient complicates injury management. For example, cardiopulmonary disease increases risks associated with general anesthesia and surgery. These risks must be taken into account when weighing treatment options.

Wrist fractures are most often treated with closed reduction followed by splinting or casting for 6 weeks. Some wrist fractures require surgical intervention.

Compression fractures of the spine without neurologic compromise often can be treated with rest and pain medication

Table 2 Modifying the Home Environment to Prevent Falls

Stairs	Bathroom	Kitchen	Living Room	Bedroom	Footwear
Keep adequately lit	Use a night light	Avoid climbing to reach high shelves	Leave open pathways	Use a night light	Wear low-heeled shoes
Remove clutter	Use rugs with nonskid backing	Arrange cabinets so frequently used items are easily accessible	Remove low tables and footrests	Remove throw rugs and extension cords	Ensure shoes have nonskid soles
Cover with carpet or nonslip tread	Install handrails in the shower	Clean up spills immediately	Keep cords out of walkways	Avoid beds that are too high or too low	Avoid shoes with heavy soles
Install steady handrails	Use a rubber mat on shower floor				
	Leave door unlocked				

followed by short-term bracing and early mobilization. Follow-up with a spine specialist is encouraged, for although it is rare, neurologic damage can occur. Severe collapse (compression) of the vertebral body may require surgical stabilization even in the absence of neurologic deformity.

Most hip fractures require surgical intervention. Morbidity and mortality have been shown to increase significantly with a surgical delay of more than 3 days following injury. After surgery, early mobilization and appropriate rehabilitation are essential.

It is crucial to coordinate the patient's care with the patient, the patient's family, and the patient's primary care physician (if the primary care physician is not the treating physician), to ensure early mobility, adequate control of any pre-existing medical conditions, and continued supervision and follow-up care. These simple measures may prevent a loss of independence, which can lead to devastating psychiatric, social, and physical consequences for the elderly patient.

Referral Decisions/Red Flags

Referral descisions depend on the specific injury; however, referral is indicated if the patient has a loss of distal pulses, evidence of nerve damage (failure to use certain muscle groups or changes in sensation), evidence of brain bleeds, displaced or open fractures, deformity, or increasing pain despite appropriate care. It also is important to note that elder abuse is increasing.

Therefore, if the circumstances surrounding the fall are suspect or the injuries do not fit the proposed mechanism of injury, it is appropriate to seek intervention by a social worker to investigate the possibility of abuse or neglect.

Fibromyalgia Syndrome

Definition

Fibromyalgia syndrome (FMS) is a chronic, non–life-threatening condition characterized by generalized pain, fatigue, and tender areas in the soft tissues. The joints, however, are spared. It is the second most common disorder encountered by rheumatologists, with rheumatoid arthritis being the first. Women between 20 and 60 years of age are primarily affected. The exact cause of FMS is unknown. In the past, many physicians questioned the validity of a diagnosis of FMS, resulting in a delay in care. Increasing evidence suggests, however, that genetic and environmental factors (**Table 1**) are responsible for FMS, and the diagnosis is becoming more widely accepted. Unfortunately, no cure is available for this often debilitating disease.

ICD-9 Code
729.1 Myalgia and myositis, unspecified

Clinical Symptoms

Prejudices should always be set aside in the evaluation of these patients. A careful history and thorough examination is much more valuable than advanced imaging and laboratory tests in arriving at the correct diagnosis. Patients typically report "hurting all over all the time." In 1992, the American College of Rheumatology established the following criteria for the diagnosis of FMS:

- Widespread pain in all four quadrants of the body, usually waxing and waning, that has been present continuously for 3 months. Pain is considered widespread when all of the following are present: pain in the left side of the body, pain in the right side of the body, pain above the waist, and pain below the waist. In addition, axial skeletal pain must be present (neck, anterior chest, or thoracic or low back). Low back pain is considered pain below the waist.
- Pain and tenderness at 11 or more of 18 tender point sites (9 pairs) on digital palpation with an approximate force of 4 kg (enough force to cause the examiner's nail bed to blanch). A dolorimeter is an examination tool that applies

Table 1 Current Theories of Causation for Fibromyalgia Syndrome

Hyperexcitability of central nervous system pain receptors, termed *central sensitization*

Abnormal central processing of nociceptive input

Dysfunction of hypothalamic-pituitary-adrenal axis, specifically dopaminergic neurotransmission

Table 2 Tender Point Sites

Location	Characteristics
Posterior	
Occiput	Bilateral, at the occipital muscle insertions
Supraspinatus	Bilateral, at origins, above the scapular spine near the medial border
Trapezius	Bilateral, at the midpoint of the upper border
Gluteal	Bilateral, in upper outer quadrants of buttocks in anterior fold of muscle
Greater trochanter	Bilateral, posterior to the trochanteric prominence
Anterior	
Low cervical	Bilateral, at the anterior aspects of the intertransverse spaces at C5-7
Second rib	Bilateral, at the second costochondral junctions, just lateral to the junctions on upper surfaces
Lateral epicondyle	Bilateral, 2 cm distal to the epicondyles
Knee	Bilateral, at the medial fat pad proximal to the joint line

(Reproduced with permission from the Arthritis Foundation, Atlanta, GA.)

exactly 4 kg of pressure. For a tender point to be considered positive, the patient must state that the palpation was "painful" in contrast to "tender" (**Table 2**).

A wide variety of symptoms and conditions can accompany FMS; these are listed in **Table 3**. The history should always include questions about a patient's diet, exercise regimen, medication list, allergies, and perpetuating factors.

An important distinction should be made between FMS and myofascial pain syndrome (MPS). MPS involves trigger points, which, like FMS tender points, have reproducible tenderness with pressure at the muscular and fascial sites; unlike FMS, however, with MPS, pain is also experienced distally, at a zone of referred pain. Trigger points are found in firm, elongated bands in muscle fibers and are associated with a local twitch response. This response is an involuntary, transient contraction of the bands and can be elicited by snapping or pinching. A comprehensive list of differences between the two syndromes is in **Table 4**.

Tests

Physical Examination

Examination reveals tenderness to palpation over 11 or more of the 18 tender point sites (**Figure 1**). These tender points are limited to the soft tissues (muscle, tendon, ligament, or bursa); examination of the joints is normal. Additionally, a patient's gait and posture should be evaluated. Patients often report a sensation of swelling, tingling, or numbness, but objective and

Table 3 Symptoms and Conditions Associated With Fibromyalgia Syndrome

Associated Symptoms

Sleep disturbances

Stiffness

Bursitis and tendinitis

Short-term memory loss

Fatigue

Mood changes: depression, anxiety

Headaches: migraines, tension

Substernal chest pain

Urinary frequency and urgency

Parasthesias in hands/feet

Associated Conditions

Restless legs syndrome (RLS)

Temporomandibular joint syndrome

Silicone breast implant syndrome

Irritable bowel syndrome

Premenstrual syndrome

Dysmenorrhea

Cystitis

Mitral valve prolapse

Myofascial pain syndrome

Systemic lupus erythematosus

Table 4 Differences between Fibromyalgia Syndrome and Myofascial Pain Syndrome

Characteristic	FMS	MPS
Point type	Tender	Trigger
Twitch response	None	Local
Sex predilection	Females	None
Pain	Diffuse	Localized or regional
Associated symptoms	Associated with fatigue	None
Associated entities	Associated conditions	None
Response	None	Responds to manual muscle therapies

FMS = fibromyalgia syndrome, MPS = myofascial pain syndrome.

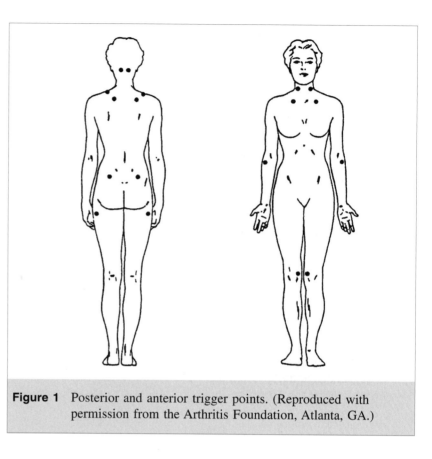

Figure 1 Posterior and anterior trigger points. (Reproduced with permission from the Arthritis Foundation, Atlanta, GA.)

Table 5 Laboratory Findings Associated With Fibromyalgia Syndrome

Reduced central serotonin

Elevated nerve growth factor

Elevated substance P

Reduced insulin-like growth factor 1, implicated in reduced stage 4 (delta) sleep

other neurologic findings are usually absent. Chest pain, shortness of breath, and palpitations are common, and studies to rule out serious cardiac problems should be pursued. Upon auscultation, a midsystolic click followed by a late systolic murmur heard best at the apex, consistent with mitral valve prolapse, may be appreciated.

Diagnostic Tests

Imaging and laboratory studies should be ordered to evaluate coexisting conditions and rule out other disease processes. Although no laboratory test can definitively diagnose FMS, recent research suggests that several laboratory findings are associated with FMS (**Table 5**).

Differential Diagnosis

- AIDS (blood test)
- Bursitis or tendinitis (usually single joint or extremity)
- Complex regional pain syndrome (usually a single extremity)
- Hypothyroidism (abnormal thyroid function tests)
- Lyme disease (serology test)
- Multiple sclerosis (abnormal MRI of the brain)
- Polymyalgia rheumatica (elevated erythrocyte sedimentation rate)
- Polymyositis (skin rash)
- Rheumatoid arthritis (positive rheumatoid factor)
- Systemic lupus erythematosus (antinuclear antibodies, elevated erythrocyte sedimentation rate)
- Tenosynovitis (single focus, associated with tendon motion)

Adverse Outcomes of the Disease

The chronic pain associated with FMS can result in depression, anxiety, and inactivity. The multiple tests ordered and the multiple clinicians consulted to make the correct diagnosis can be expensive.

Treatment

Patients should be advised that FMS is not a life-threatening or progressive disease. No cure is available, but symptomatic relief is possible. The optimal treatment program is multifaceted and should include a team consisting of the patient, a physician, psychologist, physical and massage therapists, and an exercise physiologist.

To date, the FDA has not approved a drug specifically for the treatment of FMS. Available treatment modalities are listed in **Table 6**. FMS patients are usually very sensitive to medication, and adverse effects are common, so pharmacologic therapy should begin with low doses. Narcotics should be used only rarely, and steroids should be avoided. Antidepressants, anticonvulsants, nonbenzodiazepine hypnotics, muscle relaxants, dopamine agonists, and NSAIDs can be effective. NSAIDs accompanied by a tricyclic antidepressant may offer some analgesia. Amitriptyline in doses of 10 to 50 mg or cyclobenzaprine in doses of 10 to 40 mg taken at bedtime can be useful. Fluoxetine taken in the morning is useful to reduce severe depression. The nonnarcotic analgesic tramadol taken in divided doses of 50 to 400 mg/day has been shown to help the pain in FMS. Topical agents such as capsaicin cream applied to the tender point areas and even guaifenesin may be beneficial. For sleep initiation, trazadone at a starting dose of 25 mg is

SECTION 1 GENERAL ORTHOPAEDICS

Table 6 Treatment Modalities for Fibromyalgia Syndrome

Medicinal	Antidepressants
	Anticonvulsants
	Nonbenzodiazepine hypnotics
	Benzodiazepines
	Muscle relaxants
	Dopamine agonists
	NSAIDs
	Topical agents
	Alternative therapies
Mechanical	Injections
	Massage
	Rehabilitation
	Stretching
	Exercise
Psychologic	Cognitive or behavioral therapy
	Support groups
Other	Electrical stimulation
	Cryotherapy
	Heat therapy

helpful, and for sleep maintenance, selective-serotonin reuptake inhibitors are effective. Tricyclics are the most efficacious for sleep maintenance, but some patients cannot tolerate them. Tiagibine (titrated from 2 to 12 mg) and gabapentin also can be useful for sleep maintenance. If the patient has concomitant restless legs syndrome (RLS) or mitral valve prolapse, low-dose clonazepam (0.125 or 0.25 mg) may be taken in the evening. Pramipexole also may be used to treat RLS. Alternative therapies, including vitamins, minerals, herbs, and supplements, have a limited role.

Injections, when combined with massage, rehabilitation, and stretching, are effective for providing mechanical disruption (myolysis) of tender points. Needling and infiltration with a local anesthetic (usually lidocaine; saline if the patient is allergic) is most effective. Steroids are generally not indicated or recommended. When properly administered, injections lead to pain reduction, improvement in range of motion and exercise tolerance, and enhanced circulation. These injections are contraindicated in the setting of a local or systemic infection, a bleeding disorder, or the use of anticoagulation medication.

Patients with FMS should be enrolled in a rehabilitation program, sometimes combined with cognitive and behavioral therapy. Stretching programs increase flexibility, and massage is helpful. Electrical stimulation, cryotherapy, and heat may be helpful. Initiation of an aerobic exercise program to increase cardiac fitness is recommended. The patient should begin slowly and increase gradually to build endurance while minimizing pain. The patient's target regimen should be 20 to 30 minutes of aerobic exercise 4 to 5 times per week. Aquatic exercise is well tolerated and helpful for some patients. Referral to a dietitian for weight-loss supervision often is indicated. Many patients will benefit from participation in FMS support groups, which are a useful source of information and encouragement. Many larger medical centers have established FMS clinics, which use a multidisciplinary approach in the treatment of these patients.

Adverse Outcomes of Treatment

Patients can become dependent on narcotics and tranquilizers. Medications also have side effects, including drowsiness, dry mouth, change in appetite, and constipation. Tachyphylaxis (decreased response) can develop with long-term use of amitriptyline and/or cyclobenzaprine.

Referral Decisions/Red Flags

Severe symptoms that interfere with the patient's ability to work or the presence of serious psychiatric problems indicate the need for evaluation at an FMS treatment center.

Fracture Evaluation and Management Principles

Definition

Bones form the framework of the human body and provide many functions, including stability, mobility, hematopoiesis, and protection of vital organs. Bone has a hard outer layer known as the cortex and a softer inner layer known as cancellous bone. The periosteum is a thick layer that covers the cortex and contains vessels, nerve endings, and cells capable of fracture repair. The endosteum is the inner lining of the cancellous bone (**Figure 1**).

Long bones grow through specialized regions known as a physis. The physis is very vascular and is prone to infections and fractures. The metaphysis consists largely of spongy cancellous bone and is the region most susceptible to compression fractures. The diaphysis has thick cortical bone and provides most of the structural support.

Figure 1 Anatomy of long bones.

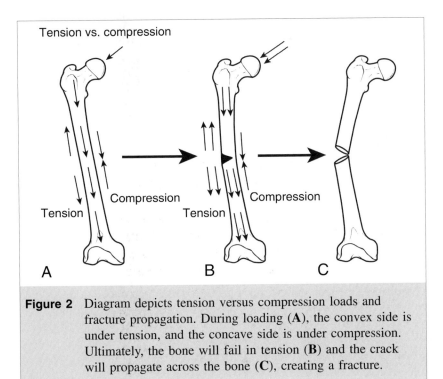

Figure 2 Diagram depicts tension versus compression loads and fracture propagation. During loading (**A**), the convex side is under tension, and the concave side is under compression. Ultimately, the bone will fail in tension (**B**) and the crack will propagate across the bone (**C**), creating a fracture.

A fracture is defined as a disruption in the continuity or structural integrity of bone. A fracture occurs when the stress applied to the bone is greater than the bone's intrinsic strength. Bone is able to withstand very high compressive forces, but it is susceptible to breaks from tension and torsion (**Figure 2**).

Fractures involve not only injury to bone but also injury to the surrounding soft tissues, including the periosteum, muscles, and surrounding vessels. A fracture that compromises the skin and results in bone exposure is called an open fracture (**Figure 3**).

Fractures are classified by location, orientation and extent of fracture lines, amount of displacement, and skin integrity (**Figures 4** and **5**).

Clinical Symptoms

Patients with acute fractures present with pain, swelling, and decreased function. Pain is worsened by movement and may limit weight-bearing capacity. Displaced fractures commonly produce visible deformity in the injured extremity. Stress fractures present more insidiously, with pain during weight bearing. Numbness and tingling also can be present, suggesting injury to nerves or vessels.

Closed
The skin over and near the fracture is intact

Open
The skin over and near the fracture is lacerated or abraded by the injury

Figure 3 Diagram shows closed and open fractures, showing the integrity of the skin and soft-tissue envelope around the fracture. (Reproduced from Johnson TR, Steinbach LS, eds: *Essentials of Musculoskeletal Imaging.* Rosemont, IL, American Academy of Orthopaedic Surgeons, 2004, p 40.)

Nondisplaced
A fracture in which the fragments are in anatomic alignment

Displaced
A fracture in which the fragments are no longer in their usual alignment

Angulated
A fracture in which the fragments are malaligned

Bayonetted
A fracture in which the distal fragment longitudinally overlaps the proximal fragment

Distracted
A fracture in which the distal fragment is separated from the proximal fragment by a gap

Figure 4 Types of fracture displacement. Bayonetted fractures are also called "shortened" fractures. For angulated fractures, valgus angulation is when the distal fragment is displaced away from the midline; varus angulation is when the distal fragment is displaced toward the midline. (Reproduced from Johnson TR, Steinbach LS, eds: *Essentials of Musculoskeletal Imaging.* Rosemont, IL, American Academy of Orthopaedic Surgeons, 2004, p 40.)

SECTION 1 GENERAL ORTHOPAEDICS

Transverse
A fracture that is perpendicular to the shaft of the bone

Comminuted
A fracture in which there are more than two fracture fragments

Oblique
An angulated fracture line

Segmental
A type of comminuted fracture in which a completely separate segment of bone is bordered by fracture lines

Spiral
A multiplanar and complex fracture line

Intra-articular
The fracture line crosses the articular cartilage and enters the joint

Torus
An incomplete buckle fracture of one cortex, often seen in children

Greenstick
An incomplete fracture with angular deformity, seen in children

Impaction
A fracture that occurs when one bone hits or "impacts" an adjacent bone

Compression
A type of impaction fracture that occurs in the vertebrae, resulting in depression of the end plates

Depression
A type of impaction fracture that occurs in the knee when the femoral condyle strikes the softer tibial plateau

Stress (Fatigue)
A fracture in normal bone that has been subjected to repeated or cyclical loads that in and of themselves are not sufficient to cause a fracture

Stress (Insufficiency)
A fracture in weakened bone that has been subjected to a load insufficient to fracture normal bone

Pathologic
A fracture through bone weakened by tumor, metabolic bone disease, or osteoporosis

Figure 5 Types of fractures and orientations of fracture lines. (Reproduced from Johnson TR, Steinbach LS, eds: *Essentials of Musculoskeletal Imaging.* Rosemont, IL, American Academy of Orthopaedic Surgeons, 2004, p 41.)

Figure 6 Radiographs demonstrate fractures stabilized with a plate-and-screw construct (**A**), pins (**B**), and an intramedullary implant (**C**).

Tests

Physical Examination

Fracture evaluation begins with a history and physical examination. The extremity, including the bones and joints above and below the injury, should be inspected for swelling, ecchymosis, deformity, and skin integrity. Lacerations and abrasions in the vicinity of the fracture should be inspected closely, as their presence may indicate an open fracture. Open fractures require expedient care and evaluation by a specialist.

On physical examination, the extremity should be palpated for tenderness, crepitus, and compartment tightness. Extreme swelling in a fractured extremity may suggest impending compartment syndrome (see page 669). The surrounding joints should be evaluated and taken through passive motion to assess stability. Neurologic and vascular status should be evaluated and documented.

Diagnostic Tests

Radiographs are an important initial diagnostic test for the evaluation of suspected fractures (**Figure 6**). At minimum, AP and lateral projections are required. Imaging should always include the joints above and below the injury. Oblique views also may be required for further evaluation.

CT is indicated for evaluating bony anatomy. It is often used for fractures with suspected joint involvement or bone loss and for bones difficult to visualize on plain radiographs (spine, scapula, foot, hand). MRI is indicated to evaluate soft-tissue injury and may be necessary for nondisplaced or stress fractures, which are difficult to view on radiographs.

See Imaging Principles and Techniques, page 128, for further details.

Differential Diagnosis

- Infection (fever; tenderness; elevated erythrocyte sedimentation rate, C-reactive protein level, and white blood cell count; no history of trauma)
- Joint dislocation (deformity, tenderness, abnormal joint alignment on radiographs)
- Sprain/strain (tenderness, normal radiographs)
- Tumor (insidious pain, swelling, possible mass, possible radiographic findings)

Adverse Outcomes of the Disease

A fracture that does not heal properly may result in a delayed union, a nonunion, or a malunion. Delayed unions are fractures that heal at a slower rate; nonunions are fractures that do not heal. Malunions are fractures that heal in unacceptable alignment, compromising the function of the extremity.

Fractures extending into the joint may result in joint stiffness and contractures. Osteonecrosis occurs from a compromised blood supply and is more likely to develop in bones that have a tenuous blood supply, such as the talus, scaphoid, and femoral head.

Fractures can result in damage to surrounding nerves and blood vessels. In severe fractures, limb viability and function may be threatened. Open fractures may develop soft-tissue loss, infection, or osteomyelitis. Compartment syndrome is a serious complication that should be considered in any injured extremity with pain with passive stretching of the involved muscles and significant swelling.

Treatment

Once a fracture is identified, a specialist should be notified to determine the need for manipulation, reduction, and urgency of stabilization. Treatment is guided by the bone involved, the fracture type, and the degree of displacement. In general, fractures require immobilization. Fractures of the extremities are commonly immobilized with a cast, splint, or sling. Axial fractures, such as those in the hip, pelvis, and spine, require bed rest and avoidance of weight-bearing activities prior to evaluation and intervention by a specialist.

SECTION 1 GENERAL ORTHOPAEDICS

Acute fracture reduction is not necessary in fractures that are nondisplaced or minimally displaced. Displaced and angulated fractures require early reduction. In some fractures, acceptable alignment and stability may be achieved definitively following reduction.

Splints and casts should always be applied loosely to allow room for swelling. Immobilization is then continued until fracture healing is achieved. Displaced and unstable fractures often require surgery for closed or open reduction and placement of a fixation device. Open reduction entails the anatomic restoration of the fracture site. Following fracture reduction, implants such as plates, screws, pins, or intramedullary devices may be needed to maintain stability (**Figure 6**).

Open fractures require urgent treatment. Acute surgical care of open fractures requires copious irrigation of wounds and application of appropriate dressings. The extremity is initially splinted for stability to prevent further injury. Appropriate intravenous antibiotics and tetanus prophylaxis should be administered, and a specialist should be notified for urgent surgical intervention.

Once the fracture unites and achieves adequate stability, rehabilitation may be necessary because immobilization may lead to muscle atrophy and joint stiffness. Different fractures and stabilization methods require specific rehabilitation protocols under the supervision and prescription of the treating specialist.

Table 1 Factors That Influence Fracture Healing

Factors That Improve Stability or Prognosis

Skeletal immaturity: thick periosteum, potential for remodeling, faster healing

Nondisplaced fractures

Single bone fracture of forearm (radius/ulna) or lower leg (tibia/fibula)

Thoracic spine fractures (support of rib cage provides added stability)

Factors That Worsen Stability or Prognosis

Skeletal maturity: little remodeling ability, thin periosteum, slower healing

Marked displacement or segmental (indicates soft-tissue stripping)

Intra-articular fractures

Nerve or vascular injury

Compartment syndrome

Osteonecrosis

Oblique fracture patterns

Adverse Outcomes of Treatment

Most fractures unite uneventfully, but certain factors can influence healing (**Table 1**). Inadequate reduction may lead to malunion. Fracture immobilization may lead to stiffness and contractures. Posttraumatic arthritis may develop from fractures involving joints. Other possible complications include vascular and nerve injury, amputation, compartment syndrome, osteonecrosis, or, if the fracture involves a joint surface, posttraumatic accidents.

Referral Decisions/Red Flags

Patients with open, displaced, unstable, or irreducible fractures, suspected compartment syndrome, nerve injury, or vascular injury require further evaluation and treatment.

Fracture Healing

Definition

Following fracture, bone has the inherent capacity for complete structural regeneration (healing) in an appropriate environment. Healing is a complex biologic cascade mediated by a variety of cells and proteins. Most fractures heal or unite uneventfully; however, certain factors make fractures more susceptible to complications during healing (see sidebar: **Risk Factors for Impaired Fracture Healing**).

Fracture healing is determined by a combination of clinical and radiographic evidence. Clinical evidence of union includes the absence of tenderness and motion at the fracture site. Radiographic union is determined by the amount of bridging callus or obliteration of the fracture line.

Principles of Fracture Healing

Fracture healing involves three overlapping phases (**Figure 1**). The first phase (inflammation) begins with bleeding from the fracture site and surrounding soft tissues. This peaks after several days, during which time numerous bioactive cells migrate to the fracture site hematoma under the direction of cell mediators. Granulation tissue is formed during this phase.

During the second phase (repair), new blood vessels are formed and deliver cells essential to the healing process. Necrotic tissue and debris is removed by phagocytes, and fibroblasts begin to produce collagen. Soft cartilaginous callus is produced first and is then mineralized. Mineralized callus is then slowly converted to woven bone (immature bone).

The final phase (remodeling) overlaps with the repair phase and can continue for several months. During this phase, woven bone is replaced by more mature lamellar bone. Typically, union occurs around 6 to 10 weeks; however, the remodeling process can last for months.

Risk Factors for Impaired Fracture Healing

Smoking

Indolent infection

Inadequate immobilization

Malnutrition

NSAID use

Significant soft-tissue injury

A   B   C

Figure 1 Stages of secondary fracture healing. **A,** Inflammatory phase: migration of bioactive cells. **B,** Repair phase: formation of bridging callus. **C,** Remodeling phase: remodeling of the fracture.

Primary Fracture Healing Pattern

Primary or intramembranous fracture healing involves a direct reestablishment of the bony cortex following fracture. Primary healing requires very small gaps and occurs almost exclusively following surgical anatomic restoration of the fracture fragments with rigid internal fixation. Under these ideal conditions, osteoclasts on one side of the fracture show a tunneling resorptive response, allowing direct bone healing across the fracture. With primary healing, no intermediate callus forms (**Figure 2**).

Secondary Fracture Healing Pattern

Secondary or enchondral fracture healing involves indirect bone healing through a cartilaginous callus intermediate (**Figure 3**). This type of healing does not require absolute stability, but rather relative stability, which allows controlled fracture motion. Examples of this type of fixation include a splint, a cast, or certain types of intramedullary fixation devices. During this type of healing, the periosteum serves as the predominant source of progenitor cells that differentiate into cells necessary for healing.

Impaired Fracture Healing Pattern

Malunion

Malunion is defined as an inadequately aligned union of a fracture and is commonly a result of inadequate fracture reduction, immobilization, or possible surgical error in alignment during fixation. Each bone has defined ranges for acceptable alignment. Alignment outside this range results in loss of function and poor cosmesis.

Delayed Union and Nonunion

Delayed union is a prolonged time to union. Healing beyond 16 to 20 weeks typically is considered delayed. Nonunion is failure of normal fracture healing and is defined as (1) a fracture that has not healed following 6 months of treatment, or (2) a fracture that demonstrates no healing progress on radiographs for three consecutive months. Delayed unions and nonunions present clinically with persistent pain. They result from a compromised biologic environment, infection, insufficient immobilization, inadequate reduction, or extensive surgical disruption of the surrounding vascular supply. Risk factors for nonunion are listed in the **Sidebar**.

Treatment of nonunions varies based on the etiology of the nonunion (**Table 1**). Hypertrophic nonunions have abundant callus but lack adequate stability. Too much motion prevents callus from properly consolidating. Atrophic nonunions result from a poor biologic environment or inadequate blood supply.

Figure 2 Primary fracture healing. **A,** Diagram illustrates primary fracture healing. **B,** Radiograph demonstrates healing without fracture callus following rigid fixation. This is indicative of intramembranous healing.

Figure 3 Radiographs of a tibia fracture treated nonsurgically. Note the exuberant callus present at the healed fracture site. (Reproduced from Sarmiento A, Latta LL: Functional fracture bracing. *J Am Acad Orthop Surg* 1999;7:66-75.)

Table 1 Classification of Nonunions

Type	Cause	Treatment
Hypertrophic	Inadequate stability	Revision to more stable fixation
Atrophic	Inadequate biologic conditions	Bone grafting
Fibrous	Inadequate reduction Inadequate biologic conditions Inadequate stability	Débridement, bone grafting
Oligotrophic	Inadequate reduction	Revision of reduction
Septic	Infection	Débridement, antibiotics

Fibrous nonunions lack radiographic evidence of complete healing but clinical union has been attained. This is due to the formation of a stable fibrous connection between fragments. Oligotrophic nonunions result from inadequate reduction, most often during rigid internal fixation.

Rigid fixation requires a very small fracture gap for primary healing to occur. If too large a gap is present, primary healing will not occur. Chronic bacterial infection can prevent healing and lead to a septic nonunion.

Nonsurgical Treatment

Nonsurgical management is appropriate for stable fracture patterns that can be immobilized with a splint or cast. Fractures treated in this manner should have follow-up radiographs to assess healing and maintenance of acceptable alignment. Loss of reduction or a lack of healing may require surgical intervention. Electrical and ultrasound stimulation may be used as an adjunct to enhance the healing of fractures prone to nonunion as well as delayed unions and established nonunions.

Surgical Treatment

Surgical treatment of fractures is indicated for unstable fractures and fractures that fail to respond to nonsurgical treatment. Surgery may range from closed reduction with percutaneous pinning to allograft reconstructions for massive bone defects.

Open fractures require urgent irrigation and débridement to minimize the development of infection. Intra-articular fractures often require open treatment to reduce the articular cartilage as a way of minimizing future posttraumatic arthritis.

Malunions may require an osteotomy, or bone cuts, to restore the anatomic alignment of the bone. Nonunions from infection are treated with extensive débridement of infected bone and tissue followed by intravenous antibiotics and delayed reconstruction.

Bone grafting is often necessary in the treatment of nonunions as well as for fractures with bone loss. Available graft properties and graft options are shown in **Tables 2** and **3**. Autograft and allograft tissue have osteoinductive and osteoconductive properties. Autograft is considered the reference standard and may be harvested from the patient's iliac crest, proximal tibia, or, less commonly, local bone near the surgical site. Allograft tissue is taken from cadavers and has a very small risk of bacterial or viral disease transmission. Newer processing procedures have decreased this risk dramatically. Demineralized bone matrix is an allograft product processed to remove calcium hydroxyapatite without disrupting the osteoinductive proteins or osteoconductive substrate. Recombinant human bone morphogenetic protein is a potent osteoinductive agent useful for treating difficult nonunions and open fractures. Osteoconductive synthetic bone substitutes, including calcium phosphate, also are available for situations involving bone loss or poor bone production.

Table 2 Properties of Bone Grafts

Graft Type	Description
Osteogenic	Contains cells capable of bone formation
Osteoinductive	Induces mesenchymal cells to differentiate into osteoblasts
Osteoconductive	Provides structural stability and forms a scaffold on which bone-forming cells can build

Table 3 Descriptions of and Indications for Bone Grafts

Type	Properties	Advantages	Disadvantages
Autogenous bone	Osteogenic Osteoconductive Osteoinductive	Reference standard	Donor site morbidity, limited supply
Allograft bone	Osteoconductive	Structural grafts	Disease transmission, infection
Synthetic bone substitutes	Osteoconductive	Large supply for filling voids, high compressive strength	Nonstructural graft
Demineralized bone matrix	Osteoconductive Osteoinductive	Bioactive, fills voids	Disease transmission, expensive
Recombinant bone proteins	Osteoinductive	Improves fracture and wound healing	Expensive

Fracture Splinting Principles

Splinting of fractures, dislocations, or tendon ruptures often is required as part of initial emergency management. A well-applied splint reduces pain, bleeding, and swelling by immobilizing the injured part. Splinting also helps prevent a number of problems:

- Further damage of muscles, nerves (including the spinal cord), and blood vessels by the sharp ends of fractured bones
- Laceration of the skin by sharp fracture ends
- Constriction of vascular structures by malaligned bone ends
- Further contamination of an open wound

General Principles of Splinting

1. Remove clothing from the area of any suspected fracture or dislocation to inspect the extremity for open wounds, deformity, swelling, and ecchymosis.
2. Note and record the pulse, capillary refill, and neurologic status distal to the site of injury.
3. Cover all wounds with a dry, sterile dressing before applying a splint. If further evaluation is necessary, notify the receiving physician of all open wounds.
4. Ensure that the splint immobilizes the joints above and below the suspected fracture.
5. With injuries in and around the joint, ensure that the splint immobilizes the bones above and below the injured joint.
6. Pad all rigid splints to prevent local pressure.
7. During application of the splint, use your hands to minimize movement of the limb and to support the injury site until the splint has set and the limb is completely immobilized.
8. Align a severely deformed limb with constant gentle manual traction so that it can be incorporated into a splint.
9. If you encounter resistance to limb alignment when you apply traction, splint the limb in the position of deformity.
10. When in doubt, splint.

Materials

Although prefabricated plastic, fabric, and metal splints are available, they generally are unsatisfactory except for very brief periods of emergency treatment. If a splint is expected to remain in place for more than a few hours, custom application of a well-padded plaster or fiberglass splint is preferred. Plaster is

Table 1 Splinting Materials

Thumb/Finger	Wrist and Forearm	Arm	Long Leg Splint	Short Leg Splint
1 to 2 rolls 4″ cast padding (adults) or 3″ cast padding (children)	2 rolls 4″ cast padding (adults) or 3″ cast padding (children)	2 or 3 rolls 4″ cast padding (adults) or 3″ cast padding (children)	3 to 4 rolls 6″ cast padding	2 rolls 4″ to 5″ cast padding
4″ × 15″ splints, six thicknesses (adults), or 3″ roll folded into splint of appropriate length (children)	5″ × 30″ splints, six thicknesses (adults), for sugar tong; or 4″ × 15″ splints, six thicknesses (children), for simple dorsal or volar splint	5″ × 30″ splints, six thicknesses (adults), or 4″ roll folded to necessary length (children)	3 to 4 rolls 5″ or 6″ wide plaster or 5″ × 45″ plaster splints	12 to 14 thicknesses of 5″ × 30″ or 5″ × 45″ plaster strips
2″ or 3″ elastic bandage	2″ or 3″ elastic bandage	3″ or 4″ elastic bandage	One roll each of 4″ and 6″ elastic bandages	One 3″ to 4″ wide roll of plaster
Tepid water (≈24°C)	Tepid water (≈24°C)	Tepid water (≈24°C)	One bucket of tepid water (≈24°C)	One roll 4″ elastic bandage
Nonsterile gloves	Nonsterile gloves	Nonsterile gloves	Nonsterile gloves	One bucket of tepid water (≈24°C)
				Nonsterile gloves

cheaper, but fiberglass is lighter, stays cleaner, and is more durable. Caution: Many-layered "homemade" splints or thick commercial plaster splints can generate enough heat to burn the patient. See **Table 1** for the materials needed for splinting. Store these materials in a dry cabinet or closet.

Splinting the Upper Extremity
Fractures or Injuries of the Hand or Wrist

1. Position the patient supine or sitting and have an assistant hold the patient's thumb and/or index fingers.

2. Loosely wrap cast padding from the palm to the elbow, making sure that there are three layers of padding at any bony prominence.

3. Place a 4″ × 15″ preassembled splint in the palm and carry it up the volar aspect of the forearm to just below the elbow (**Figure 1A**). If the injury involves the thumb, wrap it separately with 2″ or 3″ of cast padding.

4. Place the splint on the volar or radial aspect and fold the plaster around the thumb, extending across the wrist to the proximal forearm. Leave the dorsal or ulnar side open for swelling (**Figure 1B**).

Figure 1   Splinting an injury of the hand or wrist. **A,** Begin in the palm and extend up the volar surface of the forearm to below the elbow. **B,** Apply the splint along the volar aspect of the thumb, extending across the wrist to the proximal forearm.

5. Wrap the cast padding loosely over the plaster. Wrap an elastic bandage loosely over the cast padding as you mold the splint.

6. Trim the palmar portion of the splint back to the distal palmar flexion crease, proximal to the metacarpophalangeal (MCP) joint.

Fractures or Injuries of the Forearm and Elbow

1. With the patient sitting or supine, have an assistant support the patient's hand with the elbow flexed to 90°. If sitting, the patient should lean slightly to the affected side so that the elbow falls away from the body.

2. Loosely wrap cast padding from the palm to above the elbow, taking care to avoid creating a constriction in the antecubital fossa. Make sure that there are three layers of padding at any bony prominence, such as the wrist and elbow.

3. For a sugar tong spint, begin the splint in the palm, carry it up the forearm to the elbow, around the posterior elbow, then distally on the extensor aspect of the forearm to the dorsum of the hand (**Figure 2**). Use multiple 4″ × 15″ preassembled splints or a 5″ × 30″ preassembled splint if that size is appropriate.

4. Wrap cast padding loosely over the plaster, then wrap an elastic bandage loosely over the cast padding as you mold the splint.

5. Trim the palmar portion of the splint back to the distal palmar flexion crease, proximal to the MCP joint.

Figure 2 Splinting an injury of the elbow and forearm. **A,** Begin in the palm and extend proximally around the posterior elbow. **B,** Complete the splint distally on the extensor aspect of the forearm to the dorsum of the hand.

Figure 3 Splinting an injury of the humerus. **A,** Begin the splint below the axilla, extending it under the elbow, then up the lateral aspect of the arm. **B,** For unstable humeral fractures, continue the splint over the top of the shoulder.

Fractures or Injuries of the Humerus

1. With the patient sitting, have an assistant support the patient's hand with the elbow flexed to 90°. The patient should lean slightly to the affected side so that the elbow falls away from the body.

2. Loosely wrap cast padding from the palm to the upper arm. Begin the splint below the axilla, carry it under the elbow, then up the lateral aspect of the arm.

3. For unstable humeral fractures, use an elephant ear splint: continue the splint over the top of the shoulder, cover the plaster with a layer of cast padding, and then loosely wrap the entire arm with an elastic bandage (**Figure 3**).

GENERAL ORTHOPAEDICS

SECTION 1

Figure 4 Proper positioning of a sling to maintain the elbow at 90°.

4. For lower humeral fractures or elbow injuries, use a coaption splint: end the splint below the lateral shoulder, cover the plaster with a layer of cast padding, and then loosely wrap the entire arm with an elastic bandage. Provide the patient with a strap sling that loops around the wrist, then around the neck, and back to the wrist (**Figure 4**). The sling should be long enough to allow the elbow to be maintained at 90°.

5. Make sure that the sling has padding at the neck and wrist; these straps do not slide at night and can be adjusted for different arm lengths.

Patient Instructions

Patients should be advised to protect the splint for 24 hours, until the plaster cures and hardens. Fiberglass splints harden faster than plaster splints. A splinted arm should not be placed on any plastic-covered surfaces (including pillows) until the plaster has cooled. Patients also should be reminded to watch for changes in skin color (circulation), sensation, and motion in the hand.

Splinting the Lower Extremity
Long Leg Splint

1. For unstable fractures of the leg or ankle, a long leg splint with the knee flexed slightly (25° to 30°) and the ankle flexed 90° should be used.

2. The patient should be supine, with the buttock on the affected side at the edge of the table, allowing the entire leg to hang suspended as an assistant holds the patient's forefoot. Ask the patient to allow the heel to sink so that the foot will be maintained at 90° during splinting.

3. Use either a stirrup-type splint or a long posterior splint. For a stirrup splint, have an assistant hold the patient's forefoot as you wrap the leg with three layers of 6″ cast padding. Place extra padding over the kneecap and lateral knee (fibular head).

4. Begin the 5″ × 45″ plaster splint (10 to 12 thicknesses) on the lateral aspect of the thigh, extend it down the lateral aspect of the leg, under the heel, and then back up the medial side (**Figure 5A**).

5. Start a second splint medially and extend it beneath the foot and up the lateral side.

6. Apply a layer of cast padding over the plaster, and wrap a 5″ or 6″ elastic bandage over the padding as you mold the splint.

7. Ensure that the knee is positioned in slight flexion (approximately 25° to 30°) and the foot is positioned at 90° to the tibia (**Figure 5B**).

Avoid folds in the plaster over the area of the peroneal nerve below the lateral knee (fibular head) or around the ankle.

Figure 5 Long leg splint. **A,** Begin the splint on the lateral aspect of the thigh, extending it down the lateral aspect of the leg, under the heel, and then back up the medial side. **B,** Maintain the knee in 25° to 30° of flexion and the ankle at 90° as the splint hardens.

Preassembled foam-padded splints are convenient, but use them with caution, as they may develop folds or ridges in critical areas.

Use tepid or cool—never hot—water when applying the splint. The heat generated by the reaction of the plaster, if coupled with the use of hot water, can seriously burn the skin. For the same reason, place the leg on a cloth (not plastic) pillow and leave it uncovered for about 10 minutes following application to allow better heat convection.

Hold the splint in place with a loosely applied elastic bandage or bias-cut stockinet, rolled on with almost no tension. As the splint hardens, maintain the ankle at 90°. Mold or support the splint with the flat of the hand—only while it hardens—to avoid causing dents. Dents not only make the splint uncomfortable but can cause cast sores or peroneal nerve palsy and foot drop.

Short Leg Splint

1. With the patient sitting, have an assistant hold the forefoot to maintain the ankle at 90°. Wrap the foot, ankle, and leg loosely with three thicknesses of cast padding.
2. Use either 5″ × 45″ cast padding or fashion a splint with 4″ or 5″ rolls folded to length.
3. Begin the splint laterally, three fingerbreadths below the knee flexion crease, and extend it down and wrap it under the heel and then up the medial side of the leg (**Figure 6A**).
4. Apply the splint like a stirrup, extending material under the foot, covering the heel and arch.
5. Place a single layer of cast padding over the splint, and loosely wrap a 4″ elastic bandage to secure the splint as you mold it to the extremity.
6. Maintain the ankle at 90° as the splint hardens (**Figure 6B**).

Figure 6 Short leg splint. **A,** Begin the splint laterally, three fingerbreadths below the knee flexion crease, and extend it down and wrap it under the heel and then up the medial side of the leg. **B,** Maintain the angle of the ankle at 90° as the splint hardens.

An additional splint may be placed posteriorly if needed. Leave the plaster open in front and/or back, so the patient can unwrap the elastic bandage and spread the splint if needed to accommodate swelling.

Postoperative Shoe

A commercially available firm-soled, wide shoe with Velcro straps can be used to support fractures of the midfoot and forefoot (**Figure 7**). An elastic bandage is frequently wrapped around the foot before applying the shoe. A bulky sock can be substituted for the elastic bandage.

Figure 7 Postoperative shoe used for fractures of the midfoot or forefoot.

Patient Instructions

Patients should be advised to keep the injured leg elevated to the level of the heart as much as possible. Sitting in a reclining chair with a pillow beneath the leg is useful for this. In addition, ice bags should be kept on the injured leg as much as possible for 2 to 3 days after the injury to reduce pain and minimize swelling.

If the pain becomes much worse, the foot begins to feel numb or like it is "going to sleep," or the patient cannot move his or her toes up and down, the splint should be loosened by unwrapping the elastic bandage and tearing the padding down the front of the leg. If the leg does not feel better in 20 to 30 minutes, the patient should be advised to call the doctor because problems with circulation to the leg may be developing, which can have serious consequences.

The splint must be kept dry. To bathe, the patient should place a plastic bag or commercially available cast cover over the leg, prop the leg on the side of the tub, and then fill the tub, keeping the splinted leg out of the water. The patient should not shower.

The patient should be advised to contact the physician if the splint feels as though it is chafing or digging into the skin. The patient also should be reminded to watch for changes in skin color (circulation), sensation, and motion in the foot.

Adverse Outcomes of Treatment

Compartment syndrome, burns, nerve compression injuries, and pressure sores can occur in splinted upper or lower extremities. Plantar flexion contractures of the ankle can develop if the ankle is splinted for prolonged periods with the ankle plantar flexed beyond the neutral position.

Imaging: Principles and Techniques

Imaging studies are essential in the evaluation and management of musculoskeletal pathology. Each imaging modality provides unique and valuable information (Table 1). Prior to ordering imaging studies, a thorough history and physical examination should be performed to formulate a working diagnosis. This will help guide imaging selection. In general, the most basic imaging should be ordered first, and if further information is needed, more invasive and advanced imaging studies may be necessary. *Essentials of Musculoskeletal Imaging,* another volume in this series, describes appropriate imaging studies for more than 300 musculoskeletal conditions.

Radiography

Radiographic images are obtained by projecting x-ray beams through a subject onto an image detector. As the beam traverses the tissues, radiation is absorbed, which decreases the amount of radiation projected onto the detector. Decreased-intensity radiation produces a bright (or white) image on the x-ray film (**Figure 1**).

Radiographs are effective for the intial evaluation of musculoskeletal pathology. Radiographic evaluation should include a minimum of two views of the bone in perpendicular planes (AP and lateral). In fracture evaluation, imaging of the

Table 1 Imaging Modalities

Modality	Advantages	Disadvantage
Radiography	Simple, inexpensive, readily available, easily interpreted	Radiation, poor tissue contrast, relies on tech for adequate images, two-dimensional
CT	Three-dimensional capability, axial imaging, high bony detail, rapid	Highest radiation, motion and metal artifact, poor soft-tissue contrast
MRI	Superior contrast resolution	Expensive, motion and metal artifact, interacts with metals in body, not always available
Arthrography	Combined with other modalities to improve contrast	Invasive, allergic reactions
Scintigraphy (bone scan)	Images metabolic activity, especially in bones	Nonspecific, poor detail, radiation exposure
Ultrasonography	Very safe, inexpensive	Small field of view, technician- and radiologist-dependent, artifacts

Figure 1 Examples of radiographs. **A,** Distal tibia fracture (Reproduced from Bedi A, Le TT, Karunakar MA: Surgical treatment of nonarticular distal tibia fractures. *J Am Acad Ortho Surg* 2006;14:406-416.) **B,** Radius and ulna fracture (Reproduced from Ring D, Jupiter JB, Waters PM: Monteggia fractures in children and adults. *J Am Acad Ortho Surg* 1998;6:215-224.) **C,** Distal humerus fracture. (Reproduced from Anglen J: Distal humerus fractures. *J Am Acad Ortho Surg* 2005;13:291-297.)

joints above and below the area of interest is done to assess for joint dislocations or associated fractures. In specific scenarios, such as wrist, elbow, pelvic, and ankle fractures, specialized views should be obtained (**Table 2**). Views of the contralateral asymptomatic limb may be beneficial in children with suspected physeal injuries and for comparison of irregularities, which may be benign variants.

Lead shields should be used whenever possible to protect patients from radiation exposure, especially women of childbearing age and children.

Indications

The most common indications for radiographic imaging include:

- Deformity of a bone or joint
- Pain or decreased motion of a bone or joint
- Unexplained or disproportionate localized tenderness
- Abnormal asymmetry or mass
- Evaluation for foreign bodies

Table 2 Radiographic Views Commonly Ordered to Evaluate Various Anatomic Regions

Anatomic Region	Radiographic Views
Upper Extremity	
Fingers	PA, lateral and obliques with fingers separated
Hand	PA, lateral (obliques)
Wrist	PA, lateral with wrist in neutral position (consider scaphoid views for anatomic snuffbox tenderness)
Forearm	AP, lateral
Elbow	AP in supination, lateral in 90° flexion (consider radial head views for direct tenderness over radial head)
Humerus	AP, lateral
Shoulder	AP in internal and external rotation, scapular-Y lateral, axillary lateral view (for all trauma/suspected dislocations), consider zanca view for AC joint pathology
Lower Extremity	
Hip	AP in internal rotation, cross-table lateral or frog-lateral
Femur	AP, lateral
Knee	AP, lateral; consider ordering weight-bearing, flexed weight-bearing AP and lateral views and Merchant/skyline views (patellofemoral) for arthritis evaluation
Tibia/fibula	AP, lateral
Ankle	AP, lateral, mortise
Foot	AP, lateral, internal oblique (weight bearing views for Lisfranc injury, alignment abnormalities)
Calcaneus	AP, lateral, Harris axial view
Toes	AP, lateral, obliques
Axial Skeleton	
Cervical spine	AP, lateral (trauma series should also include odontoid view and C7 swimmer's view; consider lateral flexion/extension views for patients with rheumatoid arthritis and suspected instability)
Thoracic spine	AP, lateral
Lumbar spine	AP, lateral
Pelvis	AP (consider Judet views for acetabular fractures, inlet/outlet views for pelvic ring injuries)

AC = acromioclavicular.

Computed Tomography

CT offers detailed axial and three-dimensional imaging by detecting variable tissue absorption of x-rays, much like plain radiographs (**Figure 2**). A computer manipulates and reconstructs the data into contiguous axial images as well as multiplanar reconstructions. CT is useful for detailed examination of bone, and it is the best modality for evaluating intra-articular and complex fractures such as those in the

Figure 2   Depressed tibial plateau frature. **A,** AP view of the knee shows an irregularity of the lateral tibial plateau (arrows) consistent with a fracture. **B,** Coronal reformatted CT scan of the knee shows depression of the posterior lateral articular surface (black arrows) consistent with a fracture. Note the two-intra-articular fracture fragments about the tibia (white arrows). Note the bony detail of fracture pattern seen on CT. (Reproduced from Johnson TR, Steinbach LS, eds: *Essentials of Musculoskeletal Imaging.* Rosemont, IL, American Academy of Orthopaedic Surgeons, 2004, p 501.)

scapula, spine, and pelvis. Three-dimensional CT reconstructions provide spatial information, which is useful in surgical planning. Soft-tissue evaluation is limited; however, the addition of IV contrast dye can be used to evaluate tumors and other soft-tissue masses. CT myelography is typically used for evaluation of spinal cord and nerve root pathology in patients following surgical instrumentation. IV contrast is contraindicated in certain patients with kidney disease, and a small percentage of patients may have an allergy to the dye. CT also can be used to guide difficult joint aspirations. The major drawback of CT imaging is that it subjects patients to considerable radiation exposure. Claustrophobic patients and those with a larger body habitus may be unsuitable for this imaging modality because of the enclosed space of the CT scanner.

SECTION 1 GENERAL ORTHOPAEDICS

Figure 3 Fracture of the femoral neck seen on MRI but not on radiograph. **A,** AP view of the left femur does not reveal a fracture line. **B,** A T1-weighted MRI of the same patient shows the low–signal intensity fracture line across the left femoral neck (arrow). (Reproduced from Johnson TR, Steinbach LS, eds: *Essentials of Musculoskeletal Imaging.* Rosemont, IL, American Academy of Orthopaedic Surgeons, 2004, p 435.)

Indications

The most common indications for CT imaging include:

- Complex or intra-articular fracture evaluation
- Preoperative planning to evaluate bone fragment size and location
- Evaluation of bone tumors
- Bone and joint aspirations/injections

Magnetic Resonance Imaging

MRI uses a powerful magnet to align the hydrogen atoms of water, which are present in varying concentrations in tissues. Radiofrequency (RF) fields are used to alter the alignment of these atoms, producing a magnetic field detectable by the scanner. MRI provides the most detail for evaluation of soft tissues and the spine. MRI also is useful to evaluate tumors and certain bone conditions such as osteonecrosis, osteomyelitis, and stress fractures (**Figure 3**). MRI should not be used as an initial screening study because of its high cost. MRI may be used to further clarify a particular problem. Radiologists have several

Table 3 Signal Intensities for Selected Structures on Different MRI Sequences

Structure	T1-weighted; short TR/short TE	Proton-density; long TR/short TE	T2-weighted; long TR/long TE
Fat[a]	Bright	Bright	Intermediate
Fluid[b]	Dark	Intermediate	Bright
Fibrocartilage[c]	Dark	Dark	Dark
Ligament, tendon[d]	Dark	Dark	Dark
Muscle	Intermediate	Intermediate	Dark
Bone marrow	Bright	Intermediate	Dark
Nerve	Intermediate	Intermediate	Intermediate

TR = repetition time (short, < 600 to 700 msec; long, > 2,000 msec), TE = echo time (short, < 20 to 30 msec; long, ≥ 90 msec).

[a] Includes yellow marrow. Signal will be dark if fat-supressed techniques (eg, fat-saturation, short tau inversion recovery [STIR]) are used.

[b] Includes edema, most tears, and most cysts.

[c] Includes labrum, menisci, and triangular fibrocartilage.

[d] Signal may be increased because of artifacts (eg, magic angle artifact seen in the rotator cuff or the ankle tendons).

(Reproduced from Johnson TR, Steinbach LS, eds: *Essentials of Musculoskeletal Imaging.* Rosemont, IL, American Academy of Orthopaedic Surgeons, 2004, p 12.)

different techniques available to further enhance the information provided by MRI, including T1-weighted, T2-weighted, fat suppression, and short tau inversion recovery (STIR) sequences (Table 3). Gadolinium-based contrast agents can be injected into a joint or delivered intravenously to provide further contrast detail.

In the presence of metal, MRI is rarely ordered because of the metal artifact created. Caution should be used when ordering an MRI in patients who have implanted ferromagnetic metal in their body that may heat up, malfunction (cardiac pacemakers), or dislodge (aneurysm clips in the brain) when placed in a strong magnetic field. Common metals used for orthopaedic stabilization such as titanium are nonferromagnetic and are typically safe for MRI; however, images lose value in the presence of these materials because they are blurred by artifact. Care should be taken to avoid delivering contrast in patients with kidney disease or contrast material allergy. Open MRI scanners are available for those who are claustrophobic and for those who have a larger body habitus.

Indications

The most common indications for MRI include:

- Spinal column pathology
- Evaluation of soft-tissue involvement of tumors
- Tendon and ligamentous injuries
- Meniscal and cartilaginous injuries

Figure 4   Examples of arthrography of the radiocarpal joint. **A,** Preinjection PA view shows a wide scapholunate interval (arrows), suspicious for scapholunate dissociation and tear. **B,** PA view obtained after injection of iodinated contrast medium into the radiocarpal joint (long arrow) of the same wrist shows the flow of the contrast medium through the defect in the scapholunate ligament (short arrows) into the midcarpal joint (arrowhead). (Reproduced from Johnson TR, Steinbach LS, eds: *Essentials of Musculoskeletal Imaging.* Rosemont, IL, American Academy of Orthopaedic Surgeons, 2004, p 20.)

- Stress and occult fractures
- Early osteonecrosis
- Osteomyelitis

Arthrography

Arthrography is the imaging of a joint following the injection of contrast medium. This provides further information about joint congruity and the capsule, cartilage, and surrounding soft tissues (**Figure 4**). Contrast also enhances the differentiation of tissues in and around the joint. Delivering contrast is invasive and subjects the patient to a small risk of joint infection. Patients may have an allergic reaction to the material.

Indications

Common indications for arthrography include:

- Evaluating hip reduction in pediatric hip dysplasia (with fluoroscopy)
- Interosseous ligament tears in the wrist (with radiography and/or MRI)
- Shoulder and hip labral tears (with MRI)

| Perfusion image | Blood-pool image | Delayed image |

Figure 5 Images from a three-phase bone scan of a tibial stress fracture. Perfusion image shows relatively increased radiotracer flow (arrow) to the symptomatic right leg. Blood-pool image shows relatively increased tracer delivery (gray arrowhead) to the right leg. Note extensive soft-tissue activity (white arrowheads) during this phase and early accumulation of radiotracer in the right tibial stress fracture (black arrow). Delayed image shows clearance of the soft-tissue uptake compared with the blood-pool image. The stress fracture is clearly visible as a linear band of increased uptake in the tibia (arrow). (Reproduced from Johnson TR, Steinbach LS, eds: *Essentials of Musculoskeletal Imaging.* Rosemont, IL, American Academy of Orthopaedic Surgeons, 2004, p 17.)

Scintigraphy (Bone Scan)

A bone scan, like other scintigraphic studies, detects the distribution of a radioactive agent throughout the body after the agent is injected intravenously. The agent (typically technetium Tc 99m–methylene diphosphonate for bone studies) emits gamma radiation, which is then detected by a scintillation camera to form two-dimensional images. In the case of bone scans, the radioactive agent localizes to areas of increased bone deposition and therefore correlates with metabolic bone activity. Bone scans are sensitive but not specific for bone lesions.

During a three-phase bone scan, the camera detects emission at different times following administration of the contrast agent. This technique is helpful in evaluating fractures and infections (**Figure 5**). Special tracers can be ordered specifically for evaluation of infection (indium and indium-tagged white blood cells).

Indications

The most common indications for a bone scan include:

- Occult fractures
- Infections
- Inflammatory disorders
- Tumors
- Metabolic bone diseases

Ultrasonography

Use of ultrasonography (also called ultrasound) in the evaluation of the musculoskeletal system has increased because of its low cost and safety. Ultrasound relies on the interaction of pulsed sound waves with tissue interfaces. When sound waves bounce off certain structures, echoes are produced. Different tissue characteristics produce specific echo patterns. Echoes are then picked up by a transducer and converted into images and viewed. Ultrasound is noninvasive and the equipment is easy to transport. The major downside is that it is highly technician-dependent and technically difficult to perform and interpret.

Indications

The most common indications for ultrasonography include:

- Infantile hip dysplasia (**Figure 6**)
- Pediatric joint effusions
- Rotator cuff pathology
- Achilles tendon tears
- Soft-tissue masses
- Fluid collections

Figure 6 Coronal ultrasonogram of pediatric hip dysplasia demonstrates the cartilaginous femoral head (black arrows), labrum (white arrows), and alpha angle (arrowhead). IL = iliac wing, AR = bony acetabular roof. (Reproduced from Johnson TR, Steinbach LS, eds: *Essentials of Musculoskeletal Imaging*. Rosemont, IL, American Academy of Orthopaedic Surgeons, 2004, p 801.)

Infection: Osteomyelitis

Synonym

Bone infection

Definition

Osteomyelitis is defined as infection in bone. Osteomyelitis can occur in both pediatric and adult patients. In pediatric patients, the usual etiology of infection is hematogenous, with the highly vascular metaphysis of long bones the most common anatomic area of presentation. Almost half of pediatric osteomyelitis occurs in patients younger than 5 years. In adult patients, osteomyelitis usually occurs from inoculation of organisms through either open fractures or following surgical fixation of fractures.

Clinical Symptoms

In pediatric patients, osteomyelitis is often difficult to diagnose. Neonates can present with vague symptoms of malaise, including pseudoparalysis, excessive crying, local swelling, and pain with palpation at the affected site. In older children and adults, acute osteomyelitis clinically presents with fever and pain and swelling at the infected site. In patients with either previous open fractures or following surgical stabilization of fractures, osteomyelitis presents with drainage or significant delay in fracture healing.

Tests

The leukocyte count is usually elevated in acute osteomyelitis, but may be normal in chronic osteomyelitis or in patients with immune supression. Two markers of inflammation, the erythrocyte sedimentation rate and the C-reactive protein level, are typically elevated in acute and chronic osteomyelitis and therefore can be used as markers of the disease process. Radiographic diagnosis of osteomyelitis is difficult. Plain radiographs show focal osteopenia, soft-tissue swelling, periosteal elevation, and focal lucency around surgical implants. Plain radiographs have a sensitivity of only 14% and a specificity of 76% for osteomyelitis. CT better demonstrates cortical bony details and can detect the presence of early cortical erosions associated with osteomyelitis. MRI reliably detects marrow changes associated with osteomyelitis (**Figure 1**). Nuclear medicine imaging has high sensitivity but low specificity for diagnosing osteomyelitis, so it is not always productive in differentiating osteomyelitis from other clinical entities (**Figure 2**). The gold standard for diagnosing osteomyelitis is either open biopsy or aspiration, preferably performed on patients prior to the initiation of antibiotics. In pediatric patients, the most common organism is *Staphyloccus aureus*, followed by group A beta-hemolytic streptococci. *Haemophilus influenza*, a previously prevalent organism in pediatric osteomyelitis, has a diminishing prevalence secondary to immunization. In adult osteomyelitis, the most common infecting organism is *S aureus*, followed by *Pseudomonas aeruginosa*. In significantly immunocompromised patients, atypical organisms may be the infecting agent.

Differential Diagnosis

Several clinical conditions can be confused with osteomyelitis. Neuropathic arthropathy, a progressive destructive condition associated with denervated limbs, can be confused radiographically with osteomyelitis. Certain tumors, especially tumors that produce lytic lesions in bones, also can mimic osteomyelitis radiographically. Biopsy or aspiration confirms the diagnosis.

Figure 1 MRI shows features consistent with chronic intramedullary osteomyelitis.

Figure 2 Bone scan in a patient with osteomyelitis shows increased uptake at the metaphysis of the right distal femur. (Reproduced from Johnson TR, Steinbach LS, eds: *Essentials of Musculoskeletal Imaging*. Rosemont, IL, American Academy of Orthopaedic Surgeons, 2004, p 829.)

Adverse Outcomes of the Disease

Many advancements have been made in the diagnosis and treatment of osteomyelitis; nonetheless, 5% to 33% of cases remain refractory to treatment. Refractory osteomyelitis is often related to the patient's overall medical status. Diabetes mellitus, peripheral vascular disease, smoking, malnutrition, and immunosupression are related to failure of treatment. Occasionally, refractory osteomyelitis can be treated with long-term suppressive antibiotic therapy. Amputation may be required in some cases. Rarely, a chronic osteomyelitic sinus will undergo metaplasia and develop squamous cell carcinoma, called a Marjolin ulcer.

Treatment

Treatment of osteomyelitis is different than the treatment of other infections. Bacteria adhere to avascular bone by a glycocalyx that makes antibiotic treatment largely ineffective without débridement of the osteomyelitic bone. Therefore, surgical excision of osteomyelitic bone is absolutely necessary. Antibiotic therapy, either parenterally or locally by antibiotic-impregnated methylmethacrylate beads, is effective following adequate débridement. Bony reconstruction can proceed once the infection is eradicated.

Referral Decisions/Red Flags

In pediatric patients, focal extremity tenderness or fever warrants referral. In adult patients, drainage following surgery for fracture indicates the need for further evaluation.

Infection: Septic Arthritis

ICD-9 Code

711.0
Pyogenic arthritis

Synonyms

Pyogenic arthritis

Suppurative arthritis

Definition

Septic arthritis, also called pyogenic or suppurative arthritis, describes an infection of the joint space. Septic arthritis can affect a variety of joints throughout the body and may occur from direct inoculation, hematogenous spread from concomitant infectious processes, or extension from a contiguous bone infection. Several infectious agents (including bacteria, viruses, mycobacteria, and fungi) can cause septic arthritis; however, *Staphylococcus aureus* is the most common source of acute bacterial arthritis in adults and children older than 2 years and may result in rapid joint destruction. Common sites for septic arthritis include the knee, hip, shoulder, elbow, and wrists. Certain host conditions, such as IV drug abuse, predispose uncommon locations such as the sternoclavicular and sacroiliac joints, to infection with *Pseudomonas aeruginosa*.

Septic arthritis in children, described more fully in Pediatric Orthopaedics—Septic Arthritis, page 1170, most commonly results from hematogenous spread. Seeding of the joint may occur, however, from metaphyseal osteomyelitis, particularly if the metaphysis is intra-articular, as it is in the shoulder, elbow, hip, and ankle. In adults, immunocompromised or immunosuppressed patients as well as those with joint-damaging conditions such as rheumatoid arthritis and systemic lupus erythematosus are at increased risk for septic arthritis.

Periprosthetic joint infection may result from intraoperative contamination, local infection, or hematogenous spread. Periprosthetic joint infection is separated into three main categories: acute postoperative, hematogenous, and chronic infection (**Table 1**).

Table 1 Classification of Periprosthetic Joint Infection

Type	Duration
Acute postoperative	Within 3 weeks of joint replacement surgery
Hematogenous	Within 3 weeks of hematogenous seeding
Chronic infection	More than 3 weeks from joint replacement or hematogenous seeding

Table 2 Key Patient History Points for Septic Arthritis

Number of joints involved

Underlying joint disease or trauma

Prior illnesses or infections

Previous intra-articular injections or joint surgery

Intravenous drug abuse

Time of onset

Clinical Symptoms

A thorough history is necessary when evaluating a patient with a suspected septic joint. Key points to elucidate from the patient's history are listed in **Table 2**.

A high index of suspicion for septic arthritis is required when examining young patients presenting with joint pain. Symptoms may be mild in the early stages, and children will commonly report a vague history of trauma that can confuse the picture. A common scenario is a previously ambulatory child who now refuses to bear weight or move the symptomatic extremity. Other children with septic arthritis will have symptoms of systemic infection such as fever, tachycardia, irritability, and decreased appetite. In addition, it is important to note that knee pain may reflect hip joint pathology.

Joint pain, swelling, and limited range of motion are the most common symptoms and are accompanied by redness and warmth of the joint in question. However, these signs may be muted in elderly or immunocompromised patients who are unable to mount the appropriate inflammatory response to infection. Patients with periprosthetic joints should be carefully evaluated for new-onset pain and swelling, as this should always raise the suspicion of infection.

Tuberculous and fungal infections are typically indolent in their presentation. Gonococcal joint infections from *Neisseria gonorrhoeae* are more common in young, sexually active patients, who present with multiple joint arthralgias and skin lesions.

Tests

Physical Examination

The evaluation of a patient with a suspected septic joint begins with a history and physical examination to identify any possible sources of infection such as breaks in the skin and penetrating injuries, as well as skin and tooth abscesses. All joints should be inspected, palpated, and examined for range of motion. Joint tenderness, effusion, and erythema with marked limitation in passive range of motion are the hallmark clinical signs of septic arthritis. Patients with septic arthritis guard the affected joint and report severe pain with joint motion. The affected joint may be held in flexion secondary to the painful joint effusion. The hip will generally be flexed and abducted.

Diagnostic Tests

Laboratory tests for septic arthritis include a white blood cell (WBC) count with differential, erythrocyte sedimentation rate (ESR), and C-reactive protein (CRP) level. These tests are very sensitive but are nonspecific and may not distinguish between infection and other inflammatory processes. The WBC count and ESR may be normal initially, and normal levels do not preclude the diagnosis of septic arthritis. The CRP level increases in response to infection, rising earlier than ESR (within 6 to 8 hours) and normalizing more rapidly. Therefore, monitoring CRP is of value in assessing response to therapy.

Joint fluid aspirate should be evaluated for crystal analysis, Gram stain, cell count, and cultures with sensitivities. Most joints are easy to aspirate; however, ultrasonographic guidance may facilitate aspiration in difficult joints. Analysis of the synovial fluid with a WBC count of more than 50,000/mm^3 is indicative of infectious arthritis. The glucose level is typically low, and the protein may be elevated.

Blood cultures should be performed and may help identify the causative organism. If gonococcus is suspected, throat cultures, cervical cultures in females, or urethral cultures in males should be obtained. In addition, the laboratory should be notified if *Haemophilus influenza, N gonorrheoae,* or *Kingella kingae* are suspected, as these cultures require special considerations. In the setting of chronic infections, cultures should include studies for acid-fast and fungal organisms. Lyme disease titers should be added in regions where the disease is endemic.

AP and lateral radiographs should be obtained. Radiographs usually are normal but may show soft-tissue swelling around the joint and widening of the joint space. In patients with prosthetic joints, radiographs may reveal radiolucent lines around the prosthesis, which is suggestive of loosening. Ultrasonography is particularly helpful in detecting joint effusion and fluid collection in the surrounding soft tissues. MRI may be useful in excluding adjacent osteomyelitis. A technetium Tc 99m bone scan may be obtained and is useful in identifying the site of infection. Equal uptake on both sides of the joint is suggestive of septic arthritis, but it is difficult to differentiate osteomyelitis from septic arthritis.

Differential Diagnosis

- Acute rheumatic fever (migratory arthralgia, carditis, increased antistreptolysin titer, group A streptococcal infection)
- Bursitis (effusion of the bursa overlying the joint, usually does not limit range of motion, typically afebrile unless infected)
- Crystal-induced arthritis (gout, calcium pyrophosphate dihydrate deposition disease, painful joint, history of flare-ups and normal WBC count)
- Hemarthrosis (hemophilia or traumatic effusions)
- Juvenile rheumatoid arthritis (morning stiffness, usually mild joint swelling, multiple joint involvement)
- Lyme disease (indolent onset, erythema migrans, cardiac and neurologic manifestations)
- Osteoarthritis (evident on radiographs)
- Rheumatoid arthritis (morning stiffness, symmetric involvement, positive rheumatoid factor, elevated ESR, elevated leukocyte count in synovial fluid analysis)
- Transient synovitis of the hip (painful joint with prior respiratory infection, afebrile)

Adverse Outcomes of the Disease

Irreversible damage to the joint can occur without or, in some cases, despite proper treatment. Major complications of septic arthritis include degenerative joint disease, soft-tissue injury and contractures, osteomyelitis, and fibrous or bony ankylosis. The most serious associated outcomes are sepsis and death.

Treatment

Once septic arthritis is diagnosed, empiric IV antibiotic therapy should be initiated following the collection of synovial fluid and blood cultures. Administering antibiotics prior to obtaining cultures may decrease the likelihood of identifying the infecting organism. Empiric antibiotic coverage is based on patient-specific factors (Table 3).

Emergent surgical decompression and lavage of a septic joint is the cornerstone of successful treatment. In special situations where the patient may not be medically fit for surgery, it may be necessary to perform serial needle aspiration and lavage. The affected extremity should be splinted to rest the soft tissues following surgical intervention. Clinical improvement (afebrile, increased range of motion, and decreased swelling and pain) as well as CRP levels should be monitored postoperatively for resolution. The antimicrobial regimen is adjusted according to

Table 3 Causative Organisms and Empiric Antibiotic Regimens for Septic Arthritis

Age/Category	Likely Organism	Initial Antibiotic Regimen
Neonate	S aureus, group B Streptococcus	Oxacillin + gentamicin
Child < 5 years	S aureus, group A Streptococcus	Second-generation cephalosporin
	Streptococcus pneumoniae	
	K kingae	
	H influenzae	
Child 5 years to adolescence	S aureus	Oxacillin
Adolescence to adults	N gonorrhoeae, S aureus	Ceftriaxone (third-generation cephalosporin)
Older adults	S aureus	Oxacillin or cefazolin, aminoglycoside
IV drug abuse	P aeruginosa, Serratia marcesens	IV aminoglycoside + antipseudomonal cephalosporin (ceftazidime, cefepime, cefoperazone)
Prosthetic joint	S epidermidis, S aureus	Vancomycin

culture and sensitivity results, and an infectious disease consultation should be obtained. Intravenous antibiotics are typically transitioned to oral antibiotics with a total therapy duration of 4 to 6 weeks in uncomplicated infections.

In patients with a periprosthetic joint infection, surgical decisions are based on how long the infection has been present. In the acute setting, an attempt at surgical débridement and prosthesis retention should be made. A chronic periprosthetic infection may require staged revision surgery or possibly prosthetic joint removal and fusion. Antibiotics are then generally administered for 4 to 6 weeks.

Adverse Outcomes of Treatment

Patients may have allergic reactions or adverse drug interactions related to certain antibiotic regimens. Strict adherence to aseptic technique must be followed during joint aspiration to avoid inoculating a joint that is not infected.

Referral Decisions/Red Flags

Patients with a swollen, painful joint with markedly decreased range of motion should be strongly suspected of having septic arthritis and require emergent evaluation by a specialist. An erythematous or swollen joint without limited range of motion may represent overlying cellulitis or septic bursitis. This scenario would preclude arthrocentesis because such action could spread infection from overlying tissues to the joint.

Lyme Disease

Synonym

Lyme arthritis

ICD-9 Code

088.81
Lyme disease

Definition

Lyme disease is a multisystem illness caused by the spirochete *Borrelia burgdorferi* that is borne by the deer tick *Ixodes dammini* (**Figure 1**). Lyme disease was first described in 1977 as Lyme arthritis when a group of children in Connecticut suffered from symptoms similar to juvenile rheumatoid arthritis. Lyme disease is the most prevalent vector-borne illness in the United States, with an infection rate of 7.9 cases per 100,000 persons according to the Centers for Disease Control (CDC). The incidence is highest in the Northeast (Maryland to northern Massachusetts), the upper Midwest (Wisconsin and Minnesota), and the far West (northern California and Oregon) (**Figure 2**). Lyme disease has been reported in 49 states, as well as in Asia and Europe. Two additional pathogenic species, *B afzelii* and *B garinii*, are endemic in both Europe and Asia.

Clinical Symptoms

The clinical symptoms associated with Lyme disease have been divided into three distinct phases: early localized, early disseminated, and late disease. The characteristic feature of early localized disease is the characteristic skin lesion, erythema migrans (**Figure 3**). Erythema migrans lesions typically occur within 1 month of a tick bite and occur in 80% of patients infected with Lyme disease. The lesions expand over the course of days or weeks reaching a diameter of up to 20 cm. Erythema migrans lesions are classically described as displaying central clearing, but this has been reported in only 9% of lesions. In the early localized phase, patients may report symptoms similar to a viral syndrome including fatigue, anorexia, headache, neck stiffness, myalgias, arthralgias, and fever. The early disseminated phase typically occurs weeks to several months after the tick bite and can include cardiac or neurologic involvement. The three most common neurologic abnormalities are meningitis, cranial neuropathy, and radiculopathy. Bell palsy (paralysis of the facial nerve) is the most common neurologic manifestation. Pericarditis and AV heart block are the common cardiac manifestations of early disseminated Lyme disease. Ocular manifestations have been described in the early disseminated phase. Conjunctivitis is the most common manifestation and has been reported in 10% of patients. Arthritis and neurologic

Figure 1 Photograph of *Ixodes dammini*, the deer tick that transmits Lyme disease. (Reproduced with permission from the U.S. Department of Agriculture, Washington, DC. http://www.ars.usda.gov/is/graphics/photos/mar98/k8002-3.htm. Photo by Scott Bauer.)

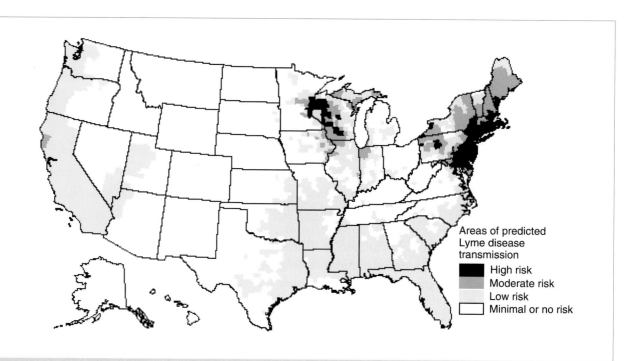

Figure 2 Approximate risk of Lyme disease in the United States by county. The true relative risk in any given county compared with other counties might differ from that shown here and might change from year to year. Risk categories are defined at www.cdc.gov. Information on risk distribution within states and counties is best obtained from state and local public health authorities. (Reproduced with permission from the Centers for Disease Control and Prevention, Atlanta, GA. http://www.cdc.gov/mmwr/preview/mmwrhtml/rr4807a2.htm. Accessed July 19, 2010.)

Figure 3 Appearance of a lesion that developed after a bite by a tick harboring *Borrelia burgdorferi*. (Reproduced from Browner BD, Pollak AN, Gupton CL, eds: *Emergency Care and Transportation of the Sick and Injured*, ed 8. Boston, MA, Jones and Bartlett, 2002, p 427.)

symptoms are manifestations of late Lyme disease and occur several months to years after the tick bite; 60% of untreated patients develop joint pain and swelling within several months of infection. Intermittent or persistent arthritis in large joints is commonly seen several months after infection in untreated patients. The knee is the most commonly affected joint. Lyme encephalopathy, characterized by mild cognitive difficulties, occurs in the late phase. Radicular pain and distal paresthesias also have been associated with late Lyme disease. In Europe, cutaneous manifestations have been associated with Lyme disease, but these symptoms have not been reported in the United States.

Tests

Physical Examination

Patients with the characteristic erythema migrans skin lesion and constitutional symptoms should be examined for synovitis and restricted joint motion. The axilla, inguinal region, and popliteal fossa are common locations for tick bites. Twenty-five percent of patients with early Lyme disease recall a tick bite.

Diagnostic Tests

Early Lyme disease can be diagnosed based on clinical examination and the presence of an erythema migrans lesion. In patients with no erythema migrans lesion but clinical features consistent with Lyme disease, serologic studies can be used to confirm the diagnosis. Patients should not be treated for Lyme disease based on serologic test results alone. When a patient begins to manifest symptoms of the early disseminated phase of Lyme disease, serologic tests are positive for both immunoglobulin M (IgM) and immunoglobulin (IgG) *Borrelia* antibodies. Enzyme-linked immunosorbent assay (ELISA) is the initial serologic test, but it has a high false-positive rate: 5% of the normal population has a positive ELISA. If the ELISA is positive or equivocal, Western blot for IgM and IgG *Borrelia* antibodies is ordered to confirm the diagnosis. Polymerase chain reaction can be run on synovial or cerebrospinal fluid for *Borrelia* DNA, but this is not recommended because of a high false-positive rate and low sensitivity.

Differential Diagnosis

- Acute rheumatic fever (serologic tests, distinctive rashes)
- Idiopathic Bell palsy (physical examination)
- Meningitis (lumbar puncture)
- Multiple sclerosis (abnormal MRI of the brain)
- Peripheral neuritis (specific nerve involvement)
- Reiter syndrome (iritis, urethritis)

Adverse Outcomes of the Disease

Lyme disease can be complicated by arthritis in major weight-bearing joints, facial paralysis, chronic fatigue, concentration defects, cardiac conduction block, and peripheral neuritis.

Prevention and Treatment

People in high-risk areas should wear long-sleeved shirts tucked into trousers with the trouser legs tucked into socks when in heavily wooded areas. Most important, the skin and clothing should be checked for ticks. Insect repellants can be used to minimize the risk of tick bites. If the tick is removed within 24 to 36 hours, the risk of Lyme disease is minimal. Ticks should be removed by grasping the tick close to the skin with tweezers and applying steady, straight traction. Heat and chemicals should not be used to remove ticks from the skin.

When diagnosed early, Lyme disease can be treated effectively with antibiotics. Doxycycline 100 mg twice a day for 10 to 30 days, or amoxicillin 500 mg three times a day for 10 to 30 days has been shown to be effective. For children younger than 8 years, amoxicillin 20 mg/kg in divided doses is indicated.

Adverse Outcomes of Treatment

Allergic reactions or adverse drug interactions to antibiotics can occur.

Referral Decisions/Red Flags

Patients with suspected Lyme disease may require evaluation by an infectious disease specialist.

Osteoporosis

Synonyms

Porous bone disease

Weak bone disease

ICD-9 Codes

733.00
Osteoporosis, unspecified

733.01
Senile osteoporosis

Definition

Osteoporosis is a disease characterized by low bone mass leading to microarchitectural deterioration. As a result, increased fragility of the bone and an increased risk of fracture exist. Other adverse outcomes include deformity, pain, loss of independence, and premature death, particularly following hip fracture. Approximately 10 million Americans older than 50 years have osteoporosis, and the disease is associated with 1.5 million fractures and health care costs of $18 billion per year. Although osteoporosis has long been considered an inevitable consequence of aging, the natural history can be altered by diet and treatment strategies.

Osteoporosis is defined as primary (type I or II) or secondary. Type I osteoporosis, frequently called postmenopausal osteoporosis, is six times more common in women than in men. Estrogen deficiency in women and testosterone deficiency in men lead to trabecular bone loss. These patients commonly present with vertebral compression fractures or fractures of the distal radius (**Figure 1**). Type II osteoporosis, previously called senile osteoporosis, is twice as frequent in women as in men, and it occurs more commonly in individuals older than 70 years. Altered calcium metabolism and intrinsic problems in bone formation lead to a decrease in the formation of new bone. Hip and pelvic fractures are common in this group. In secondary osteoporosis (male-to-female ratio, 65:45), an identifiable agent or disease process causes bone loss.

Clinical Symptoms

Osteoporosis frequently is not recognized until a patient seeks medical attention for back pain, fracture, loss of height, or spinal deformity (**Figure 2**). Over the past decade, however, with the greater availability of dual-energy x-ray absorptiometry (DEXA) and quantitative ultrasonography, screening examinations for osteoporosis, especially in women with risk factors, is becoming more common. **Table 1** summarizes risk factors for osteoporotic fractures. Recently, the World Health Organization (WHO) developed the fracture risk assessment tool

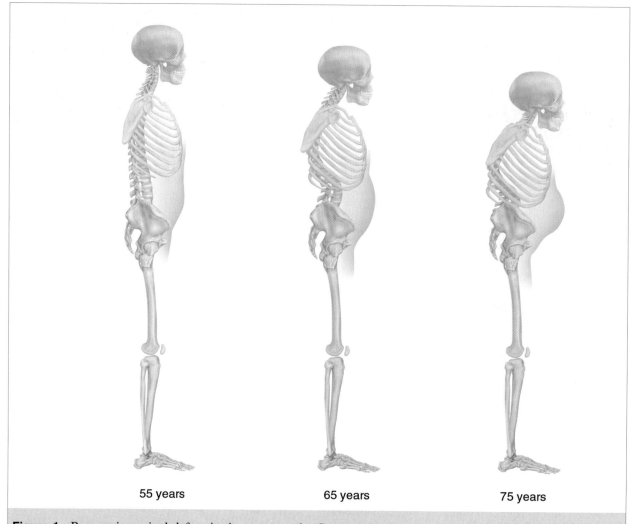

55 years   65 years   75 years

Figure 1 Progressive spinal deformity in osteoporosis. Compression fractures of thoracic vertebrae lead to loss of height and progressive thoracic kyphosis (dowager's hump). The lower ribs eventually rest on the iliac crests, and downward pressure on the viscera causes abdominal distention.

(FRAX), which merges bone density and other factors to establish the 10-year fracture risk assessment.

Secondary osteoporosis is seen commonly in patients undergoing long-term steroid therapy. It also is seen in a wide range of disorders such as hormone abnormalities (hyperthyroidism, hyperparathyroidism), neoplastic disorders (multiple myeloma), metabolic abnormalities (osteomalacia), and connective tissue diseases (osteogenesis imperfecta). Most men who have osteoporosis have secondary osteoporosis.

Osteoporosis is a serious problem for patients who require prolonged immobilization.

Figure 2 **A,** Radiograph of the forearm and wrist of a 74-year-old woman who fell on her outstretched hand, sustaining a fracture of the distal radius and ulna (white arrow). Carpometacarpal arthritis of the thumb (black arrow) is an incidental finding. **B,** Radiograph of the right foot and ankle of an 82-year-old woman who sustained fractures of the necks of metatarsals 2 through 5 (arrows). In both patients, the generalized lack of bone mineral density (BMD) is suggestive of osteopenia or frank osteoporosis, and further studies to evaluate BMD are indicated.

Table 1 Risk Factors for Osteoporotic Fracture

Nonmodifiable

Personal history of fracture as an adult*

History of fracture in a first-degree relative*

Caucasian or Asian descent (recent data suggest that African Americans and Hispanic Americans are at a significant risk, as well)

Advanced age

Female sex

Dementia

Poor health/fragility**

Potentially modifiable

Current cigarette smoking*

Low body weight (<127 lb)*

Estrogen deficiency

Early menopause (age <45 years) or bilateral ovariectomy

Prolonged premenopausal amenorrhea (>1 year)

Low calcium intake (lifelong)

Use of certain medications such as corticosteroids and anticonvulsants

Alcoholism

Impaired eyesight despite adequate correction

Recurrent falls

Inadequate physical activity

Poor health/fragility**

* These items are major factors in determining the risk of hip fracture, independent of bone density.

** Note that poor health and fragility may or may not be modifiable and thus occur under both headings.

(Adapted from *National Osteoporosis Foundation: Physician's Guide to the Prevention and Treatment of Osteoporosis.* Washington, DC, National Osteoporosis Foundation, 1998.)

Tests

Physical Examination

The physical examination is normal in the early stages. In advanced disease, findings may include tenderness to palpation over an area of fracture, spinal deformity, loss of height (often more than 2 inches), lax abdominal musculature with a protuberant abdomen, hypermobility, and exaggerated thoracic kyphosis (dowager hump).

Female athletes, particularly those participating in endurance activities, gymnastics, skating, and dance, may develop low bone density and subsequent stress or overt fractures because of overtraining, inadequate diet, and menstrual cessation. It is imperative to thoroughly question female athletes about their menstrual history and to question all athletes about their diet and exercise habits.

Diagnostic Tests

Diagnostic tests are performed to identify the presence and severity of the disease, measure response to therapeutic interventions, and rule out secondary causes of osteoporosis.

Because no specific measurement exists for bone strength, bone mineral density (BMD) is used as a surrogate. DEXA is currently the reference standard for BMD measurement (**Figure 3**). This quick, painless test helps estimate bone strength and predict future fracture risk. It is fast, reproducible, and involves very low radiation exposure. Bone mass is reported as a real density and compared with both peers (Z score) and young healthy individuals (T score). Z and T scores represent standard deviations (SDs) lower than the comparison group. Bone density is characterized by the lowest value at either the spine, femoral neck, trochanter, or total femur. Values of 0 to −1 are normal; −1 to −2.5 indicate osteopenia; lower than −2.5 indicates osteoporosis. DEXA currently is the best test for monitoring the results of osteoporosis treatment. For reasons of cost, speed, and availability, however, quantitative ultrasonography may be used as a screening tool in younger patients.

Because osteoporosis typically is a "silent" disease, the decision to test should be based on a patient's risk profile. The National Osteoporosis Foundation (NOF) recommends BMD testing for the following individuals:

- All women 65 years or older, regardless of risk factors
- Postmenopausal women younger than 65 years who have one or more of the following risk factors: family history of osteoporosis, personal history of low-trauma fracture older than 45 years, current cigarette smoker, or low body weight (less than 127 pounds)

Patient: Sample, Report
Birth Date: 5/21/1941 61.9 years
Height / Weight: 65.0 in. 123.0 lbs.
Sex / Ethnic: Female White

Facility ID:
Physician:
Measured: 4/15/2004 9:11:44 AM (7.51)
Analyzed: 4/15/2004 9:17:03 AM (7.51)

Total Body Bone Density

Reference: Total

Region	BMD [1] (g/cm²)	Young-Adult [2] T-Score	Age-Matched [3] Z-Score
Total	1.276	1.9	3.3

COMMENTS: Family history of hip Fx

A

B

Image not for diagnosis
Printed: 4/15/2003 9:36:08 AM (7.51) 76:0.15:153.85:31.2 0.00:-1.00
4.80x12.99 12.2:%Fat=32.5%
0.00:0.00 0.00:0.00
Filename: samplr_hde22h001.dfb
Scan Mode: Standard

1 -Statistically 68% of repeat scans fall within 1SD (± 0.010 g/cm² for Total Body Total)
2 -NHANES/USA, Total Body Reference Population, Ages 20-40
3 -Matched for Age, Weight (females 25-100 kg), Ethnic

Figure 3   A dual-energy x-ray absorptiometric scan (**A**) and report (**B**) for a 61-year-old white woman. The report provides a reference database of BMD as a function of age. The middle line is the mean BMD, and the lines above and below the line represent 1 standard deviation (SD) above and below the mean, respectively. Findings are compared with young adults (T scores) and with age-matched adults (Z scores). The World Health Organization (WHO) bases management guidelines on T scores. According to WHO, a T score of −1.0 SD or higher is normal; a T score between −1.0 and −2.5 indicates osteopenia; and a T score of −2.5 SD or lower indicates osteoporosis.

- Men with a history of a low-trauma fracture or of treatment with a gonadotropin-releasing hormone (GnRH) agonist for prostate cancer
- Individuals with primary hyperparathyroidism, who are undergoing long-term glucocorticoid treatment, with diseases or conditions known to cause bone loss, or using medications known to cause bone loss.

Osteoporosis may be either high-turnover osteoporosis (increased rate of absorption) or low-turnover osteoporosis (decreased rate of bone formation). The cross-linked N-telopeptide (NTx) test measures bone collagen breakdown products, with a high NTx level indicating high turnover and a low NTx level indicating low turnover. Tests to rule out secondary causes of osteoporosis include a complete blood cell count, erythrocyte sedimentation rate, C-reactive protein level, serum protein level, and immunoelectrophoresis (serum/urine) to rule out a bone marrow disorder. Thyroid function tests and parathyroid hormone (PTH) level tests are performed to rule out hyperthyroidism or hyperparathyroidism. Cushing disease and diabetes are ruled out by patient history. Tests performed for serum levels of calcium, phosphorus, alkaline phosphatase, and 25-hydroxyvitamin D (along with PTH levels) rule out osteomalacia. Other studies include renal and liver function tests and a 24-hour urine calcium test.

Differential Diagnosis

- Disuse osteopenia (history of prolonged immobilization or bed rest)
- Multiple myeloma (anemia, elevated erythrocyte sedimentation rate, bone pain, immunoelectrophoresis results)
- Osteomalacia (deformity, renal osteodystrophy) (bone pain, low hydroxyvitamin D level, high intact PTH level, elevated alkaline phosphatase, low calcium, low urinary calcium)
- Poor imaging technique on radiographs (overpenetration) (overpenetration may be suspected when soft tissues are not visible on radiographs; all radiographic diagnoses optimally confirmed by DEXA)
- Primary osteoporosis (type I or type II) (by exclusion, all low-energy fracture patients, a loss of more than 2 inches in height)
- Secondary osteoporosis (history, occurs in men)

Adverse Outcomes of the Disease

Adverse outcomes of osteoporosis include fracture, deformity, chronic pain, social withdrawal, loss of independence, and death, particularly following hip fracture.

Treatment

Prevention

Because peak bone mass is achieved in patients younger than 25 to 28 years, women should be encouraged to maximize bone formation during youth through proper diet and exercise and minimize bone loss during adulthood. Recommendations for the general population include an adequate intake of calcium and vitamin D, regular weight-bearing exercise, and avoidance of tobacco use and alcohol abuse.

Table 2 Dietary Reference Intake Values for Calcium by Life-stage Group

Life-stage Group	Adequate Calcium Intake (mg/day)
Males and Females	
0 to 6 months	210
6 to 12 months	270
1 through 3 years	500
4 through 8 years	800
9 through 13 years	1,300
14 through 18 years	1,300
19 through 30 years	1,000
31 through 50 years	1,000
51 through 70 years	1,200
>70 years	1,200
Women only	
Pregnancy	
≤18 years	1,300
19 through 50 years	1,000
Lactation	
≤18 years	1,300
19 through 50 years	1,000

(Adapted from *National Osteoporosis Foundation: Physician's Guide to the Prevention and Treatment of Osteoporosis.* Washington, DC, National Osteoporosis Foundation, 1998.)

Older patients should be educated about the importance of maintaining their body weight and reducing their risk factors for falls by walking for exercise, avoiding long-acting benzodiazepams, minimizing caffeine intake, and treating impaired visual function (**Table 1**).

Standards for the optimal type and duration of exercise have not been established. The ideal exercise program includes impact-loading exercise (such as walking), strength training, and balance training (such as tai chi).

Recommendations for calcium intake are listed in **Table 2**. Most Americans consume far less calcium than is recommended, particularly in their elder years. Calcium supplements are frequently required. The two main forms of calcium are carbonate and citrate. Carbonate requires an acid environment to dissolve; H2 blockers and indigestion impair its availability. Citrate forms dissolve at all pH levels and decrease the risk of kidney stones. As a consequence, citrate is preferred to carbonate unless chewed.

Vitamin D is essential for intestinal absorption of calcium, and requirements increase with age. Because skin production of this vitamin decreases even with adequate sun exposure, 25(OH) vitamin D levels should be higher than 15 ng/mL to avoid insufficiency, and some are even recommending levels should be higher than 30 ng/mL. Current recommendations for vitamin D intake are under review; 800 to 1,200 IU/day appear to be appropriate. Higher replacement is required in the face of vitamin D insufficiency. Fractures resulting from falls can be decreased by 20% with a minimum vitamin D intake of 800 IU/day. A combination of vitamin D and calcium can decrease the risk of hip fracture in the elderly by approximately 25%.

Intervention

In the best circumstances, treatment of osteoporosis is initiated before a fracture occurs. Physicians should encourage all patients to follow the prevention strategies listed above. The NOF recommends pharmacologic intervention for osteoporosis in white women whose BMD scores are 2 SDs lower than those of a "young healthy" adult in the absence of risk factors and in women whose BMD scores are 1.5 SDs lower than those of a "young healthy" adult if other risk factors are present. The NOF also notes that white women older than 70 years with multiple risk factors (especially those with previous fractures not occurring in the hip or spine) are at high enough risk of fracture to initiate treatment without BMD testing. Currently, the FRAX provides an estimated fracture risk for an individual (**Table 2**).

All interventions include appropriate calcium and vitamin D intake. Treatment classes include antiresorptive agents (bisphosphonates [alendronate, risedronate], SERMS [selective estrogen receptor modulators], calcitonin), prescribed for patients with high NTx levels; and anabolic agents (intermittent PTH), prescribed for patients with low NTx levels. Bisphosphonates decrease the fracture risk in all bones at least 50%. For individuals who cannot tolerate oral bisphosphonates, intravenous forms are efficacious in protecting bone mass. Bisphosphonates are indicated for all forms of osteoporosis, glucosteroid use, and acute fractures. Although estrogen prevents fractures, it is no longer recommended by the FDA for the treatment of osteoporosis because of its increased risk for myocardial infarct, stroke, breast cancer, and possibly dementia. Raloxifene is a selective estrogen receptor modulator (SERM) that enhances spinal bone mass and decreases vertebral fractures, but it does not prevent hip fractures. Calcitonin gives minor spinal fracture protection and possibly some pain relief, but it affords no protection against nonvertebral fracture.

Anabolic agents are recommended for low-turnover states, failures of bisphosphonates, premenopausal women, and in the setting of impaired fracture healing. Intermittent PTH (1 to 34 amino acids) is given only subcutaneously and results in marked enhancement of bone mass, fracture protection comparable to bisphosphonates, and enhancement of fracture healing. It is contraindicated in children, patients who have undergone prior radiation, and patients with Paget disease.

Adverse Outcomes of Treatment

Estrogen hormone replacement therapy is associated with an increased risk of breast cancer, heart disease, and deep vein thrombosis. Side effects can include vaginal bleeding, breast tenderness, mood disturbances, and gallbladder disease. Consequently, estrogen is not recommended for osteoporosis. Bisphosphonates must be administered on an empty stomach, and some patients report upper gastrointestinal disturbance. Also, some animal studies suggest a delay of maturation during fracture healing. Calcitonin has fewer side effects but is minimally effective and used only for the spine. Raloxifene has been shown to increase the risk of deep vein thrombosis at the same rate as estrogen, and it provides no hip fracture protection. It also causes hot flashes and does not treat menopausal symptoms. PTH may cause cramps and orthostatic hypotension in the very elderly.

Referral Decisions/Red Flags

Osteoporosis and fragility fractures are not inevitable in any age group. All appropriate patients should be referred for BMD testing and offered treatment.

Many physicians may feel uncomfortable evaluating BMD studies, ruling out secondary causes of osteoporosis, or initiating pharmacologic treatment. Referral to an osteoporosis specialist may be appropriate.

Overuse Syndromes

ICD-9 Code

729.5
Pain in limb

Synonyms

Cumulative trauma disorder
Occupational arm pain
Occupational stress syndrome
Repetitive strain injury
Work-related pain disorder

Definition

Overuse syndrome is an umbrella term that encompasses many specific diagnoses. These conditions typically result from repetitive motions, stresses, or sustained exertion of a particular body part. Overuse conditions can affect muscles, tendons, nerves, or bones, but most commonly involve the musculotendinous unit and the surrounding soft tissues. Overuse syndromes can occur in the upper or lower extremities. **Table 1** lists some of the most common forms of tendinitis seen with overuse injuries and their anatomic locations.

A wide population is at risk; however, overuse conditions commonly affect athletes, laborers, or workers with repetitive, stressful movements. At least 25% of adult athletes have experienced overuse injuries. Sporting activities typically associated with overuse injuries include baseball, dancing,

Table 1 Most Common Diagnoses and Locations of Chronic Tendinitis

Diagnosis	Location
Rotator cuff tendinitis	Supraspinatus tendon insertion
Lateral epicondylitis (tennis elbow)	Common wrist extensor tendon origin
de Quervain disease and trigger finger	Sheath/pulley of abductor pollicis longus and long finger flexors
Hamstring tendinitis	Hamstring tendon origin
Quadriceps tendinitis	Quadriceps tendon insertion
Patellar tendinitis (jumper's knee)	Patellar tendon origin
Achilles tendinitis	Sheath, midsubstance, or calcaneal insertion
Posterior tibial tendinitis	Midsubstance

(Reproduced from Almekinders LC: Tendinitis and other chronic tendonopathies. *J Am Acad Orthop Surg* 1998;6:157-164.)

tennis, golf, rowing, and long-distance running. In the workplace, contributing factors may include repetitive tasks, forceful exertions, and exposure to vibration or cold temperatures, awkward postures, or poor ergonomic environment. Injury also can occur, or be exacerbated by incorrect mechanics or kinematics during activities. Certain jobs and occupations seem to predispose workers to overuse syndromes. Professional musicians, grocery store checkers, computer keyboard operators, and dental hygienists are particularly susceptible.

Overuse tendon injuries can be related to several extrinsic and intrinsic factors (**Table 2**).

Overuse syndromes are typically secondary to repetitive microtrauma, which can produce either acute inflammation or a chronic degenerative state. Reactive or acute inflammatory overuse syndromes are a result of repetitive microtrauma that produces fatigue and inflammation. This is termed *tendinitis* and represents infiltration of the tendon or epitendinous covering with inflammatory cells and mediators. In the acute setting, the injury typically is not associated with degeneration to the musculotendinous unit. A persistent inflammatory state, however, can eventually lead to tissue breakdown over time. Chronic tendon injuries are a degenerative process rather than an inflammatory process. The term *tendinosis* defines chronic degeneration without inflammation of the tendon, epitendon, or tendon-bone interface secondary to prolonged microtrauma. Inflammation can be involved in the initial stages; however, later stages demonstrate failed healing and disruption of the tendon structure. Degeneration often occurs in areas of diminished blood flow, and age appears to be an important factor associated with tendon injuries.

Clinical Symptoms

Overuse syndromes develop over time and patients may not report their problems early, in anticipation that the condition will improve. Symptoms include pain, fatigue, numbness, swelling, or any combination thereof. With repetitive microtrauma—induced overuse syndromes, pain is usually localized to the tendinous insertion and exacerbated with muscle stretch or contraction. With chronic, degenerative overuse syndromes, rupture can cause significant pain and dysfunction. In syndromes affecting nerve tissue, there will be numbness and/or tingling in the distribution of that particular nerve. Over time, muscle weakness or muscle atrophy may develop secondary to nerve compression.

In exertional compartment syndrome, the patient may report worsening pain with activity or exercise. The only relieving factor may be extended rest from the activity. The patient also

Table 2 Factors in Chronic Tendon Problems

Extrinsic Factors

Repetitive mechanical load

Increased duration

Increased frequency

Increased intensity

Technique errors

Equipment problems

Footwear

Raquet size

Running surface

Protective gear

Intrinsic Factors

Anatomic factors

Malalignment

Inflexibility

Muscle weakness

Muscle imbalance

Decreased vascularity

Age-related factors

Tendon degeneration

Decreased healing response

Increased tendon stiffness

Decreased vascularity

Systemic factors

Inflammatory enthesopathy

Quinolone-induced tendinopathy

(Reproduced from Almekinders LC: Tendinitis and other chronic tendonopathies. *J Am Acad Orthop Surg* 1998;6:157-164.)

GENERAL ORTHOPAEDICS

SECTION 1

may report numbness in the foot, swelling in the lower leg, and pain that is aggravated by passive stretch of the ankle joint. Stress fractures demonstrate exquisite bony tenderness and localized pain at the site of the fracture. Pain typically is worsened with activity.

History and Physical Examination

Patients should be questioned specifically about sporting activities, job-related tasks, exposures, and recent changes in activity level. With regard to occupational overuse syndromes, job satisfaction, working conditions, exposure to repetitive and forceful exertions, vibration, or cold temperature should be investigated. It also is important to identify the type of industry and job specificity, as the incidence of overuse syndromes is higher for certain industries and occupations, such as meat packers, assembly line workers, grocery store cashiers, and clerical workers.

Physical examination should be thorough and comparison should be made with the contralateral extremity. Inspect the injured extremity for signs of swelling, erythema, pallor, or muscle atrophy. After inspection, palpate the area of complaint to determine the area of maximal tenderness. This will help shorten your differential diagnosis. Next, range of motion should be tested both passively and actively and compared with the contralateral extremity. Strength is assessed, paying particular attention to pain with resistance. A thorough neurovascular examination should also be conducted. For example, in de Quervain tenosynovitis, the patient will report pain when moving the thumb and will have tenderness to palpation over the radial-dorsal aspect at the base of the first metacarpal when moving the thumb because this is the location of the inflamed tendons (**Figure 1**). Flexion of the thumb with ulnar deviation of the wrist typically reproduces the pain (a positive Phalen test).

Diagnostic Tests

Diagnostic evaluation begins with radiographic evaluation of the affected extremity, although plain radiographs are typically normal. Radiographs can help rule out fractures, joint pathology, masses, or lesions. Radiographs also may demonstrate calcifications within the tendon, or bone spurs at the tendon insertion sites in cases of chronic tendinosis. (**Figure 2**)

Bone scans or MRIs may be necessary to identify a stress fracture. Bone scans can detect occult, osseous pathology; MRIs are important for both osseous and soft-tissue pathologies that are not adequately visualized on plain radiographs. **Figure 3** shows a tibial stress fracture seen on MRI that was not seen on initial radiographs of the tibia. MRI also is useful to diagnose

Figure 1 Anatomic drawing of the first dorsal compartment shows tendon insertion points involved in de Quervain tenosynovitis. APL = abductor pollicis longus, EPB = extensor pollicis brevis, EPL = extensor pollicis longus. (Reproduced from Ilyas AM, Ast M, Schaffer AA, Thoder J: De Quervain tenosynovitis of the wrist. *J Am Acad Orthop Surg* 2007;15:757-764.)

Figure 2 Lateral radiograph of chronic Achilles tendinosis shows calcification (arrow).

Figure 3 Sagittal MRI shows tibial stress fracture (arrow).

certain tendon tears or areas of chronic tendon injury, but should be ordered with discretion. **Figure 4** demonstrates an Achilles tendon injury seen on MRI.

Nerve compression syndromes can be evaluated with nerve conduction velocity (NCV) studies or electromyelographic (EMG) studies. NCVs or EMGs are ordered to rule out carpal

Figure 4 Sagittal MRI demonstrates Achilles tendon injury. Note the fluid (white area) within the tendons.

tunnel syndrome or ulnar nerve entrapment at the elbow. A NCV will show latency in conduction of nervous impulses, and an EMG will show decreased electric potential produced by particular muscle cells, which may present as muscle atrophy or weakness in chronic nerve compression syndromes.

Exertional compartment syndrome can be confirmed by measuring compartment pressures before and after exercise. Intracompartmental pressure measurements that confirm the diagnosis of chronic exertional compartment syndrome are as follows: at rest, greater than 15 mm Hg; 1 minute after exercise, greater than 30 mm Hg; 5 minutes after exercise, greater than 20 mm Hg.

Differential Diagnosis

- Angina with referred arm pain (abnormal electrocardiogram)
- Claudication (decreased peripheral pulses)
- Deep vein thrombosis (abnormal venogram, Doppler ultrasonogram)
- Fibromyalgia (11 of 18 tender points in four body quadrants)
- Herniated cervical or lumbar disk (abnormal spine radiographs, myelogram, and MRI)
- Tendon rupture
- Tumor

Adverse Outcomes of the Disease

With these disorders, patients often lose time from work or sport and may experience psychologic changes. In chronic conditions, especially those arising from work injuries, patients may become dependent upon pain medication. Persistent activity in patients with tendinosis can result in tendon ruptures. Continued activity in athletes with stress fractures can result in a truly displaced fracture. Finally, persistent pressure on nerves in carpal tunnel syndrome, cubital tunnel syndrome, or compartment syndrome can result in irreversible damage.

Treatment

Most overuse syndromes are mild and resolve spontaneously with time and rest. With overuse injuries in the workplace, satisfactory outcomes for many depend on the cooperative efforts of the employer, the insurance carrier, and a physician-directed health care team including rehabilitation specialists. A case manager, such as an occupational health nurse, can be invaluable in coordinating the efforts of these groups to return the patient to work.

Initial treatment should include protection, ice, and rest of the affected extremity. A progressive exercise program that includes eccentric strengthening has shown to be helpful in tendinitis. At the workplace, modify tasks, work schedules, and possible vocational changes should be considered if the symptoms persist.

NSAIDs and analgesic creams are beneficial in reducing pain associated with these conditions. Corticosteroid injections can be helpful in carpal tunnel syndrome, plantar fasciitis, lateral epicondylitis, and chronic tendinosis of the shoulder. Narcotics should be avoided because of the possibility of addiction. Antidepressants can be a useful adjunct if depression is a significant part of the clinical picture.

Although surgery may be indicated, it is seldom urgent and the results of surgery have been found to be less predictable in patients with workplace-associated overuse injuries. In workplace overuse injuries, lack of job satisfaction, depression, and litigation also are important predictors of recovery.

Overuse syndromes associated with running are very common in both the young and old. **Figure 5** is an algorithm that can be used for the work-up of a runner who presents with leg pain.

Adverse Outcomes of Treatment

Drug dependence on narcotics or antidepressants is possible. If the patient has undergone multiple ill-advised surgeries, persistently tender scars may be left. Patients may become depressed and lose conditioning if they are unable to perform their sport. It is important to keep patients physically active in alternative activities, such as swimming, which do not aggravate the injured area.

Referral Decisions/Red Flags

Persistent pain despite appropriate care merits referral to a specialist for further evaluation. In the workplace, once the diagnosis of overuse syndrome is suspected, treatment by a team of health care professionals may be helpful in managing these difficult problems.

SECTION 1 GENERAL ORTHOPAEDICS

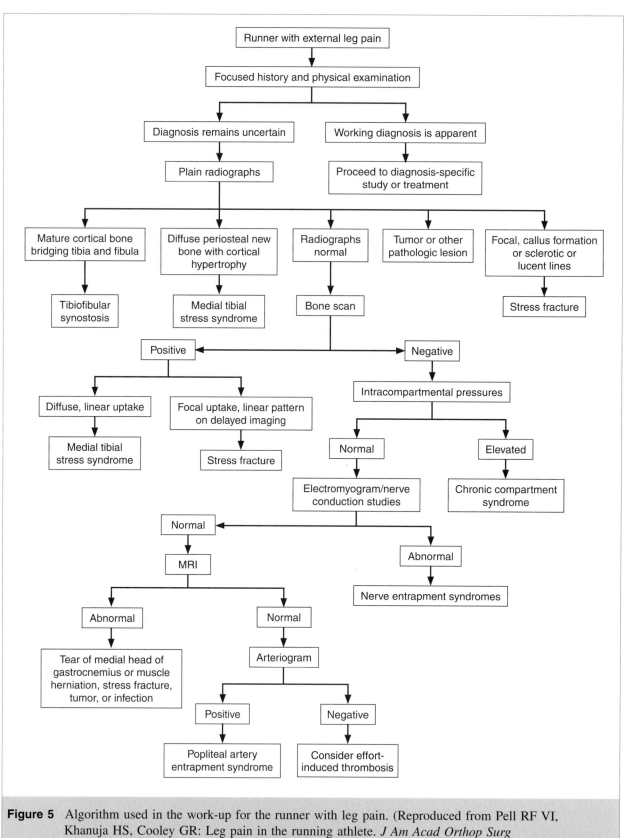

Figure 5 Algorithm used in the work-up for the runner with leg pain. (Reproduced from Pell RF VI, Khanuja HS, Cooley GR: Leg pain in the running athlete. *J Am Acad Orthop Surg* 2004;12:396-404.)

Pain: Nonorganic Symptoms and Signs

Synonyms

Functional overlay

Psychosomatic illness

ICD-9 Code

ICD-9 lists psychophysiologic disorders according to body system.

Definition

Patient responses or symptoms that do not fit known patterns of illnesses or injury are considered nonorganic. These physical signs were described early in the 20th century following the development of the Compensation Acts and the development of the medicolegal arena. These findings are not considered malingering; rather, they often are the way in which some patients communicate their perception of the seriousness of their problem or that they are not receiving the care they think they need. True malingering is rare and typically is a manifestation of bizarre social behavior.

Nonorganic findings should not be construed as indicating a lack of concomitant disease because significant underlying pathology can be present. Nonorganic findings occur three to four times more often in situations where workers' compensation and litigation are issues. They are often a clue that further psychologic assessment should be pursued. A standard examination is valuable preoperatively to determine and arrange postoperative pain expectations and treatment requirements. Additionally, with a thorough history and physical examination that includes a few of the standardized tests detailed below, dealing with unrealistic expectations prior to treatment initiation may save the clinician and patient a few ill emotions at the end of the day.

Clinical Symptoms

It should be assumed that all patients with pain have a physical source and it is only human nature to have an emotional and behavioral reaction to that pain. The clinician should always be cognizant of external factors that may influence the patient's presentation, including compensation, family, or employment issues. Nonorganic physical signs are most recognizable in relation to low back pain, most notably the five signs of Waddell, originally described in 1979 (see **Sidebar: Waddell Signs**).

Waddell Signs

Overreaction to examination

Simulation testing (axial loading, rotation)

Distraction with straight-leg raising and other tests

Regional symptoms of weakness and sensation

Tenderness (superficial and nonanatomic)

Waddell considered three or more signs as clinically significant. Pain or symptoms that appear to "travel" from one side or area of the body to another in a nonanatomic fashion and global pain are characteristic. Nonsegmental numbness (numbness that does not fit a nerve root or peripheral nerve pattern) also occurs.

Tests

Physical Examination

Exaggerated responses: Light touch causes a jerk or withdrawal. Other findings include grimacing, groaning, and grabbing the affected extremity during examination when no obvious trauma or medical problem exists.

Axial loading (low back pain): With the patient standing, place both hands on the head and push down, asking if it causes pain. Low back pain elicited in this position is a nonorganic finding; however, neck pain may be a legitimate finding.

Axial rotation (spine): With the patient's hands on the iliac crests, grasp and rotate the pelvis, asking the patient if this causes pain. This maneuver should not elicit back pain, since the motion occurs at the hips, not in the back. Because this test may be positive in 20% of patients, it is not as sensitive in identifying nonorganic behavior as are exaggerated responses and axial loading.

Flip sign: This sign is elicited with the patient seated and leaning slightly forward, with his or her hands on the edge of the examination table. While asking if the patient has knee problems, lift the foot and extend the knee. This maneuver increases tension on the sciatic nerve, and patients with lower lumbar herniated disks or other similar conditions will involuntarily "flip" back against the wall, reporting back and leg pain. A negative flip sign in the presence of a supine straight-leg raising test that produces leg and back pain at less than 45° of leg elevation is a significant nonorganic finding, as these maneuvers are the same test.

Distraction: A provocative test (such as palpation) may be negative when the patient is distracted with conversation, but positive when attention is drawn to the test or body part.

Giving way: During muscle testing, a nonorganic finding is a lack of sustained effort. Typically, the patient "gives way" or "lets go" in a ratchety, uneven pattern. Another variant is the patient who gives a poor effort on muscle testing and then, with coaxing, may intermittently contract the muscle, then let go.

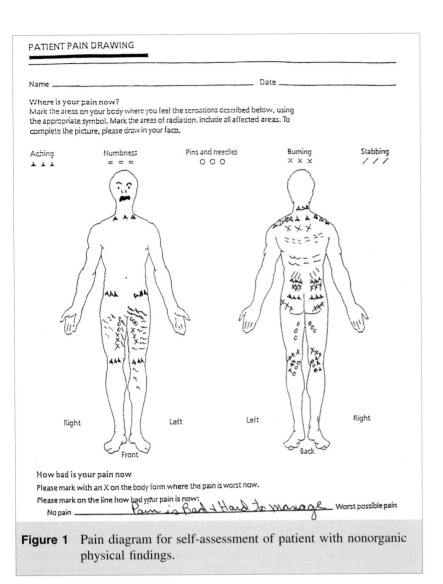

Figure 1 Pain diagram for self-assessment of patient with nonorganic physical findings.

Stocking or nonanatomic numbness: Some patients report hypoesthesia that affects the extremity in a circumferential (stocking-glove) distribution or covers nonanatomic patterns. Patients with diabetes mellitus or multiple sclerosis may develop sensory abnormalities in a stocking-glove or nonsegmental pattern.

Pain diagram: On a diagram of the body, ask the patient to draw representations of symptoms, using marks such as dashes, slashes, or Xs, etc. Bizarre drawings do not indicate malingering or mental disease. Many people have perceptual disorders that blunt the scientific validity of these drawings, but they often yield insight into how pain is perceived by patients and what areas of the body they believe are related in their current problem (**Figure 1**).

The kneeling bench test of Burns: This is another test of exaggerated response. Ask a patient who reports back pain to kneel on a stool. Hold the patient's ankles to ensure confidence and ask the patient to bend forward and touch the floor. Patients who are exaggerating symptoms will bend forward a few degrees and then grab their back, saying they cannot bend. Note that these patients are already bending forward significantly.

A thorough neurologic examination is always required to give the above-mentioned tests perspective and to rule out concomitant disease.

Diagnostic Tests
None

Differential Diagnosis

- Acute injury (withdrawal from a painful examination maneuver may be an appropriate response)
- Diabetes mellitus (stocking-type peripheral neuropathy)
- Multiple sclerosis (bizarre sensory patterns that are not segmental)
- Stroke or other central lesions with altered sensory appreciation

Treatment

Rule out serious disorders that may be masked by these symptoms and discuss the absence of specific disorders with the patient. Because patients with this condition often are indirectly indicating that they are not getting the support or help they need, discuss psychologic and social support interventions and inquire about contributing factors such as occupational stress and marital difficulties.

Adverse Outcomes of Treatment

Failure to identify an associated serious condition is possible. Patients should always be screened for constitutional symptoms including fevers, chills, night sweats, unexpected weight loss, and incontinence. These alert the physician to other entities including infection, malignancy, and neural compression.

Referral Decisions/Red Flags

True diminished pinprick or light touch sensation with or without areflexia, brisk reflexes, clonus, spasticity, or a positive Babinski reflex usually indicates neurologic involvement.

Preoperative Evaluation of Medical Comorbidities

Definition

Surgical risk is the likelihood of an adverse outcome or death for a given surgery and associated anesthesia. A thorough preoperative evaluation allows both the orthopaedic surgeon and patient to make a more informed decision regarding the timing and tactics for surgical management of musculoskeletal problems.

The patient and the intensity of the procedure must be evaluated to accurately assess the need for a high-risk protocol. The patient's medical comorbidities, including both the severity and effect on surgical risk, need to be assessed. Additionally, consideration should be given as to whether these factors are modifiable. The procedure itself also is important to consider not only in terms of the complexity of procedure, but also the timing (ie, whether the surgery is elective, urgent or emergent) (**Table 1**).

Table 1 Classification of Orthopaedic Procedures

Parameter	Elective	Necessary	Emergent
Time frame for intervention	At the patient's request and convenience, depending on surgeon availability	Poorly defined, case independent	Within hours or even minutes, depending on the situation
Success of nonsurgical options	Variable, depending on the procedure	Usually poor	Usually poor or even fatal to the patient or limb
Importance relative to other surgical cases	Equal to other elective cases; secondary to necessary or emergent cases	Secondary only to emergent cases	Highest importance; warrants "bumping" of nonemergent cases
Timing and extent of medical evaluation	May schedule in conjuction with the patient's primary care physician	Should be performed expediously, but also be as thorough as possible	If condition permits, should be performed emergently and only include life or limb-saving tests or procedures
Examples	Total joint arthroplasty, anterior cruciate ligament reconstruction, ganglion cyst excision, carpal tunnel release, bunionectomy	Fixation of hemiarthroplasty for hip fracture, treatment of unstable fractures or dislocations failing closed reduction	Fasciotomy for compartment syndrome, stabilization of open book pelvis, treatment of open fracture

(Adapted from Bushnell BD, Horton JK, McDonald MF, Robertson PG: Perioperative medical comorbidities in the orthopaedic patient. *J Am Acad Orthop Surg* 2008;16:217-227.)

Table 2 Clinical Predictors of Increased Perioperative Cardiovascular Risk

Major Clinical Predictors

Unstable coronary syndromes

Uncompensated congestive heart failure

Significant arrhythmias

Sever valvular disease

Clinical Risk Factors

History of ischemic heart disease

History of cerebrovascular disease

History of compensated or prior congestive heart failure

Diabetes mellitus

Renal insufficiency

(Adapted from Vaccarro AR: *Orthopaedic Knowledge Update*, ed 8. Rosemont, IL, American Academy of Orthopaedic Surgeons, 2005.)

General Principles

Preoperative testing should be tailored to the group of patients that are more likely to have an abnormal result and only should be ordered if the result will affect management. This helps to avoid both unnecessary cost and delay in surgical treatment.

Cardiac

In 2007, the American College of Cardiology and the American Heart Association issued guidelines for the cardiac evaluation of patients undergoing noncardiac surgery. The guidelines divide cardiac issues into major clinical predictors and clinical risk factors are shown in **Table 2**.

Pulmonary

Routine chest radiographs are not recommended for all patients but should be obtained for a clinically significant subset (**Table 3**). Elective surgery should be delayed for active respiratory infections and acute exacerbations of obstructive lung disease. Conflicting evidence exists regarding the timing of smoking cessation and lowering risk of pulmonary complications, but an 8-week period of abstinence is probably ideal.

Renal

In patients who have chronic kidney disease, the leading cause of death is cardiac, and a full cardiac assessment is indicated for these patients. Particular attention needs to be paid to volume

Table 3 Recommendations for Preoperative Testing

Preoperative Test	Characteristics
Hemoglobin	Anticipated blood loss or symptoms of anemia
White blood cell count	Symptoms of infection, myeloproliferate disorder, or myelotoxic medications
Platelet count	History of bleeding, diathesis, myeloproliferate disorder, or myelotoxic medications
Partial thromboplastin time	History of bleeding
Electrolytes	Renal insufficiency, congestive heart failure, medications that affect electrolytes
Renal function	Hypertension, older than 50 years, cardiac disease, major surgery, anticipated use of medications that may affect renal function
Glucose	Obesity or known diabetes
Electrocardiogram	Men older than 40 years, women older than 50 years, known coronary artery disease, diabetes or hypertension
Chest radiograph	Older than 50 years, known cardiac or pulmonary disease, symptoms or examination suggestive of cardiac or pulmonary disease

(Adapted from Vaccarro AR: *Orthopaedic Knowledge Update*, ed 8. Rosemont, IL, American Academy of Orthopaedic Surgeons. 2005.)

status, electrolytes, acid/base status, anemia, bleeding diatheses, and blood pressure. In the face of acute or chronic renal failure, the use of nephrotoxins, such as NSAIDs, some antibiotics, angiotensin-converting enzyme inhibitors, and radiocontrast, should be minimized.

Diabetes

Diabetic patients are at an increased risk of many postoperative complications, including infection, metabolic/electrolyte abnormalities, renal issues, and cardiac issues. Hyperglycemia significantly impairs wound healing and the ability to fight infection. Additionally, patients are at significant risk for hypoglycemia in the perioperative period, making strict glucose control critical. Preoperative evaluation should include evaluating recent blood glucose and hemoglobin A1C measurements. A reasonable hemoglobin A1C target value is less than 7%. For patients taking oral hypoglycemics, they should withhold their medications in the 24 hours prior to surgery. For insulin-dependent diabetics, they should take one half to two thirds of their normal dose. The American Diabetes Association recommends a preprandial blood glucose level of 90 to 130 mg/dL for all hospitalized patients.

Rheumatologic Disease

For the patient with rheumatologic disease, there are several additional factors to consider. Bleeding times may be prolonged by the use of salicylates or NSAIDs. Additionally, patients who

Table 4 Risk Factors for Malnutrition

Prior surgery

Gastrointestinal disease

Advanced age

Depression

Poverty

Recent weight loss

Systemic disease

Alcohol abuse

Medications that interfere with eating/appetite

(Adapted from Bushnell BD, Horton JK, McDonald MF, Robertson PG: Perioperative medical comorbidities in the orthopaedic patient. *J Am Acad Orthop Surg* 2008;16: 217-227.)

have taken systemic steroids for more than a week in the 6 months preceding surgery may need a stress dose of steroids to decrease the risk of adrenal suppression. A typical regimen begins with 100 mg of IV hydrocortisone every 8 hours on the day of surgery, followed by 50 mg IV every 8 hours on postoperative day 1, 25 mg IV every 8 hours on postoperative day 2, 25 mg IV every 12 hours on postoperative day 3, and ends by resuming the patient's maintenance dose on postoperative day 4. Anesthesia in patients with rheumatoid arthritis can be challenging due to either cervical instability or cricoarytenoid arthritis (seen in up to 50% of patients). Evaluation performed with lateral, flexion, and extension radiographic views of the cervical spine is needed preoperatively to assess for atlantoaxial instability. Although an anterior atlantodental interval of more than 3 mm or subaxial subluxation of more than 3 mm have been classically used as markers of instability, recent studies suggest that a posterior atlantodental interval of less than 14 mm or a subaxial space available for the cord measuring less than 14 mm may be more accurate predictors of paralysis.

Nutrition

Nutrition plays an important role in wound healing and fighting infection. Risk factors for malnutrition are listed in **Table 4**. A body mass index less than 20, total cholesterol less than 160 mg/dL, and an albumin less than 3.3 mg/dL are all markers of malnutrition that have correlated with increased mortality. In these patients, maintenance fluids should contain carbohydrates; nothing-by-mouth (NPO) periods should be minimized; and protein supplements and vitamins should be given in the perioperative period. Conversely, obesity also increases the

Table 5 Risk Factors for Venous Thromboembolism

Surgery

Trauma (major or lower extremity)

Immobility, paresis

Malignancy

Cancer therapy (hormonal, chemotherapy, or radiotherapy)

Previous venous thromboembolic disease

Increasing age

Pregnancy and the postpartum period

Estrogen-containing oral contraception or hormone replacement
therapy

Selective estrogen receptor modulators

Acute medical illness

Heart or respiratory failure

Inflammatory bowel disease

Nephrotic syndrome

Myeloproliferative disorders

Paroxysmal nocturnal hemoglobinuria

Obesity

Smoking

Varicose veins

Central venous catheterization

Inherited or acquired thrombophilia

(Adapted from Bushnell BD, Horton JK, McDonald MF, Robertson PG: Perioperative
medical comorbidities in the orthopaedic patient. *J Am Acad Orthop Surg* 2008;16:
217-227.)

perioperative risk of complications including higher rates of
prosthetic failure, infection, hardware failure, and fracture
malunion. One study found a relative risk of deep vein
thrombosis (DVT) of 2.5 in obese patients compared with
nonobese patients.

DVT Prophylaxis

An important part of perioperative management of the
orthopaedic patient is appropriate DVT prophylaxis. Venographic
studies have shown an absolute risk of DVT of 40% to 60% in
patients who have undergone hip or knee arthroplasty. Although
the majority of these are asymptomatic, they have the potential
to lead to a pulmonary embolism, a potentially fatal
complication. Patients who are either hypercoagulable, have
endothelial damage, or experience decreased activity are at
increased risk of DVT (Table 5). Recommendations for

prophylaxis after orthopaedic procedures have been issued by the American Academy of Chest Physicians and the American Academy of Orthopaedic Surgeons. The majority of symptomatic DVTs occur following hospitalization and the risk remains elevated for 8 weeks.

Rehabilitation and Therapeutic Modalities

Definition

Rehabilitation is an important component of successful management of musculoskeletal health and musculoskeletal injuries or surgery. Rehabilitation has evolved into an evidence-based multidisciplinary profession with advancements in kinesiology, physiology, and soft-tissue management. The main objective of rehabilitation is to return the patient to maximum function as quickly and safely as possible following injury or surgery. The physician should be involved in the patient's rehabilitation program and maintain communication with the rehabilitation specialist to ensure optimum recovery following a musculoskeletal injury or surgery.

Conditioning exercises are often a part of the rehabilitation plan. Although the goal of rehabilitation is to return an injured person to a preinjury state, the goal of conditioning, whether for a healthy or injured individual, is to facilitate an improvement in strength, speed, balance, and overall cardiovascular fitness.

Rehabilitation

Evaluation by the physician and rehabilitation specialist is essential to identify a patient's specific impairments or weaknesses. Following the evaluation, a problem list (or list of impairments or weaknesses) is created and serves to generate treatment goals for the patient (Table 1). The goals of rehabilitation are specific for each patient and often include the following: decreasing inflammation, increasing joint range of motion (ROM) and flexibility, and increasing muscle strength as well as neuromuscular function, proprioception, and balance.

Table 1 Guidelines for Exercise Prescription

Match goals to exercise preferences

Set realistic and achievable goals

Provide regular follow-up to monitor progress; think of exercise as a medication

Review goals regularly and adjust accordingly

Involve family members; encourage the individual to exercise with other people

(Reproduced from Ashe MC, Khan KM: Exercise prescription. *J Am Acad Orthop Surg* 2004;12:21-27.)

SECTION 1 GENERAL ORTHOPAEDICS

Table 2 Guidelines for Athletic Injury Rehabilitation

Phase	Pathologic Process	Functional Goals	Rehabilitation
I - Acute injury	Tissue injury (hematoma, edema, inflammation, necrosis)	Protection; limit injury, swelling, and pain	PRICE (protection, rest, ice, compression, elevation)
II - Initial rehabilitation	Fibroblastic stage, decreasing inflammation, edema waning, minimal tensile strength (0%–15%)	Progressive pain-free ROM	Active/assisted ROM, limited short-arc resistance, cold, gentle isometrics, early aerobics
III - Progressive rehabilitation	Early tissue repair, primitive collagen and early tissue maturation, moderate tensile strength (15%–50%)	Improve ROM, increase strength, limited activity skills, ongoing protection	Passive and active ROM and stretching, progressive resistive exercises with isotonic and/or isokinetic exercise, increased aerobic activities
IV - Integrated functions	Mature collagen, tissue characteristics evident, tensile strength improved (50%–90%)	Increase skills and strength, enhance flexibility	Advanced progressive resistive exercises, flexibility exercises, coordination training, proprioceptive training
V - Return to sport	Tissue remodeling, tissue characteristics maturing, tensile strength increased (90%–99%)	Maximize skills, simulated participation, prevent reinjury	Maintain strength and flexibility, advanced coordination activities, protect previously injured area from reinjury

ROM = range of motion.
(Adapted with permission from Skerker RS, Schulz LA: Principles of rehabilitation of the injured athlete, in Pappas AM, Walzer J, eds: *Upper Extremity Injuries in the Athlete*. New York, NY, Churchill Livingstone, 1995, p 31; and Morgan WJ, Slowman LS: Acute hand and wrist injuries in athletes: Evaluation and management. *J Am Acad Orthop Surg* 2001;9:389-400.)

The end goals of rehabilitation may range from the ability to successfully perform activities of daily living to returning to a high level of athletic participation. Rehabilitation generally progresses in stepwise fashion through five main phases (Table 2).

Restoring full ROM is a primary goal of rehabilitation. Flexibility exercises, passive low-load prolonged stretching, and manual therapy are the most successful approaches to restoring full ROM. Flexibility exercises should be performed daily by those recovering from an injury. Stretching techniques include static (slow, gentle stretching), ballistic (quick, repetitive stretching), and proprioceptive neuromuscular function (PNF; a slow stretch followed by isometric contraction against a partner's resistance for 5 to 10 seconds followed by relaxation and slow stretch). Caution should be taken during ballistic stretching, as injury can result. Hence, many rehabilitation specialists prefer static and PNF stretching techniques (Figure 1).

As ROM improves, it is important to strengthen the muscles surrounding the joint and to improve muscle endurance. Three general types of exercises can be used: isometric, isotonic, and isokinetic, so named based on the type of muscle contraction

Figure 1   Commonly used stretching exercises for the muscles of the upper and lower extremities. **A,** Ankle roll—Loosen the tibiotalar and subtalar joints by placing toes on the ground and gently rolling the ankle. **B,** Plantar fascia and calf—Stand back several feet from a fence/wall, place toes against the object, and lean forward. Hold for 30 seconds. Repeat with opposite extremity. **C,** Alternate calf stretch—Lean forward on hands, gently arching back while keeping foot flat on the ground, and slowly lift the other leg. Hold for 30 seconds and switch legs. **D,** Standing quadriceps stretch—Stand on one leg (may brace yourself against a stationary object), bend knee toward your buttock, and grasp ankle. Hold for 30 seconds. Repeat with opposite leg. **E,** Lower body and hip stretch—Slowly bend forward at the hips. Keep knees slightly bent during the stretch so that the lower back is not stressed. Let the neck and shoulders relax. Bend to the point where you feel a stretch in the back of the legs. Hold for 30 seconds. **F,** Calf, hamstring and spine stretch—Stand with your legs crossed. Keep your feet together and your legs straight. Slowly bend forward toward your toes. Hold for 30 seconds. Repeat with opposite leg crossed in front. **G,** Low back, hips, and hamstring stretch—Stand with feet at a comfortable distance apart. To stretch the inside of your upper legs and hips, slowly lean forward from the hips, trying to touch the ground in front of you (upper). Hold for 15 seconds. Then slowly reach both hands toward the right ankle (lower). Hold for 30 seconds. Repeat, reaching for left ankle.

elicited (Table 3). Isometric exercises produce a muscle contraction without measurable change in joint angle. They are often indicated early in a rehabilitation program when muscle contraction is desired without excessive stress on the joint. An example of isometric exercise is a patient or rehabilitation specialist applying a force to the forearm with the elbow at 90° of flexion while the patient resists or pushes against the applied force. Isotonic exercises consist of a fixed resistance applied to a joint while it moves through an ROM. These exercises can be

SECTION 1 GENERAL ORTHOPAEDICS

Figure 1 (continued) **H,** Side stretch—Stand with your weight evenly distributed and your feet shoulder width apart. Place one hand at your side and the other above your head, leaning to the opposite side. Hold for 30 seconds. Repeat three times on each side. **I,** Trunk rotation—Stand with your weight evenly distributed and your feet shoulder width apart. Slowly rotate your upper body to one side while keeping your hips still. Hold for 30 seconds. Alternate sides. Repeat 10 times. May also be performed in a seated position with good posture. **J,** Low back and hamstring stretch—Sit with legs straight out in front of you. Reach forward with both hands toward your feet. Hold for 30 seconds. Feel the stretch at the back of the thighs. Try not to bend at the knees. Can do with one knee bent out to side (figure-of-4 position). **K,** Groin and low back stretch—Sit on floor, place the soles of your feet together, and drop your knees toward the floor. Place your forearms on the insides of your knees and gently push your knees toward the floor. Lean forward, bringing your chin to your feet. Hold for 30 seconds. **L,** Crossover arm—Grasp the elbow of one arm with your opposite hand and pull the arm across the front of your chest. **M,** Overhead arm—Raise your injured arm above your head, as high toward the ear as possible, and bend the elbow with the palm up. Use your opposite hand to help pull the arm toward the ear. Hold for 30 seconds and then relax. Perform 25 times, 3 times per day. **N,** Front of shoulder—Put arms behind your back, shoulder width apart. Move hands slowly toward each other and hold for 30 seconds.

further classified as concentric (contraction occurs as the muscle shortens) or eccentric (contraction occurs as the muscle lengthens). Isotonic exercises are used as the rehabilitation program advances to increase muscle strength and endurance. An example is a bicep curl performed with a dumbbell. Isokinetic exercises consist of a varied resistance applied to a joint moving at a constant rate of speed. These exercises can be performed manually by the rehabilitation specialist or with specialized equipment. Isokinetic exercises can be used to decrease the stress on a muscle or joint at points of the ROM

Table 3 Muscle Contraction Terminology

Type of Muscle Contraction	Definition	Indications	Example
Isometric	A muscle contraction that produces force without a measurable change in the joint angle.	Increasing strength at a specific point in the ROM.	The patient or therapist applies a force to the patient's forearm at 90° of elbow flexion. This produces a contraction of the biceps without moving the joint.
Isotonic	A manual or mechanical resistance remains constant while the joint moves through some ROM (may be concentric or eccentric).		
Concentric	An isotonic contraction that occurs as the muscle shortens.	Important for producing acceleration of a body segment.	Patient performs a bicep curl with resistance from full extension to full elbow flexion.
Eccentric	An isotonic contraction that occurs as the muscle lengthens.	Important for deceleration of a body segment and shock absorption.	Patient lowers a heavier weight from full elbow flexion to extension.
Isokinetic	A muscle contraction that occurs at a constant rate of speed.	Strengthening throughout the ROM.	Therapist applies manual accommodating resistance throughout elbow ROM. This can be performed concentrically or eccentrically.

ROM = range of motion.

where the joint may be less capable of producing a strong counterforce (ie, at the beginning or end of the ROM vs the mid range). Isokinetic exercise is frequently used following an injury or surgery to test muscular strength.

As progress in rehabilitation advances, strength training with heavier weights and lower repetitions may be initiated as long as no pain is present during the exercise. Strengthening exercises for rehabilitation should be performed 4 or 5 days per week. Both closed chain and open-chain exercises are utilized to improve strength and function during the rehabilitation program (Table 4). Closed-chain exercises are generally safer and are used at the beginning of a rehabilitation program. The patient generally begins closed-chain exercises with use of both limbs and smaller joint ROM, progresses to a larger ROM, and then performs the exercises using a single (involved) limb. Open-chain exercises are used to strengthen a particular muscle or muscle group, such as a muscle that has atrophied from disuse or immobilization. Open-chain exercises can place greater stress on a joint, so these exercises should begin with low weight and

Table 4 Open- Versus Closed-Chain Exercises

Exercise	Characteristics	Examples
Open chain	Distal segment is free; non–weight bearing; muscle contraction is primarily concentric; proprioceptive carryover to functional activities is questionable	Isometrics; straight-leg raises; stationary bike; terminal knee extension
Closed chain	Distal segment is not free; partial weight bearing; muscle contraction includes concentric, eccentric, isometric, and isotonic; movements are functional; significant proprioceptive carryover to functional activities	Partial weight bearing: mini wall squats, proprioceptive exercises with BAPS board Full weight bearing: elliptical machine, agility drills, step ups, mini wall squats

BAPS = biomechanical ankle platform system.

a higher number of repetitions and advance accordingly.

Proprioception (awareness of the body's position in space) exercises must be included in any rehabilitation program, especially those for lower extremity injuries, so the patient can regain and enhance neuromuscular control. Initially, the patient simply stands on one leg, then progresses to maintaining balance with eyes closed or while standing on an unstable or soft surface.

After normal ROM, strength, and neuromuscular control/ balance are achieved, the patient can progress to activity-specific exercises designed to achieve the end goals of rehabilitation. For athletes, this would include sport-specific exercises, such as change-of-direction ("cutting") activities, jumping, and throwing. General physical conditioning also may be included in the rehabilitation plan at this point. For a discussion of general physical conditioning and detailed exercise plans for the conditioning of the shoulder, hip, knee, foot, and lumbar spine, see the chapter on Musculoskeletal Conditioning: Helping Patients Prevent Injury and Stay Fit, page 183.

Therapeutic Modalities

Rehabilitation specialists use therapeutic modalities to decrease pain and inflammation following an acute injury or surgery. Certain modalities also can be utilized to reestablish neuromuscular control in atrophied muscles and are a useful adjunct with strengthening exercises. For example, good evidence exists that high-frequency electrical stimulation used in conjunction with a closed kinetic chain anterior cruciate ligament rehabilitation program enhances quadriceps strength. Transcutaneous electrical nerve stimulation (TENS) is designed to help control pain through a proposed spinal cord gating mechanism and can be useful to prepare the soft tissue prior to manual therapy or passive and active stretching exercises.

Table 5 Therapeutic Modalities, Exercises, and Equipment

Symptoms and Physical Findings	Treatment	Exercises	Equipment	Comments
Acute swelling	Ice, EGS	In uninjured areas only	Compression, braces, and splints for immobilization	
Chronic inflammation	Ice, phonophoresis, iontophoresis, NSAIDs	Stretching, joint mobilization, isometric, and short-arc strengthening	Tape, soft braces neoprene sleeves	
Restricted joint motion with inflammation	Ice	Isometric strengthening, active exercises in ROM without pain	Compression wraps, functional braces	Assess for intra-articular pathology
Restricted joint motion without inflammation	Heat, ultrasound	Active ROM, passive ROM, and active-assist ROM exercises	Progressive splints to maintain motion, night splints	Rule out systemic disease, CRPS
Joint instability	None, unless swelling present	Strengthening in ROM without pain, closed-chain kinetic exercises, proprioception exercises	Immobilize acute injury, functional braces later	Distinguish between static and functional instability
Muscle atrophy	EGS	PREs	Weights and tubing for home exercise program	Distinguish between disuse and neurologic injuries
Muscle imbalances	Objective measurement	Selective strengthening exercises		Distinguish between disuse and neurologic injuries
Loss of flexibility with injury	Ice, EGS, ultrasound	Static stretching, massage, PREs	Compression with and without immobilization	
Loss of flexibility without injury		Active stretching, with and without assistance, massage, myofascial release		Address underlying cause of muscle tightness
Proprioceptive deficit		Balance and proprioceptive exercises, functional exercises	Neoprene sleeve for warmth, neoprene sleeve or wrap for tactile input, balance board	Modified Romberg test

EGS = electric galvanic stimulation, ROM = range of motion, CRPS = chronic regional pain syndrome, PRE = passive resistance exercise.

Therapeutic ultrasound can be utilized to increase tissue elasticity, increase blood flow to tissues, and promote good alignment of scar tissue. Low-level or cold laser therapy has become more popular as a technique to promote tissue healing by increasing cell metabolism. Table 5 lists the indications for various therapeutic modalities, exercises, and equipment.

SECTION 1 GENERAL ORTHOPAEDICS

Table 6 Contraindications to Exercise

Absolute

Recent myocardial infarction

Ischemic electrocardiographic changes

Unstable angina

Uncontrolled arrhythmia

Third-degree heart block

Acute congestive heart failure

Relative

Uncontrolled hypertension

Valvular heart disease

Cardiomyopathies

Complex ventricular ectopy

Uncontrolled metabolic disease

(Reproduced from Galloway MT, Jokl P: Aging successfully: The importance of physical activity in maintaining health and function. *J Am Acad Orthop Surg* 2000;8:37-44.)

Adverse Outcomes of Treatment

Untimely or overaggressive therapy may disrupt the healing process, as can therapy that does not respect weight-bearing limitations. Additional contraindications to rehabilitation exercises are listed in **Table 6**.

Preparation for activity-related emergencies, preparticipation physical exams, and proper hydration and nutrition must also be instituted for competitive athletes to prevent possible adverse outcomes from conditioning and rehabilitation programs.

Referral Decisions/Red Flags

Complex problems, lack of progression, or the need for special rehabilitation equipment indicates referral to a rehabilitation specialist. Patients who are not able to undergo therapy on their own or who desire to return to a high level of athletic competition also benefit from referral. When ordering rehabilitation, the physician should specify the diagnosis and the limitations of the patient.

Musculoskeletal Conditioning: Helping Patients Prevent Injury and Stay Fit

Over the past 50 to 75 years, the United States has experienced a shift in lifestyle. Once a society in which most individuals worked in physically stressful jobs (eg, farming, steelmaking, road and railroad building); walked to work, to visit friends, and to shop; and climbed stairs rather than riding elevators, ours is now a society in which individuals may sit in offices during most of their workday and drive to their activities. The mental stresses may be great, but the physical stresses of most jobs are small. Yard and household chores have also become physically less demanding, thanks to technologic advances: lawn mowers are motorized, and sweepers, floor waxers, dishwashers, and clothes washers have replaced manual activities for these tasks.

Unfortunately, as physical inactivity has become more common, health issues associated with this inactivity have become all too prominent. Obesity and associated diseases such as heart disease, diabetes mellitus, and hypertension have been reported to be "epidemic" in the United States.

One responsibility of a physician is to educate patients on the importance of physical activity as a part of a healthy lifestyle. Such an exercise prescription typically includes not only instruction in a general aerobic exercise program for cardiovascular fitness (such as swimming, cycling, or walking) but also exercise to strengthen areas weakened by injury or inactivity or areas that would be particularly challenged by a new activity. For example, a 50-year-old man who wishes to play tennis or a 45-year-old woman who recently secured a job as a painter would benefit from both cardiovascular exercise to increase endurance and specific exercises for conditioning the shoulders and trunk. A body made fit by musculoskeletal stretching, strengthening, and proprioceptive exercises is less likely to sustain injury during sport- or work-related activities or daily activities such as gardening or housekeeping. This chapter provides examples of these exercises.

A conditioning program for either the body as a whole or a specific targeted anatomic area of the body consists of three basic phases: stretching exercises to restore range of motion, strengthening exercises to improve muscle power, and proprioceptive exercises to enhance balance and agility.

Stretching and strengthening exercises are generally begun first, followed by proprioceptive exercises. Patient handouts are provided on the DVD for the stretching and strengthening exercises, and additional proprioceptive exercises for beginners are described in the text. Plyometric exercises may also be added for power after basic strength and flexibility have been achieved. Advanced proprioceptive exercises and plyometric exercises should be done under the supervision of a rehabilitation specialist (eg, physical therapist, athletic trainer, or occupational therapist) or other exercise professional (eg, strength and conditioning personal trainer).

The goal of a conditioning program is to enable people to live a fit and healthier lifestyle by being more active. A well-structured conditioning program will also prepare the individual for participation in sports and recreational activities. The greater the intensity of the activity that the individual wishes to engage in, the greater the intensity of the conditioning that will be required. If the individual attends supervised rehabilitation (including all specialists listed above) for instruction in a conditioning routine rather than using only an exercise handout such as provided here, the focus should be on developing and committing to a home exercise fitness program.

Conditioning exercises follow, arranged by anatomic area. Musculoskeletal conditioning of the shoulder is discussed first, followed by the hip, knee, foot and ankle, and lumbar spine. Each section describes a home exercise program and includes patient exercise handouts that may be printed out from the DVD that accompanies this book.

Shoulder Conditioning

The shoulder is a complex structure that allows movement in many different planes. The muscles of the shoulder most important in overhead sports activities such as tennis, baseball, and swimming are the glenohumeral and scapular rotators. Strengthening the scapular stabilizers, as well as the rotator cuff and deltoid muscles, is important because strong, coordinated function of all shoulder muscle groups helps stabilize the glenohumeral joint and helps prevent injury when the individual engages in activities such as gardening, housekeeping, or work- or sport-related activities that involve repetitive upper extremity motion. Also, increased strength in these muscles translates into a higher velocity tennis serve or baseball pitch.

Proprioceptive or balance exercises help train the joints of the upper extremity to perceive joint positions and hence enhance the individual's perception of the position of the body in space. Examples of proprioceptive exercises for the shoulder are scapular retraction done while lying on an exercise ball or push-ups performed on an air mattress or with each hand on a small ball instead of the floor. These exercises should be done only after adequate flexibility and strength have been achieved. Also, instruction and supervision in such exercises is required to ensure that they are performed safely.

For individuals beginning a new sport activity, once the prescribed goals of strengthening, stretching, and proprioceptive conditioning have been met, a period of sport-specific training should begin. During this period, the patient would perform the actions normally required by the sport with gradually increasing intensity and duration.

Forcing stretching or strengthening to the point of pain is always deleterious and should be avoided. Progress is achieved by performing these exercises frequently (2 to 4 times per day, 7 days per week) and making small gains. The patient should be instructed to call the physician if the exercises cause pain.

Strengthening Exercises

Exercises to strengthen the deltoid and rotator cuff muscles can be done most easily using commercially available elastic therapy bands. These are available in different thicknesses, which provide different amounts of resistance. The same exercises can also be performed with pulleys or free weights. It usually takes 2 to 3 weeks to progress from one band or weight to the next. For strength training, the patient should perform 3 sets of 8 repetitions, progressing to 3 sets of 12 repetitions. Once 12 repetitions are reached, the resistance should be increased and the repetitions started over at 8. However, the patient should be advised not to progress to the next level of resistance if he or she still has difficulty at the current level or if pain develops when trying the new one. The patient should also be instructed to continue stretching exercises during this stage so that the hard-won gains in range of motion are not lost.

Stretching Exercises

The capsule and muscles of the posterior shoulder may be tight, especially in the individual who participates in repetitive overhead activities, including overhead throwing sports and swimming. Crossover arm stretches are helpful to relax these muscles. Static stretching should be done to increase the flexibility of the muscles surrounding the shoulder. A static stretch is performed at the end of the available range of painless motion of the muscle and joint.

Proprioceptive Exercises

In addition to strength, the athlete requires balance and power. Neuromuscular training, which improves the communication between the muscles and the proprioceptors, includes balance

SECTION 1 GENERAL ORTHOPAEDICS

and perturbation exercises. Balance involves the visual, vestibular, and proprioceptive systems. With balance training, the athlete consciously attempts to hold a posture for 30 to 60 seconds.

Proprioceptive exercises for the shoulder involve weight bearing through the arms. For example, push-ups performed with the hands on an exercise ball are an excellent advanced exercise for improving dynamic scapular stabilization. For the novice, standing push-ups done against a wall provide good proprioceptive training. To perform this exercise, the individual should stand several feet away from a wall with a 5″ or 7″ exercise ball in each hand. Leaning toward the wall, place the balls on the wall and move them up and down with the eyes closed to increase position sense. Then do push-ups against the wall with the hands on the balls, bending and extending at the elbow.

Home Exercise Program for Shoulder Conditioning

- When performing the stretching exercises, you should stretch slowly to the limit of motion, taking care to avoid pain. If you experience pain with the exercises, call your physician.
- For the exercises that use a stick, you may use a yardstick or stick of similar size.

Strengthening and Stretching Exercises for the Shoulder

Exercise	Muscle Group	Number of Repetitions/Sets	Number of Days per Week
Strengthening			
External rotation	Infraspinatus Teres minor	8 repetitions/3 sets, progressing to 12 repetitions/3 sets	3
Standing row	Middle trapezius Rhomboid	8 repetitions/3 sets, progressing to 12 repetitions/3 sets	3
Internal rotation	Pectoralis major and minor Subscapularis	8 repetitions/3 sets, progressing to 12 repetitions/3 sets	3
Bent-over horizontal abduction	Middle and lower trapezius	8 repetitions/3 sets, progressing to 12 repetitions/3 sets	3
Elbow flexion	Biceps	8 repetitions/3 sets, progressing to 12 repetitions/3 sets	3
Elbow extension	Triceps	8 repetitions/3 sets, progressing to 12 repetitions/3 sets	3
External rotation with arm abducted 90°	Infraspinatus Teres minor	8 repetitions/3 sets, progressing to 12 repetitions/3 sets	3
Stretching			
Pendulum	General	10 repetitions/2 sets, progressing to 15 repetitions/3 sets	5 to 6
Passive internal rotation	Subscapularis Pectoralis major and minor	4 sets	5 to 6
Passive external rotation	Infraspinatus Teres minor	4 sets	5 to 6
Crossover arm stretch	Posterior deltoid	4 sets	5 to 6

Strengthening Exercises

External Rotation

- Make a 3-foot-long loop with the elastic band and tie the ends together. Attach the loop to a doorknob or other stable object.
- Standing with your side to the wall, hold the loop, as shown in the start position.
- Keeping your elbow close to your side, rotate the arm outward slowly and then slowly return to the start position.
- Repeat on the other side.
- Perform 3 sets of 8 repetitions, progressing to 3 sets of 12 repetitions, 3 days per week.

Start   45°   Finish

Standing Row

- Make a 3-foot-long loop with the elastic band and tie the ends together. Attach the loop to a doorknob or other stable object.
- Standing facing the wall, hold the loop as shown in the start position.
- Keeping your arm close to your side, slowly pull the arm straight back and then slowly return to the start position.
- Repeat on the other side.
- Perform 3 sets of 8 repetitions, progressing to 3 sets of 12 repetitions, 3 days per week.

Start   Finish

Internal Rotation

- Make a 3-foot-long loop with the elastic band and tie the ends together. Attach the loop to a doorknob or other stable object.
- Standing with your side to the wall, hold the loop as shown in the start position.
- Keeping your elbow close to your side, rotate the arm across your body slowly and then slowly return to the start position.
- Repeat on the other side.
- Perform 3 sets of 8 repetitions, progressing to 3 sets of 12 repetitions, 3 days per week.

Start   Finish

Bent-Over Horizontal Abduction

- Stand next to a table.
- Bend at the waist with your side supported on the table and the other arm hanging straight down and holding a light weight (up to 5 lb).
- Keeping the arm straight, slowly raise the hand up to eye level and then slowly lower it back to the starting position.
- Repeat on the other side.
- Perform 3 sets of 8 repetitions, progressing to 3 sets of 12 repetitions, 3 days per week.

Elbow Flexion

- Stand with your weight evenly distributed over both feet.
- Holding a light weight (up to 5 lb) and keeping the arm close to the side, slowly bend the elbow up toward the shoulder as shown; hold for 2 seconds, slowly return to the starting position, and then relax.
- Repeat on the other side.
- Perform 3 sets of 8 repetitions, progressing to 3 sets of 12 repetitions, 3 days per week.

Elbow Extension

- Stand with your weight evenly distributed over both feet.
- Holding a light weight (up to 5 lb), raise your arm with the elbow bent and with your opposite hand supporting your elbow. Slowly straighten the elbow overhead, hold for 2 seconds, and then slowly lower the arm to the starting position.
- Repeat on the other side.
- Perform 3 sets of 8 repetitions, progressing to 3 sets of 12 repetitions, 3 days per week.

External Rotation With Arm Abducted 90°

- Make a 3-foot-long loop with the elastic band and tie the ends together. Attach the loop to a doorknob or other stable object.
- Standing facing the wall, hold the loop as shown in the start position, with the arm held straight out from the shoulder and the elbow bent 90°.
- Keeping the shoulder and elbow level, slowly rotate the hand up from the elbow, and then slowly return to the start position.
- Perform 3 sets of 8 repetitions, progressing to 3 sets of 12 repetitions, 3 days per week.

Stretching Exercises

Pendulum

- Lean forward, supporting the body with one arm and relaxing the muscles of the other arm so that it hangs freely.
- Gently move the arm in forward-and-back, side-to-side, and circular motions.
- Repeat on the other side.
- Perform 2 sets of 10 repetitions, progressing to 3 sets of 15 repetitions, 5 to 6 days per week.

Passive External Rotation

- Grasp the stick with one hand and cup the other end of the stick with the other hand.
- Push the stick horizontally as shown, keeping the elbow against the side of the body so that the arm is passively stretched to the point of feeling a pull without pain.
- Hold for 30 seconds and then relax for 30 seconds.
- Repeat on the other side.
- Perform 4 sets, 5 to 6 days per week.

Start   Finish

Passive Internal Rotation

- Behind your back, grasp the stick with one hand and lightly grasp the other end of the stick with the other hand.
- Pull the stick horizontally as shown so that the arm is passively stretched to the point of feeling a pull without pain.
- Hold for 30 seconds and then relax for 30 seconds.
- Repeat on the other side.
- Perform 4 sets, 5 to 6 days per week.

Start   Finish

Crossover Arm Stretch

- Gently pull the elbow of one arm across the chest as far as possible without feeling pain.
- Hold the stretch for 30 seconds and then relax for 30 seconds.
- Repeat on the other side.
- Perform 4 sets, 5 to 6 days per week.

Conditioning of the Hip

The muscles of the hip and pelvis are important in walking and running activities. Both the shoulder and the hip are ball-and-socket joints, but because of its anatomy, the hip is more stable than the shoulder. An exercise program for conditioning of the hip should include an active warm-up; stretching, strengthening, and proprioceptive exercises; and, once basic stretching and strengthening have been achieved, plyometrics for power.

Active Warm-Up

The hip muscle groups are large and require an adequate warm-up, such as riding on a stationary bicycle or jogging for 10 minutes to raise the core body temperature. In addition, dynamic stretching exercises such as leg swings can be used to warm up the synovial fluid in the hip joint and actively stretch the muscles before activity.

Strengthening Exercises

Exercises that isolate muscle contraction and do not stimulate co-contractions are important for strengthening the hip muscles. In general, weight-bearing exercises produce co-contractions, and non–weight-bearing exercises do not. Co-contractions are important for stabilizing the joint that is being strengthened. Strengthening of the large hip muscle groups requires heavier weights and few (6 to 12) repetitions. After beginning with a weight that allows the patient to perform 6 to 8 repetitions initially, working up to 12 repetitions should be the goal of the strengthening phase. The exercises described below isolate the gluteus medius (posterior fibers), the gluteus maximus, and the internal and external rotators, which often are weak and therefore contribute to hip pathology.

Static Stretching Exercises

Static stretching should be done to increase the flexibility of the muscles surrounding the hip. A static stretch is performed at the end of the available range of painless motion of the muscle and joint.

Proprioceptive Conditioning and Plyometrics

In addition to strength, the athlete requires balance and power. Neuromuscular training, which improves communication between the muscles and the proprioceptors, includes balance and perturbation exercises as well as plyometrics. Balance involves the visual, vestibular, and proprioceptive systems. With balance training, the athlete consciously attempts to hold a posture for 30 to 60 seconds. These exercises might include balancing on one leg or balancing on one leg while touching the other foot to different points on the ground within reach. With perturbation training, the athlete stands on an unstable surface

SECTION 1 GENERAL ORTHOPAEDICS

such as a balance board while it is being perturbed by an outside force. Jumping exercises, such as jumping forward and backward over a barrier, are a basic form of plyometrics. These should be attempted only by individuals with full range of motion and adequate strength in the hip, pelvic and abdominal, and back muscles. These types of plyometric and proprioceptive exercises should be supervised by a rehabilitation specialist or other exercise professional.

Home Exercise Program for Hip Conditioning

- Before beginning the conditioning program, warm up the muscles and the hip joint by riding a stationary bicycle or jogging for 10 minutes and performing leg swings as follows: While standing, swing one leg forward and backward 10 times and then side-to-side 10 times. Repeat with the opposite leg. Place one hand against a wall for balance if needed.

- When performing the stretching exercises, you should stretch slowly to the limit of motion, taking care to avoid pain. If you experience pain with the exercises, call your physician.

- After performing the active warm-up and strengthening exercises, static stretching exercises should be performed to maintaining or increase flexibility.

Exercise	Muscle Group	Number of Repetitions/Sets	Number of Days per Week
Strengthening			
Hip extension (prone)	Gluteus maximus	6 to 8 repetitions, progressing to 12 repetitions	2 to 3
Side-lying hip abduction	Gluteus medius	6 to 8 repetitions, progressing to 12 repetitions	2 to 3
Internal hip rotation	Medial hamstrings	6 to 8 repetitions, progressing to 12 repetitions	2 to 3
External hip rotation	Piriformis	6 to 8 repetitions, progressing to 12 repetitions	2 to 3
Stretching			
Seat side straddle	Adductor muscles Medial hamstrings Semitendinosus Semimembranosus	4 repetitions/2 to 3 sets	Daily
Modified seat side straddle	Hamstrings Adductor muscles	4 repetitions/2 to 3 sets	Daily
Leg stretch	Hamstrings	4 repetitions/2 to 3 sets	Daily
Sitting rotation stretch	Piriformis External rotators Internal rotators	4 repetitions/2 to 3 sets	Daily
Knee to chest	Posterior hip muscles	4 repetitions/2 to 3 sets	Daily
Leg crossover	Hamstrings	4 repetitions/2 to 3 sets	Daily
Cross overstand	Hamstrings	4 repetitions/2 to 3 sets	Daily
Iliotibial band stretch	Tensor fascia	4 repetitions/2 to 3 sets	Daily
Quadriceps stretch (prone)	Quadriceps	4 repetitions/2 to 3 sets	Daily

Strengthening Exercises

Hip Extension (Prone)

- Lie face down with a pillow under your hips and one knee bent 90°. Elevate the leg off the floor, lifting the leg straight up with the knee bent.
- Lower the leg to the floor slowly, to a count of 5. Ankle weights should be used. Start with weight light enough to allow 6 to 8 repetitions and work up to 12 repetitions.
- Repeat on the other side.
- Perform the exercise 2 to 3 days per week.
- Once you have worked up to 12 repetitions, add as much weight as can be lifted only 8 times, working up to 12 repetitions again. Continue this cycle of adding weight and increasing repetitions.

Side-Lying Hip Abduction

- Lie on your side while cradling your head in your arm. Bend the bottom leg for support.
- Slowly move the top leg up and back to 45°, keeping the knee straight. Lower the leg slowly, to a count of 5, and relax it for 2 seconds. Ankle weights should be used, starting with weight light enough to allow 6 to 8 repetitions, working up to 12 repetitions.
- Repeat on the other side.
- Perform the exercise 2 to 3 days per week.
- Once you have worked up to 12 repetitions, add as much weight as can be lifted only 8 times, working up to 12 repetitions again. Continue this cycle of adding weight and increasing repetitions.

Internal Hip Rotation

- Lie on your side on a table with a pillow between your thighs. Bend the top leg 90° at the hip and 90° at the knee.
- Start with the foot of the top leg below the level of the top of the table; lift to the finish position, which is rotated as high as possible.
- Lower the leg slowly, to a count of 5. Ankle weights should be used, starting with weight light enough to allow 6 to 8 repetitions, working up to 12 repetitions.
- Repeat on the other side.
- Perform the exercise 2 to 3 days per week.
- Once you have worked up to 12 repetitions, add as much weight as can be lifted only 8 times, working up to 12 repetitions again. Continue this cycle of adding weight and increasing repetitions.

External Hip Rotation

- Lie on your side on a table with the bottom leg bent 90° at the hip and 90° at the knee.
- Start with the foot below the level of the top of the table; lift to the finish position, which is rotated as high as possible.
- Lower the leg slowly, to a count of 5. Ankle weights should be used, starting with weight light enough to allow 6 to 8 repetitions, working up to 12 repetitions.
- Repeat on the other side.
- Perform the exercise 2 to 3 days per week.
- Once you have worked up to 12 repetitions, add as much weight as can be lifted only 8 times, working up to 12 repetitions again. Continue this cycle of adding weight and increasing repetitions.

Start

Finish

Stretching Exercises

Seat Side Straddle

- Sit on the floor with your legs spread apart.
- Place both hands on the same ankle and bring your chin as close to your knee as possible. Hold the stretch for 30 seconds and then relax for 30 seconds.
- Repeat on the other side.
- Repeat the sequence 4 times, performing 2 to 3 sets daily.

Modified Seat Side Straddle

- Sit on the floor with one leg extended to the side and the other leg bent as shown.
- Place both hands on the ankle of the extended leg and bring your chin as close to your knee as possible. Hold the stretch for 30 seconds and then relax for 30 seconds.
- Reverse leg positions and repeat on the other side.
- Repeat the sequence 4 times, performing 2 to 3 sets daily.

Leg Stretch

- Sit on the floor with your legs straight and your hands grasping the calf of one leg.
- Slowly lift and pull the leg toward your ear, keeping your back straight and the other leg flat on the floor or bent slightly if necessary for comfort. Hold the stretch for 30 seconds and then relax for 30 seconds
- Repeat with the other leg.
- Repeat the sequence 4 times.
- Perform 2 to 3 sets daily.

Sitting Rotation Stretch

- Sit on the floor with both legs straight out in front of you.
- Cross one leg over the other, place the elbow of the opposite arm on the outside of the thigh, and support yourself with your other arm behind you.
- Rotate your head and body in the direction of the supporting arm. Hold the stretch for 30 seconds and then relax for 30 seconds.
- Reverse positions and repeat the stretch on the other side.
- Repeat the sequence 4 times.
- Perform 2 to 3 sets daily.

Knee to Chest

- Lie on your back on the floor with your knees bent and your heels flat on the floor.
- Grasp one knee and slowly bring it toward your chest as far as it will go. Hold the stretch for 30 seconds and then relax for 30 seconds.
- Repeat with the other leg; then do both legs together.
- Repeat the sequence 4 times.
- Perform 2 to 3 sets daily.

Leg Crossover

- Lie on the floor with your legs spread and your arms at your sides.
- Keeping the leg straight, bring your right toe to your left hand.
- Try to keep the other leg flat on the floor, but you may bend it slightly if needed for comfort. Hold the stretch for 30 seconds and then relax for 30 seconds.
- Repeat with the left leg and the right hand.
- Repeat the sequence 4 times. Perform 2 to 3 sets daily.

Crossover Stand

- Stand with your legs crossed, with your feet close together and your legs straight.
- Slowly bend forward and try to touch your toes. Hold the stretch for 30 seconds and then relax for 30 seconds.
- Repeat with the position of the legs reversed.
- Repeat the sequence 4 times.
- Perform 2 to 3 sets daily.

Iliotibial Band Stretch

- Stand next to a wall for support.
- Begin with your weight distributed evenly over both feet, and then cross one leg behind the other.
- Lean the hip of the crossed-over leg toward the wall until you feel a stretch on the outside of the leg. Hold the stretch for 30 seconds and then relax for 30 seconds.
- Repeat on the opposite side.
- Repeat the sequence 4 times.
- Perform 2 to 3 sets daily.

Quadriceps Stretch (Prone)

- Lie on your stomach with your arms at your sides and your legs straight.
- Bend one knee up toward your buttocks and grasp the ankle with the hand on the same side.
- Pull on the ankle. Hold the stretch for 30 seconds and then relax for 30 seconds.
- Repeat on the opposite side.
- Repeat the sequence 4 times.
- Perform 2 to 3 sets daily.

SECTION 1 GENERAL ORTHOPAEDICS

Conditioning of the Knee

The knee has both dynamic and static stabilizers. Muscles provide dynamic stability to the knee joint and the patellofemoral articulation. Strengthening the quadriceps and hamstrings muscle groups provides dynamic stability to the knee. In addition, the hip muscles, such as the gluteus maximus, the gluteus medius, and the internal and external rotators, help to control the movements of the femur and the position of the patellofemoral articulation. Conditioning of the knee should focus on three phases: strengthening, stretching, and neuromuscular (proprioceptive) training. Plyometrics (power training) would be added for the competitive athlete after basic strength and flexibility have been achieved. Advanced proprioceptive exercises and plyometric exercises should be done under the supervision of a rehabilitation specialist or other exercise professional.

Strengthening Exercises

Exercises to strengthen the quadriceps and hamstrings can be performed conveniently with progressively heavier ankle weights. The resistance training must be progressive so that the muscle is constantly stimulated to grow. Forward lunges (for the quadriceps), hamstring curls, side-lying hip abductions, and hip extensions are good strengthening exercises. The patient should begin with a weight that allows 6 to 8 repetitions and should work up to 12 repetitions. After reaching 12 repetitions with a given weight, the patient should add weight and drop back to 6 to 8 repetitions.

Stretching Exercises

The effectiveness of strengthening exercises for the quadriceps muscle group may be compromised if the range of motion of the knee is limited. Stretching the soft tissues to gain range of motion, especially after trauma or periods of immobilization, can be very effective in gaining range of motion. Hamstring stretching exercises such as leg crossovers and crossover standing increase the range of motion at the knee and hip during functional activities such as walking and running.

Once the patient has achieved normal range of motion and strength, sport-specific or work-specific training should begin. The knee musculature needs to be strong and powerful, and protective reflexes need to be optimized to reduce the risk of injury during sporting maneuvers such as sudden changes in direction while running.

Proprioceptive Training

Proprioceptive training is important for balance. Balance, or postural control, is the result of the integration of visual, vestibular, and proprioceptive afferent inputs. The goal of proprioceptive training is to enhance the activity of the proprioceptors, thereby improving their ability to protect ligaments of the knee. Several commercial devices, such as tiltboards and proprioceptive disks, are available for proprioceptive training. Advanced balance training should be performed under the supervision of a physical therapist, athletic trainer, or other exercise specialist.

Plyometric Exercises

Explosive power of the lower leg is necessary for a high level of athletic performance. Plyometrics and explosive weight training facilitate the development of power in the quadriceps, hamstrings, and gluteal muscles. Examples of plyometric exercises are jumping rope and jumping from side to side over a 6-inch-high barrier. More advanced exercises should be performed under the supervision of a physical therapist, athletic trainer, or other trained professional.

Home Exercise Program for Knee Conditioning

- Before beginning the conditioning program, warm up the muscles by riding a stationary bicycle or jogging for 10 minutes.
- After the active warm-up and the strengthening exercises, stretching exercises should be performed to maintaining or increase flexibility. When performing the stretching exercises, you should stretch slowly to the limit of motion, taking care to avoid pain.
- If you experience pain with exercising, call your doctor.

Strengthening and Stretching Exercises for the Knee

Exercise	Muscle Group	Number of Repetitions/Sets	Number of Days per Week
Strengthening			
Forward lunge	Quadriceps	Work up to 3 sets of 10 repetitions	3
Hamstring curl	Hamstrings	10 repetitions/5 sets/3 times per day	3
Side-lying hip abduction	Gluteus medius	6 to 8 repetitions, progressing to 12 repetitions	3
Hip extension (prone)	Gluteus maximus	6 to 8 repetitions, progressing to 12 repetitions	3
Stretching			
Leg stretch	Hamstrings	3 to 6 repetitions/3 sets	Daily
Leg crossover	Hamstrings	3 to 6 repetitions/3 sets	Daily
Crossover stand	Hamstrings	3 to 6 repetitions/3 sets	Daily
Straight-leg raise	Quadriceps	Work up to 3 sets of 10 repetitions	Daily
Straight-leg raise (prone)	Gluteus maximus	Work up to 3 sets of 10 repetitions	Daily
Wall slide	Quadriceps Hamstrings	Work up to 3 sets of 10 repetitions	Daily

Strengthening Exercises

Forward Lunges

- Stand up with the feet about 3 to 4 feet apart and with the forward foot pointing forward and the back foot angled to provide support.
- Lunge forward, bending the forward knee and keeping the back and the back leg straight. You should feel a slight stretch in the left groin area. Do not let the forward lunging knee pass beyond the toes.
- Hold the stretch for 5 seconds.
- Repeat with the opposite leg.
- Work up to 3 sets of 10 repetitions, 3 days per week.

Hamstring Curls

- Stand on a flat surface with your weight evenly distributed over both feet. Hold onto the back of a chair or the wall for balance.
- Raise the heel of one leg toward the ceiling. Hold this position for 5 seconds and then relax.
- Perform 5 sets of 10 repetitions, 3 times per day.

Side-Lying Hip Abduction

- Lie on your side, cradling your head in your arm. Bend the bottom leg for support.
- Slowly move the top leg up and back to 45°, keeping the knee straight. Hold this position for 5 seconds.
- Slowly lower the leg and relax it for 2 seconds.
- Ankle weights should be used, starting with light enough weight to allow 6 to 8 repetitions, progressing to 12 repetitions. Then return to 6 to 8 repetitions and add weight.
- Repeat on the opposite leg.
- Perform the exercise 3 times per week.

Hip Extension (Prone)

- Lie face down with a pillow under your hips and one knee bent 90°.
- Elevate the leg off the floor to a count of 5, lifting the leg straight up with the knee bent.
- Ankle weights should be used, starting with light enough weight to allow 6 to 8 repetitions, working up to 12 repetitions. Then return to 6 to 8 repetitions and add weight.
- Repeat on the opposite leg.
- Perform the exercise 3 times per week.

Stretching Exercises

Leg Stretch

- Sit on the floor with your legs straight in front of you and place your hands on the backs of your calves. For comfort, you may slightly bend the leg not being stretched.
- Slowly lift and pull one leg toward your ear, keeping your back straight. Hold the stretch for 5 seconds.
- Alternate from side to side.
- Repeat the exercise with each leg 3 to 6 times.
- Perform the exercise daily.

Leg Crossover

- Lie on the floor with your legs spread and your arms out to the sides.
- Bring your right toe to your left hand, keeping the leg straight.
- Hold the stretch for 5 seconds.
- Alternate from side to side.
- Repeat the exercise with each leg 3 to 6 times. For comfort, you may slightly bend the leg not being stretched.
- Perform the exercise daily.

Crossover Stand

- Stand with your legs crossed.
- Keeping your feet close together and your legs straight, slowly bend forward toward your toes. Hold the stretch for 5 seconds.
- Repeat with the opposite leg crossed in front.
- Perform 3 sets of 3 to 6 repetitions daily

Straight-Leg Raise

- Lie on the floor with one leg straight and the other leg bent.
- Tighten the thigh muscle of the straight leg and slowly raise it 6 to 10 inches off the floor. Hold this position for 5 seconds. Repeat with the opposite leg.
- Work up to 3 sets of 10 repetitions.
- Perform the exercise daily.

Straight-Leg Raise (Prone)

- Lie on the floor on your stomach with your legs straight.
- Keeping the leg straight, tighten the hamstrings of one leg and raise the leg as high as you can. Hold this position for 5 seconds.
- Repeat with the opposite leg.
- Work up to 3 sets of 10 repetitions.
- Perform the exercise daily.

Wall Slides

- Stand with your back against a wall and your feet about 1 foot from the wall.
- Tuck your pelvis under so that your lower back is flat against the wall.
- Stop when your knees are bent 90°. The knees should not pass beyond the toes.
- Hold for 5 seconds and then relax. Work up to 3 sets of 10 repetitions.
- Perform the exercise daily.

SECTION 1 GENERAL ORTHOPAEDICS

Conditioning of the Foot and Ankle

The foot is the first part of the lower kinetic chain to hit the ground during weight-bearing activities and is therefore the first input to the neuromuscular system of the lower kinetic chain. Dynamic joint stability is critical for injury prevention and improved performance during sports activities. Whether an individual experiences a single-episode lateral ankle sprain or develops chronic ankle instability most likely depends on rehabilitation of the individual's proprioception.

Strengthening Exercises
Strengthening exercises for the foot and ankle include calf raises, ankle dorsiflexion/plantar flexion, and ankle inversion/eversion exercises.

Stretching Exercises
Perform stretching to maintain or increase flexibility. Heel cord stretches performed with the knee both straight and bent are good stretching exercises for the gastrocnemius-soleus muscle complex.

Toe Strengthening Exercises
The toe strengthening program is helpful for patients with the particular conditions listed, including bunions, hammer toes, plantar fasciitis, and toe cramps.

Proprioceptive Exercises
Optimizing the proprioceptive system is important in preventing injuries such as ankle sprains in both athletes and nonathletes. Balance, or postural control, is the result of the integration of visual, vestibular, and proprioceptive afferent inputs. The goal of proprioceptive training is to enhance the activity of the proprioceptors, thereby improving their ability to protect the ligaments of the foot and ankle. Several commercial devices, such as tiltboards and proprioceptive disks, are available for proprioceptive training. Perturbation training is another way to optimize the proprioceptive system, especially in athletes. Perturbation exercises are performed on an unstable surface with perturbing forces applied in all directions. Perturbation training and advanced balance training should be performed under the supervision of a rehabilitation specialist or other exercise professional.

Plyometrics

Explosive power is necessary for a high level of athletic performance. Plyometrics facilitate the development of power. Examples of plyometric exercises are jumping rope and jumping from side to side over a 6-inch-high barrier. More advanced exercises should be performed under the supervision of a rehabilitation specialist or other trained exercise professional.

SECTION 1 GENERAL ORTHOPAEDICS

Home Exercise Program for Foot and Ankle Conditioning

- Performing active warm-up exercises prior to athletic activities is important for optimal neuromuscular control and for maintaining normal range of motion.

- Before beginning the conditioning program, warm up the muscles of the lower extremities by riding a stationary bicycle or jogging for 10 minutes and performing leg swings as follows: While standing, swing one leg forward/backward 10 times and then side-to-side 10 times. Repeat with the opposite leg. Place one hand against a wall for balance if needed.

- Perform the exercises indefinitely or as directed by your physician. Contact your physician if the exercises cause pain.

Strengthening and Stretching Exercises for the Foot and Ankle

Exercise	Muscle Group	Number of Repetitions/Sets	Number of Days per Week
Strengthening			
Calf raises	Gastrocnemius-soleus complex	10 repetitions/3 sets	3
Ankle dorsiflexion/plantar flexion	Anterior tibialis Gastrocnemius-soleus complex	10 repetitions/3 sets	3
Ankle eversion/inversion	Posterior tibialis Peroneus longus and peroneus brevis	10 repetitions/3 sets	3
Stretching			
Heel cord stretch	Knee straight: Gastrocnemius Knee bent: Soleus	4 to 5 repetitions/ 2 to 3 sets	Daily

Toe Strengthening Program

Exercise	Recommended For	Repetitions or Duration	Number of Days Per Week
Toe squeeze	Hammer toes, toe cramps	10 repetitions	Daily
Big toe pulls	Bunions, toe cramps	10 repetitions	Daily
Toe pulls	Bunions, hammer toes, toe cramps	10 repetitions	Daily
Golf ball roll	Plantar fasciitis, arch strain, foot cramps	2 minutes	Daily
Marble pickup	Pain in ball of foot, hammer toes, toe cramps	Until all marbles have been picked up	Daily
Towel curls	Hammer toes, toe cramps, pain in ball of foot	5 repetitions	Daily

Strengthening Exercises

Calf Raises

- Stand with your weight evenly distributed over both feet. Hold onto the back of a chair or the wall for balance.
- Lift one foot so that all your weight is on the other foot.
- Then lift the heel off the floor as high as you can.
- Repeat on the other side.
- Work up to 3 sets of 10 repetitions.
- Perform the exercise 3 days per week.

Ankle Dorsiflexion/Plantar Flexion

- Find a position where your weight is off your feet, such as lying on a bed or on the floor with your legs straight out in front of you.
- For dorsiflexion, wrap an elastic band or tubing around your foot and anchor the other end to a door or bedpost or have someone hold it. Pull your toes toward you; then return slowly to the starting position. Repeat 10 to 15 times.
- For plantar flexion, wrap an elastic band or tubing around your foot and hold the other end in your hand. Gently point your toes; then return slowly to the starting position. Repeat 10 to 15 times.
- Perform 3 sets of 10 repetitions; 3 days per week.

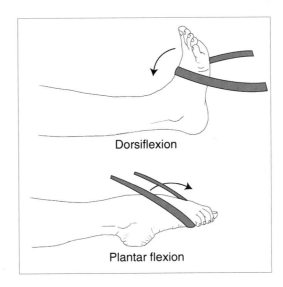

Dorsiflexion

Plantar flexion

Ankle Eversion/Inversion

- Find a position where your weight is off your feet, such as lying on a bed or on the floor with your legs straight out in front of you.

- For inversion, wrap an elastic band or tube around the inside of your foot and anchor the other end to a door or bedpost or have someone hold it. Pull your foot inward against the resistance; then return slowly to the starting position. Repeat 10 to 15 times.

- For eversion, wrap an elastic band or tube around the inside of your foot and anchor the other end to a door or bedpost or have someone hold it. Pull your foot outward against the resistance; then return slowly to the starting position. Repeat 10 to 15 times.

Strengthening Exercises

Heel Cord Stretch

- Support yourself against a wall with your feet pointed straight ahead.
  Stretch with knee straight: Keeping the heel in contact with the ground and the knee straight, place the foot as far back as possible until a stretch is felt in the calf.
  Stretch with knee flexed: Same position but bend the knee of the leg being stretched.

- Hold the stretch for 30 seconds; then relax for 30 seconds.

- Repeat on the other side.

- Perform 2 to 3 sets of 4 to 5 repetitions of each exercise daily.

Toe Strengthening Exercises

Toe Squeeze

- Place small sponges or corks between the toes.

- Squeeze and hold for 5 seconds.

- Repeat 10 times.

Big Toe Pulls

- Place a thick rubber band around both big toes and pull the big toes away from each other and toward the small toes.
- Hold for 5 seconds.
- Repeat 10 times.

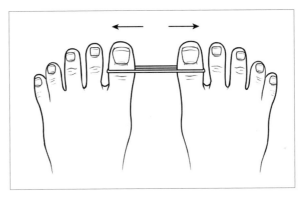

Toe Pulls

- Put a thick rubber band around all your toes and spread them.
- Hold this position for 5 seconds.
- Repeat 10 times.

Golf Ball Roll

- Roll a golf ball under the ball of your foot for 2 minutes to massage the bottom of the foot.

Marble Pickup

- Place 20 marbles on the floor. Pick up one marble at a time and put it in a small bowl.
- Repeat until you have picked up all 20 marbles.

Towel Curls

- Place a small towel on the floor and curl it toward you, using only your toes. You can increase the resistance by putting weight on the end of the towel.
- Relax and repeat 5 times.

SECTION 1   GENERAL ORTHOPAEDICS

Conditioning of the Spine

Conditioning of the lumbar spine to prevent low back pain should include strengthening and stretching exercises, to improve range of motion. The focus of conditioning should be on a daily home exercise program. Because little or no muscle damage occurs with isometric exercises (unlike the concentric and eccentric exercises involved with strength training), recovery from isometric training occurs within several hours, and so isometric exercises may and should be done every day.

Strengthening Exercises

The four muscle groups that protect the spine from daily overuse and trauma include the abdominals, the quadratus lumborum (two groups, one on each side of the spine), and the back extensors. The back extensors are important because poor endurance of these muscle groups has been found in patients with low back pain. Isometric exercises for these muscle groups, such as the bird dog exercise, have an important stabilizing effect on the spine.

The quadratus lumborum is an important lateral stabilizer of the trunk. A strengthening exercise for this muscle is the side bridge, which should be repeated on both sides for maximum and symmetric lateral stability.

The abdominals are important to stabilization of the lumbar and thoracic spine. The four major muscle groups that make up the abdominals are the transverse abdominus, the internal and external obliques, and the rectus abdominus. The transverse abdominus muscle is a stabilizer of the lumbar spine through its attachment to the thoracolumbar fascia. Traditional sit-ups have been found to greatly increase the load on the lumbar disks and therefore should be avoided by patients with low back pain. A safe exercise is abdominal bracing, which activates all the abdominal muscles, including the transverse abdominus, and does not stress the lumbar spine. This exercise does not activate the transverse abdominus if a pelvic tilt is performed.

Stretching Exercises

Stretching exercises for the trunk and pelvis are helpful for improving range of motion. The cat back stretch and the kneeling back extension exercises are excellent stretching exercises for the spine in general. Flexibility of the hamstring muscles is also important for improving the mobility of the lumbar spine and reducing stress on the lumbar spine. The seat side straddle, modified seat side straddle, sitting rotation stretch, and leg crossover are all excellent stretching exercises for the lumbothoracic spine.

Home Exercise Program for Lumbar Spine Conditioning

- Perform the exercises in the order listed.
- If any of the exercises cause pain, call your doctor.

Strengthening and Stretching Exercises for the Lumbar Spine

Exercise Type	Muscle Group/ Area Targeted	Number of Repetitions	Number of Days per Week
Strengthening Exercises			
Side bridges	Quadratus lumborum	5	Daily
Abdominal bracing	Abdominals	5	Daily
Bird dog	Back extensors	5	Daily
Stretching Exercises			
Cat back stretch	Middle and low back	10	Daily
Kneeling back extension	Low back	10	Daily
Seat side straddle	Adductor muscles Medial hamstrings Semitendinosus Semimembranosus	10	Daily
Modified seat side straddle	Adductor muscles Hamstrings	10	Daily
Sitting rotation stretch	Piriformis External rotators Internal rotators	10	Daily
Leg crossover	Hamstrings	10	Daily

Strengthening Exercises

Abdominal Bracing

- Lie on your back on the floor with your arms at your sides, your knees bent, and your feet flat on the floor.
- Contract your abdominal muscles so that your stomach is pulled away from your waistband.
- Hold this position for 15 seconds.
- Perform 5 repetitions daily.

Side Bridges

- Lie on your side on the floor (for beginners, the knees may be bent 90°).
- With your elbow bent at 90°, lift your body off the floor as shown, keeping your body straight.
- Hold this position for 15 seconds and then repeat on the other side. The goal is to hold this position for 150 seconds total on each side.
- Perform 5 repetitions daily.

Bird Dog

- Kneel on the floor on your hands and knees.
- Lift your right arm straight out from the shoulder, level with your body, at the same time you lift your left leg straight out from the hip.
- Start by holding this position for 15 seconds. The goal is to hold this position for 150 seconds (30 years or older) or 170 seconds (younger than 30 years) total.
- Repeat with the opposite arm and leg.
- Perform 5 repetitions daily.

Stretching Exercises
Cat Back Stretch

- Kneel on your hands and knees in a relaxed position.
- Raise your back up like a cat and hold for 30 seconds.
- Relax for 30 seconds.
- Repeat 10 times daily.

Kneeling Back Extension

- Crouch on your hands and knees.
- First rock forward onto your extended arms, allowing your back to sag. Hold for 5 seconds.
- Then rock back and sit on your bent knees with your arms extended and your head tucked in. Hold for 5 seconds.
- Repeat 10 times daily.

Seat Side Straddle

- Sit on the floor with your legs spread apart.
- Place both hands on the same ankle and bring your chin as close to your knee as possible.
- Hold the maximum stretch for 30 seconds and then relax for 30 seconds.
- Repeat on the other side.
- Repeat the sequence 10 times daily.

Modified Seat Side Straddle

- Sit on the floor with one leg extended to the side and the other leg bent as shown.
- Place both hands on the ankle of the extended leg and bring your chin as close to your knee as possible.
- Hold the maximum stretch for 30 seconds and then relax for 30 seconds.
- Reverse leg positions and repeat on the other side.
- Repeat the sequence 10 times daily.

SECTION 1 GENERAL ORTHOPAEDICS

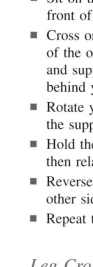

Sitting Rotation Stretch

- Sit on the floor with both legs straight out in front of you.
- Cross one leg over the other, place the elbow of the opposite arm on the outside of the thigh, and support yourself with your other arm behind you.
- Rotate your head and body in the direction of the supporting arm.
- Hold the maximum stretch for 30 seconds and then relax for 30 seconds.
- Reverse positions and repeat the stretch on the other side.
- Repeat the sequence 10 times daily.

Leg Crossover

- Lie on the floor with your legs spread and your arms at your sides.
- Keeping the leg straight, bring your right toe to your left hand.
- Try to keep the other leg flat on the floor, but you may bend it slightly if needed for comfort.
- Hold the maximum stretch for 30 seconds and then relax for 30 seconds.
- Repeat with the left leg and the right hand.
- Repeat the sequence 10 times daily.

Rehabilitation: Canes, Crutches, and Walkers

Canes, crutches, and walkers (assistive devices) progressively reduce weight-bearing stresses on the lower extremities and also augment balance and stability during walking. As such, these devices are helpful in the treatment of arthritic conditions and lower extremity injuries.

Canes

Canes are lightweight and are easily stored. For long-term use, a spade handle is easier on the hand than the standard crook handle (**Figure 1** and **Table 1**). A "quad," or four-footed cane, has four prongs at its base; it is more cumbersome than a single-tipped cane but provides a wider base of support and can be quite useful to patients after a stroke when they have only one functional upper extremity.

A cane should be used on the contralateral side to maximize stress reduction.

A cane that is too long creates excessive flexion of the elbow and increases the demand on the triceps muscle, a major stabilizer of the upper extremity when using a cane. A cane that is too short provides inadequate support and compromises walking. The optimal length of a cane will position the elbow in 20° to 30° of flexion when the tip of the cane is placed approximately 6″ in front of and 6″ lateral to the little toe.

Figure 1 Appropriate cane walking in a patient with an injured right leg.

Table 1 Patient Guide to Using a Cane

General Guidelines

Prepare residence by removing small rugs, foot stools, electrical cords, or other ground level objects that may cause falls.

Organize everyday necessities on main level of residence to prevent unnecessary stair climbing.

Equip bathroom with shower tub seat, raised toilet seat, grab bars, and nonslip bath mats.

Positioning

Height should reach wrist crease when standing, elbow slightly bent, held in hand opposite of injured leg

Walking

Cane and injured leg strike ground simultaneously; initiate step with injured leg and finish with healthy leg

Stairs

Grasp handrail with free hand, if possible
Up: step up on healthy leg followed by injured leg
Down: place cane on step first followed by injured leg then good leg and body weight

Figure 2 Appropriate crutch walking in a patient with an injured left leg.

Crutches

Crutches offer more support than a cane (**Figure 2** and **Table 2**), but less than a walker and come in several designs:

- Wooden axillary—satisfactory for short-term use, economic
- Aluminum axillary—durable for long-term use in chronic conditions, easily adjustable (**Figure 3**)

Table 2 Patient Guide to Using Crutches

General Guidelines

Prepare residence by removing small rugs, foot stools, electrical cords, or other ground level objects that may cause falls

Organize everyday necessities on main level of residence to prevent unnecessary stair climbing

Equip bathroom with shower tub seat, raised toilet seat, grab bars, and nonslip bath mats

Positioning

Crutch tip 4″ to 6″ in front of little toe
Top of crutches 2″ below armpits when standing
Hand grips even with hips
Elbows slightly bent at 25°
Absorb weight with hands so crutch does not touch armpit
Do not wrap towels around armpit pad

Walking

Advance both crutches 1 foot
Shift body weight to crutches
Take forward step with healthy leg

Stairs

Grasp handrail in one hand and crutch in other hand or use both crutches

Up: supporting body weight with crutch, step up on healthy leg while injured leg is raised behind you, then advance crutches

Down: advance crutches first to lower step followed by body weight shift and step with healthy leg

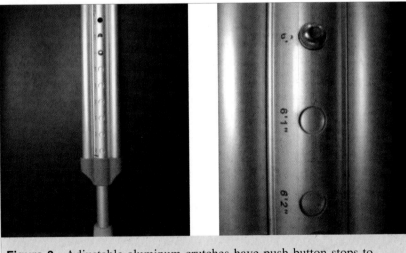

Figure 3   Adjustable aluminum crutches have push-button stops to adjust for height range of generally 6 to 8 inches (eg, 5'2″ to 5'10″)

SECTION 1   GENERAL ORTHOPAEDICS

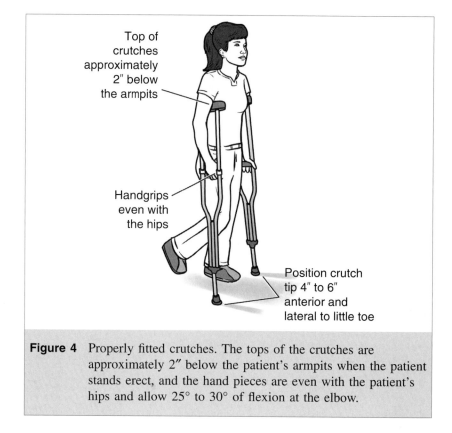

Figure 4 Properly fitted crutches. The tops of the crutches are approximately 2″ below the patient's armpits when the patient stands erect, and the hand pieces are even with the patient's hips and allow 25° to 30° of flexion at the elbow.

- Hyperbaric stainless steel crutches—used by patients heavier than 280 lb
- Forearm—extend only to forearm, less bulky design for patients with chronic conditions, require better balance and upper body strength
- Platform—transmit forces through forearm, useful in patients with arthritic or traumatic conditions of hand or wrist

Patients should be properly fitted for and instructed in the use of crutches (**Figure 4**). Crutches that are too long or that are used improperly can cause axillary artery or venous thrombosis or a brachial plexus compression neuropathy (primarily the radial nerve). The hand piece should be positioned to provide optimal function of the triceps and latissimus dorsi muscles. Depending on the height of the patient, position the crutch tip 4″ to 6″ anterior and lateral to the little toe. In that position, adjust the length of the crutch to allow approximately 2″ of clearance between the anterior axillary fold and the top of the crutch. Adjust the hand piece to position the elbow in 25° to 30° of flexion. As a general guideline, the length of the crutch should be 77% of the patient's height. Caution the patient against wrapping towels around the axillary pad.

Gait techniques for crutches are described in **Table 3**. Following injury to the lower extremity, the technique most commonly prescribed is a non–weight-bearing, swing-through

Table 3 Gait Patterns Used With Crutches

Gait Pattern	Instructions
Swing-to	Advance both crutches. Lift the body to advance both feet on line with the crutches
Swing-through	Advance both crutches. Lift the body to advance both feet beyond the crutches
Non–weight-bearing, swing-through	Advance both crutches
Four-point	Move one crutch forward, then advance the opposite foot, followed by the ipsilateral crutch, then the contralateral foot (three points of contact are always maintained).
Alternating two-point	Advance one crutch and the contralateral foot at the same time. Shift weight and advance the other foot and crutch (a progression of the four-point gait).

Figure 5 Appropriate walker use in a patient with an injured right leg.

gait. Walking on level ground using this method is easy to teach because it involves simply advancing both crutches, followed by a forward step with the uninjured leg. Ascending or descending steps is more difficult, but the key is to advance the crutches first when going down stairs and to advance the sound leg first when going up. A training session with a rehabilitation specialist often is helpful. Toe-touch weight bearing with crutches, if the injury permits, may be easier for the patient and demands less upper body strength than non–weight-bearing crutch walking.

Walkers

Walkers have four points of contact and provide greater support and balance than either cane or crutch (**Figure 5** and **Table 4**).

Table 4 Patient Guide to Using a Walker

General Guidelines

Prepare residence by removing small rugs, foot stools, electrical cords, or other ground level objects that may cause falls

Organize everyday necessities on main level of residence to prevent unnecessary stair climbing

Equip bathroom with shower tub seat, raised toilet seat, grab bars, and nonslip bath mats

Positioning

Height should reach wrist crease when standing

Elbows slightly bent at 30°

Grip with both hands to support some of your weight

Walking

Place walker one step ahead of you

Initiate step with injured leg and walk into walker

Do not step all the way to front bar

Take small steps when turning

Stairs

Never use a walker to climb stairs

The bulkiness of a walker is its major disadvantage. Some walkers fold, making storage in cars easier, but these models are more fragile. Rolling walkers require less energy to use but are less stable. If balance is adequate, a rolling walker may be advantageous for a patient with significant cardiopulmonary restrictions. The same principles used for fitting crutches apply for adjusting the height of a walker (ie, the hand grip should be positioned to allow 30° flexion at the elbow when the patient is in a neutral standing position).

Sports Medicine Evaluation and Management Principles

Definition

Sports medicine is a comprehensive term describing a branch of medicine involved in prevention, diagnosis, management, and rehabilitation of sport- and exercise-related injuries and disorders. Sports medicine is a multidisciplinary field encompassing disciplines such as rehabilitation, athletic training, nutrition, exercise physiology, and psychology. In addition, primary care, internal medicine, and medical and surgical specialties have roles in the management of sports-related problems.

Being a team physician is a complex task. The role of the team physician includes performing a preparticipation evaluation. Determining readiness for participation and implementing injury prevention programs is vital to decreasing game time injuries. Team physicians should also provide medical coverage for high-risk practices and competitions, visit the training room regularly to evaluate and monitor problems, and arrange appropriate referrals. Open lines of communication between parents, coaches, and administrators are a necessity and injuries should be properly documented. Physicians providing care to athletes must always place the medical well-being of the athlete above the needs of the team.

General Issues of Importance in Sports Medicine

It is important for physicians responsible for covering sports practices and games to formulate administrative medical supervision plans and implement an emergency response plan that must be made available to the entire athletic and sports medicine staff. An individual who is qualified to administer cardiopulmonary resuscitation and first aid should be available at all practices and games. The emergency plan should address and designate who calls 911 in an emergency, who attends to the athlete, where the emergency response equipment is kept, and what equipment is available.

The team physician should appreciate the importance of sports and fitness participation to athlete-patients and communicate their commitment to helping them return to participation as effectively and safely as possible. Competitive athletes and serious fitness participants need a prompt diagnosis and treatment plan; they (and their parents, if applicable) also need to know the prognosis. If the athlete is part of a team, all concerned must understand the diagnosis, prognosis, and the anticipated lost playing time as soon as possible so that appropriate team planning can be initiated.

Communication plays a critical role. Prompt, authoritative, and efficient communication among parents, coaches, trainers, and involved colleagues is essential. An immediately available sports injury report form with multiple copies can help.

Personal coverage of competitions is optimal for team physicians, but is not always feasible. When not physically present, a team physician needs to be available for timely communication with coaches, trainers, parents, or athletes. The physician should provide a team approach to the care of the athlete. Coordinated involvement of all concerned with the athlete and the team (athletes, parents, coaches, trainers, colleagues, and therapists) optimizes outcomes.

Another unique aspect of sports medicine, particularly in high-profile athletes, is the public's interest in the status of the injured athlete. Treating physicians frequently are approached by the media for information about prominent athletes who are injured. It is important to protect physician-patient confidentiality. A practical, successful approach is to prepare a brief factual statement that includes no confidential details. This statement can be released upon request, with the proviso that any additional information has to come from the athlete.

Within sports medicine, more nonsurgical illnesses and injuries are encountered than surgical ones. Nonsurgical treatment does not mean "no treatment." Aggressive nonsurgical treatment, often engaging a team of specialists including internists, family physicians, rehabilitation specialists, psychologists, and nutritionists is frequently the norm in sports medicine. Understanding the injury and the necessary steps for a safe and effective return to competition is essential. Some therapeutic regimens apply to all sports and fitness activities; others are sport- or position-specific.

Any injury, even a successfully treated injury, may impact greatly on an athlete's career and life. Hence, a major focus of the sports medicine team is establishing injury prevention programs. Educating athletes on the importance of prevention should include the following:

- Good hygiene (eg, not sharing towels and water bottles)
- Properly fitted and well-maintained protective equipment
- Appropriate hydration and nutrition for sport success
- The perils of using banned performance-enhancing substances (a prime responsibility of the sports medicine physician)

The sports medicine team is responsible for developing sport- and age-appropriate conditioning programs for off-season, preseason, and in-season injury prevention (**Table 1**).

Table 1 Prevention Strategies in Sports Medicine

Sports Injury Prevention Strategies

Planning and administration of sports programs

Preparticipation physical examination (PPE)

Perform strengthening and endurance training exercises to condition and maintain muscles used in sports

Always perform appropriate warm-up exercises

Gradually increase practice time and intensity to acclimate to full speed

Stretching should be done before and after to increase flexibility

Hydrate before, during, and after exercise

Decrease intensity during high heat/humidity periods

Rest periodically during practice and games to reduce fatigue

Gear and protective equipment should be appropriately fitted

Emphasize proper technique during practice to avoid game time injury

Take time for recovery

Special Considerations for Adolescent Athletes

Determine the young athlete's level of interest

Provide adequate adult supervision

Avoid strict and intense training to prevent early overuse injuries

Tailor rules to specific age groups

Opponents should be appropriately matched

Keep strengthening exercises light and focus on cross-training

Adjust playing field or court to accommodate for different ages

Clinical Symptoms

Symptoms for athletes are exactly the same for nonathletes in situations of sprains/strains, tendinitis, ruptures, or fractures. Certain injuries such as turf toe, myositis ossificans, knee ligament injuries, and shoulder and elbow tendonitis are more common in athletics.

Tests

Preparticipation physical evaluation (PPE) is mandated to ensure that an athlete is capable of performing in his or her sport safely and to identify those at risk for injury. History, physical examination, and appropriate laboratory studies and radiographs are needed, as indicated for specific situations. If warning signs for cardiac disease are present, additional history or physical examination should be performed, and an electrocardiogram or echocardiogram should be obtained. Cardiac studies can be added as part of the PPE but these tests have a large false-positive rate, and the cost-benefit ratio should be considered.

Treatment

Sports-oriented rehabilitation is a graduated progression, as outlined in the rehabilitation section of this book. The final

Table 2 Return to Running Program

Returning From Lower Extremity Injury

Begin with straight-line jogging

Progress from jogging to ½ speed, then to ¾ speed, and then to full-speed sprinting as tolerated.

Agility drills are added in the same speed progression as with running

Jumping and plyometric activity

Sport-specific and position-specific drills

phases focus on sport- and position-specific exercises. The principles of protection, rest, ice, compression, and elevation (PRICE) should be followed. Pain-control modalities such as ice, electrical stimulation, and ultrasound are a useful adjunct. Joint range of motion, muscle flexibility, strengthening, endurance training, and functional and aerobic activities are initiated as tolerated. Pain is often useful in guiding these activities. In order to maintain aerobic fitness, athletes are encouraged to engage in alternative activities that do not aggravate or jeopardize their injury.

Functional rehabilitation begins following adequate healing and when joint motion, muscle flexibility, strength, balance, and endurance are adequate. Examples of a gradual return to sports programs for throwing and running athletes are given in **Tables 2** and **3**.

For all athletes, a gradual return to play should include transitioning from light or partial practice to full practice as tolerated. A helpful guideline is to require at least two full practices without restriction or problems before returning to full competition. This helps the athlete, coaches, and family know that the athlete is truly ready to return to competition effectively and safely.

Team physicians should be competent in the basic evaluation and treatment of the concussed player. A concussion is defined as a trauma-induced complex type of neurologic and physiologic process affecting the brain. Symptoms include headaches, nausea, blurred vision, confusion, amnesia, difficulty processing information, and lack of consciousness (Table 4).

Evaluation of the concussed athlete should include a detailed recount of the event and symptoms, paying particular attention to the presence of amnesia and loss of consciousness. Sideline neurophysiologic function begins with a full neurologic examination and should include tests for orientation, concentration, and recall. On-the-field screening tests as well as more elaborate computerized tests are available to assess neurophysiologic function. Any loss of consciousness should prompt evaluation at a medical facility. Return to play during the same game is limited to those athletes who, after 15 to 20 minutes of rest, have minimal symptoms or have no amnesia and are without symptoms, even when physically stressed. A

Table 3 Basic Interval Throwing Program for Pitchers

Graduated Throwing Program

1. Begin with basic stretching, strengthening and proprioceptive exercises

   Once pain and inflammation subside may continue to the next phase

2. Begin interval throwing

   Jogging/warm up

   25 throws at 45 feet for 3 sets

   Advance distance each week (45, 60, 90, 120, 150 feet)

   Perform 3 times per week at each distance

   Rest 10 min between sets

   Only advance if pain-free

3. Begin throwing off the mound (180 feet)

   Jogging/warm up

   Throwing begins at 50% maximum velocity

   Begin at 15 throws and add 15 throws each week ending at 70 throws per session

   Advance 30, 60, 90 throws at 75%

   Begin adding breaking balls thrown at 50% and advance intensity weekly

   Once 70 throws is reached increase intensity to 75% maximum velocity

4. Simulated game (you must meet the following criteria to move to the next level)

   No pain or stiffness while throwing

   No pain or stiffness after throwing (mild muscle soreness acceptable)

   Good throwing motion/mechanics

   Good throwing accuracy throughout the current level

   Throws are consistently on line

   Good strength throughout the current level with little fatigue

*Timing of beginning and advancing throwing phases will vary depending on the following factors: type of injury, surgery, and age of the athlete.

Table 4 Signs and Symptoms of a Concussion

Headache

Nausea/vomiting

Sleep disturbances

Sensitivity to light

Disorientation

Memory abnormalities

Lack of coordination/delayed response

Confusion

Amnesia

Loss of consciousness

Poor concentration

Inappropriate emotions

Slurred speech

Dizziness

Fatigue

Irritability

Blurred vision

Empty stare

major concern with returning to play before the brain has physiologically recovered is the potential that a second impact, even a minor one, can result in severe consequences and even death (second impact syndrome).

Liability and Ethical Issues

Team physicians face many competing pressures from coaches, administrators, parents, and boosters to have athletes perform when they are injured. There also are times when athletes will want to perform when injured. It is important that the physician remains impartial and not stray from proper health care of the athlete. Ethical issues include the use of performance-enhancing drugs, and overzealous administration of corticosteroid injections or pain medications to promote playing while injured.

Sprains and Strains

Synonyms

- Ligament tear
- Pulled muscle
- Tendon tear

Definition

Sprains and strains are common injuries that are differentiated by the tissue involved. Sprains are injuries to ligaments and strains are injuries involving the muscle-tendon unit.

Sprains typically occur in the ankle, knee, and wrist during sports activities. As ligaments stretch beyond their normal limits, fibers begin to fail sequentially. **Table 1** illustrates the grading scheme for sprains, which is based upon the degree of injury to the ligament fibers. Classifying sprains provides useful information concerning the degree of disability, prognosis, and treatments for these injuries.

Sprains are uncommon in children with open growth plates. This is because the physis is weaker than the ligaments and will fail before the ligament does, resulting in a growth plate or physeal injury. Similarly, in patients with significant osteoporosis, the bone may fail (a fracture may occur) rather than the ligament tearing.

Strains also are common sports injuries and usually follow forceful eccentric loading of the muscle. These injuries are frequently seen in athletes who jump, kick, and run and typically occur at the myotendinous junction of muscles spanning two joints, such as the gastrocnemius, hamstring, and quadriceps muscles. Aging brings about collagen changes, resulting in decreased elasticity. This makes the muscle-tendon unit susceptible to injury. Strains are graded on the amount of musculotendinous fibers torn (**Table 2**). A complete tear of a muscle, or a grade IV strain, typically is described as a rupture.

Table 1 Classification of Sprains

Grade	Degree of Injury	Treatment Principles
I	Partial tear but no instability, or opening of the joint on stress maneuvers	Symptomatic treatment only
II	Partial tear with some instability indicated by partial opening of joint on stress maneuvers	Immobilization to protect injured part, but full healing expected
III	Complete tear with complete opening joint on stress	Immobilization or possibly repair

Table 2 Classification of Strains

Grade	Injury
I	Tear of a few muscle fibers with the fascia intact
II	Tear of moderate amount of muscle fibers with the fascia intact
III	Tear of all muscle fibers and intact fascia
IV	Tear of all muscle fibers and disrupted fascia

Clinical Symptoms

Sprains and strains typically occur acutely as a result of a traumatic event. Patients often report a popping, snapping, or tearing sensation at the time of the injury. This is typically followed by pain, swelling, stiffness, and difficulty bearing weight. Injury to these structures causes bleeding, and ecchymosis can appear within 24 to 48 hours.

Physical Examination

The injured extremity should be examined for swelling, tenderness, and ecchymosis. These findings may not be well defined in deep muscle injuries, or in sprained joints covered by muscles. The injured area should be palpated for the site of maximal tenderness. Examination findings should always be compared with the contralateral or uninjured extremity.

With a sprain, the joint should be examined to determine stability and the degree of injury. This may be difficult as patients will typically guard the injured extremity because of pain. Some ligamentous injuries require specific clinical maneuvers to determine injury and instability. Tests for specific joints can be found in the corresponding chapters of this text.

With strains, the examiner should gently attempt to stretch the injured muscle, palpating for a defect in the injured muscle. Distinguishing a partial from a complete rupture of the muscle is important but may be difficult initially if swelling obscures the palpable defect. The inability of the patient to actively contract the muscle to move a joint suggests a complete rupture, but pain also can limit function in grade I and II injuries. An MRI may be needed to quantify the degree of muscle injury.

Diagnostic Tests

Radiographs should be obtained if a fracture is suspected. Radiographic evaluation can demonstrate musculotendinous avulsion injuries or signs of ligamentous injury, or it can be used in a stressed manner for evaluation of suspected physeal injuries. Patients with grade IV strains, grade III sprains or strains, or severe grade II sprains or strains require further evaluation.

Table 3 Ottawa Ankle Rules

Ankle Sprains

Pain at the medial malleolus or along the distal 6 cm of the posterior/medial tibia

Pain at the lateral malleolus or along the distal 6 cm of the posterior fibula

Inability to bear weight immediately and for four consecutive steps in the emergency department

Foot Sprains

Pain in the midfoot and at the base of the fifth metatarsal

Pain in the midfoot and at the navicular bone

Inability to bear weight immediately and for four consecutive steps in the emergency department

Figure 1 Lateral radiograph of the knee in a 19-year-old man obtained 4 weeks after a football injury to the posterior thigh shows fluffy calcifications (arrow) in the posterior thigh musculature consistent with early myositis ossificans. (Reproduced from Lieberman JR, ed: *AAOS Comprehensive Orthopaedic Review.* Rosemont, IL, American Academy of Orthopaedic Surgeons, p 456.)

The Ottawa ankle rules (**Table 3**) are useful to determine if a patient with a suspected foot or ankle sprain requires radiographs on initial evaluation. Radiographs should be obtained if abnormal alignment, pain over the malleoli or midfoot areas, or any of the Ottawa findings is present.

In all suspected sprains and strains, radiographs should be obtained if pain or swelling increases with appropriate care, or if pain and swelling persists after 7 to 10 days of appropriate management.

MRI is the most sensitive test for evaluating soft-tissue injuries. MRI should be used sparingly; however, it is useful when confirmation or grading is necessary. MRI also is valuable for the evaluation of suspected ruptures or severe sprains.

Differential Diagnosis

- Fracture (evident on radiographs)
- Soft-tissue contusion (swelling, no palpable defect)

Adverse Outcomes of the Disease

Ligamentous laxity or chronic injuries may lead to joint instability. Joint instability can lead to accelerated degenerative changes in the involved joint. Prolonged injury or muscle rupture can lead to muscle atrophy, weakness, loss of range of motion, and disability. Complex regional pain syndrome (CRPS) can develop after seemingly minor strains or sprains (see page 67). Compartment syndrome occasionally can occur (see page 58). Myositis ossificans, which is ossification in the muscle, can form in the muscle following severe strains (**Figure 1**).

Treatment

Protection, rest, ice, compression, and elevation (PRICE) is the mainstay of treatment. Cryotherapy should be instituted early. NSAIDs also are useful for analgesia and to decrease inflammation.

Table 4 Treatment Protocol for Hamstring Strains

Phase	Time	Goals	Treatment
I: Acute	3 to 5 days	Control pain and edema	Rest, ice, compression, elevation
	1 to 5 days	Limit hemorrhage and inflammation	Immobilization in extension, NSAIDs
	After 1 to 5 days	Prevent muscle fiber adhesions	Pain-free PROM (gentle stretching),
	Up to 1 week	Normal gait	AAROM (crutches)
II: Subacute	Day 3 to >3 weeks	Control pain and edema	Ice, compression, and electrical stimulation
		Full AROM	
		Alignment of collagen	Pain-free pool activities
		Increase collagen strength	Pain-free PROM, AAROM
		Maintain cardiovascular conditioning	Pain-free submaximal isometrics, stationary bike
			Well-leg stationary bike, swimming with pull buoys, upper body exercise
III: Remodeling	1 to 6 weeks	Achieve phase II goals	Ice and compression
		Control pain and edema	Ice and electrical stimulation
		Increase collagen strength	Prone concentric isotonic exercises, isokinetic exercise
		Increase hamstring flexibility	
		Increase eccentric loading	Moist heat or exercise prior to pelvic-tilt hamstring stretching
			Prone eccentric exercises, jump rope
IV: Functional	2 weeks to 6 months	Return to sport without reinjury	Walk/jog, jog/sprint, sport-specific skills and drills
		Increase hamstring flexibility	Pelvic-tilt hamstring stretching
		Increase hamstring strength	Prone concentric and eccentric exercises
		Control pain	Heat, ice, and modalities; NSAIDs as needed
V: Return to competition	3 weeks to 6 months	Avoid reinjury	Maintenance stretching and strengthening

AAROM = active-assistive range of motion, AROM = active range of motion, PROM = passive range of motion.

Concentric high speeds at first, proceeding to eccentric low speeds.

(Adapted from Clanton TO, Coupe KJ: Hamstring strains in athletes: Diagnosis and treatment. *J Am Acad Orthop Surg* 1998;6:237-248.)

In general, minor sprains can be treated with elastic compression bandages, bracing, or a brief period of immobilization. If necessary, strain injuries should be immobilized in a position where the muscle is stretched to help minimize bleeding from the injured muscle. Rehabilitation is often helpful in assuring a successful recovery. An example of a treatment protocol following a significant muscle strain of the lower extremity is illustrated in **Table 4.**

Adverse Outcomes of Treatment

Inadequate immobilization or unsupervised rehabilitation may lead to worsening of the condition. Overemphasis on treatment in the suggestible patient can lead to chronic impairment and disability, particularly in workers' compensation situations. Surgical intervention may result in scarring, infection, or postoperative arthrofibrosis.

Referral Decisions/Red Flags

Patients with grade IV strains, grade III sprains or strains, or severe grade II sprains or strains require further evaluation. Patients with symptoms disproportionate to their injury can be at risk for chronic conditions or CRPS. Equivocal radiographs should be repeated if necessary.

Tumors of Bone

Synonyms

- Bone lesion
- Neoplasm

Definition

A tumor can be defined as "a swollen or distended part" or abnormal tissue that possesses no physiologic function. Consequently, the term *bone tumor* can be used to describe benign neoplastic, malignant neoplastic, and even nonneoplastic inflammatory and traumatic conditions. The word *tumor*, however, is synonymous with cancer to many people and especially to patients. Physicians must be careful of the manner in which they explain to patients that an abnormality has been found involving a bone. In many cases, a common benign abnormality is discovered on a radiograph or bone scan that sets off a series of additional but unnecessary studies and concerns. It is important that when a bone tumor or bone lesion is discovered that the lesion be evaluated expediently and appropriately. In most cases, a diagnosis can be rendered by an experienced observer with only a radiograph and without the need for additional advanced imaging. Experienced observers rely on prior experience and pattern recognition. Pattern recognition aims to categorize the appearance of a bone lesion and thereby determine the next best course of action. The most basic categories that should be used when evaluating a bone lesion are benign or malignant. Characteristics or patterns that favor a benign or malignant diagnosis are listed in **Table 1**.

Clinical Symptoms

Typically, malignant bone tumors present with a history of a dull aching pain that progresses over time. It may or may not be associated with a soft-tissue mass. Symptoms are typically exacerbated with activity indicative of a lesion that has weakened the structural integrity of the bone. Benign bone tumors may or may not be symptomatic depending on the type of tumor and the stage. Benign bone tumors are staged as follows:

- Stage 1: Latent
- Stage 2: Active
- Stage 3: Aggressive

Like malignant bone tumors, benign tumors that weaken the bone typically present with pain that is exacerbated with

Table 1 Characteristics or Patterns of Bone Tumors
Benign
Well-defined
Nonaggressive
Without cortical destruction or periosteal reaction
Malignant
Lytic
Destructive
Permeative
Ill-defined
Aggressive
Moth-eaten
Cortical destruction
Periosteal reaction

activity. Most benign tumors that do not weaken the bone remain asymptomatic. Important exceptions to this generalization include osteoid osteoma and osteochondroma. Constitutional symptoms such as fever, malaise, and weight loss are absent in patients with benign tumors and are a very late presentation in patients with primary malignant bone tumors. Constitutional symptoms in patients with a bone lesion favor a diagnosis of metastatic disease, lymphoma, or infection.

Tests

History and Physical Examination

The three common clinical scenarios by which a bone tumor is discovered are as follows:

- As an incidental finding. This occurs when an imaging study is performed for an unrelated reason and a bone lesion or abnormality is discovered.
- When a patient is symptomatic and an imaging study is performed, and a bone lesion or abnormality is discovered.
- When a bone lesion is discovered as part of the evaluation of a patient with a known history of cancer.

The first scenario is the most common one; most cases will be benign, and no further tests are needed. In the second scenario, it is necessary to determine if the radiographic finding is related to the patient's symptoms or is actually an incidental finding. Obtaining a history and physical examination will direct the physician to the most logical and appropriate next step in many cases. The history should include the patient's age, past medical history, family history, location and character of symptoms, and aggravating and alleviating factors. When a metastatic lesion is suspected, the history and physical examination should include an inquiry regarding the five most common primary sites of cancer that metastasize to bone: breast, lung, kidney, thyroid, and prostate. These primary sites account for more than 85% of skeletal metastases.

Diagnostic Tests

The radiograph is the single most valuable imaging study for evaluating a bone lesion. In most cases, a determination can be made about the likelihood of the lesion being benign or malignant, and in many cases is either pathonemonic or highly suggestive of a definitive diagnosis. The need for and selection of additional imaging studies should be determined after a differential diagnosis is established from the initial radiographs. Commonly used diagnostic tests include CT and MRI. The role of CT and/or MRI in evaluating a bone lesion will depend on what specific information is being sought. MRI is superior to CT for visualizing the soft tissues and marrow infiltrative processes. CT is superior to MRI for visualizing bone detail, such as cortical continuity, erosion, or endosteal scalloping. A technetium Tc 99 bone scan uses a radioactive technetium isotope bound to the ligand methylene-diphosphonate. In situations where more active bone turnover exists, the bone scan will be hot, or more active than normal. Bone scans are generally sensitive for infection, trauma, and tumor, but they are not specific and do not indicate if the activity is related to trauma, infection, or tumor. Bone scans also are useful to determine if a patient with a primary cancer has skeletal metastases.

In patients older than 40 years with a suspected malignant bone tumor, the most likely diagnosis is metastatic tumor or myeloma. If a primary site can not be found after obtaining a thorough history and physical examination, patients should undergo a CT scan of the chest, abdomen, and pelvis. A bone scan should be obtained to see if there are additional bone lesions that may be more appropriate for biopsy. Additional tests such as upper and lower endoscopy, indirect laryngoscopy, and even mammography are not necessary.

Blood Tests

In patients with aggressive bone lesions the differential diagnosis will include metastatic tumor, primary malignant bone tumor, and infection. In patients older than 40 years, the most likely diagnosis of an aggressive bone lesion will be metastases or myeloma. Serum tests that are sometimes helpful in narrowing a differential diagnosis include complete blood cell count, erythrocyte sedimentation rate, and C-reactive protein level (possible infection). In patients older than 40 years, blood tests to indicate myeloma should be performed, including serum protein electrophoresis (SPEP) and urine protein electrophoresis (UPEP). In most cases, additional blood tests will not obviate the need for a biopsy of suspected malignant bone lesions.

Biopsy

A biopsy is indicated when the diagnosis remains uncertain after appropriate history, physical examination, and review of laboratory and imaging studies. The most common methods used to biopsy bone include closed-needle biopsy and open-bone biopsy. Each method has advantages and disadvantages, but it is recommended that patients with bone tumors be evaluated by an orthopaedic surgeon prior to obtaining a biopsy.

Differential Diagnosis

The differential diagnosis depends on the patient's age, location of the lesion, and most importantly, the pattern appearance seen on radiographs. In most cases of benign bone tumors the diagnosis can be made based on characteristics of the plain radiograph without the need for additional imaging (**Figure 1**).

Figure 1 An expansile, multiloculated lesion without periosteal new bone, marked cortical thinning, and a small, nondisplaced fracture are essentially diagnostic for a unicameral bone cyst.

Figure 2 AP radiograph demonstrates a destructive, ill-defined lesion in the metaphysis of a skeletally immature individual with cortical breakthrough, new periosteal bone, and matrix formation (bone-forming malignant tumor). This is almost certainly an osteosarcoma based on the radiographs.

In cases of malignant tumors, age becomes a major factor in determining the differential diagnosis (**Figure 2**).

Table 2 provides a list of common benign bone tumors.

Adverse Outcomes of the Disease

Benign tumors that are latent may cause symptoms and limit function. Benign active and aggressive lesions can cause pathologic fracture and loss of function. Malignant tumors that are metastatic cause pain, disability, and loss of function. With immobility comes the risk of hypercalcemia and pneumonia.

Table 2 Benign Bone Tumors

Tumor Type	Age Range of Occurrence, in Years	Location	Characteristic Radiographic Appearance	Unique Clinical or Radiographic Feature
Osteochondroma	Childhood and young adult	Metaphysis of long bone	Bone arising from stalk or "bump" on bone	Normal-appearing bone growing from the surface of bone
Chondroblastoma	Childhood and young adult	Epiphysis of long bone	Well defined, with sclerotic border, may have cortical breakthrough	Epiphyseal location
Chondromyxoid fibroma	Adolescence	Eccentric, metaphyseal	Well defined, with internal calcifications	Favored location: tibia
Enchondroma	15-40	Hands and fingers, metaphysis of long bones	Lucent in hands and fingers; matrix calcification in long bones	Metaphysis of long bones, usually incidental finding
Osteoblastoma	10-35	Posterior elements of the spine, metaphysis of long bone	May be lytic, sclerotic, or mixed	Proclivity for the posterior elements of the spine
Osteoid osteoma	10-35	Long bones and posterior elements of the spine	Sclerotic, with small (<1-cm) lucent nidus	Distinct nidus, best seen with CT; typical night pain that is responsive to NSAIDs and/or aspirin
Eosinophilic granuloma	5-10 (rare in patient older than 30)	Vertebrae, long or flat bone	Spine lesions: vertebra plana. In long bones lytic and may appear aggressive	Vertebra plana in a child; may involve more than one bone
Fibrous dysplasia	Late childhood through adulthood; polyostotic fibrous dysplasia present earlier	Any bone (ie, ribs, femur, tibia, maxilla, mandible, humerus)	Lytic, may expand the bone with thinning of the cortex	Ground-glass appearance on radiograph
Nonossifying fibroma	3-30	Femur and tibia are most common	Lytic, well-defined, thin, lobulated margin	Eccentric, involves cortex and expands into medullary cavity
Fibrous cortical defect	4-15	Distal femur and tibia	Radiolucent, well-defined, confined to cortex with sclerotic border	Well-defined cortical lesion with sclerotic borders less than 4 cm
Aneurysmal bone cyst	Younger than 30	Any bone; most commonly in vertebra, femur, and tibia	Eccentric, lytic, expansile	Fluid levels seen on CT or MRI
Giant cell tumor	20-40	Distal femur, proximal tibia, distal radius, proximal humerus, pelvis, sacrum	Eccentric, lytic epiphyseal/metaphyseal long bones	Lytic lesion extending from subchondral bone to metaphysic; may erode beyond cortex
Simple bone cyst (unicameral bone cyst)	Younger than 20	80% proximal humerus or proximal femur	Central medullary lytic lesion, may expand bone and be multicystic	Fallen-leaf sign is pathonemonic

Treatment

Many benign tumors may be observed and require no treatment. Active and aggressive lesions are managed surgically with a goal of minimizing local recurrence while maximizing function. Primary malignant tumors in children are usually treated with systemic chemotherapy and surgery. The majority of primary malignant bone tumors are successfully treated with limb-sparing surgery. The treatment of metastatic bone tumors includes radiation, chemotherapy, and surgery. Bisphosphonates play a vital role in the management of patients with established bone metastases.

Referral Decisions/Red Flags

Further evaluation by a specialist is recommended for a suspicious bone or soft-tissue mass, unusual pain or night pain, constitutional symptoms associated with bone pain, lytic or blastic changes in bone, soft-tissue calcification, or periosteal reaction on radiographs.

PAIN DIAGRAM
Shoulder

Cervical radiculopathy
(see Spine section)
Frozen shoulder

Acromioclavicular injuries

Fracture of the clavicle

Rotator cuff tear
Shoulder instability

Posterior

Anterior

Fracture of
the scapula

Cervical
radiculopathy
(see Spine section)

Impingement syndrome
Rotator cuff tear
Frozen shoulder
Arthritis of the shoulder
Fracture of the proximal
    humerus
Thoracic outlet syndrome

Fracture of the humeral shaft
Rupture of the proximal biceps tendon

Rotator cuff tear
Impingement syndrome
Frozen shoulder
Cervical radiculopathy
(see Spine section)

Lateral

Shoulder

Section Editor

Leesa M. Galatz, MD

Associate Professor
Shoulder and Elbow Service
Department of Orthopaedic Surgery
Washington University School of Medicine
St. Louis, MO

Contributor

Michael Huxford, MEd, ATC, CSCS

Sports Medicine Coordinator
Rehabilitative Services
Institute for Sports Medicine
Children's Memorial Hospital
Chicago, IL

ANATOMY OF THE SHOULDER

Trapezius muscle

Levator scapulae muscle

Rhomboid minor muscle

Rhomboid major muscle

Acromion

Deltoid muscle

Supraspinatus muscle

Spine of scapula

Infraspinatus fascia

Infraspinatus muscle

Teres minor muscle

Teres major muscle

Latissimus dorsi muscle

Long head

Lateral head

Triceps brachii muscle

Triangle of auscultation

Posterior View

Acromion

Coracoid process

Coracoacromial ligament

Pectoralis minor tendon (cut)

Subdeltoid bursa

Subscapularis muscle

Greater tubercle,

Lesser tubercle of humerus

Musculocutaneous nerve (cut)

Coracobrachialis muscle

Intertubercular tendon sheath

Circumflex scapular artery (cut)

Deltoid muscle (reflected)

Teres major muscle

Latissimus dorsi muscle

Pectoralis major muscle (reflected)

Anterior circumflex humeral artery

Acromial angle

Acromion

Coracoid process

Clavicle

Biceps brachii muscle

Long head

Short head

Supraglenoid tubercle

Superior angle

Superior border

Anatomic neck

Suprascapular notch

Brachial artery (cut)

Greater tubercle

Neck

Median nerve (cut)

Lesser tubercle

Medial border

Brachialis muscle

Surgical neck

Glenoid cavity of scapula

Subscapular fossa

Lateral cutaneous nerve of forearm

Intertubercular sulcus

Head of humerus

Bicipital aponeurosis

Crest of greater tubercle

Infraglenoid tubercle

Biceps brachii tendon

Crest of lesser tubercle

Lateral border

Brachioradialis muscle

Deltoid tuberosity

Humerus

Inferior angle

Pronator teres muscle

Scapula

Flexor carpi radialis muscle

Anterior Arm

Medial supracondylar ridge

Lateral supracondylar ridge

Humerus and Scapula Anterior Views

Condyles

Medial

Lateral

Radial fossa

Lateral epicondyle

Medial epicondyle

Capitellum

Trochlea

Coronoid fossa

Overview of the Shoulder

This section of *Essentials of Musculoskeletal Care* focuses on the conditions that commonly affect the shoulder in adults. These include acute injuries (fractures, dislocations, and acute tendon ruptures), chronic or repetitive injuries (impingement syndrome and most rotator cuff tears and biceps tendon ruptures), and degenerative, inflammatory, or idiopathic conditions (glenohumeral and acromioclavicular [AC] arthritis, adhesive capsulitis [frozen shoulder]). Most shoulder disorders are diagnosed from a history, a thorough physical examination, and radiographs.

A concise differential diagnosis often is achieved after evaluating the symptoms in the context of their chronicity and the patient's age. The chief symptom is usually related to pain or instability. Decreased motion, power, or function sometimes accompanies pain or instability but only rarely is the chief symptom.

Pain

Patients with acute symptoms (less than 2 weeks' duration) usually have sustained an injury such as a fracture or a dislocation, a rotator cuff tear, or a biceps tendon rupture. Common physical findings include local tenderness, deformity, swelling, and ecchymosis. Determining the mechanism and magnitude of the injury and the anatomic location of the symptoms helps in making the diagnosis. For example, a football player who has severe pain and deformity at the superior aspect of the shoulder after falling directly on that shoulder most likely has an AC joint separation.

Similarly, for patients with chronic shoulder pain, knowledge of the activities related to the onset of symptoms and the location and character of symptoms often leads to the correct diagnosis. Pain localized to the top of the shoulder suggests AC joint arthritis or chronic AC separation. This pain often is exacerbated by cross-body adduction in the horizontal plane. Pain from subacromial bursitis, frozen shoulder, or rotator cuff pathology is typically referred to the lateral deltoid region and may radiate to the lateral aspect of the upper arm. Overhead activities most commonly exacerbate this pain. In contrast, shoulder pain arising from cervical nerve root irritation usually follows a dermatomal distribution, is associated with numbness and/or tingling, and is often relieved by placing the forearm on top of the head. Degenerative arthritis of the glenohumeral joint may cause pain along the anterior and posterior joint lines. Both rotator cuff tears and arthritis may cause night pain, which makes sleeping on the affected side difficult.

Instability

Instability is classified by the frequency of symptomatic episodes, as well as the direction and degree of instability. An acute injury may be a first-time dislocation or a recurrent episode. The instability episode may be partial (subluxation) with spontaneous reduction, or it may be complete (dislocation). The instability can be anterior, posterior, inferior, or multidirectional. Most traumatic dislocations are anterior. Multidirectional instability should be considered when a patient presents with recurrent episodes of subluxations or dislocations and no history of significant trauma.

Range of Motion, Muscle Strength, and Function

When assessing motion, it is important to determine if there is a discrepancy between active and passive motion. Patients with rotator cuff tears lose active elevation and external rotation, although some loss of passive range of motion can occur secondary to disuse. Equal losses of active and passive range of motion may be secondary to soft-tissue contracture, as in frozen shoulder, or the result of joint incongruity from trauma or arthritis.

Muscle strength should be assessed and compared with the opposite shoulder. Tears of the rotator cuff and neurologic injury may produce weakness. Pain inhibition can affect the accuracy of muscle testing.

Functional status relates to a patient's ability to perform his or her normal activities. The level of functional disability depends on the specific type and intensity of activities the patient normally performs. Motivation and the ability to adapt to impairment also play a significant role.

Patient Age

Younger Patients

Patients younger than 30 years most commonly present with traumatic injuries or instability such as glenohumeral dislocations and AC joint separations. Impingement syndrome and rotator cuff tears rarely occur in this age group.

Middle-aged Patients

Impingement syndrome and rotator cuff tears are common in this group. These must be distinguished from the early onset of adhesive capsulitis. Often it is difficult to distinguish between impingement syndrome and early adhesive capsulitis, and, adding to the confusion, the two diagnoses often coexist. Glenohumeral dislocations are much less common and must be treated with a high index of suspicion for a concomitant rotator cuff tear (50% of patients older than 40 years will have an acute tear).

Older Patients

Patients older than 50 years commonly have symptoms related to rotator cuff dysfunction. Rotator cuff disease can run the spectrum from acute tendinitis and chronic tendinopathy to partial-thickness and full-thickness rotator cuff tears. Rotator cuff tears and degenerative arthritis of the AC joint, the glenohumeral joint, or both also are common in this group. Acute pain following a fall in an elderly, frail patient with osteoporosis should raise suspicion for a fracture of the proximal humerus.

Musculoskeletal Conditioning of the Shoulder

A conditioning program consists of three basic phases: stretching exercises, to improve range of motion; strengthening, to improve muscle power; and proprioception, to enhance balance and agility. In addition, the exercise session should begin with an active warm-up, and plyometric exercises may be added for power after basic strength and flexibility have been achieved. Patient handouts are provided here for the stretching and strengthening exercises. Advanced proprioceptive exercises and plyometric exercises should be done under the supervision of a rehabilitation specialist or other exercise professional.

The goal of a conditioning program is to enable people to live a more fit and healthy lifestyle by being more active. A well-structured conditioning program also will prepare the individual for participation in sports and recreational activities. The greater the intensity of the activity that the individual wishes to engage in, the greater the intensity of the conditioning that will be required. If the individual participates in a supervised rehabilitation program that provides instruction in a conditioning routine—instead of using only an exercise handout such as provided here—the focus should be on developing and committing to a home exercise fitness program. A conditioning program for the body as a whole that includes exercises for the hip, knee, foot, and spine as well as the shoulder is described in the chapter Musculoskeletal Conditioning: Helping Patients Prevent Injury and Stay Fit, beginning on page 183.

The shoulder is a complex structure that allows movement in many different planes. The muscles of the shoulder most important in overhead sports activities such as tennis, baseball, and swimming are the glenohumeral and scapular rotators.

SECTION 2 SHOULDER

Strengthening the scapular stabilizers, as well as the rotator cuff and deltoid muscles, is important because strong, coordinated function of all shoulder muscle groups helps stabilize the glenohumeral joint and helps prevent injury when the individual engages in activities such as gardening, housekeeping, or work- or sport-related activities that involve repetitive upper extremity motion. Also, increased strength in these muscles translates into a higher velocity tennis serve or baseball pitch.

Proprioceptive or balance exercises help train the joints of the upper extremity to perceive joint positions and hence enhance the individual's perception of the position of the body in space. Examples of proprioceptive exercises for the shoulder are scapular retraction done while lying on an exercise ball or push-ups performed on an air mattress or with each hand on a small ball instead of the floor. These exercises should be done only after adequate flexibility and strength have been achieved. Also, instruction and supervision in such exercises is required to ensure that they are performed safely.

For individuals beginning a new sport activity, once the prescribed goals of strengthening, stretching, and proprioceptive conditioning have been met, a period of sport-specific training should begin. During this period, the patient would perform the actions normally required by the sport with gradually increasing intensity and duration.

Forcing stretching or strengthening to the point of pain is always deleterious and should be avoided. Progress is achieved by performing these exercises frequently (2 to 4 times per day, 7 days per week) and making small gains. The patient should be instructed to call the physician if the exercises cause pain.

Strengthening Exercises

Exercises to strengthen the deltoid and rotator cuff muscles can be done most easily using commercially available elastic therapy bands. These are available in different thicknesses, which provide different amounts of resistance. The same exercises can also be performed with pulleys or free weights. It usually takes 2 to 3 weeks to progress from one band or weight to the next. For strength training, the patient should perform 3 sets of 8 repetitions, progressing to 3 sets of 12 repetitions. Once 12 repetitions are reached, the resistance should be increased and the repetitions started over at 8. However, the patient should be advised not to progress to the next level of resistance if he or she still has difficulty at the current level or if pain develops when trying the new one. The patient should also be instructed to continue stretching exercises during this stage so that the hard-won gains in range of motion are not lost.

Stretching Exercises

The capsule and muscles of the posterior shoulder may be tight, especially in the individual who participates in repetitive overhead activities, including overhead throwing sports and swimming. Crossover arm stretches are helpful to relax these muscles. Static stretching should be done to increase the flexibility of the muscles surrounding the shoulder. A static stretch is performed at the end of the available range of painless motion of the muscle and joint.

Proprioceptive Exercises

In addition to strength, the athlete requires balance and power. Neuromuscular training, which improves the communication between the muscles and the proprioceptors, includes balance and perturbation exercises. Balance involves the visual, vestibular, and proprioceptive systems. With balance training, the athlete consciously attempts to hold a posture for 30 to 60 seconds.

Proprioceptive exercises for the shoulder involve weight bearing through the arms. For example, push-ups performed with the hands on an exercise ball are an excellent advanced exercise for improving dynamic scapular stabilization. For the novice, standing push-ups done against a wall provide good proprioceptive training. To perform this exercise, the individual should stand several feet away from a wall with a 5″ or 7″ exercise ball in each hand. Leaning toward the wall, place the balls on the wall and move them up and down with the eyes closed to increase position sense. Then do push-ups against the wall with the hands on the balls, bending and extending at the elbow.

SECTION 2 SHOULDER

Home Exercise Program for Shoulder Conditioning

- When performing the stretching exercises, you should stretch slowly to the limit of motion, taking care to avoid pain. If you experience pain with the exercises, call your doctor.
- For the exercises that use a stick, you may use a yardstick or stick of similar size.

Strengthening and Stretching Exercises for the Shoulder

Exercise	Muscle Group	Number of Repetitions/Sets	Number of Days per Week
Strengthening			
External rotation	Infraspinatus Teres minor	8 repetitions/3 sets, progressing to 12 repetitions/3 sets	3
Standing row	Middle trapezius Rhomboid	8 repetitions/3 sets, progressing to 12 repetitions/3 sets	3
Internal rotation	Pectoralis major and minor Subscapularis	8 repetitions/3 sets, progressing to 12 repetitions/3 sets	3
Bent-over horizontal abduction	Middle and lower trapezius	8 repetitions/3 sets, progressing to 12 repetitions/3 sets	3
Elbow flexion	Biceps	8 repetitions/3 sets, progressing to 12 repetitions/3 sets	3
Elbow extension	Triceps	8 repetitions/3 sets, progressing to 12 repetitions/3 sets	3
External rotation with arm abducted 90°	Infraspinatus Teres minor	8 repetitions/3 sets, progressing to 12 repetitions/3 sets	3
Stretching			
Pendulum	General	10 repetitions/2 sets, progressing to 15 repetitions/3 sets	5 to 6
Passive internal rotation	Subscapularis Pectoralis major and minor	4 sets	5 to 6
Passive external rotation	Infraspinatus Teres minor	4 sets	5 to 6
Crossover arm stretch	Posterior deltoid	4 sets	5 to 6

SECTION 2 SHOULDER

Strengthening Exercises

External Rotation

- Make a 3-foot-long loop with the elastic band and tie the ends together. Attach the loop to a doorknob or other stable object.
- Standing with your side to the wall, hold the loop, as shown in the start position.
- Keeping your elbow close to your side, rotate the arm outward slowly and then slowly return to the start position.
- Repeat on the other side.
- Perform 3 sets of 8 repetitions, progressing to 3 sets of 12 repetitions, 3 days per week.

Start   Finish

Standing Row

- Make a 3-foot-long loop with the elastic band and tie the ends together. Attach the loop to a doorknob or other stable object.
- Standing facing the wall, hold the loop as shown in the start position.
- Keeping your arm close to your side, slowly pull the arm straight back and then slowly return to the start position.
- Repeat on the other side.
- Perform 3 sets of 8 repetitions, progressing to 3 sets of 12 repetitions, 3 days per week.

Start   Finish

SECTION 2   SHOULDER

Internal Rotation

- Make a 3-foot-long loop with the elastic band and tie the ends together. Attach the loop to a doorknob or other stable object.
- Standing with your side to the wall, hold the loop as shown in the start position.
- Keeping your elbow close to your side, rotate the arm across your body slowly and then slowly return to the start position.
- Repeat on the other side.
- Perform 3 sets of 8 repetitions, progressing to 3 sets of 12 repetitions, 3 days per week.

Start   Finish

Bent-Over Horizontal Abduction

- Stand next to a table.
- Bend at the waist with your side supported on the table and the other arm hanging straight down and holding a light weight (up to 5 lb).
- Keeping the arm straight, slowly raise the hand up to eye level and then slowly lower it back to the starting position.
- Repeat on the other side.
- Perform 3 sets of 8 repetitions, progressing to 3 sets of 12 repetitions, 3 days per week.

SECTION 2 SHOULDER

Elbow Flexion

- Stand with your weight evenly distributed over both feet.
- Holding a light weight (up to 5 lb) and keeping the arm close to the side, slowly bend the elbow up toward the shoulder as shown; hold for 2 seconds, slowly return to the starting position, and then relax.
- Repeat on the other side.
- Perform 3 sets of 8 repetitions, progressing to 3 sets of 12 repetitions, 3 days per week.

Elbow Extension

- Stand with your weight evenly distributed over both feet.
- Holding a light weight (up to 5 lb), raise your arm with the elbow bent and with your opposite hand supporting your elbow. Slowly straighten the elbow overhead, hold for 2 seconds, and then slowly lower the arm to the starting position.
- Repeat on the other side.
- Perform 3 sets of 8 repetitions, progressing to 3 sets of 12 repetitions, 3 days per week.

SECTION 2 SHOULDER

External Rotation With Arm Abducted 90°

- Make a 3-foot-long loop with the elastic band and tie the ends together. Attach the loop to a doorknob or other stable object.
- Standing facing the wall, hold the loop as shown in the start position, with the arm held straight out from the shoulder and the elbow bent 90°.
- Keeping the shoulder and elbow level, slowly rotate the hand up from the elbow, and then slowly return to the start position.
- Perform 3 sets of 8 repetitions, progressing to 3 sets of 12 repetitions, 3 days per week.

Stretching Exercises

Pendulum

- Lean forward, supporting the body with one arm and relaxing the muscles of the other arm so that it hangs freely.
- Gently move the arm in forward-and-back, side-to-side, and circular motions.
- Repeat on the other side.
- Perform 2 sets of 10 repetitions, progressing to 3 sets of 15 repetitions, 5 to 6 days per week.

Passive External Rotation

- Grasp the stick with one hand and cup the other end of the stick with the other hand.
- Push the stick horizontally as shown, keeping the elbow against the side of the body so that the arm is passively stretched to the point of feeling a pull without pain.
- Hold for 30 seconds and then relax for 30 seconds.
- Repeat on the other side.
- Perform 4 sets, 5 to 6 days per week.

Start   Finish

Passive Internal Rotation

- Behind your back, grasp the stick with one hand and lightly grasp the other end of the stick with the other hand.
- Pull the stick horizontally as shown so that the arm is passively stretched to the point of feeling a pull without pain.
- Hold for 30 seconds and then relax for 30 seconds.
- Repeat on the other side.
- Perform 4 sets, 5 to 6 days per week.

Start   Finish

Crossover Arm Stretch

- Gently pull the elbow of one arm across the chest as far as possible without feeling pain.
- Hold the stretch for 30 seconds and then relax for 30 seconds.
- Repeat on the other side.
- Perform 4 sets, 5 to 6 days per week.

SECTION 2 SHOULDER

Physical Examination of the Shoulder

Inspection/Palpation

Anterior View

With the patient standing, inspect for abnormal contours and bony prominences. An acromioclavicular separation produces a "step-off" deformity with prominence of the distal clavicle. An anterior shoulder dislocation produces a prominent posterior acromion and anterior fullness of the deltoid, and the arm typically is held in slight abduction and external rotation. By contrast, with a posterior dislocation, the coracoid and anterior acromion are prominent, there is posterior fullness, and the arm is held in adduction and internal rotation.

Posterior View

With the patient standing, note symmetry of shoulder heights and contours (the dominant shoulder often rests slightly lower than the opposite shoulder). Look for muscle atrophy, particularly of the trapezius, deltoid, and infraspinatus muscles. Diminished posterior contour from neck to shoulder indicates atrophy of the trapezius. With atrophy of the supraspinatus/infraspinatus muscles, loss of lateral shoulder contour occurs at the deltoid, and a prominent scapular spine can be seen.

Acromioclavicular Joint

To evaluate the acromioclavicular joint, palpate the distal clavicle and the acromion for tenderness or spurs. Tenderness usually is most pronounced at the posterior joint interval and is exaggerated when the patient horizontally adducts the arm toward the opposite shoulder.

Subacromial Bursa

To evaluate the subacromial bursa, palpate the anterolateral portion of the acromion, moving down toward the deltoid until you feel the acromiohumeral sulcus. Tenderness in this area usually is related to subacromial bursitis or a rotator cuff tear (supraspinatus tendon).

Long Head of the Biceps Tendon

To evaluate the long head of the biceps tendon, palpate over the humeral head in the region of the bicipital groove. With tendinitis, there is tenderness and swelling, and the area of tenderness should move with the humeral head as the shoulder is rotated.

Range of Motion

Flexion

Normal shoulder motion is a composite movement that couples glenohumeral motion with movement of the scapula on the thorax. Scapular movement is derived from motion of the acromioclavicular and sternoclavicular joints. Shoulder mobility is efficiently assessed by measuring four ranges of motion: flexion, external rotation with the arm at the side, external rotation with the arm in 90° of abduction, and internal rotation.

To evaluate shoulder flexion, place the patient's arm at the side **(A)**. Ask the patient to raise the arm in the sagittal plane **(B)**, and then measure active and passive motion in reference to the thoracic spine. Normal shoulder flexion is 160° to 170°.

External Rotation, Arm at the Side

To evaluate external rotation, place the patient's arm at the side, held comfortably against the thorax, the elbow flexed to 90°, and the forearm parallel to the sagittal plane of the body **(A)**. Measure external rotation by evaluating the maximum lateral rotation of the arm **(B)**.

External Rotation, Arm Abducted 90°

To evaluate external rotation, a goniometer is needed. The patient's arm is abducted 90°, the arm is aligned with the plane of the scapula, the elbow is flexed 90°, and the forearm is parallel to the floor **(A)**. Measure external rotation in this position by evaluating how many degrees the forearm moves away from the previous parallel position **(B)**. Limited external rotation in this position is seen in some athletes who emphasize strengthening exercises without including an appropriate stretching program and in patients who have had reconstructive surgery of the shoulder.

Internal Rotation

To evaluate internal rotation, ask the patient to place the arm behind the back and reach as high as possible. Note the highest midline spinous process that can be reached by the hitch-hiking thumb. This maneuver is simple and easy to reproduce, but it represents a composite motion that depends on shoulder extension as well as scapular protraction and elbow, wrist, and thumb motion. Young adults typically can reach beyond the inferior tip of the scapula (approximately at the T7 level). Internal rotation may be severely limited in patients with adhesive capsulitis or degenerative arthritis. In these patients, the thumb may reach only to the sacrum, gluteal region, or greater trochanter.

Muscle Testing

Deltoid

To test the deltoid muscle, place the patient's arm in 90° of abduction with the elbow flexed 90° and the forearm parallel to the floor. Push down on the distal arm as the patient resists this pressure. This position also activates the supraspinatus and, to some degree, the other rotator cuff muscles. The anterior deltoid is isolated by moving the arm forward. The posterior deltoid is isolated by moving the arm backward and then performing the muscle test.

Supraspinatus

To evaluate the supraspinatus, place the patient's arm in 90° of abduction, 30° of horizontal abduction, and internal rotation with the elbow extended. Push down on the distal arm as the patient resists this pressure.

Infraspinatus and Teres Minor

Test strength in the infraspinatus and the teres minor by placing the patient's arm at the side in neutral rotation and with the elbow flexed. Support the elbow and instruct the patient to maintain this position while you apply moderate to firm pressure at the distal forearm, attempting to internally rotate the arm.

Hornblower's Test

To evaluate the teres minor, the hornblower's test is helpful. Support the patient's arm abducted to 90° in the scapular plane with the elbow flexed to 90°. Ask the patient to rotate the arm externally 90° against resistance. A positive sign is the inability to maintain the externally rotated position, and the arm drops back to neutral position.

Subscapularis (Gerber Lift-off Test)

Test subscapularis strength and possible tendon rupture by asking the patient to place a hand behind the back, palm facing away from the body, and then lift it away from the back against resistance.

Serratus Anterior

Test serratus anterior strength by asking the patient to elevate the arm as you depress the arm with one hand and palpate the scapula with the other. With normal strength of the serratus anterior, the scapula remains in position on the chest wall. Winging and prominence of the vertebral border occurs with a weak serratus anterior muscle. Stretch or avulsion injuries of the long thoracic nerve with resultant paralysis of the serratus anterior also cause winging of the scapula and fatigue with overhead activities.

Rhomboid

Test rhomboid function by asking the patient to place both hands on the iliac crests. Push the patient's arm forward with your hand at the elbow and palpate the vertebral border of the scapula with the other hand. An intact rhomboid maintains the scapula against the chest wall.

SECTION 2 SHOULDER

Special Tests

Neer Impingement Sign

The Neer impingement sign is helpful to evaluate the shoulder for impingement or rotator cuff tear. Place one hand on the posterior aspect of the scapula to maintain it in the anatomic position and use your other hand to take the patient's internally rotated arm by the wrist and place it in full flexion. This maneuver compresses the greater tuberosity against the anterior acromion and elicits discomfort in patients who have a rotator cuff tear or rotator cuff tendinitis. It may also be painful in patients with adhesive capsulitis, interior instability, or arthritis.

Hawkins Impingement Sign

The Hawkins impingement sign reinforces a positive Neer impingement sign. Flex the patient's shoulder to 90°, flex the elbow to 90°, and place the forearm in neutral rotation. Support the elbow and then internally rotate the humerus. Pain elicited with this test is indicative of rotator cuff tear or rotator cuff tendinitis.

Cross-Body or Horizontal Adduction Test

To perform the cross-body adduction test, flex the patient's shoulder to 90° and then horizontally adduct the arm across the patient's body. Pain over the acromioclavicular joint suggests arthritis of this joint but also is indicative of other acromioclavicular joint pathology, such as a sprain or separation.

SECTION 2 SHOULDER

Apprehension Sign for Anterior Instability

With the patient supine, place the patient's arm in 90° of abduction with the elbow flexed 90°. Gently externally rotate the forearm to 90°. Patients with anterior instability may display apprehension and report a sense of impending dislocation. A report of pain without apprehension is less specific.

Sulcus Sign

With the patient's arm relaxed at the side, place one hand on the posterior scapula and use your other hand to apply traction to the patient's arm in an inferior direction. In patients with inferior shoulder laxity, this maneuver causes inferior subluxation of the humeral head and a widening of the sulcus between the humerus and acromion. A visible dimple is a positive sulcus sign.

Jerk Test for Posterior Instability

To perform the jerk test for posterior instability, place the patient's arm in 90° of flexion and maximum internal rotation with the elbow flexed 90° **(A)**. Adduct the arm across the body in the horizontal plane while applying an axial load at the elbow to push the humerus in a posterior direction **(B)**. If this maneuver causes a posterior subluxation or dislocation, the humeral head can be felt to "clunk" or jerk back into the joint as the arm is then horizontally abducted.

Acromioclavicular Injuries

Synonyms

Acromioclavicular separation

Shoulder separation

Definition

Acromioclavicular (AC) injuries commonly result from a fall onto the tip of the shoulder. A common example is a fall off a bicycle. When the acromion is driven into the ground, variable degrees of ligamentous disruption occur.

These injuries can be classified as one of six types based on the severity of injury and the degree of clavicular separation (**Figure 1**). In type I injuries, the AC joint ligaments are partially disrupted and the strong coracoclavicular (CC) ligaments are intact. As a result, there is no superior separation of the clavicle from the acromion. In type II injuries, the AC ligaments are torn and the CC ligaments are intact. As a result,

Type I

Type II

Type III

Type IV

Type V

Type VI

Conjoined tendon
of biceps and
coracobrachialis

Figure 1   Classification of acromioclavicular separations. (Adapted with permission from Rockwood CA Jr: Subluxation and dislocations about the shoulder, in Rockwood CA Jr, Green DP, eds: *Rockwood and Green's Fractures in Adults*, ed 3. Philadelphia, PA, JB Lippincott, 1988.)

SECTION 2   SHOULDER

there is partial separation of the clavicle from the acromion. The joint is unstable in the anterior-posterior direction and slightly unstable in the vertical direction. In type III injuries, the CC ligaments are completely disrupted, and there is complete separation of the clavicle from the acromion. Types IV through VI are uncommon. In these injuries, the periosteum of the clavicle and/or the deltoid and trapezius muscles also are torn, causing wide displacement.

Clinical Symptoms

Patients report pain over the AC joint and pain on lifting the arm. With type III through VI injuries, an obvious deformity is present.

Tests

Physical Examination

The patient supports the arm in an adducted position, and any motion, especially abduction, causes pain. Tenderness to palpation can be elicited over the AC joint. The distal end of the clavicle may be prominent and slightly superior to the acromion in type II injuries, and there is an obvious deformity in type III through VI injuries. Elevating the arm or depressing the clavicle will temporarily reduce the AC joint, except in type IV and V injuries, in which there is soft-tissue interposition. Type VI injuries are exceedingly rare.

Diagnostic Tests

AP radiographs of both shoulders will confirm type II through VI AC separations.

Type I injuries are sprains; therefore, patients have pain and tenderness, but radiographs are normal.

In type II injuries, some AC joint widening is seen on radiographs, but the distance between the clavicle and coracoid remains normal.

In type III injuries, complete displacement of the clavicle above the superior border of the acromion is seen, as is a 30% to 100% increase in the CC interspace. These injuries are reducible with gentle upward pressure under the elbow.

In type IV injuries, superior displacement of the clavicle may be seen on AP radiographs; an axillary lateral view will clearly show the predominantly posterior displacement.

In type V injuries, the CC interspace is more than twice as large as the opposite shoulder without the application of weights. These injuries are not reducible.

Type VI injuries are rare. With these injuries, the distal end of the clavicle lies in either the subacromial space or the subcoracoid space.

Differential Diagnosis

- Fracture of the acromion (evident on radiographs)
- Fracture of the end of the clavicle (evident on radiographs)
- Rotator cuff tear (most tenderness over the greater tuberosity, not the AC joint; no visible deformity or radiographic findings)

Adverse Outcomes of the Disease

Deformity, weakness on lifting the arm, chronic shoulder pain, and numbness in the arm are possible. Arthritis of the AC joint may eventually develop.

Treatment

Nonsurgical treatment of type I and II injuries consists of wearing a sling for a few days until the pain subsides. Ice is helpful for the first 48 hours, and analgesics can be used to control severe pain. Patients may resume everyday activities as pain allows, with a full return to normal activities and sports within 4 weeks. Treatment of type III injuries is controversial. Many type III injuries can be treated nonsurgically with good functional results. However, surgical repair may be considered in a young manual laborer who does heavy overhead work.
Type IV, V, and VI injuries require evaluation for surgical repair.

Rehabilitation Prescription

The functional goal of rehabilitation for a patient with an AC injury is to reduce the pain, protect the joint from further damage, and restore function. After the shoulder has been immobilized in a sling for an appropriate period of time, a home exercise program that includes basic pain-free exercises to promote rotation of the glenohumeral joint should be started (see page 276). Exercises for the scapular rotators also are initiated, especially scapular retractions and protractions. The patient should be able to perform the exercises without pain.

Rehabilitations should begin if the patient continues to report pain or limited mobility after performing the home exercise program for 2 to 3 weeks. The prescription should include evaluation of the strength of the glenohumeral and scapular rotators and the mobility of the AC joint. The rehabilitation specialist also should supervise the home exercise program to ensure that the patient is using proper technique and is not experiencing pain. Mobilization of the AC joint is indicated if joint motion is limited.

Adverse Outcomes of Treatment

Following prolonged immobilization in a sling, stiffness may develop; use of a sling or tape also may cause skin breakdown. AC arthritis can be a late sequela of any grade of injury, regardless of treatment.

Referral Decisions/Red Flags

Patients with type IV, V, or VI injuries; some athletes (baseball throwers and football quarterbacks on an individual basis); and laborers with type III injuries may be candidates for early surgical repair. Injuries that remain painful warrant further evaluation.

Home Exercise Program for Acromioclavicular Injuries

- Perform the exercises in the order listed.
- To prevent inflammation, apply ice, such as a bag of crushed ice or frozen peas, to the shoulder for 20 minutes after performing all the exercises.
- You should not experience any pain with the exercises. If you are unable to perform any of the exercises because of pain or stiffness, call your doctor.

Exercise Type	Muscle Group	Number of Repetitions/Sets	Number of Days per Week	Number of Weeks
External rotation	Infraspinatus Teres minor	8 to 10 repetitions/2 sets, progressing to 15 repetitions/3 sets	3	2 to 3
Internal rotation	Subscapularis Teres major	8 to 10 repetitions/2 sets, progressing to 15 repetitions/3 sets	3	2 to 3
Scapular retraction/ protraction	Middle trapezius Serratus	8 to 10 repetitions/2 sets, progressing to 15 repetitions/3 sets	3	2 to 3

External Rotation

- Lie on your side on a firm, flat surface with the unaffected arm under you, cradling your head.
- Hold the injured arm against your side as shown, with the elbow bent at a 90° angle.
- Slowly rotate the arm at the shoulder, keeping the elbow bent and against your side, to raise the weight to a vertical position; then slowly lower the weight to the starting position to a count of 5.
- Begin with weights that allow 2 sets of 8 to 10 repetitions (approximately 1 to 2 pounds), and progress to 3 sets of 15 repetitions.
- Add weight in 1-pound increments to a maximum of 5 pounds, starting over at 2 sets of 8 to 10 repetitions each time weight is added.
- Perform the exercise 3 days per week, continuing for 2 to 3 weeks.

Start

Finish

SECTION 2 SHOULDER

Internal Rotation

- Lie on your side on a firm, flat surface with the affected arm under you and with a pillow or folded cloth under your head to keep your spine straight.
- Hold the injured arm against your side as shown, with the elbow bent at a 90° angle.
- Slowly rotate the arm at the shoulder, keeping the elbow bent and against your torso, to raise the weight to a vertical position; then slowly lower the weight to the starting position.
- Begin with weights that allow 2 sets of 8 to 10 repetitions, and progress to 3 sets of 15 repetitions.
- Add weight in 1-pound increments to a maximum of 5 pounds, starting over at 2 sets of 8 to 10 repetitions each time weight is added.
- Perform the exercise 3 days per week, continuing for 2 to 3 weeks.

Start

Finish

Scapular Retraction/Protraction

- Lie on your stomach on a table or bed with the injured arm hanging over the side.
- Keeping the elbow straight, lift the weight slowly by moving the scapula toward the opposite side as far as possible. Do not shrug the shoulder. Then return slowly to the starting position.
- Begin with a weight that allows 2 sets of 8 to 10 repetitions without pain. Progress to 3 sets of 15 repetitions.
- Add weight in 1-pound increments to a maximum of 5 pounds, starting over at 2 sets of 8 to 10 repetitions each time weight is added.
- Perform the exercise 3 days per week, continuing for 2 to 3 weeks.

SECTION 2 SHOULDER

Arthritis of the Shoulder

Synonym

Glenohumeral arthritis

Definition

Arthritis of the shoulder is characterized by destruction of joint cartilage with pain and loss of joint space and function (**Figure 1**). Like arthritis in other joints, glenohumeral arthritis generally affects patients older than 50 years and occurs as a result of many etiologies, including osteoarthritis, rheumatoid arthritis, and posttraumatic arthritis. Less common causes include osteonecrosis, infection, seronegative spondyloarthropathies, and rotator cuff tear arthropathy (a type of arthritis that results from large, long-standing rotator cuff tears) (**Figure 2**).

Clinical Symptoms

Patients report diffuse or deep-seated pain but most often localize the worst pain to the posterior aspect of the shoulder. Initially, the pain is aggravated by any strenuous activity. As the disease progresses, any movement of the shoulder causes pain, and rest and night pain are reported.

ICD-9 Codes

714.0
Rheumatoid arthritis

715.01
Osteoarthrosis, generalized, shoulder region

715.11
Primary osteoarthritis, shoulder

715.21
Secondary osteoarthritis, shoulder (rotator cuff arthropathy)

715.91
Osteoarthrosis, unspecified whether generalized or localized, shoulder region

716.11
Traumatic arthropathy, shoulder

716.81
Other specified arthropathy, shoulder region

716.91
Arthropathy, unspecified, shoulder

SECTION 2 SHOULDER

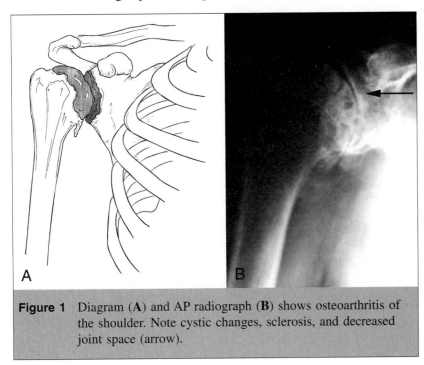

Figure 1 Diagram (**A**) and AP radiograph (**B**) shows osteoarthritis of the shoulder. Note cystic changes, sclerosis, and decreased joint space (arrow).

Figure 2 Radiograph of shoulder with end-stage rotator cuff arthropathy demonstrates superior migration of the humeral head.

Figure 3 Radiograph of shoulder demonstrates superior migration of the humeral head secondary to a chronic rotator cuff tear.

Along with pain, range of motion is progressively limited. Activities of daily living, such as dressing, combing the hair, and reaching overhead, are increasingly difficult.

Osteoarthritis involves a single joint in an older patient, whereas multiple and symmetric joint involvement and a positive rheumatoid factor suggest rheumatoid arthritis. There is no apparent relationship between the development of osteoarthritis in the shoulder and the patient's previous level of physical activity. A history of previous fracture or dislocation, however, suggests posttraumatic arthritis or osteonecrosis. Superior migration of the humeral head (**Figure 3**) develops in association with long-standing rotator cuff tears, which results in eccentric loading of the glenoid and leads to rotator cuff tear arthropathy.

Tests

Physical Examination

Examination may reveal generalized atrophy of the muscles about the shoulder. Swelling within the shoulder joint is not common; when present, it is difficult to detect. Palpation elicits tenderness over the front and back of the shoulder. Bone-on-bone crepitus is commonly present with rotation or flexion of the shoulder. Range of motion is usually decreased. Patients with concomitant rotator cuff tears often have less active than passive range of motion.

Diagnostic Tests

AP and axillary radiographic views of the shoulder are indicated. The axillary view most reliably demonstrates the joint space narrowing that is indicative of cartilage destruction. Other radiographic findings that support a diagnosis of osteoarthritis include flattening of the humeral head, an inferior osteophyte, and posterior erosion of the glenoid. Rheumatoid arthritis is suggested by the presence of periarticular erosions, osteopenia, and central wear of the glenoid. Superior migration of the humeral head suggests a large rotator cuff deficiency.

Differential Diagnosis

- Adhesive capsulitis (normal radiographs)
- Charcot joint (gross destruction of the joint without trauma and relatively little pain)
- Fracture of the humerus (history of trauma, evident on radiographs)
- Herniated cervical disk (unilateral or bilateral radicular pain, positive Spurling test)
- Infection (acute onset, systemic symptoms, elevated WBC)

- Rotator cuff tear (normal radiographs, pain mostly with overhead use)
- Tumor of the shoulder girdle (variable presentation, radiographic lesion)

Adverse Outcomes of the Disease

Chronic shoulder pain and loss of strength and motion can develop. Severe loss of strength and motion can be difficult to recover, even with joint arthroplasty surgery.

Treatment

Nonsurgical treatment is recommended initially, including use of NSAIDs and application of heat and/or ice to relieve symptoms, and gentle stretching exercises to preserve motion. A trial of glucosamine and/or chondroitin sulfate can be considered, but their efficacy has not been definitively established. Activity modifications are beneficial in reducing pain. Corticosteroid injections may provide relief, particularly in some patients with inflammatory (rheumatoid) arthritis. Corticosteroid injections should be limited to 2 to 3 per joint, as cortisone can have a detrimental effect on rotator cuff tendons.

For advanced arthritis, total shoulder replacement or hemiarthroplasty (the choice of which procedure to use remains controversial) offers a very satisfactory solution, even in younger patients (30 to 50 years of age) who do not use their shoulders for strenuous activities. Manual laborers may be better served by glenohumeral arthrodesis because the heavy demands placed on their shoulders often lead to early loosening of the prosthetic components.

Adverse Outcomes of Treatment

Addiction to narcotic pain medication is a possibility, so narcotics should be used only for short-term postoperative pain relief; alternatives should be considered when treating patients with chronic pain secondary to arthritis. NSAIDs may cause gastric, renal, and hepatic complications. Corticosteroid injection has a small risk of causing an infection in the joint that may preclude or compromise later joint arthroplasty. Patients who undergo shoulder replacement surgery may experience perioperative complications, including limb thrombophlebitis and possible embolus.

SECTION 2 SHOULDER

Referral Decisions/Red Flags

Patients with intolerable shoulder pain and/or a progressive loss of motion that does not respond to at least 3 months of nonsurgical treatment require further evaluation. In some cases, surgery may be indicated.

Burners and Other Brachial Plexus Injuries

Synonyms

Brachial plexopathy

Stingers

Definition

Brachial plexus injuries include a broad array of neurologic dysfunction around the shoulder, ranging from momentary paresthesias to flail upper extremity. The mechanism of injury is equally diverse, from high-energy motor vehicle crashes, falls from a height, and gunshot wounds to lower energy injuries such as athletic injuries.

Burners or stingers (transient brachial plexopathy) are transient stretch injuries to the upper trunk of the brachial plexus involving the C5 and C6 nerve roots. The most common mechanism of injury is a traction force that occurs when the shoulder is forcefully depressed and the head and neck are tilted toward the opposite side or by compression of the upper plexus between a shoulder pad and the scapula. These injuries are relatively common among college and professional athletes in contact sports, especially American football.

Brachial plexus injuries involving axonal disruption are further categorized as occurring proximal to the dorsal root ganglion in the spinal foramen (preganglionic) or anywhere distal to the ganglion (postganglionic) (**Figure 1**). This distinction is important because surgical repair is not possible and the prognosis for recovery is poor for preganglionic root avulsions.

Clinical Symptoms

Symptoms of a brachial plexus injury depend on the position of the plexus when it is injured. The mechanism of injury to the upper and middle trunks (C5, C6, and C7, respectively) involves a direct blow to the top of the shoulder accompanied by tilt of the head in the opposite direction, causing traction on the plexus with the arm adducted at the side. Lower trunk injuries (C8, T1) occur when these nerves are stretched with the arm abducted, as when grabbing onto a ledge when falling from a height. Injuries involving the entire plexus result from extreme traction from high-energy trauma.

ICD-9 Codes
353.0 Brachial plexus lesions
723.4 Brachial neuritis or radiculitis NOS
953.4 Injury to nerve roots and spinal plexus, brachial plexus

SECTION 2 SHOULDER

Figure 1 The brachial plexus. (Adapted from Thompson WO, Warren RF, Barnes RP, Hunt S: Shoulder injuries, in Schenck RC Jr, ed: *Athletic Training and Sports Medicine*, ed 3. Rosemont, IL, American Academy of Orthopaedic Surgeons, 1999, pp 219-291.)

A typical presentation is a football player injured by a direct blow to the head, neck, or shoulder. The classic symptom is sharp, burning shoulder pain that radiates down the arm in the affected nerve root distribution. Weakness is common, and the patient often is seen holding the affected arm, which often is hanging at the side. Burners last seconds to minutes, although some lasting several weeks have been reported.

Tests
Physical Examination

A neurologic examination is the cornerstone of an accurate diagnosis. At a minimum, sensation to light touch, motor power, and deep tendon reflexes should be tested. Deficits should be mapped out by nerve root and peripheral nerve distribution. The neurologic examination also includes evaluation of the lower extremities because spasticity or weakness in the ipsilateral leg suggests a concomitant spinal cord injury.

Injuries to C8 and T1 are more likely to be preganglionic, which is confirmed by the presence of an ipsilateral ptosis, myosis, anhydrosis, and enophthalmos (Horner syndrome). Because the dorsal scapular nerve and the long thoracic nerve arise from the C5 and C5 through C7 nerve roots, respectively, intact function of the rhomboids and serratus anterior muscles in upper plexus injuries indicates that the injury is distal to these nerves and hence is postganglionic.

Examination of the neck (with cervical spine precautions if indicated) and shoulder, as well as a general examination, is indicated to rule out associated injuries such as cervical spine fractures or disk herniations; clavicle, scapula, or humerus fractures; and scapulothoracic dissociation.

As with other plexus injuries, the sideline evaluation of a burner should include the cervical spine and a neurologic examination of the extremities. Bilateral upper extremity burners or radicular symptoms into the legs should be treated as a spinal cord injury until proven otherwise.

Diagnostic Tests

Radiographs should be obtained if injury to the cervical spine or shoulder girdle is suspected. Although some controversy still exists, many experts suggest that anyone experiencing a burner or stinger should be evaluated with cervical spine radiographs, including flexion and extension lateral views, to rule out instability, congenital anomaly, or cervical stenosis (assessed by the relative width of the cervical body and the spinal canal). MRI is helpful in patients with abnormal plain radiographs or when symptoms persist.

Differential Diagnosis

- Cervical spine fracture or instability (evident on radiographs)
- Peripheral nerve injury (isolated weakness or sensory deficit confined to a specific nerve distribution)
- Transient quadriplegia (neurapraxia of the cervical spinal cord producing bilateral paresthesias and weakness)

Adverse Outcomes of the Disease

Burners resolve spontaneously, although recurrent episodes may suggest cervical stenosis and an associated increased risk for catastrophic spinal cord injury. Depending on the location and severity of a brachial plexus injury, persistent pain, sensory loss, paresthesias, and weakness, paralysis, or even amputation is possible.

SECTION 2 SHOULDER

Treatment

Resolution of pain and neurologic symptoms, as well as a normal neurologic examination and full range of cervical spine motion, is required before an athlete with a burner is allowed to return to play. Athletes with prolonged or bilateral symptoms or recurrent episodes should not return to play without further evaluation.

Treatment options for more severe brachial plexus injuries vary, including nonsurgical measures and a variety of surgical repair and reconstruction procedures. Nonsurgical management is aimed at strengthening and stretching exercises and splinting to maintain passive range of motion of the joints affected by muscle paralysis or weakness, protection of anesthetic areas of skin, and pain relief. Referral to a pain clinic is often helpful in this regard.

Adverse Outcomes of Treatment

The effectiveness of therapy, splinting, and pain control must be monitored frequently. Although surgical techniques are continuously evolving, the prognosis for severe brachial plexus injuries, especially root avulsions, remains guarded.

Referral Decisions/Red Flags

Any injury that is persistent, recurrent, bilateral, or associated with other concomitant injuries requires further evaluation. Cervical spine precautions should be followed if a cervical injury is suspected.

SECTION 2 SHOULDER

Fracture of the Clavicle

Synonym

Collarbone fracture

Definition

Clavicle fractures are the most common bony injury. The most commonly used classification of clavicle fractures is based on anatomic location (middle third, distal third, proximal third) rather than treatment rationale (**Figure 1**). The most common location of injury is the middle third of the clavicle . Approximately 80% occur in this location, 15% occur in the distal third, and 5% involve the proximal third.

Clinical Symptoms

Patients typically report a history of significant injury, such as falling on the shoulder or being struck over the clavicle with a heavy object. Shoulder motion and strength are limited by pain in the affected extremity. A bony deformity is often seen, as well as shoulder droop.

ICD-9 Codes

810.00
Fracture of clavicle, closed, unspecified part

810.01
Closed fracture of clavicle, sternal end

810.02
Closed fracture of clavicle, shaft

810.03
Closed fracture of clavicle, acromial end

810.11
Open fracture of clavicle, sternal end

810.12
Open fracture of clavicle, shaft

810.13
Open fracture of clavicle, acromial end

SECTION 2 SHOULDER

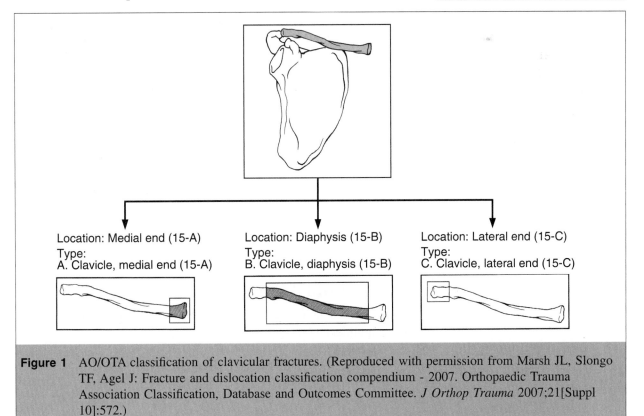

Location: Medial end (15-A)
Type:
A. Clavicle, medial end (15-A)

Location: Diaphysis (15-B)
Type:
B. Clavicle, diaphysis (15-B)

Location: Lateral end (15-C)
Type:
C. Clavicle, lateral end (15-C)

Figure 1 AO/OTA classification of clavicular fractures. (Reproduced with permission from Marsh JL, Slongo TF, Agel J: Fracture and dislocation classification compendium - 2007. Orthopaedic Trauma Association Classification, Database and Outcomes Committee. *J Orthop Trauma* 2007;21[Suppl 10]:572.)

Figure 2 AP view shows a fracture of the middle third of the clavicle.

Tests

Physical Examination

Examination typically reveals an obvious deformity, or bump, at the fracture site. Gentle pressure over the fracture site will elicit pain, and a grinding sensation can be felt when the patient attempts to raise the arm. The skin may appear tented over a fracture fragment, but the fragment rarely penetrates the skin to create an open fracture. Assess neurologic function distal to the fracture, including the axillary, musculocutaneous, median, ulnar, and radial nerves. Check the radial pulse and capillary refill.

Diagnostic Tests

AP and 10° cephalic tilt views of the clavicle will confirm most clavicle fractures (**Figure 2**). Fractures or dislocations at the medial end of the clavicle are uncommon and are often difficult to see on plain radiographs, so if there is a high index of suspicion for a clavicle fracture, CT should be ordered.

Differential Diagnosis

- Acromioclavicular separation (deformity near the tip of the shoulder)
- Sternoclavicular dislocation (deformity at the sternoclavicular junction)

Adverse Outcomes of the Disease

Nonunion is rare, occurring in 1% to 4% of patients. Some degree of malunion is common, and a visible lump can occur, even when the fracture is well approximated. This lump may be of cosmetic concern to some patients but has little functional significance. Neurovascular complications may occur on an early or delayed basis. Rarely, clavicle fractures can result in shoulder deformity.

Treatment

Most midshaft clavicle fractures are treated nonsurgically. Treatment with a figure-of-8 strap should be followed closely for possible neurovascular compression or skin breakdown from strap compression overlying the fracture site. Support for 3 to 4 weeks is adequate for a child younger than 12 years, whereas 6 to 8 weeks may be required for an adult. After 2 to 3 weeks, the patient is encouraged to begin gentle shoulder exercises as pain allows. Surgical treatment should be considered for severely shortened middle third fractures, open fractures, or fractures associated with neurovascular injury or severe injury to the ipsilateral chest, such as rib fractures or flail chest. Fractures with scapulothoracic dissociation or floating shoulder (ipsilateral clavicle and scapular fracture) also should be considered for surgical intervention. Fractures of the distal third of the clavicle just medial to the coracoclavicular ligaments in which the medial part of the clavicle is significantly superiorly displaced are associated with a higher rate of nonunion because the proximal fragments buttonhole through the fascia.

Adverse Outcomes of Treatment

Pressure over the nerves and vessels in the armpit from a tight clavicle strap may cause numbness and paresthesias in the arm, which are usually transient but may persist. Surgical treatment of clavicle fractures is associated with a high complication rate. The particular complication depends on the type of surgery but could include infection, neurovascular injury, hardware complication, or skin breakdown.

Referral Decisions/Red Flags

Painful nonunion after 4 months of treatment requires further evaluation. Patients with widely displaced lateral or midshaft clavicle fractures or with segmental fractures have a greater risk of nonunion and should be evaluated for possible surgical treatment.

SECTION 2 SHOULDER

Fracture of the Humeral Shaft

ICD-9 Codes

812.21
Fracture of shaft of humerus, closed

812.31
Fracture of shaft of humerus, open

Definition

Fractures of the humeral shaft often result from a direct blow to the arm, such as occurs in a motor vehicle accident, or from a fall on the outstretched hand (**Figure 1**). These fractures also can result from sports activities involving a fall or a direct blow. Most of these fractures can be treated nonsurgically, with a rate of union of nearly 100%.

Clinical Symptoms

Severe pain, swelling, and deformity are characteristic of a displaced fracture of the humerus. With gentle palpation and movement of the arm, it is often possible to detect motion at the fracture site. Radial nerve injuries are associated with this fracture. If the radial nerve has been injured, patients are unable to extend the wrist or fingers and may have loss of sensation over the back of the hand. Rarely, the nerve becomes trapped within the fracture (**Figure 2**).

Figure 1 Midshaft humeral fracture.

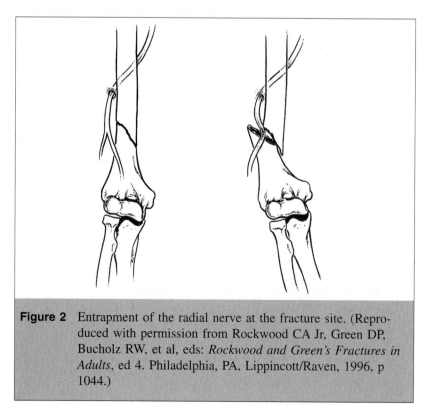

Figure 2 Entrapment of the radial nerve at the fracture site. (Reproduced with permission from Rockwood CA Jr, Green DP, Bucholz RW, et al, eds: *Rockwood and Green's Fractures in Adults*, ed 4. Philadelphia, PA, Lippincott/Raven, 1996, p 1044.)

Referra

Patients
fracture:
associat
soon as

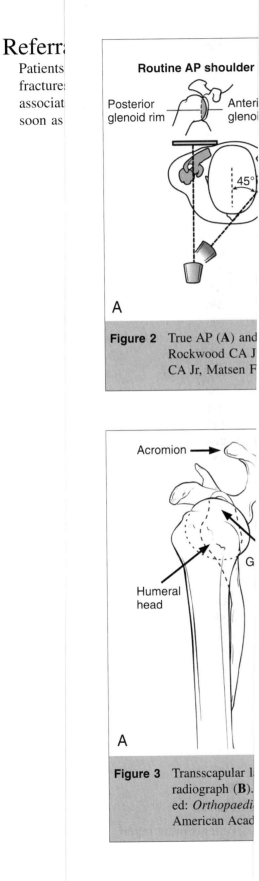

Routine AP shoulder

Posterior
glenoid rim

Anteri
gleno

45°

A

Figure 2 True AP (**A**) and
Rockwood CA J
CA Jr, Matsen F

Acromion

G

Humeral
head

A

Figure 3 Transscapular l
radiograph (**B**).
ed: *Orthopaedi*
American Acad

Tests

Physical Examination

Examination reveals marked swelling and contusion. Look for puncture wounds in the skin near the fracture site, as these indicate an open fracture. Assess neurologic function distal to the fracture, including the median, radial, and ulnar nerves. Check the radial pulse and record the color and temperature of the hand. The shoulder and elbow should be evaluated for pain, tenderness, and swelling or deformity because concomitant injury proximal or distal to the shaft fracture can be easily missed in the acute setting.

Diagnostic Tests

AP and lateral radiographs confirm the diagnosis. These views also should include both the shoulder and elbow joints.

Differential Diagnosis

- Fracture of the distal humerus (evident on radiographs)
- Fracture of the proximal humerus (evident on AP and lateral radiographs)
- Ruptured biceps tendon (swelling localized to biceps muscle)

Adverse Outcomes of the Disease

Radial nerve injury, indicated by weakness in the wrist or finger or thumb extensors and numbness in the first dorsal web space, is possible. Injury to the brachial plexus or vascular system also may occur. Healing of the fracture with angulation is common but results in little functional impairment unless the angulation is severe. Nonunion is possible but uncommon. Persistent stiffness in the shoulder and elbow may be a problem.

Treatment

Most humeral shaft fractures are treated nonsurgically, with up to 20° of apex anterior or apex lateral angulation being acceptable. Fractures with minimal shortening (2 cm or less) can be treated with a U-shaped coaptation splint for 2 weeks (**Figure 3**), followed by a humeral fracture brace (**Figure 4**). A coaptation splint is applied as follows: place 12 thicknesses of plaster or a commercially available prepackaged splint in a U-shaped fashion. Begin at the axilla, being careful that the medial end of the splinting material is not at the level of the fracture, and continue around the elbow, extending to the top of the shoulder. Splint material is held in place with an elastic bandage. A collar and cuff made from stockinette can be used to support the forearm and wrist. Alternatively, a simple sling can

Figure 3 Coaptation splint.

Figure 4 Humeral fracture brace.

SECTION 2 SHOULDER

Fracture of the Scapula

SECTION 2 SHOULDER

SECTION 2 SHOULDER

SECTION 2 SHOULDER

ICD-9 Codes

811.00
Fracture of scapula,
unspecified part, closed

811.01
Fracture of scapula, acromial
process, closed

811.02
Fracture of scapula, coracoid
process, closed

811.03
Fracture of scapula, glenoid
cavity and neck of scapula,
closed

811.09
Fracture of scapula, other,
closed

811.10
Fracture of scapula,
unspecified part, open

811.11
Fracture of scapula, acromial
process, open

811.12
Fracture of scapula, coracoid
process, open

811.13
Fracture of scapula, glenoid
cavity and neck of scapula,
open

811.19
Fracture of scapula, other,
open

Synonyms

Fracture of the acromion
Fracture of the coracoid process
Fracture of the shoulder blade
Glenoid fracture

Definition

Scapular fractures result from high-energy trauma such as
motorcycle accidents or falls from a significant height. These
fractures may involve the body of the scapula, the glenoid, the
acromion, or the coracoid process (**Figure 1**). Ninety percent of
patients with scapular fractures have associated injuries,
including rib fractures, which are the most common;
pneumothorax; pulmonary contusion; and head, spinal cord, and
brachial plexus injuries. Because of these associated injuries,
scapular fractures are often missed on initial examination.

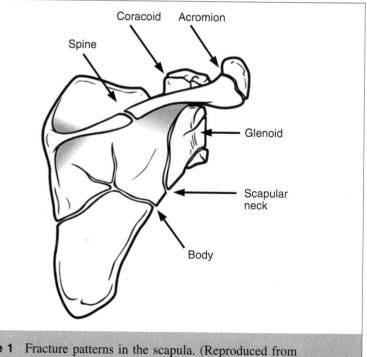

Figure 1   Fracture patterns in the scapula. (Reproduced from
Zuckerman JD, Koval KJ, Cuomo F: Fractures of the
scapula. *Instr Course Lect* 1993;42:271-281.)

Figure 2 Oblique view of the shoulder demonstrates a fracture of the body of the scapula (black arrow).

Clinical Symptoms

Pain and tenderness about the back of the shoulder are the most common symptoms. The patient typically holds the arm securely at the side, and any attempts to actively move the extremity result in pain.

Tests

Physical Examination

Skin abrasions, swelling, and ecchymosis over the back of the shoulder are common. Tenderness to gentle palpation over the back of the shoulder or acromion suggests a possible scapular fracture.

Diagnostic Tests

Radiographic visualization of scapular fractures can be difficult. An AP view of the shoulder and a chest radiograph should be obtained. If the patient is cleared to sit upright, a transscapular lateral or oblique radiograph can be helpful in the diagnosis of a displaced scapular body fracture (**Figure 2**). The axillary view is more useful in revealing acromial and coracoid fractures. Poorly visualized fractures and any fracture involving the glenoid should be further evaluated with CT.

Differential Diagnosis

- Acromioclavicular (AC) separation (maximum tenderness over the AC joint)

SECTION 2 SHOULDER

- Fracture of the proximal humerus (radiograph needed to confirm diagnosis)
- Fracture of the rib (evident on plain radiographs of the chest)
- Os acromiale (nontender, no history of trauma, incidental finding on radiographs)
- Shoulder dislocation (deformity of the anterior and lateral shoulder, evident on radiographs)

Adverse Outcomes of the Disease

Persistent loss of motion and chronic pain are possible. Malunion is common but usually asymptomatic. Complications such as suprascapular nerve injury or impingement syndrome are rare.

Treatment

Nonsurgical treatment using a sling is adequate for most patients, followed by early range of motion as tolerated, usually within 1 week of injury. Patients with scapular body fractures should be considered for hospital admission because of the risk of pulmonary contusion.

Adverse Outcomes of Treatment

Prolonged immobilization may result in shoulder stiffness.

Referral Decisions/Red Flags

Patients with displaced (>2 mm) fractures of the glenoid articular surface, fractures of the neck of the scapula with severe angular deformity (>30°), and fractures of the acromion process with impingement syndrome require further evaluation.

Frozen Shoulder

Synonyms

Adhesive capsulitis

Stiff shoulder

ICD-9 Codes

719.51
Stiffness of joint, not elsewhere classified, shoulder region

726.0
Adhesive capsulitis of shoulder

Definition

Adhesive capsulitis of the shoulder, commonly called frozen shoulder, is defined as an idiopathic loss of both active and passive motion. It is considered distinct from posttraumatic shoulder stiffness, a condition that is related to a significant shoulder injury or a surgical procedure.

Frozen shoulder most commonly affects patients between the ages of 40 and 60 years, with no clear predisposition based on arm dominance or occupation. It occurs more frequently in women. Diabetes mellitus, especially type 1, is the most common risk factor. Patients with diabetes tend to be more refractory to treatment, and 40% to 50% will have bilateral involvement. Other conditions related to frozen shoulder include hypothyroidism, Dupuytren disease, cervical disk herniation, Parkinson disease, cerebral hemorrhage, and tumors.

Clinical Symptoms

Patients typically progress from an early "freezing" phase of pain and progressive loss of motion to a "thawing" phase of decreasing discomfort associated with a slow but steady improvement in range of motion. The process typically takes 6 months to 2 years or more to resolve, with most patients experiencing minimal long-term pain or functional deficit, although some motion loss may remain.

Tests

Physical Examination

Examination reveals significant (at least 50%) reduction in both active and passive range of motion compared with the opposite, normal shoulder. Loss of external rotation with the arm at the side is consistent with the condition, as contracture of the coracohumeral ligament, which limits external rotation, is pathognomonic for frozen shoulder. Motion is painful, especially at the extremes. Pain and tenderness at the deltoid insertion are common. Diffuse tenderness about the shoulder also may be present.

SECTION 2 SHOULDER

Figure 1 MRI reveals the contracted capsule, which is the hallmark of a frozen shoulder, and the loss of the inferior pouch (arrow).

Diagnostic Tests

AP and axillary radiographs of the shoulder are indicated to ensure that smooth, concentric joint surfaces with an intact cartilage space are present and to rule out other pathology such as osteophytes, loose bodies, calcium deposits, or tumors. Other ancillary studies, such as arthrography or MR arthrograms, can substantiate a frozen shoulder diagnosis by demonstrating a contracted capsule and loss of the inferior pouch (**Figure 1**).

Differential Diagnosis

- Chronic posterior shoulder dislocation (evident on axillary radiographs)
- Impingement syndrome (motion preserved and pain primarily with elevation)
- Osteoarthritis (evident on radiographs)
- Posttraumatic shoulder stiffness (history of clear and significant previous trauma)
- Rotator cuff tear (normal passive range of motion)
- Tumor (rare, but evident on shoulder or ipsilateral chest radiograph)

Adverse Outcomes of the Disease

Residual pain and/or stiffness may persist for years in some patients.

Treatment

NSAIDs, nonnarcotic analgesics, and moist heat are indicated, followed by a gentle stretching program. Often ice is used after stretching to control swelling. Intra-articular injection of corticosteroid also should be considered, but multiple injections should be avoided. The injection should be performed under fluoroscopic or ultrasonographic guidance to ensure the injection is intra-articular. A transcutaneous electrical nerve stimulation (TENS) unit (applied by a physical therapist) may help control pain. The patient should be instructed in a home stretching program that is to be performed within a comfortable range. Advise patients that, on average, a recovery period of 1 to 2 years is to be expected before motion is fully restored and pain is completely relieved. Nonsurgical treatment is successful approximately 80% to 85% of the time. Surgical treatment consists of arthroscopic capsular release.

Rehabilitation Prescription

The functional goal of rehabilitation for a patient with a frozen shoulder is to reduce pain and increase mobility of the glenohumeral joint and scapula. External rotation in the adducted position tends to be the most restricted range of motion associated with frozen shoulder. Pain in the subscapularis area, localized to the scapular fossa, also is very common.

The home exercise program should include stretching into external rotation with the arm at no more than 30° to 45° of abduction (see page 294). A low-load prolonged shoulder stretching device may be ordered for home use to promote passive external rotation. Forced elevation should be avoided. Strengthening exercises are initiated after the inflammation and painful period of frozen shoulder has subsided and should include strengthening of the glenohumeral joint and scapula rotators.

The formal rehabilitation prescription should include evaluation of the mobility of the glenohumeral joint and scapula mobility and posture. Aggressive mobilization is very effective in increasing the range of motion.

Adverse Outcomes of Treatment

Therapy that is too aggressive may aggravate symptoms and/or cause a fracture of the humerus.

Referral Decisions/Red Flags

If significant improvement in pain and motion is not seen after 3 months of consistent rehabilitation, further evaluation is indicated. Indications for surgery include failure of nonsurgical treatment and patient intolerance to continued symptoms. Multiple cortisone injections should be avoided.

SECTION 2 SHOULDER

Home Exercise Program for Frozen Shoulder

- Perform the exercises in the order listed.
- Apply moist or dry heat to the shoulder for 5 or 10 minutes before the exercises and during the external rotation passive stretch.
- If you experience pain during or after the exercises, discontinue the exercises and call your doctor.

Exercise Type	Muscle Group	Number of Repetitions/Sets	Number of Days per Week	Number of Weeks
External rotation passive stretch	Anterior capsule	4 repetitions/3 sets	Daily	3 to 4
Supine forward flexion	Inferior capsule	4 repetitions/3 sets	Daily	3 to 4

External Rotation Passive Stretch

- Stand in a doorway, facing the doorjamb.
- With the affected arm held next to your side and the elbow bent 90°, grasp the edge of the doorjamb.
- Keep the hand in place and rotate your upper body as shown in the illustration.
- Hold the stretch for 30 seconds; then return to the starting position for 30 seconds.
- Perform 3 sets of 4 repetitions daily, continuing for 3 to 4 weeks.

Start   Finish

Supine Forward Flexion

- Lie on your back with your legs straight.
- With the unaffected arm, grasp the affected arm at the elbow and lift the affected arm overhead until you feel a gentle stretch.
- Hold the stretch for 15 seconds and slowly lower to starting position.
- Perform 3 sets of 4 repetitions daily, continuing for 3 to 4 weeks.

Impingement Syndrome

Synonyms

Rotator cuff tendinitis

Shoulder bursitis

ICD-9 Codes

726.10
Rotator cuff syndrome NOS

726.11
Calcifying tendinitis of shoulder

Definition

Four muscles—the infraspinatus, supraspinatus, subscapularis, and teres minor—come together to form the rotator cuff, which covers the anterior, superior, and posterior aspects of the humeral head. As these muscles assist in elevation of the arm, the rotator cuff, primarily the supraspinatus tendon, is pulled repetitively under the coracoacromial arch. The coracoacromial arch includes the coracoid process, the coracoacromial ligament, the acromion, and the acromioclavicular joint capsule (**Figure 1**).

Inflammation of the subacromial bursa and underlying rotator cuff tendons is a common cause of shoulder pain in middle-aged patients. Rotator cuff pathology spans a continuum from edema

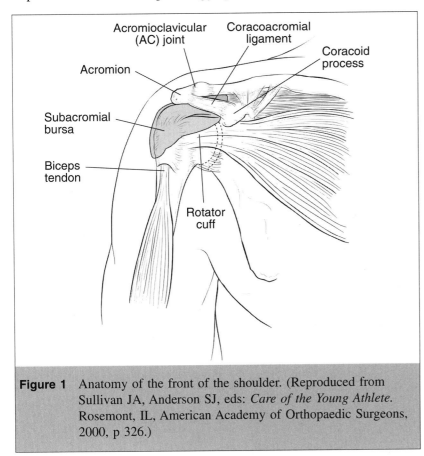

Figure 1 Anatomy of the front of the shoulder. (Reproduced from Sullivan JA, Anderson SJ, eds: *Care of the Young Athlete.* Rosemont, IL, American Academy of Orthopaedic Surgeons, 2000, p 326.)

SECTION 2 SHOULDER

Figure 2 Testing the strength of the supraspinatus.

Figure 3 Visible muscle atrophy (arrows) indicative of a rotator cuff tear.

and hemorrhage to chronic inflammation and fibrosis to microscopic tendon fiber failure progressing to full-thickness rotator cuff tears. The etiology is likely a combination of factors, including loss of microvascular blood supply to the tendon and repeated mechanical insult as the tendon passes under the coracoacromial arch.

Clinical Symptoms

Gradual onset of anterior and lateral shoulder pain exacerbated by overhead activity is characteristic. Night pain and difficulty sleeping on the affected side also are common. Atrophy of the muscles about the top and back of the shoulder may be apparent if the patient has had symptoms for several months.

Tests

Physical Examination

Palpation over the greater tuberosity and subacromial bursa commonly elicits tenderness and crepitus with shoulder motion. Pain is worse between 90° and 120° of abduction and when lowering the arm. Patients with impingement generally have positive Neer and Hawkins signs (see page 261). After these examinations are completed, a diagnostic injection can be done as follows: 10 mL of 1% plain local anesthetic is injected into the subacromial space (see page 301), followed by reexamination. Complete pain relief supports a diagnosis of impingement syndrome.

To evaluate weakness of the supraspinatus tendon, position the arm in 90° of elevation and internal rotation (thumb turned down). Ask the patient to resist while you push the arm down (**Figure 2**). Compare the result with that of the opposite shoulder. If the shoulder initially demonstrates weakness but is strong following subacromial injection, pain inhibition from inflammation and fibrosis rather than a full-thickness rotator cuff tear is the likely cause of the weakness. Muscle atrophy about the top and back of the shoulder usually indicates a rotator cuff tear (**Figure 3**).

Diagnostic Tests

AP and axillary radiographs of the shoulder are usually normal. Narrowing of the space between the head of the humerus and the undersurface of the acromion (normally >7 mm) suggests a long-standing rotator cuff tear.

Differential Diagnosis

- Acromioclavicular (AC) arthritis (tenderness over the AC joint)
- Frozen shoulder (active and passive motion loss)
- Glenohumeral arthritis (pain with any motion, evident on radiographs)
- Herniated cervical disk (associated neck stiffness, deltoid weakness with absent biceps reflex, possible sensory loss)
- Rotator cuff tear (weakness of the supraspinatus that does not improve following subacromial injection of local anesthetic)
- Suprascapular nerve entrapment (atrophy of the supraspinatus and infraspinatus muscles, negative impingement sign)

Adverse Outcomes of the Disease

Pain may be persistent or recurrent. Rotator cuff tendinitis may progress to a full-thickness tear.

Treatment

NSAIDs and rest from the offending activity may relieve an acute exacerbation of pain. The patient should begin a stretching program (see page 250) with emphasis on posterior capsule stretching. If a home exercise program performed three to four times per day for 6 weeks does not result in any improvement, a subacromial corticosteroid injection can be considered, followed by continued stretching. Steroid injections should not be repeated if the previous injection did not produce significant and sustained (4 to 6 weeks) relief. Rotator cuff weakness with impingement is often the result of subacromial bursitis, rotator cuff tendinitis, or even calcific tendinitis.

A rotator cuff strengthening program should be added to the stretching program once the shoulder is supple and pain is improved. Avoidance of repetitive overhead activities also is recommended.

Rehabilitation Prescription

The functional goal of rehabilitation for a patient with shoulder impingement should be to perform overhead activities without pain. Patients with shoulder impingement typically have a restricted glenohumeral joint capsule and weakness of the glenohumeral and scapulothoracic rotators.

A home exercise program may be initiated that includes stretching and very basic strengthening exercises (see page 299). The home program should not cause more pain, although patients may report muscle soreness and a stretching sensation that may be considered uncomfortable. Ice may be used after exercise to prevent inflammation.

Formal rehabilitation should be started within 3 to 4 weeks if the home exercise program has not increased the ability of the patient to perform overhead activities of daily living without pain. The prescription should include an evaluation of the strength of the glenohumeral and scapulothoracic rotator muscles as well as an appropriate strengthening program. In addition, mobilization of the glenohumeral and scapulothoracic joints may be very effective.

Adverse Outcomes of Treatment

NSAIDs may cause gastric, renal, or hepatic complications. Tearing of the rotator cuff and rupture of the long head of the biceps tendon may occur after repeated corticosteroid injections. The latter is more likely with more than three injections.

Referral Decisions/Red Flags

Significant weakness of the rotator cuff or failure of 2 to 3 months of rehabilitation (with or without subacromial steroid injection) is an indication for further evaluation and surgical consideration.

SECTION 2 SHOULDER

Home Exercise Program for Shoulder Impingement

- Perform the exercises in the order listed.
- Apply a bag of crushed ice or frozen peas to the shoulder for 20 minutes after performing the exercises to prevent inflammation.
- These exercises should not increase the pain in your shoulder, although you may experience muscle soreness and a stretching sensation. Call your doctor if you experience increased pain or if you do not see improvement in your ability to perform overhead activities without pain after performing the exercises for 3 or 4 weeks.

Exercise Type	Muscle Group	Number of Repetitions/Sets	Number of Days per Week	Number of Weeks
Sleeper stretch	Posterior rotator cuff Posterior inferior capsule/ glenohumeral ligament	4 repetitions/3 to 4 sets	Daily	3 to 4
External rotation	Infraspinatus Teres minor	8 repetitions/2 sets, progressing to 15 repetitions/3 sets	3 to 4	6 to 8
Internal rotation	Subscapularis Teres major	8 repetitions/2 sets, progressing to 15 repetitions/3 sets	3 to 4	6 to 8

Sleeper Stretch

- Lie on your side on a firm, flat surface with the affected shoulder under you and the arm positioned as shown, keeping your back perpendicular to the surface.
- With the unaffected arm, push the other wrist down, toward the surface. Stop when you feel a stretching sensation in the back of the affected shoulder.
- Hold this position for 30 seconds, then relax the arm for 30 seconds.
- Perform 3 or 4 sets of 4 repetitions daily, continuing for 3 to 4 weeks.

Sleeper position

Start

Finish

SECTION 2 SHOULDER

External Rotation

- Lie on your side on a firm, flat surface with the unaffected arm under you, cradling your head.

- Hold the affected arm against your side as shown, with the elbow bent at a 90° angle.

- Slowly rotate the arm at the shoulder, keeping the elbow bent and against your side, to raise the weight to a vertical position, and then slowly lower the weight to the starting position to a count of 5.

- Begin with approximately 1- to 2-pound weights that allow 2 sets of 8 repetitions, progressing to 3 sets of 15 repetitions.

- Add weight in 1-pound increments, starting over at each new weight level with 2 sets of 8 repetitions up to a maximum of 3 to 6 pounds, depending on your size and fitness level.

- Perform the exercise 3 or 4 days per week, continuing for 6 to 8 weeks.

Internal Rotation

- Lie on your side on a firm, flat surface with the affected arm under you and with a pillow or folded cloth under your head to keep your spine straight.

- Hold the affected arm against your side as shown, with the elbow bent at a 90° angle.

- Slowly rotate the arm at the shoulder, keeping the elbow bent and against your torso, to raise the weight to a vertical position, and then slowly lower the weight to the starting position.

- Begin with weights that allow 2 sets of 8 repetitions, progressing to 3 sets of 15 repetitions.

- Add weight in 1-pound increments, starting over at each new weight level with 2 sets of 8 repetitions up to a maximum of 3 to 6 pounds, depending on your size and fitness level.

- Perform the exercise 3 or 4 days per week, continuing for 6 to 8 weeks.

Procedure: Subacromial Bursa Injection

Note: Although this injection can be made from the anterior or anterolateral aspect of the shoulder, the easiest way to access the subacromial space is from the posterior aspect. The posterolateral corner of the acromion is easily palpated in most patients and serves as a reliable anatomic landmark. Also, opinions differ regarding single- versus two-needle injection techniques. Proponents of the single-needle technique believe that one needle is less painful for the patient than two. Physicians who prefer the two-needle technique point out that the smaller gauge needle is easier for patients to tolerate and that the pain of the second injection is dulled by the anesthetic. A two-syringe, two-needle technique is described on the DVD.

Step 1
Wear protective gloves during this procedure and use sterile technique.

Step 2
Seat the patient with the arm hanging down with hand in lap to distract the subacromial space. The injection site can be anterior, anterolateral, or straight posterior into the subacromial space.

Step 3
Palpate the acromion both posteriorly and laterally until the posterolateral corner is located.

Materials

- Sterile gloves
- Bactericidal skin preparation solution
- 1% lidocaine solution without epinephrine
- 2 mL of betamethasone 40 mg/mL or similar steroid
- 10-mL syringe with a 22-gauge, 1¼" needle
- 3-mL syringe with a 25-gauge, ¾" needle
- Adhesive bandage

SECTION 2 SHOULDER

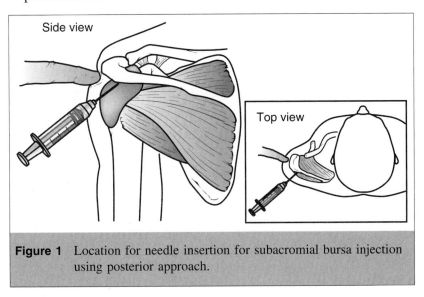

Side view

Top view

Figure 1 Location for needle insertion for subacromial bursa injection using posterior approach.

Step 4
Cleanse this area with a bactericidal solution.

Step 5
With an index finger on the lateral acromion, insert the 25-gauge needle about 1 cm below the palpating finger and raise a wheal with the local anesthetic.

Step 6
Insert the syringe with the 22-gauge needle. The site of posterior injection is 1 cm medial and inferior to the posterolateral corner of the acromion (**Figure 1**). Angle the needle superiorly approximately 20° to 30° to access the subacromial space. Inject 8 to 10 mL of the 1% lidocaine solution. If resistance is encountered while attempting to inject the solution, partially withdraw the needle and reinsert. If the needle is in the proper place, there is little resistance to injection. If you feel the needle hit bone, redirect it superiorly if the bony obstruction is thought to be the humerus, or inferiorly if the bone is thought to be the acromion.

Step 7
Detach the syringe from the needle hub, leaving the needle in the correct location. Attach the second syringe with 2 mL of corticosteroid preparation and inject it into the subacromial space. The syringe can again be exchanged and local anesthetic injected as the needle is withdrawn to avoid steroid deposition subcutaneously. This reduces the risk of fat atrophy or depigmentation in dark-skinned patients.

Step 8
Dress the puncture site with a sterile adhesive bandage.

Adverse Outcomes
A temporary increase in pain is possible, and, although rare, infection can occur. Subcutaneous atrophy and depigmentation also may occur.

Aftercare/Patient Instructions
One third of patients will experience a temporary increase in pain for 24 to 48 hours after the corticosteroid injection. Advise the patient to apply ice bags to the shoulder and take an NSAID or acetaminophen if increased pain occurs the night following the injection. Instruct the patient to resume usual activities as soon as tolerated, but no later than 24 to 48 hours after the injection.

Overhead Throwing Shoulder Injuries

Synonyms

Rotator cuff tendinitis (syndrome)

Definition

The unique anatomy of the glenohumeral joint provides multiple and extreme degrees of functional motion. All overhead athletic motions (eg, throwing a baseball) require the repeated systematic and sequential delivery of kinetic energy to the four rotator cuff muscle/tendon units (infraspinatus, supraspinatus, subscapularis, teres minor) (**Figure 1**). The primary function of these relatively small muscle/tendon units (the rotator cuff) is to precisely seat and center the humeral head in the shallow fossa of the glenoid (**Figure 2**). This working relationship between the rotator cuff and the humeral head must be operational for the larger power muscles such as the deltoid and pectoralis to

ICD-9 Codes
353.0   Thoracic outlet syndrome
718.81   Anterior instability
723.4   Suprascapular nerve entrapment
726.1   Biceps tendinitis   Rotator cuff tendinitis (syndrome)   Internal impingement
726.19   External impingement (subacromial bursitis)

Continued on next page

SECTION 2 SHOULDER

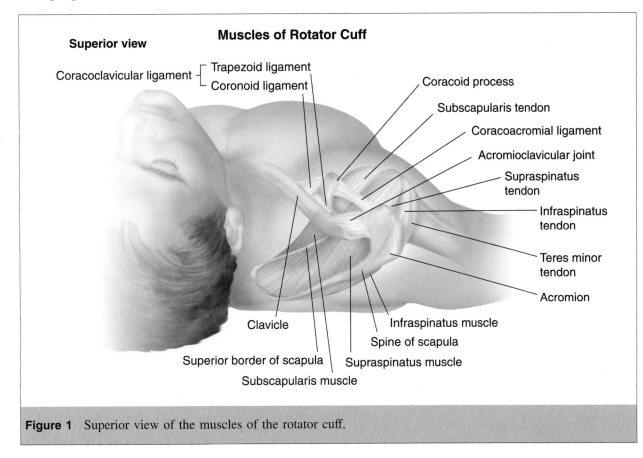

Muscles of Rotator Cuff

Superior view

Coracoclavicular ligament — Trapezoid ligament / Coronoid ligament

Coracoid process

Subscapularis tendon

Coracoacromial ligament

Acromioclavicular joint

Supraspinatus tendon

Infraspinatus tendon

Teres minor tendon

Acromion

Infraspinatus muscle

Spine of scapula

Supraspinatus muscle

Subscapularis muscle

Superior border of scapula

Clavicle

Figure 1 Superior view of the muscles of the rotator cuff.

Figure 2 Lateral view of the glenohumeral (shoulder) joint, opened.

727.61
Rotator cuff tear, nontraumatic

840.4
Rotator cuff sprain

840.7
SLAP lesion

953.4
Brachial plexus compression

955.0
Axillary nerve involvement

function effectively, resulting in the desired fluid shoulder motion. When the relationship between the rotator cuff and the humeral head malfunctions, the humeral head translocates forcefully, causing damage to surrounding structures.

Repetitive overhead throwing produces very significant dynamic stress forces on the rotator cuff–glenohumeral complex. Of the five primary phases of the optimal overhead throwing motion (**Figure 3**), late cocking, early acceleration, and follow-through are the most violent and are chiefly responsible for the inflammatory tissue response. Compression forces are experienced where the humeral head contacts the glenoid and soft tissues. Tensile forces tend to stretch, irritate, and cause plastic deformation of ligaments, tendons, and capsular tissues. As a result, with repetitive throwing, excessive wear (abuse), subacute stress accumulation (overuse), and obsessive sport participation (wearout) will invariably damage the rotator cuff–glenohumeral complex. This damage leads to malfunctioning of the rotator cuff–humeral head relationship so that the humeral head is no longer firmly seated. Given the complex anatomy and mechanism of the shoulder, combining all thrower's shoulder symptoms under rotator cuff tendinitis fails to appreciate the broad spectrum of rotator cuff–glenohumeral pathology. A clearer understanding of the mechanism, treatment,

SECTION 2 SHOULDER

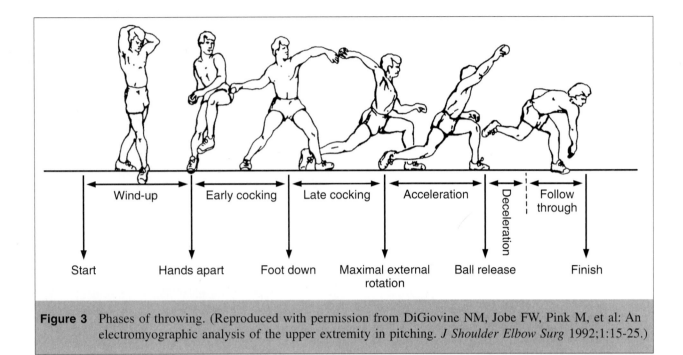

Wind-up | Early cocking | Late cocking | Acceleration | Deceleration | Follow through

Start | Hands apart | Foot down | Maximal external rotation | Ball release | Finish

Figure 3 Phases of throwing. (Reproduced with permission from DiGiovine NM, Jobe FW, Pink M, et al: An electromyographic analysis of the upper extremity in pitching. *J Shoulder Elbow Surg* 1992;1:15-25.)

and prevention of these debilitating injuries is important to guide treatment.

Rotator cuff tendinitis results from a variety of mechanisms in the thrower's shoulder. One mechanism is termed internal impingement. This develops initially as a result of the throwing arm being abducted and placed in extreme external rotation. As a consequence, the suprapinatus and infraspinatus muscles and their tendons are compressed between the posterosuperior glenoid rim, the posterior humeral head, and the greater tuberosity (**Figure 4**). External impingement occurs with excessive superior translation of the humeral head in the glenoid fossa. Such translation decreases the space available in the subacromial area, resulting in impingement of the structures that occupy this space, most notably the subacromial bursa and the tendons of the rotator cuff.

In throwers, repetitive hyperextension together with internal impingement (abnormal positioning of the humeral head) causes fraying of the deep layers of the infraspinatus, ultimately leading to a partial-thickness tear. A similar situation is seen on the articular surface of the supraspinatus. With continued throwing, partial-thickness tears may proceed to full-thickness tears, but full-thickness tearing is usually the result of a nonthrowing injury.

If the athlete with a dysfunctional rotator cuff–glenohumeral complex continues to pitch without resting the shoulder, the relatively unrestrained humeral head will translate (migrate) and abut the glenoid labrum, and compression and shear forces will cause roughening, fraying, and tearing of the fibrocartilaginous

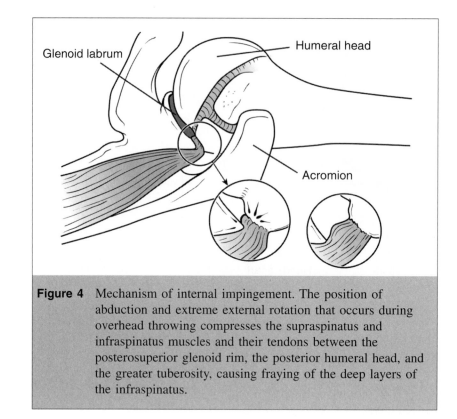

Figure 4 Mechanism of internal impingement. The position of abduction and extreme external rotation that occurs during overhead throwing compresses the supraspinatus and infraspinatus muscles and their tendons between the posterosuperior glenoid rim, the posterior humeral head, and the greater tuberosity, causing fraying of the deep layers of the infraspinatus.

labrum. More significant forces may result in superior labrum anterior-to-posterior (SLAP) detachment with or without the biceps tendon remaining intact. The exact etiology is controversial, but some authors believe SLAP lesions develop from traction of the biceps. Others believe that the extreme external rotation that occurs during overhead throwing causes the lesion (ie, the labrum is "peeled back" by the rotating humeral head). Loss of the anchoring function of the biceps results in increased stress on the inferior glenohumeral ligament. The anterior band of the inferior glenohumeral ligament and the anterior capsule serve as static restraints to anterior translation of the humeral head. When the static restraints become dysfunctional and the dynamic muscle restraints are insufficient, anterior instability results.

Biceps tendinitis may present in the throwing athlete as anterior shoulder pain that increases with activity. Palpation of the biceps tendon in its groove on the front of the humerus typically reproduces the patient's discomfort.

Brachial plexus compression, thoracic outlet syndrome, and axillary nerve involvement should be considered when a thrower has atypical shoulder symptoms.

In a patient with significant atrophy of the infraspinatus muscle, consider the possibility of suprascapular nerve entrapment. Electromyographic and nerve conduction velocity studies are diagnostic.

Clinical Symptoms

Stage I—"Sore Shoulder" Syndrome

Initially, the athlete reports aching and soreness deep in the anterior shoulder when throwing certain pitches (usually sliders and curveballs) or after pitching a few innings. The athlete also reports a decrease in pitch velocity and accuracy and difficulties with activities of daily living. The situation improves with rest, and the athlete is able to continue to pitch.

Stage II—Profound Pathologic Pain

In this stage, the aching and soreness of stage I has gradually progressed to pain, predominantly located in the posterior shoulder, that prevents full abduction and external rotation (the throwing motion). A period of rest is no longer effective. Sleeping on the affected shoulder produces night pain, and pain medication is requested.

Tests

Physical Examination

Inspect the fully exposed trunk for muscle asymmetry, atrophy, and obvious deformity. Examine the skin for abrasion, rashes, and boils, and especially note ecchymosis or swelling. Dominant arm hypertrophy may be evident.

Palpate the shoulder area systematically, searching for tenderness in the scapular support muscles as well as the supraspinatus and infraspinatus area, posterior capsule, quadrilateral space, and posterior deltoid. Anteriorly, palpate the muscles about the humeral head, the rotator cuff attachment to the greater and lesser tuberosity, the bicipital groove, and the deltoid and pectoralis muscles. Note any tenderness of the acromioclavicular and sternoclavicular joints, clavicle, and adjacent neck structures. Similarly palpate the upper arm, elbow, forearm, wrist, and hand.

Evaluate full range of passive motion of the shoulder in forward flexion, abduction, external rotation with the arm at the side, and internal rotation (hitchhiking thumb up the back). (For these and other tests, see pages 256-262). Repeat the examination while providing active resistance, and compare the results with the opposite extremity. Active resistance to full range of motion should also be evaluated in the biceps, triceps, forearm muscles, and intrinsic muscles of the hand.

Generalized musculoskeletal laxity is indicated by the ability to actively hyperextend the elbows, wrist, and fingers. Inferior shoulder laxity is exhibited as the sulcus, or sag, sign. Perform the lift-off test bilaterally to compare subscapularis strength. With the patient supine and with the elbow flexed 90°, measure external rotation at 30°, 90°, and at full overhead, also comparing with the opposite extremity. Also perform the cross-chest maneuver. To evaluate anterior instability, the shoulder is abducted to about 150°, and pressure is applied anteriorly and then posteriorly to the humeral head to estimate the amount of translation and firmness of resistance.

Pain that limits motion, especially in forward flexion, is an indication of impingement. If application of anterior pressure to the humeral head relieves the pain, internal impingement may be suspected.

With the patient in the prone position, scapular protraction, tilt, and retraction are assessed. Winging may be tested by having the patient perform a standing push-up against the wall. Alternatively, have the patient perform a seated press. For the seated press, the patient, who is seated in a chair without arms, grips the seat of the chair on either side and, by extending the arms at the elbows, attempts to lift his or her body up off the chair.) Axillary nerve irritation on deep palpation of the quadrilateral space indicates compression by the posterior capsule and pectoralis minor. Likewise, if pressure on the posterior capsule produces localized discomfort, capsulitis should be suspected. Also with the patient in the prone position, allow the arm to hang freely over the edge of the table and then forward flex it to 90°; pain in the anterior shoulder is indicative of rotator cuff tendinitis.

With the patient seated and the elbow flexed 90°, abduct the arm to 90°. While one hand of the examiner stabilizes the scapula, rotate the arm forcefully posteriorly (exteriorly). If the pain of throwing is reproduced, the pathology may be subacromial bursitis. With the arm in the same position, apply internal rotation pressure. If this maneuver produces pain, rotator cuff tendinitis should be suspected. Crepitus noted in the subacromial space with rotation of the arm in abduction is a probable indication of subacromial bursitis.

Provocative testing to produce pain at a specific shoulder location is very sensitive but is not specific. Impingement is indicated by positive Hawkins and Neer impingement tests (see page 261).

Diagnostic Tests

Radiographs provide additional information. Evidence of sclerosis on AP internal and external rotation views represents contact erosive areas on the greater tuberosity of the humeral head and the posterior glenoid rim.

An additional diagnostic tool is the subacromial injection (9 mL lidocaine/1 mL dexamethasone). Alleviation of the patient's pain supports a diagnosis of subacromial bursitis. In addition, gadolinium-enhanced MRI may be helpful to establish a working diagnosis, especially if lateral pathology is suspected.

Differential Diagnosis

- Acromial abnormalities (radiographic findings)
- Anterior instability (apprehension with abduction and external rotation of the shoulder)
- External impingement (positive impingement test)
- Internal impingement (pain with the cocking motion of throwing)
- Labral pathology (labral defect apparent on MRI)
- Rotator cuff tendinitis (pathology) (weakness on testing, positive MRI)
- SLAP lesion (may be seen on MRI with contrast; arthroscopy is diagnostic)

Adverse Outcomes of the Disease

Athletes with the shoulder symptoms described in this chapter are usually unable to participate effectively in their sport because effective pitching requires an intact rotator cuff–glenohumeral complex and pain-free motion.

Treatment

Stage I—Sore Shoulder Syndrome

Initially, the athlete with stage I disease is placed on active rest (activity modification). No overhead weight training or throwing of any object is allowed, but daily core stability work, leg work, and running for cardiovascular endurance are encouraged. Dynamic stabilization of the humeral head by rehabilitation of the rotator cuff muscles is undertaken. Stabilization is followed by strengthening of the rotator cuff muscles with isometric exercises. Basic rehabilitation includes internal and external rotation of the shoulder with the elbow at the side, using elasticized bands of increasing stiffness. Riding a stationary bicycle or an elliptical trainer with arms that move alternately also is advised. A rope-and-pulley system to increase range of motion can be used at home. Ice bags may be applied locally for pain, and rehabilitation specialists may apply electrical modalities. Initial time away from throwing is about 10 days, or until the shoulder is free from soreness. Then a published protocol of interval throwing, which must be supervised and followed closely, is begun.

SECTION 2 SHOULDER

Stage II—Pathologic Pain

In the overhead thrower with stage II disease (ie, profound pathologic pain that prevents the athlete from competing), rehabilitation must be instituted in a very precise, scientific, and individualized manner. This is necessary because pain is an indication that tissue injury (inflammation) is already established.

First, upper body activity is controlled and modified to reestablish dynamic stability and muscle balance and to improve flexibility. Rehabilitation specialists, using hands-on methods, initiate the basic rotator cuff protocols as outlined previously. They also use electrical stimulation and ultrasound modalities and proprioception techniques. As pain permits, isotonic muscle strengthening and neuromuscular control exercises are begun. Core stabilization, which includes leg work, is coupled with a well-structured shoulder exercise program.

Referral Decisions/Red Flags

Referral is indicated if painful overhead motion persists after an initial trial of rehabilitation exercises, especially if labral pathology is suspected.

Rotator Cuff Tear

Synonyms

Musculotendinous cuff rupture

Rotator cuff rupture

Rotator cuff tendinitis

Definition

The rotator cuff is composed of four muscles: the supraspinatus, the infraspinatus, the subscapularis, and the teres minor (see the illustration on page 303). These muscles form a cover around the head of the humerus and function to rotate the arm and stabilize the humeral head against the glenoid.

Rotator cuff tears occur with acute injury, but most are the result of age-related degeneration, chronic mechanical impingement, and altered blood supply to the tendons. Tears generally originate in the supraspinatus tendon and may progress posteriorly and anteriorly (**Figure 1**). Full-thickness tears are uncommon in individuals younger than 40 years but are present in 25% of individuals older than 60 years. Most older people with rotator cuff tears are asymptomatic or have only mild, nondisabling symptoms.

Clinical Symptoms

Patients often report chronic shoulder pain for several months and a specific injury that triggered the onset of the pain. Night pain and difficulty sleeping on the affected side are characteristic. Common symptoms include weakness, catching, and grating, especially when raising the arm overhead.

Tests

Physical Examination

The back of the shoulder may appear sunken, indicating atrophy of the infraspinatus muscle following a long-standing cuff tear. Passive range of motion is near normal, but active range of motion may be limited. With large tears, the patient cannot raise the arm when asked to do so but can only shrug, or "hike," the shoulder (**Figure 2**). The patient also cannot hold the arm elevated when it is lifted by the examiner parallel to the floor. Some patients, however, maintain remarkably good active motion despite large cuff tears. As the patient raises the arm, a grating sensation about the tip of the shoulder can be felt. Tenderness to palpation over the greater tuberosity is usually present as well.

Figure 1 Coronal oblique MRI of the shoulder demonstrates a rotator cuff tear (arrows).

SECTION 2 SHOULDER

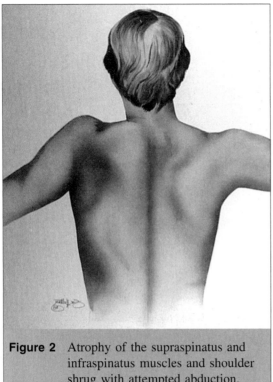

Figure 2 Atrophy of the supraspinatus and infraspinatus muscles and shoulder shrug with attempted abduction. (Reproduced with permission from Rockwood CA Jr: Subluxations and dislocations about the shoulder, in Rockwood CA Jr, Green DP, eds: *Rockwood and Green's Fractures in Adults*, ed 2. Philadelphia, PA, JB Lippincott, 1984, pp 722-805.)

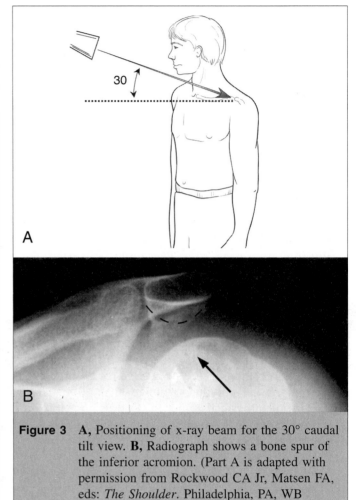

Figure 3 **A,** Positioning of x-ray beam for the 30° caudal tilt view. **B,** Radiograph shows a bone spur of the inferior acromion. (Part A is adapted with permission from Rockwood CA Jr, Matsen FA, eds: *The Shoulder*. Philadelphia, PA, WB Saunders, 1990.)

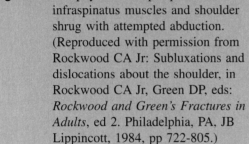

Diagnostic Tests

A 30° caudal tilt view will often show a spur projecting down from the inferior surface of the acromion (**Figure 3**). Often a coracoacromial arch view (outlet view) is needed to show a hooked acromion, indicative of this spur (**Figure 4**). The presence of a spur does not necessarily indicate a rotator cuff tear, however. Soft-tissue imaging is necessary to confirm the diagnosis. With large, long-standing tears, AP radiographs may reveal a high-riding humerus relative to the glenoid, indicative of rotator cuff arthropathy (**Figure 5**).

If the diagnosis is equivocal or if surgical treatment is being considered, MRI is the imaging study of choice because it can provide additional information on the status of the muscle and on the size of full-thickness and some partial-thickness tears. Ultrasonography, in experienced hands, also is useful and accurate in evaluating the rotator cuff.

Differential Diagnosis

- Acromioclavicular joint arthritis (localized pain and tenderness and preserved motion)
- Cervical spondylosis (neck stiffness, absent biceps reflex, sensory changes)
- Frozen shoulder (restricted active and passive motion)
- Glenohumeral joint arthritis (evidence of arthritis on radiographs)
- Impingement syndrome/cuff tendinitis (similar pain, but preserved active motion)
- Pancoast tumor (venous distention, pulmonary changes, or bony metastases)
- Thoracic outlet syndrome (ulnar nerve paresthesias, worse with "military brace" position)

Figure 4 Outlet view demonstrates a hooked acromion (arrow).

Adverse Outcomes of the Disease

Loss of shoulder motion (especially the ability to lift the arm overhead), chronic pain, and/or weakness in the affected arm is possible. Long-standing large tears sometimes lead to joint degeneration.

Treatment

Nonsurgical treatment includes NSAIDs, rehabilitation with strengthening and stretching exercises (see page 250), and avoiding overhead activities. Corticosteroid injections should be used judiciously. The steroid injection may decrease inflammation of an associated subacromial bursitis and provide short-term pain relief, but it also weakens the tendon. Repeated injections may ultimately accelerate propagation of the rotator cuff tear. Therefore, patients should never receive more than two or three subacromial injections. If they are not effective, additional injections are unlikely to help.

In general, patients with significant symptoms and failed rehabilitation over 3 to 6 months should be considered candidates for surgery. One exception to this rule is the patient who has an acute traumatic cuff tear, in which case rotator cuff repair is best performed acutely or no later than within 6 weeks of injury. If an acute tear is neglected longer than this, it may propagate and become retracted and much harder to repair. Another possible exception is a rotator cuff tear in a younger patient (younger than 55 years). Tears can enlarge with time and become more difficult to repair. Therefore, consideration should be given to surgical repair in younger patients of working age with repairable tears.

Figure 5 AP view of shoulder shows high-riding humeral head (arrow), indicative of rotator cuff arthropathy.

SECTION 2 SHOULDER

Rehabilitation Prescription

The functional goal of rehabilitation for a patient with a rotator cuff tear is to reduce pain, increase strength, increase the range of motion of the involved shoulder, and restore function. Stiffness of the glenohumeral joint and poor scapulothoracic mobility may be present, secondary to a period of immobilization. Rehabilitation should not involve forcing the shoulder into passive or active elevation. It is very important to avoid further damage to the rotator cuff. Instructions to the patient regarding a home exercise program should emphasize that the patient should experience no pain during or after the exercises. The home exercise program (see page 315) begins with light weights and high repetitions to increase range of motion and progresses to heavier weights and fewer repetitions to strengthen the rotator cuff and the scapula rotators. Active elevation should be avoided.

Formal rehabilitation should be prescribed immediately for athletes or if the patient does not progress on the home program. Poor progress would include the presence of pain and/or stiffness during or after the exercises. In addition, formal rehabilitation is indicated when, upon reevaluation by the physician in 3 to 4 weeks, muscle strength or range of motion has not improved. The prescription should include an evaluation of glenohumeral and scapula rotator muscle strength and initiation of an appropriate strengthening program. Pain-relieving modalities such as interferential current, ultrasound, or heat also may help to prepare the soft tissues for mobilization and strengthening.

Adverse Outcomes of Treatment

NSAIDs may cause gastric, renal, or hepatic complications. Corticosteroid injections may result in a transient increase in pain because of the injection itself and degeneration of cuff tissue. Repair of large rotator cuff tears has a high incidence of failure, though the débridement alone may relieve persistent pain.

Referral Decisions/Red Flags

Failure of 6 weeks of nonsurgical treatment is an indication for further evaluation.

Home Exercise Program for Rotator Cuff Tear

- Perform the exercises in the order listed.

- Apply a bag of crushed ice or frozen peas to the shoulder for 20 minutes after performing both exercises to prevent any further inflammation or pain.

- You should not experience pain with any of the exercises. If pain or stiffness occurs that prevents you from performing any of the exercises correctly, call your doctor.

Exercise Type	Muscle Group	Number of Repetitions/Sets	Number of Days per Week	Number of Weeks
Trapezius strengthening	Middle and posterior deltoid Supraspinatus Middle trapezius	20 repetitions/3 to 4 sets, decreasing to 8 to 10 repetitions/3 to 4 sets as weight is added, then progressing to 15 repetitions/3 sets	3 to 5	3 to 4
Internal and external rotation at 90° or 45° elevation	*Internal rotation:* Anterior deltoid Pectoralis Subscapularis Latissimus *External rotation:* Posterior deltoid Infraspinatus Teres minor	20 repetitions/3 to 4 sets, decreasing to 8 to 10 repetitions/3 to 4 sets as weight is added, then progressing to 15 repetitions/3 sets	3 to 5	3 to 4

Trapezius Strengthening

- Stand next to a bench or chair with your knee and hand (on the unaffected side) resting on the bench. The other hand should be at your side, palm facing the body.

- As you lift the arm slowly, rotate the hand to the thumb-up position, stopping when the arm is parallel to the floor.

- Slowly lower the arm to the original position to a count of 5.

- Begin with a light enough weight to allow 3 to 4 sets of 20 repetitions without pain.

- Decrease the repetitions to 8 to 10 and add no more than 2 to 3 pounds of weight so that the last few repetitions are difficult but pain free.

- Progress to 3 sets of 15 repetitions at each weight increment.

- Perform the exercise 3 to 5 times per week, continuing for 3 to 4 weeks.

Top view

Start   Finish

SECTION 2 SHOULDER

Internal and External Rotation

- Lie on your back on the floor or a bed.
- Extend your arm straight out from the shoulder and bend the elbow 90°.
- Keeping your elbow bent, slowly move your arm in the arc shown in the illustration.
- Change the angle of the arm to 45° if you experience pain at 90°.
- Begin with a light enough weight to allow 3 to 4 sets of 20 repetitions without pain.
- Decrease the repetitions to 8 to 10 and add no more than 2 to 3 pounds of weight so that the last few repetitions are difficult but pain free.
- Progress to 3 sets of 15 repetitions at each weight increment, with maximum weight approximately 5 to 7 pounds.
- Perform the exercises 3 to 5 times per week, continuing for 3 to 4 weeks.

SECTION 2 SHOULDER

Rupture of the Proximal Biceps Tendon

Definition

Rupture of the biceps tendon usually involves the proximal long head of the biceps. Most often, ruptures occur in older adults who have a long history of shoulder pain secondary to rotator cuff disease, either inflammation or a tear. The long head of the biceps tendon ascends in the intertubercular groove and is intra-articular for its proximal 3 cm. The shoulder capsule is continuous with the biceps tendon sheath; therefore, inflammatory changes in the shoulder can affect the tendon as well. Its anatomic position predisposes the tendon to attritional changes, and the tendon ultimately ruptures, often as a result of a trivial event.

Rupture of the proximal biceps tendon is uncommon in young adults but may occur in athletic individuals involved in weight lifting or throwing sports. Rupture of the distal biceps tendon also may occur but is less common (see page 389).

ICD-9 Codes
727.62 Nontraumatic rupture of tendons of biceps (long head)
840.8 Sprain of other specified site of shoulder and upper arm
840.9 Sprains and strains of shoulder and upper arm, unspecified site

Clinical Symptoms

Sudden pain in the upper arm, often accompanied by an audible snap, is often reported. Subsequently, patients notice a bulge in the lower arm. Pain in the acute stage is often mild.

Tests

Physical Examination

Examination reveals a bulge in the lower arm, which results from the muscle belly of the biceps retracting into the lower arm after the long head ruptures (**Figure 1**). A defect also can be palpated proximally. Acutely, ecchymosis can be seen tracking down the middle and lower arm.

The bulge can be accentuated by having the patient contract the biceps against resistance with the elbow flexed or by doing the Ludington test. (For this test, the patient puts his or her hands behind the head and flexes the biceps muscle.) Gentle pressure over the bicipital groove of the humerus with the arm in 10° of internal rotation will elicit acute pain (**Figure 2**).

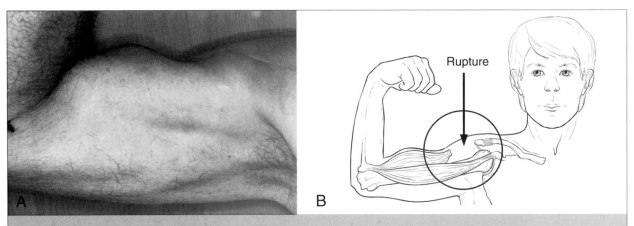

Figure 1 Rupture of the proximal biceps tendon made more obvious by attempted contraction. **A,** Clinical photograph. **B,** Drawing showing the underlying anatomy.

Figure 2 Palpation of the bicipital groove.

Diagnostic Tests

AP and axillary radiographs of the shoulder are useful to rule out a fracture but are not helpful in confirming a diagnosis of a ruptured biceps tendon. For patients with a previous history of disabling shoulder pain, a shoulder arthrogram or MRI should be considered to rule out a rotator cuff tear.

Differential Diagnosis

- Dislocated biceps tendon (tenderness over the bicipital groove, but no distal muscle bulge)
- Distal biceps rupture (pain and ecchymosis distally with high-riding muscle belly, often missed until late)
- Glenohumeral arthritis (pain in the joint exacerbated with motion, evident on radiographs)
- Impingement syndrome (can coexist with biceps tendon rupture)
- Rotator cuff tear (often coexists with biceps tendon rupture)
- Rupture of the pectoralis major muscle (abnormal muscle contour apparent in anterior axillary fold)

Adverse Outcomes of the Disease

Patients can lose approximately 10% of elbow flexion and forearm supination strength (the motion required to use a manual screwdriver). Cosmetic deformity of the arm in the form of a bulge in the lower arm also may be of concern to the patient.

Treatment

Nonsurgical treatment is effective for most patients, resulting in little loss of function and acceptable cosmetic deformity. Most patients regain full range of motion and normal elbow flexion strength with an exercise program consisting of range of motion and strengthening as pain allows. Patients with persistent shoulder pain and young athletes require evaluation for a concomitant rotator cuff tear.

In young athletes and in adults younger than 40 years who work as heavy laborers and need the extra strength for lifting, surgical repair of the biceps tendon should be considered.

Adverse Outcomes of Treatment

Functional improvement from surgery is often modest, and postoperative stiffness is a potential concern. Bodybuilders may trade a distal muscle bulge for a surgical scar with little subjective cosmetic improvement.

Referral Decisions/Red Flags

Young patients who are heavy laborers and older patients with a concomitant rotator cuff tear and persistent symptoms require further evaluation.

SECTION 2 SHOULDER

Shoulder Instability

Synonyms

Dislocation
Multidirectional instability
Recurrent dislocation
Subluxation

Definition

With its shallow glenoid and loose capsule, the shoulder joint has exceptional mobility. As a corollary, instability is also most common at the shoulder. Patients with shoulder instability have recurrent episodes of subluxation (the humeral head partially slips out of the socket) and/or dislocation (**Figure 1**). Instability can be anterior, posterior, inferior, or multidirectional, with anterior and multidirectional being the most common (**Figure 2**). Classically, instability is thought to lie along a spectrum, from Traumatic Unidirectional instability with a Bankart lesion (a tear of the anterior glenoid labrum) (**Figure 3**) best treated with Surgery (TUBS) to Atraumatic, Multidirectional, Bilateral signs of laxity, Rehabilitation as the preferred treatment, and Inferior capsular shift as the indicated procedure if surgery becomes necessary (AMBRI). All individuals have varying degrees of laxity (nonpathologic), which can become instability (pathologic) when affected by trauma or overuse. Posterior dislocations result from a posteriorly directed force applied when the arm is in adduction and internal rotation. This uncommon injury is associated with seizures or electric shock injuries.

Figure 1 AP views of shoulder. **A,** Nondislocated shoulder. **B,** Dislocated shoulder.

Figure 2 Relative positions of the humeral head and the glenoid with the humeral head reduced (**A**), subluxated anteriorly (**B**), and dislocated anteriorly (**C**).

Clinical Symptoms

Patients with anterior instability typically describe the sensation of the shoulder slipping out of joint when the arm is abducted and externally rotated. The initial anterior shoulder dislocation is associated with significant trauma from a fall or forceful throwing motion, but with recurrent dislocations, the patient may experience instability by simply positioning the arm overhead. With multidirectional instability, symptoms may be vague but tend to be activity related. Ask the patient whether he or she can voluntarily dislocate the shoulder, as this is an important clue. The ability to voluntarily dislocate the shoulder is quite frequently associated with a multidirectional instability component and may indicate a poor prognosis for surgical treatment. Voluntary dislocations may be associated with psychological disturbance.

Tests

Physical Examination

With an acute dislocation, any movement of the shoulder is associated with considerable pain. With an anterior dislocation, the patient supports the arm in a neutral position. Patients with a posterior dislocation hold the arm in adduction and internal

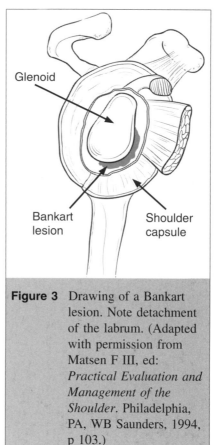

Figure 3 Drawing of a Bankart lesion. Note detachment of the labrum. (Adapted with permission from Matsen F III, ed: *Practical Evaluation and Management of the Shoulder*. Philadelphia, PA, WB Saunders, 1994, p 103.)

Figure 4 Sulcus sign. **A,** With the patient's arm relaxed at the side, the examiner applies traction in an inferior direction. **B,** Positive sulcus sign, indicative of inferior shoulder laxity.

rotation; external rotation is impossible. Neurovascular function, particularly function of the axillary nerve, should be carefully assessed before and after reduction.

Assessment of a patient believed to have recurrent instability on physical examination should include the apprehension test for anterior instability, the sulcus sign test for inferior laxity (**Figure 4**), and the jerk test for posterior instability (see page 261). The patient also should be assessed for generalized ligamentous laxity: Ask the patient to try to touch the thumb against the volar (flexor) surface of the forearm; also, bend the fingers back at the metacarpophalangeal joint to determine how far they extend past neutral with the finger and hand in a straight line. Patients with ligamentous laxity are more likely to have multidirectional instability, but other types of instability are possible.

Diagnostic Tests

AP and axillary radiographs of the shoulder should be obtained. The axillary view may show a bony defect at the anterior edge of the glenoid rim (**Figure 5**). A compression fracture of the posterior humeral head (a Hill-Sachs lesion) is created when the head is pressed against the anterior edge of the glenoid. A Hill-Sachs lesion is clear evidence of an anterior dislocation. Patients older than 40 years with a history of traumatic dislocation are also prone to tear the rotator cuff at the time of dislocation. A shoulder arthrogram or MRI may be indicated in these cases.

Posterior dislocation of the shoulder is easily missed if only an AP radiograph is obtained. If an axillary view cannot be obtained, request a transscapular lateral view.

Figure 5 Axillary view shows erosion of the glenoid rim (arrows) associated with anterior glenohumeral instability. (Reproduced from Bigliani LU, ed: *The Unstable Shoulder*. Rosemont, IL, American Academy of Orthopaedic Surgeons, 1996, p 32.)

Differential Diagnosis

- Glenohumeral arthritis (confirm with radiographs)
- Impingement syndrome (pain but no apprehension of instability)
- Rotator cuff tear (pain and weakness without apprehension)

Adverse Outcomes of the Disease

Axillary nerve injury (deltoid dysfunction and numbness over lateral arm) is not uncommon but usually resolves. Osteoarthritis of the glenohumeral joint, and/or persistent dislocation is possible. The risk of recurrent instability is greater in younger patients and in those with multiple episodes.

Treatment

Most acute shoulder dislocations can be reduced in the emergency department. There are several ways to reduce a shoulder, but only two are described here (see page 325). Patients with a first-time anterior dislocation should be immobilized in neutral arm rotation for 3 weeks, followed by a rehabilitation program that emphasizes strengthening the rotator cuff muscles, especially the subscapularis muscle (see page 250).

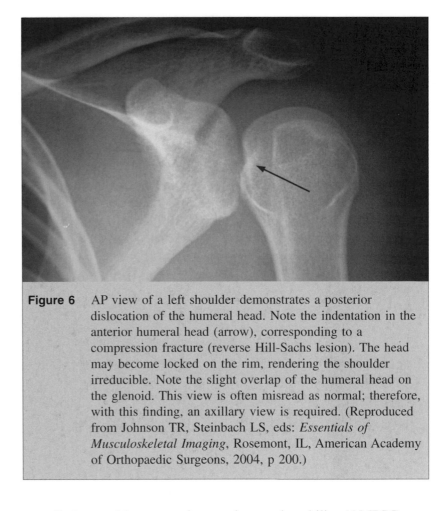

Figure 6   AP view of a left shoulder demonstrates a posterior dislocation of the humeral head. Note the indentation in the anterior humeral head (arrow), corresponding to a compression fracture (reverse Hill-Sachs lesion). The head may become locked on the rim, rendering the shoulder irreducible. Note the slight overlap of the humeral head on the glenoid. This view is often misread as normal; therefore, with this finding, an axillary view is required. (Reproduced from Johnson TR, Steinbach LS, eds: *Essentials of Musculoskeletal Imaging*, Rosemont, IL, American Academy of Orthopaedic Surgeons, 2004, p 200.)

Patients with atraumatic or voluntary instability (AMBRI) should be treated nonsurgically with the shoulder exercise program described in Musculoskeletal Conditioning of the Shoulder, page 250. Educating patients to avoid voluntarily dislocating the shoulder and to avoid positions of known instability is an important part of the treatment plan.

Adverse Outcomes of Treatment

Up to 80% of posterior dislocations are missed upon initial evaluation. **Figure 6** is a radiograph that demonstrates the classic signs of posterior dislocation.

Referral Decisions/Red Flags

Further evaluation is warranted in the following situations: when closed manipulation fails to reduce an acute dislocation; when recurrent dislocations (two or more) occur despite a 3-month trial of shoulder rehabilitation exercises; and in patients with multidirectional instability whose symptoms are intolerable and do not respond to a rehabilitation program.

Procedure: Reduction of Anterior Shoulder Dislocation

Prior to reduction, a neurovascular examination should be performed. Assess function of the axillary, musculocutaneous, median, radial, and ulnar nerves, with emphasis on evaluating the axillary nerve through voluntary isometric contraction of the deltoid and sensation over the lateral deltoid region. Obtain AP and axillary radiographs to document the dislocation and rule out any fractures that may displace during the reduction maneuver. Reducing a first-time dislocation is safely accomplished in the emergency department with a resuscitation cart available.

Establish an intravenous line, ensure that naloxone is available, and initiate pulse oximetry and cardiac monitoring if narcotics are used for anesthesia. Apply oxygen by mask or nasal cannula throughout the procedure. Fentanyl in a dose of 100 µg is given intravenously over 1 minute, and then repeated every 3 to 5 minutes until adequate sedation is achieved. The usual total dose of fentanyl is 3 µg/kg. Patients with recurrent dislocations may not require anesthesia.

Stimson Technique (Gravity-Assisted Reduction)

Step 1

Place the patient prone on a stretcher with the dislocated arm hanging off the cart. Secure the patient to the stretcher with a sheet.

Step 2

Either have an assistant sit on the floor and provide downward traction, or attach 5 to 15 lb of weight to the patient's arm (**Figure 1**). The weights should not touch the floor.

Step 3

For reduction of the left shoulder, place your left thumb on the patient's acromion and the fingers of your left hand over the front of the humeral head.

Figure 1 Stimson technique (gravity-assisted reduction with patient lying on stomach).

Figure 2 Longitudinal traction technique for shoulder reduction.

Step 4
As the muscles relax, gently push the humeral head caudally until it reduces.

Longitudinal Traction

Step 1
Place the patient supine on a stretcher with a sheet folded into a band 4" to 5" wide around the patient's chest (**Figure 2**). Stand next to the patient on the same side as the injured shoulder, at or below the level of the patient's waist.

Step 2
Position the patient's elbow in 90° of flexion to relax the biceps muscle. Have an assistant apply traction to the sheet that is wrapped around the patient's thorax while you apply a steady traction to the arm.

Step 3
Reduction may be aided if you gently rotate the arm while the longitudinal traction is applied. You usually can feel and see the shoulder reduce. Occasionally, especially in large patients, the reduction may be subtle, and you may neither feel nor see it.

Adverse Outcomes

Axillary nerve palsy may develop with reduction. Be sure to test axillary nerve function (motor and sensory) before and after the reduction. General anesthesia may be required to reduce the shoulder.

The administration of opioids such as fentanyl carries the risk of overdose. Fentanyl overdose is treated with naloxone. Initially, give 0.2 to 0.4 mg IV, and if there is no response, administer repeated doses of up to 4 to 5 mg; doses as high as 15 to 20 mg may be administered with resistant opioids such as fentanyl. First-time dislocation in a patient older than 40 years may be associated with a rotator cuff tear, so examine these patients with a high index of suspicion for a tear. Humeral fracture may result with excessive force.

Aftercare/Patient Instructions

Obtain postreduction AP and axillary radiographs to confirm the reduction. Immobilize the arm in a sling, in neutral rotation if possible, but have the patient remove the sling and extend the elbow several times daily to prevent elbow stiffness. Begin isometric exercises for the rotator cuff.

Begin strengthening exercises for the subscapularis and infraspinatus muscles at 2 to 3 weeks postreduction in the older patient and at 6 weeks in the younger patient.

Increase shoulder external rotation to 30° or 40° and shoulder flexion to 140°. This occurs at 6 weeks postreduction in patients younger than 30 years and at 3 weeks in patients older than 30 years.

Begin vigorous shoulder motion at 6 weeks postreduction in patients older than 30 years, but delay this step to 3 months for patients younger than 30 years.

The propensity for shoulder stiffness in patients older than 40 years is an advantage in regaining stability; however, these patients are more likely to sustain a rotator cuff tear at the time of the dislocation.

In the athlete, allow return to sports activities once near-full flexion and rotation of the arm and near-normal strength of the cuff have been regained.

SECTION 2 SHOULDER

Superior Labrum Anterior-to-Posterior Lesions

Synonyms

Biceps tendon labral complex injuries
SLAP lesions
Superior glenoid labrum tears

Definition

Superior labrum anterior-to-posterior (SLAP) lesions involve an injury to the superior glenoid labrum and the biceps anchor complex. The long head of the biceps tendon originates from the superior aspect of the glenoid labrum and is confluent with the labrum in this region, also called the biceps anchor. The glenoid labrum itself, which has been likened to the shoulder equivalent of the meniscus of the knee, consists of a cartilaginous lining of the glenoid, which serves to deepen the glenoid, thereby providing increased stability of the shoulder. Injuries to the labrum involve either fraying (usually degenerative in nature) or frank tears (associated with acute and chronic symptoms). Injuries that involve the superior labrum are termed SLAP lesions.

Clinical Symptoms

SLAP lesions are difficult to diagnose and are often a diagnosis of exclusion, confirmed only at the time of surgery. Symptoms may include painful popping or catching in the shoulder as well as pain with overhead activities. In a throwing athlete, symptoms may be present only with maximal effort throwing, but a thorough history may reveal an insidious onset of pain while performing overhead sports that limits performance and eventually leads to a persistent aching in the shoulder. The aching is often described as being deep inside the shoulder.

Tests

Physical Examination

Several tests are commonly used to detect SLAP lesions, but they have poor sensitivity and specificity. They include the active compression test, the crank test, the resisted supination/external rotation test, and the clunk test. They are designed to elicit pain as the lesion is compressed. For instructions on performing the active compression test (also called the O'Brien test), see page 256.

For the crank test, the arm is elevated to 160° in the scapular plane and is then loaded axially by the examiner, who then moves the arm into maximal internal and external rotation of the arm while still axially loading the shoulder. Pain or a clicking produced by the maneuver is a positive test.

The resisted supination/external rotation test attempts to mimic the "peel-back" position in an overhead thrower. For this test, the patient is placed supine with the shoulder at 90° of abduction. The elbow is flexed to 70° with the wrist in neutral rotation. The patient actively supinates against the examiner's resistance as the shoulder is slowly externally rotated to maximum external rotation. Pain at or just before maximal external rotation is a positive test.

For the clunk test, the patient is placed supine with the shoulder flexed to 180°, the elbow flexed to 90°, and the hand pointing to the floor. While holding the elbow in place, the examiner grasps the hand and uses it to internally rotate the shoulder. The clunk test is considered positive if the patient experiences a sharp pain with the internal rotation.

Diagnostic Tests

Plain radiographs should be obtained because they are part of a thorough workup of any shoulder disorder, but they cannot confirm a diagnosis of a SLAP lesion. MR arthrography (injection of contrast medium into the shoulder before the MRI is obtained) is the gold standard to evaluate for a SLAP lesion, with a sensitivity and specificity for the condition of up to 90%. MRI without contrast has a sensitivity of less than 50%.

Differential Diagnosis

- Acromioclavicular (AC) joint arthritis (tenderness over the AC joint, positive cross-body adduction test, AC pain on bench pressing)
- Biceps tendinitis (tenderness anteriorly over the biceps tendon)
- Rotator cuff disease (pain referred to lateral deltoid)
- Shoulder instability (history of shoulder "slipping out of place," positive apprehension test)
- Subacromial impingement (positive clinical impingement signs, palpable crepitus, local tenderness over rotator cuff insertion)
- Suprascapular nerve entrapment (possible wasting of infraspinatus on examination, diagnosed with electromyography)

SECTION 2 SHOULDER

Adverse Outcomes of the Disease

Continued shoulder pain and some disability with activities are possible.

Treatment

Nonsurgical care should be attempted initially. This includes NSAIDs as well as rehabilitation directed at rotator cuff and periscapular stabilization, posterior capsule stretching, and strengthening with gradual return to activities. In a throwing athlete, gradual return to activities would include the use of an interval throwing program after at least 6 weeks of rest to return the athlete to a competitive level of play in a controlled fashion. If nonsurgical care fails and symptoms persist, diagnostic shoulder arthroscopy is the only other alternative. At the time of surgery, all intra-articular pathology can be delineated and addressed.

Rehabilitation Prescription

The functional goal of rehabilitation for a patient with a SLAP lesion is to reduce pain and protect the joint from further damage. Unfortunately, many SLAP lesions do not respond well to nonsurgical treatment. The home exercise program should include stretching of the posterior structures (see page 331). In addition, deep bench presses, overhead presses, and biceps curls should be prohibited. Reaching behind and overhead activities should be limited to pain-free movement. If the patient does not respond to the home program of exercises, stretching, and activity modification, referral to a rehabilitation specialist is indicated. The rehabilitation specialist should evaluate the muscle strength and posterior capsule mobility and determine the appropriate exercises for the patient's condition.

Adverse Outcomes of Treatment

NSAIDs may cause gastric, renal, and hepatic complications. Physical therapy may not improve symptoms but has no adverse effect. The most common adverse effect following surgical repair of a SLAP lesion is shoulder stiffness.

Home Exercise Program for SLAP Lesions

- Perform the exercises in the order listed.
- Apply dry or moist heat to the shoulder before the exercises and during the sleeper stretch.
- To reduce inflammation, apply a bag of crushed ice or frozen peas to the shoulder for 15 to 20 minutes after performing both exercises.
- You should not experience pain during or after the exercises. If the exercises cause pain, call your doctor.
- Avoid activities that may cause additional damage to the labral tear, such as arm curls while lifting heavy objects (heavier than 5 pounds), overhead sports activities (a tennis serve or throwing a baseball), and reaching overhead or behind your body.

Exercise Type	Muscle Group	Number of Repetitions/Sets	Number of Days per Week	Number of Weeks
Sleeper stretch	Infraspinatus Teres minor Posterior capsule	4 repetitions/2 to 3 sets	Daily	2 to 3
External rotation	Infraspinatus Teres minor Posterior deltoid	8 to 10 repetitions/2 sets, progressing to 15 repetitions/3 sets	3	2 to 3

Sleeper Stretch

- Lie on your side on a firm, flat surface with the affected shoulder under you and the arm positioned as shown, keeping your back perpendicular to the surface.
- With the unaffected arm, push the other wrist down, toward the surface. Stop when you feel a stretching sensation in the back of the affected shoulder.
- Hold this position for 30 seconds; then relax the arm for 30 seconds.
- Perform 2 to 3 sets of 4 repetitions daily, continuing for 2 to 3 weeks.

Sleeper position

Start   Finish

SECTION 2 SHOULDER

External Rotation

- Lie on your side on a firm, flat surface with the unaffected arm under you, cradling your head.

- Hold the injured arm against your side as shown, with the elbow bent at a 90° angle.

- Slowly rotate the arm at the shoulder, keeping the elbow bent and against your side, to raise the weight to a vertical position, and then slowly lower the weight to the starting position to a count of 5.

- Begin with weights that allow 2 sets of 8 to 10 repetitions and progress to 3 sets of 15 repetitions.

- Add weight in 1-pound increments, starting over with 8 to 10 repetitions each time weight is added.

- Perform the exercise 3 days per week, continuing for 2 to 3 weeks.

Start

Finish

SECTION 2 SHOULDER

Thoracic Outlet Syndrome

Definition

Thoracic outlet syndrome (TOS) is compression of the brachial plexus and/or subclavian vessels as they exit the narrow space between the superior shoulder girdle and the first rib (**Figure 1**). These structures may be affected individually or in combination. Women between the ages of 20 and 50 years are most commonly affected.

TOS may be secondary to congenital anomalies such as a cervical rib or abnormally long transverse process of C7, or an anomalous fibromuscular band in the thoracic outlet. Posttraumatic fibrosis of the scalene muscles also is a possibility.

ICD-9 Code

353.0
Brachial plexus lesions

Clinical Symptoms

Symptoms are vague and variable. Compression of the brachial plexus accounts for most presenting symptoms and may mimic distal nerve entrapment, especially of the ulnar nerve, with little and ring finger paresthesias. Aching pain and paresthesias can extend from the neck into the shoulder, arm, medial forearm,

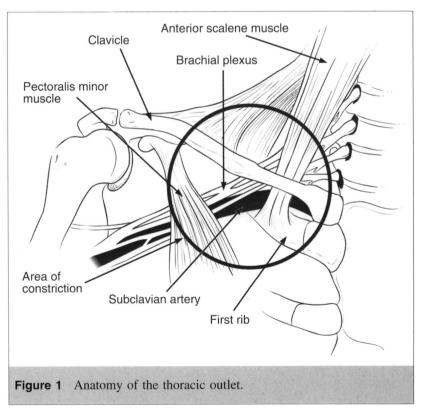

Clavicle

Anterior scalene muscle

Brachial plexus

Pectoralis minor muscle

Area of constriction

Subclavian artery

First rib

Figure 1 Anatomy of the thoracic outlet.

Figure 2 Elevated arm stress test (EAST).

and the fingers. Symptoms from vascular compression include intermittent swelling and discoloration of the arm. The aching fatigue and weakness are worse when the arm is in an overhead position. Psychological disturbances such as depression are seen with TOS, but whether they contribute to the causation or are the result of a chronically painful condition is unclear.

Tests

Physical Examination

Inspect for swelling or discoloration of the arm and palpate the supraclavicular fossa to rule out a mass lesion. Auscultation over this area may reveal a bruit, especially during the provocative maneuvers described below. Compare distal pulses with those on the opposite side. Assess sensory and motor function of the axillary, musculocutaneous, medial antebrachial cutaneous, median, radial, and—most important—ulnar nerves.

Several clinical tests have been described to diagnose TOS. Perhaps the simplest and most reproducible provocative maneuver is the elevated arm stress test (EAST) (**Figure 2**). With both shoulders abducted at least 90° and braced somewhat posteriorly, the patient opens and closes his or her fists at a moderate speed for 3 minutes. Reproduction of neurologic and/or vascular symptoms is a positive test. A sense of fatigue without neurologic or vascular symptoms is considered a negative or inconclusive test.

Diagnostic Tests

No laboratory studies currently exist to confirm the diagnosis. AP and lateral radiographs of the cervical spine identify cervical ribs or overly long C7 transverse processes. PA and lateral views of the chest help rule out an apical lung tumor or infection. MRI of the cervical spine may be needed if the patient has signs and symptoms of a cervical disk rupture or a cervical spondylosis. AP and axillary radiographs of the shoulder are indicated if the patient has shoulder symptoms. Somatosensory-evoked potentials, nerve conduction velocity studies, and ultrasonograpy are not reliable in confirming the diagnosis but can be useful in ruling out alternative diagnoses (eg, ulnar nerve entrapment).

Differential Diagnosis

- Brachial plexus neuritis (sudden onset, severe pain, proximal muscle weakness)
- Carpal tunnel syndrome (numbness on the radial side of the hand, positive Phalen maneuver)
- Herniated cervical disk (neck pain and stiffness with unilateral or bilateral pain and neurologic findings in a radicular pattern)

SECTION 2 SHOULDER

- Impingement syndrome (localized shoulder pain with positive impingement signs)
- Pancoast tumor (venous congestion, lesion on apical lordotic chest radiograph)
- Ulnar nerve entrapment (Tinel sign at elbow, abnormal nerve conduction velocity studies, no symptoms above the elbow)

Adverse Outcomes of the Disease

Weakness and loss of coordination of the upper extremity, chronic headaches, and the inability to work with the arm overhead are possible. Ulcerations on the arm and hand and the Raynaud phenomenon are rare. Serious problems such as venous thrombosis and aneurysm of the subclavian artery are uncommon but can develop.

Treatment

Most patients can be treated nonsurgically with 3 to 6 months of a home exercise program (see page 337) that emphasizes muscle strengthening and posture education exercises. Strenuous activities, such as carrying heavy objects, should be avoided, as should placing straps over the affected shoulder, including bras, purses, and seat belts. Activities that aggravate symptoms, such as prolonged overhead activities, strenuous aerobic exercises, and sleeping on the affected shoulder, should be discouraged as well.

Maintaining proper posture is important. The patient should be taught to stand up straight with the shoulders back, not slumped forward. The use of NSAIDs, muscle relaxants, and transcutaneous electrical nerve stimulation (TENS) units can help decrease the severity of the symptoms. Weight reduction, when indicated, should be encouraged as well. A multidisciplinary approach, including physical therapists, occupational therapists, and physiatrists, may be beneficial.

Because the success rate from surgery is variable and the complication rate is significant, every effort should be made to treat these patients nonsurgically.

Adverse Outcomes of Treatment

The following conditions may develop following or as a result of treatment: complex regional pain syndrome, intercostal neuroma, frozen shoulder, brachial plexus injury, or pneumothorax.

SECTION 2 SHOULDER

Referral Decisions/Red Flags

Vascular compromise with swelling and/or ulceration necessitates early consultation. Similarly, patients with TOS and a cervical rib or unusually long transverse process require early specialty evaluation when these findings are associated with loss of sensation, muscle atrophy, and weakness. Finally, failure of a well-supervised exercise program in a patient with disabling symptoms is an indication for further evaluation.

SECTION 2 SHOULDER

Home Exercise Program for Thoracic Outlet Syndrome

- The following exercises are designed to stretch the soft-tissue structures that may be compressing the neurovascular bundle.
- Perform the exercises in the order listed.
- If any of the exercises causes an increase in your symptoms, discontinue the exercises and call your doctor.

Exercise Type	Number of Repetitions/Sets	Number of Days per Week	Number of Weeks
Corner stretches	10 repetitions/2 sets	Daily	12
Neck stretches	10 repetitions/2 sets	Daily	12
Shoulder rolls	10 repetitions/2 sets	Daily	12
Neck retractions	10 repetitions/2 sets	Daily	12

Corner Stretches

- Stand in a corner with your hands against the walls at shoulder height.
- Lean into the corner until you feel a gentle stretch.
- Hold for 5 seconds.
- Perform 2 sets of 10 repetitions daily for 12 weeks.

(Adapted with permission from Visual Health Information, Tacoma, WA.)

Neck Stretches

- Place your left hand on the far side of your head and your right hand behind your back.
- Pull your head toward your shoulder until you feel a gentle stretch.
- Hold for 5 seconds.
- Switch hand positions and repeat the exercise in the opposite direction.
- Perform 2 sets of 10 repetitions daily for 12 weeks.

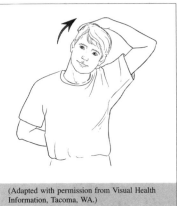

(Adapted with permission from Visual Health Information, Tacoma, WA.)

Shoulder Rolls

- Roll your shoulders up, back, and then down in a circular motion.
- Perform 2 sets of 10 repetitions daily for 12 weeks.

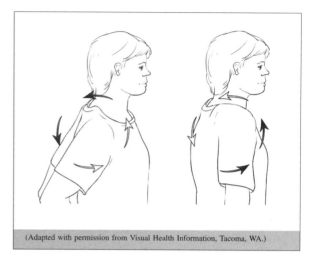

(Adapted with permission from Visual Health Information, Tacoma, WA.)

Neck Retractions

- Pull your head straight back, keeping your jaw level.
- Hold in the retracted position for 5 seconds.
- Perform 2 sets of 10 repetitions daily for 12 weeks.

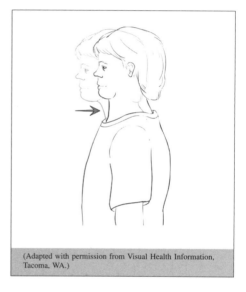

(Adapted with permission from Visual Health Information, Tacoma, WA.)

PAIN DIAGRAM
Elbow and Forearm

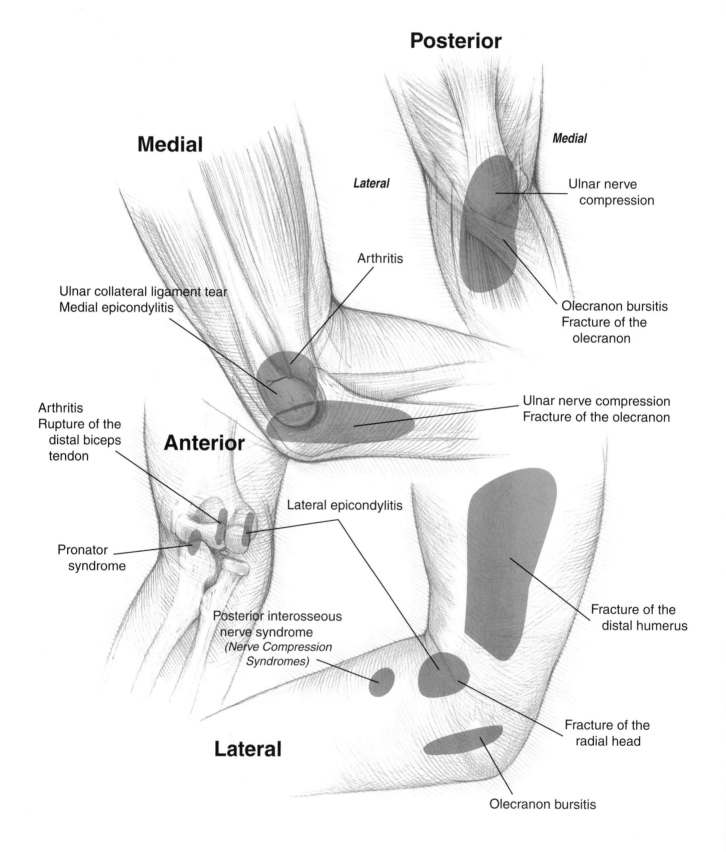

Posterior

Medial

Lateral

Ulnar nerve compression

Arthritis

Olecranon bursitis
Fracture of the olecranon

Ulnar collateral ligament tear
Medial epicondylitis

Medial

Ulnar nerve compression
Fracture of the olecranon

Arthritis
Rupture of the distal biceps tendon

Anterior

Lateral epicondylitis

Pronator syndrome

Fracture of the distal humerus

Posterior interosseous nerve syndrome
(Nerve Compression Syndromes)

Fracture of the radial head

Lateral

Olecranon bursitis

ESSENTIALS OF MUSCULOSKELETAL CARE ■ © 2010 AMERICAN ACADEMY OF ORTHOPAEDIC SURGEONS

Elbow and Forearm

Section Editor

April D. Armstrong, MD
Associate Professor
Bone and Joint Institute
Penn State Milton S. Hershey Medical Center
Hershey, PA

Contributor

Michael Huxford, MEd, ATC, CSCS
Sports Medicine Coordinator
Rehabilitative Services
Institute for Sports Medicine
Children's Memorial Hospital
Chicago, IL

ANATOMY OF THE ELBOW AND FOREARM

Muscles of the Anterior Forearm

Biceps brachii muscle

Brachial artery and median nerve

Lateral cutaneous nerve of forearm
(terminal musculocutaneous nerve)

Brachialis muscle

Biceps brachii tendon

Radial artery

Bicipital aponeurosis

Brachioradialis muscle

Extensor carpi radialis longus muscle

Extensor carpi radialis brevis muscle

Flexor pollicis longus muscle and tendon

Radial artery

Median nerve

Palmar carpal ligament (continuous with extensor retinaculum)

Thenar muscles

Palmar aponeurosis

Medial cutaneous nerve of forearm

Ulnar nerve

Triceps brachii muscle

Medial intermuscular septum

Ulnar artery

Medial epicondyle of humerus

Common flexor tendon

Pronator teres muscle

Flexor carpi radialis muscle

Palmaris longus muscle

Flexor carpi ulnaris muscle

Superficial flexor muscles

Flexor digitorum superficialis muscle

Palmaris longus tendon

Dorsal branch of ulnar nerve

Ulnar artery and nerve

Flexor digitorum superficialis tendon

Pisiform

Palmar branch of median nerve

Hypothenar muscles

Muscles of the Posterior Forearm

Triceps brachii muscle

Brachioradialis muscle

Extensor carpi radialis longus muscle

Superior ulnar collateral artery (anastomoses distally with posterior ulnar recurrent artery)

Common extensor tendon

Extensor carpi radialis brevis muscle

Extensor digitorum muscle

Extensor digiti minimi muscle

Abductor pollicis longus muscle

Extensor pollicis brevis muscle

Ulnar nerve

Medial epicondyle of humerus

Olecranon of ulna

Anconeus muscle

Flexor carpi ulnaris muscle

Extensor carpi ulnaris muscle

Extensor pollicis longus tendon
Extensor carpi radialis brevis te
Extensor carpi radialis longus te

Superficial branch of radial

Abductor pollicis longus
Extensor pollicis brevis te
Extensor pollicis longus

Anatomic snuffb

Extensor retinaculum (compartments numbered)

Dorsal branch of ulnar nerve

6 5 4 3 2 1

Extensor carpi ulnaris tendon
Extensor digiti minimi tendon
Extensor digitorum tendons
Extensor indicis tendon

5th metacarpal bone

Bones of the Elbow Joint

Right elbow

Condyle { Medial Lateral }

Lateral supracondylar ridge

Radial fossa

Lateral epicondyle

Capitellum

Head

Neck

Tuberosity

Radius

Humerus

Medial supracondylar ridge

Coronoid fossa

Medial epicondyle

Trochlea

Coronoid process

Radial notch of ulna

Tuberosity

Ulna

Humerus

Olecranon fossa

Lateral epicondyle

Olecranon

Head

Neck

Tuberosity

Groove for ulnar nerve

Ulna

Radius

Anterior View in extension

Posterior View in extension

Humerus

Radius

Humerus

Ulna

Lateral view in extension

Medial view in extension

Humerus

Lateral epicondyle

Capitellum

Head

Neck

Tuberosity

Radial notch
Coronoid process } of ulna
Trochlear notch
Olecranon

Lateral view in 90° flexion

Humerus

Medial epicondyle

Capitellum

Trochlea

Head

Tuberosity

Neck

Tuberosity

Coronoid process

Trochlear notch

Olecranon

Medial view in 90° flexion

Overview of the Elbow and Forearm

This section of *Essentials of Musculoskeletal Care* focuses on common and important conditions encountered in the elbow and forearm. Making a correct diagnosis of a condition in the elbow or forearm begins with clearly defining the nature and the anatomic location of the patient's chief symptom, which usually is related to pain, stiffness, swelling, or a combination of the three. Unlike the shoulder, the elbow has considerable articular congruency, and elbow instability is a much less common problem than shoulder instability.

The elbow joint has three distinct articulations: the ulnohumeral joint, the radiocapitellar joint, and the proximal radioulnar joint. The ulnohumeral and radiocapitellar joints provide flexion/extension of the elbow and pronation/supination of the forearm, and the proximal radioulnar joint works in conjunction with the distal radioulnar joint at the wrist to achieve forearm pronation and supination. Basic radiographic assessment consists of an AP view of the extended elbow and a lateral view with the elbow flexed to 90° and the forearm supinated. Oblique views can be helpful in identifying subtle fractures and when the elbow cannot be extended enough to obtain an AP view. The basic evaluation should include not only an assessment of the bony anatomy but also attention to the soft tissues; for example, the presence of a posterior fat pad may herald an intra-articular fracture.

Acute Pain

Acute pain and swelling after an injury can be caused by a fracture, dislocation, or tendon/ligament rupture. Important physical findings include the location of the pain and any tenderness, deformity, and ecchymosis. Pain with elbow flexion/extension suggests involvement of the ulnohumeral articulation, whereas pain with forearm pronation/supination should direct attention to the radiocapitellar and proximal radioulnar joints.

Radiographs will confirm a fracture or dislocation, although some radial head or other articular surface fractures are easily missed. Subtle radiographic signs such as bony avulsions or soft-tissue swelling seen with a fat pad sign can signal an important bony injury. Normal radiographs do not rule out the possibility of a tendon or ligament rupture, such as a distal biceps or triceps rupture.

Acute pain or swelling over the tip of the elbow may indicate acute olecranon bursitis. Intra-articular conditions, which may produce acute synovitis of the elbow, include septic arthritis (especially in IV drug abusers), rheumatoid arthritis, or other inflammatory conditions, such as crystal deposition diseases (gout, pseudogout). A thorough evaluation of all body systems is helpful, as the elbow may be only one of many joints that are involved in an inflammatory condition.

Chronic Pain

Most elbow and forearm conditions are chronic in nature (longer than 2 weeks' duration) and represent overuse injuries from work or sport. Very often a change in training habits or a change in sports equipment (for example, a tennis racket) can be identified in the patient's history. Localization of the pain and tenderness, as well as identification of the movement or position that provokes pain, is important.

Arthritis of the elbow includes posttraumatic arthritis, inflammatory (rheumatoid or crystalline) arthritis, osteoarthritis, and septic arthritis (although septic arthritis typically presents acutely). Chronic pain resulting from inflammatory elbow arthritis may be either diffuse and poorly defined or localized to the area of greatest involvement. A patient with osteoarthritis of the elbow typically presents with pain at the extremes of motion in flexion and extension. Lateral elbow pain that is exacerbated by forearm rotation is probably caused by arthritis in the radiocapitellar articulation. These lateral symptoms are often the initial presentation of rheumatoid arthritis involving the elbow or of posttraumatic arthritis after a radial head fracture. Early morning pain and stiffness and pain with weather changes are common findings in patients with any type of arthritis. Loose bodies often develop in arthritic elbows and may produce catching or locking.

Localization of Pain

Lateral Elbow

Pain and tenderness localized to the lateral epicondyle and the common extensor origin of the forearm muscles extending from it indicate lateral epicondylitis. This condition is commonly referred to as tennis elbow, although many patients with lateral epicondylitis have no history of playing tennis. The pain of lateral epicondylitis is exacerbated by forearm supination and wrist extension against resistance. Asking the patient with lateral epicondylitis to pick up a chair with the forearm pronated (the chair test) will usually elicit pain, whereas the same maneuver in the supinated position will not. When the pain and tenderness are localized about 5 cm distal to the lateral epicondyle, entrapment of the posterior interosseous branch of the radial nerve (radial tunnel syndrome) might be present. Because this nerve compression syndrome typically produces pain without distal motor or sensory deficits, distinguishing it from lateral epicondylitis sometimes is difficult. In fact, some authors think the two conditions coexist in 5% of patients. Lateral ulnar collateral ligament insufficiency also may be a source of lateral elbow pain. Lateral collateral ligament tears have been reported following repeated corticosteroid injections in the elbow for lateral epicondylitis. The patient also may describe clicking or popping of the elbow and will be reluctant to fully extend the elbow, particularly with weight bearing or when pushing up from a chair.

Medial Elbow

Pain over the medial aspect of the elbow is most commonly the result of one of two conditions: ulnar nerve entrapment or medial epicondylitis (golfer's elbow). Ulnar nerve entrapment is associated with localized pain at the elbow, usually accompanied by numbness and tingling in the little finger and ulnar half of the ring finger that is exacerbated by tapping over the nerve in the ulnar groove. Patients with medial epicondylitis have pain and tenderness over and just lateral and distal to the medial epicondyle. This pain increases with wrist flexion or forearm pronation against resistance. Ulnar neuritis may complicate medial epicondylitis in up to 20% of patients. In the overhead throwing athlete with medial elbow pain, injury to the ulnar collateral ligament must be considered.

Posterior Elbow

Posterior elbow pain usually is associated with chronic olecranon bursitis. Overhead throwing athletes may develop painful spurs on the posteromedial olecranon secondary to repetitive valgus strain (medial collateral ligament insufficiency) on the elbow during the throwing motion. Tendinitis or even frank rupture of the triceps tendon sometimes develops in weight lifters.

Anterior Elbow

Anterior elbow pain occurring acutely and associated with tenderness, ecchymosis, and change in the contour of the biceps muscle indicates a distal biceps tendon rupture. Exceedingly rare in females, this rupture typically occurs in middle-aged men who also report weak supination (screwdriver motion) following a sudden jerking movement or heavy lifting. Chronic anterior elbow discomfort may represent chronic degeneration of the biceps tendon, arthritis, synovitis, or compression of the median nerve at the elbow (pronator syndrome).

Stiffness

Normal elbow flexion/extension is from 0° (arm held out straight) to 140° to 150° of flexion. Normal forearm rotation is

ELBOW AND FOREARM

SECTION 3

from 80° of pronation to 80° of supination. The elbow has a particular predisposition to develop stiffness with arthritis, trauma, or immobilization; however, mild loss of motion causes no significant disability because most daily activities, including bringing the hand to the mouth and performing other aspects of personal hygiene, are performed in an arc of motion from 30° to 130° of flexion and 50° of pronation and supination.

Physical Examination of the Elbow and Forearm

Inspection/Palpation

Anterior View

Inspect the elbow for swelling and ecchymosis. Measure the carrying angle (the angle made by the intersection of the axes of the humerus and the forearm) with the elbow extended and the forearm supinated. Note that the normal carrying angle is a cubitus valgus of 5° to 8°. Cubitus varus (reverse carrying angle) usually results from a malunion of a supracondylar fracture of the humerus.

The biceps brachii tendon can be easily palpated in the middle of the antecubital fossa, especially when the patient flexes the elbow against resistance with the forearm supinated as shown. Absence of this normally palpable tendon with associated tenderness and ecchymosis suggests a complete biceps tendon rupture.

Lateral View

Check for an effusion by inspecting and palpating the area in the center of the triangle bounded by the lateral epicondyle of the humerus, the tip of the olecranon, and the radial head. Confirm the position of the radial head by feeling it move with forearm pronation/supination.

Palpate the area over the radial head to check for pain and crepitus. These findings, along with limited forearm rotation, suggest a radial head fracture (if acute) or arthritis (if chronic). Tenderness to palpation just distal to the lateral epicondyle indicates lateral epicondylitis. Tenderness 5 cm distal to the lateral epicondyle that is localized deep to the extensor muscles suggests entrapment of the posterior interosseous branch of the radial nerve.

Medial View

Pain and tenderness immediately distal to the medial epicondyle suggest medial epicondylitis. The ulnar nerve lies in the ulnar groove just posterior to the medial epicondyle. Palpation and light percussion in this area may produce local pain and paresthesias in the medial forearm and ulnar two fingers (the Tinel sign), in association with ulnar nerve entrapment. Tenderness elicited with specific palpation of the sublime tubercle may indicate pathology involving the ulnar collateral ligament.

Posterior View

Inspect the area over the olecranon for focal swelling and palpate for tenderness to confirm the presence of olecranon bursitis. An olecranon fracture produces a broader area of swelling with ecchymosis and a possible skin abrasion at the point of impact. Palpate just above the olecranon to identify elbow effusion. A palpable defect, particularly with slight attempts by the patient to extend the elbow, may indicate a triceps brachii tear.

Range of Motion

Flexion and Extension: Zero Starting Position

Evaluate elbow flexion and extension with the arm comfortably at the side. Observe from the lateral side. Begin the examination with the patient's elbow straight. Young children commonly hyperextend the elbow by 10° to 15°, but adults show minimal, if any, elbow hyperextension. Normal elbow range of motion is from 0° to 140° to 150° of flexion. Mild flexion contractures are of little functional consequence, as most activities of daily living are accomplished in an arc of elbow flexion from 30° to 130°.

Limitation of motion may be expressed as either "The elbow flexes from 30° to 90°," or "The elbow has a flexion contracture of 30°, with further flexion to 90°."

Forearm Rotation

Forearm rotation, which includes both pronation and supination, is a composite motion occurring at the proximal and distal radioulnar joints, as well as the radiohumeral joint. Measure forearm rotation by stabilizing the arm against the chest wall and flexing the elbow to 90°. Begin with the extended thumb aligned with the humerus (**A**). Palpate the radial and ulnar styloid as the forearm is rotated to estimate pronation and supination. Ask the patient to grasp a pencil or similar object to facilitate visual estimation of forearm rotation.

Pronation is the position in which the palm is turned down (**B**), and supination is the position in which the palm is turned up (**C**). Normal pronation and supination is approximately 80° in each direction. Many activities of daily living are accomplished in an arc of motion between 50° pronation to 50° supination. A very restricted arc of forearm rotation may be of limited consequence if shoulder mobility is normal and if the forearm is ankylosed in a neutral position.

SECTION 3   ELBOW AND FOREARM

Muscle Testing

Resisted Flexion

Test the strength of the flexors of the elbow, primarily the biceps brachii muscle, by resisting the patient's maximum effort to flex the supinated forearm. Weakness will be present with biceps tendinitis or rupture, dysfunction of the musculocutaneous nerve, or a lesion involving the C5 and C6 nerve roots.

Resisted Extension

Test the strength of the extensors of the elbow, primarily the triceps brachii muscle, by resisting the patient's maximum effort to extend the elbow with the forearm in neutral position. Weakness will be present with triceps tendinitis or rupture, or a lesion involving the C7 or C8 nerve roots.

Resisted Supination

Test the strength of the forearm supinators, the most powerful of which is the biceps brachii muscle, by grasping the patient's distal forearm, supporting the elbow with your other hand, and resisting the patient's maximum effort to turn the palm up. Weakness will be evident with rupture or tendinitis of the biceps tendon at the elbow, subluxation of the biceps tendon at the shoulder, a lesion of the musculocutaneous nerve, or a lesion involving the C5 and C6 nerve roots. Patients with lateral epicondylitis also may experience pain with this maneuver.

Resisted Pronation

Test the strength of the forearm pronators, the most powerful of which is the pronator teres muscle, by grasping the patient's distal forearm, supporting the elbow with your other hand, and resisting the patient's maximum effort to turn the palm down. Weakness will be evident with rupture of the pronator origin from the medial epicondyle, fracture of the medial elbow, or lesions involving the median nerve or the C6 and C7 nerve roots. Patients with medial epicondylitis also may experience pain with this maneuver.

Resisted Wrist Flexion

Test the strength of the wrist flexors with the patient's arm at the side, forearm supported on a table, and elbow flexed 90°, with the wrist in flexion and the fingers extended. (This position eliminates wrist flexion activity by the finger flexors.) Ask the patient to keep the wrist flexed while you push the wrist into extension. Weakness will be evident with rupture of the muscle origin, fracture of the medial elbow, medial epicondylitis, or lesions involving the ulnar nerve (C8 and T1 nerve roots) or median nerve (C6 and C7 nerve roots).

Resisted Wrist Extension

Test the strength of the wrist extensors, the most powerful of which are the extensor carpi ulnaris and extensor carpi radialis brevis muscles, with the patient's arm at the side, forearm supported on a table, and elbow flexed 90°, with the wrist in extension and the fingers in flexion. (This eliminates wrist extension activity by the finger extensors.) Ask the patient to hold the wrist in extension as you push the wrist into flexion. Weakness will be evident with rupture of the extensor origin, fracture of the lateral elbow, lateral epicondylitis, or lesions involving the radial nerve or C6 to C8 nerve roots.

Arthritis of the Elbow

Definition

Arthritis of the elbow can result from numerous pathologic conditions. These include rheumatoid arthritis (RA), nonrheumatoid inflammatory arthritis (including gout and "pseudogout"), posttraumatic arthritis, osteoarthritis (OA) (**Figure 1**), and septic arthritis. RA is the most common cause of elbow joint destruction, which nearly always develops in patients with multiple joint involvement. Concomitant wrist and hand involvement occurs in 90% of patients with RA, with shoulder involvement in 80% of these patients. An active synovitis of the elbow causes periarticular erosions and symmetric joint narrowing, similar to the effect of synovitis in other joints. Further progression causes gross destruction of the bone and soft-tissue constraints. The end result is a grossly unstable elbow.

Nonrheumatoid inflammatory arthritis of the elbow generally presents as an acute crystalline synovitis (gout or pseudogout) with acute pain, swelling, stiffness, and warmth. This is often difficult to distinguish from septic arthritis. Long-standing degenerative changes of the elbow joint are unusual in these conditions.

Posttraumatic arthritis results from primary injury to the articular cartilage at the time of trauma, as well as fracture malunion. The end result is incongruity of the articular cartilage and progressive arthritis. Because posttraumatic arthritis often presents as an isolated joint impairment in an otherwise young

Figure 1 Radiographs demonstrate elbow arthritides. **A,** Lateral view of an elbow with radiographic changes typical of OA. **B,** Lateral view of an elbow showing erosive changes of bone typical of RA.

and active patient, treatment options and the patient's expectations are often quite different from those of patients with RA.

Because the elbow is not a weight-bearing joint, OA is not nearly as common in the elbow as it is in the hip, knee, or even the shoulder, and it may not be as symptomatic. Elbow OA most often is seen in manual laborers and weight lifters, suggesting repetitive overuse as an underlying cause. Repetitive overuse of the elbow also commonly causes intra-articular loose bodies that can promote joint degeneration.

Septic arthritis results from infection (bacterial or nonbacterial) within the elbow joint producing acute pain, swelling, loss of motion, and warmth. Septic arthritis is more common in patients with RA, HIV, and other immunocompromised states, as well as in intravenous drug abusers. Septic arthritis may lead to articular cartilage destruction and ultimately to joint degeneration.

Clinical Symptoms

RA of the elbow causes pain and swelling, as it does in other joints. In the early stages, the pain may be primarily localized to the lateral side of the joint and exacerbated by forearm rotation. Advanced disease causes diffuse pain and often gross instability that makes even light household tasks impossible.

Symptoms of nonrheumatoid inflammatory arthritis include acute pain, swelling, effusion, loss of motion, and warmth, mimicking septic arthritis.

The primary symptom reported by patients with posttraumatic arthritis is either pain or stiffness, depending on the type of injury. With malunion of a radial head fracture, the pain may be isolated to the lateral side of the joint and exacerbated by forearm rotation.

OA is characterized by pain and restricted motion. Intra-articular loose bodies are associated with symptoms of catching and locking. Posterior osteophytes typically cause limited extension and pain on terminal extension. Less commonly, anterior osteophytes can cause pain and limited flexion. Pain during midrange motion and at rest are symptoms of late disease. Osteophytes on the medial side of the elbow can cause ulnar nerve irritation.

Septic arthritis generally produces acute and severe pain, stiffness, warmth, swelling, and effusion, as well as constitutional symptoms of fever, chills, and malaise.

SECTION 3 ELBOW

Tests

Physical Examination

Inspection of the rheumatoid elbow demonstrates joint swelling, best seen laterally, and occasionally rheumatoid nodules over the olecranon and extensor surface of the forearm. Tenderness may occur primarily over the radial head or may be diffuse. Range of motion and varus/valgus stability also should be assessed.

An elbow with posttraumatic arthritis or OA typically does not have an effusion. The joint lines should be palpated for tenderness, and range of motion should be measured. Gently "jogging" the joint in full extension and then full flexion will elicit impingement pain from posterior and anterior osteophytes, respectively.

Synovitis resulting from nonrheumatoid inflammatory arthritis and septic arthritis typically produces severely painful range of motion, which is restricted. A significant effusion and warmth are usually present.

Diagnostic Tests

AP and lateral radiographs of the elbow often are sufficient for diagnosis. RA produces the typical picture of osteopenia, symmetric joint narrowing, and periarticular erosions, or it may show gross joint destruction. Malunion, nonunion, and joint space narrowing are possible findings in posttraumatic arthritis. With OA, radiographs reveal osteophytes and narrowing of the joint space. Multiple loose bodies may be present in the anterior and posterior portions of the elbow. With nonrheumatoid inflammatory arthritis and septic arthritis, radiographs are usually normal acutely.

If an effusion is present, aspiration of the joint fluid may be helpful. Fluid should be examined for white blood cell (WBC) count (to differentiate between inflammatory and noninflammatory arthritis), crystals (present with nonrheumatoid inflammatory arthritis), Gram stain, and culture.

Differential Diagnosis

- Fracture of the distal humerus (evident on radiographs)
- Fracture of the radial head (evident on radiographs)
- Osteochondritis dissecans of the elbow (typically affects adolescent boys, capitellum usually involved, seen with repetitive overuse, may produce loose bodies)

Adverse Outcomes of the Disease

Progressive pain and stiffness are common to all arthritic conditions. RA can lead to an unstable, essentially flail elbow. Septic arthritis left untreated may lead to rapid joint destruction and even osteomyelitis.

Treatment

Mild limitation of elbow motion does not interfere with daily activities and is well tolerated, so treatment is often unnecessary. Modification of job or sports activities can be very helpful when symptoms warrant.

For RA, medical management should be optimized (see page 45). Intra-articular corticosteroid injection and gentle rehabilitation may be of benefit. Static and hinged splints may be helpful for some patients. Synovectomy with or without radial head excision can provide pain relief in early stages of RA that is resistant to nonsurgical management. Total elbow arthroplasty is the best option for patients with RA who have advanced joint destruction.

Nonrheumatoid inflammatory arthritis is treated medically to address the underlying pathology (eg, gout or pseudogout). Intra-articular corticosteroid injections may be helpful in episodes of acute nonrheumatoid inflammatory synovitis.

For posttraumatic arthritis and OA, nonsurgical measures are limited to analgesics and gentle stretching to preserve motion. Arthroscopic débridement and removal of loose bodies can be quite helpful. Unless the patient is elderly with a very limited activity level, total elbow replacement generally is not considered beneficial because of concern about prosthesis loosening and breakage.

Prompt treatment of septic arthritis is critical and should specifically address the causal agent. Therapy generally involves a combination of appropriate antibiotics and surgical drainage.

Adverse Outcomes of Treatment

Patients with RA require regular monitoring for side effects from NSAIDs and disease-modifying agents. Nerve injury and infection are possible with surgery. Joint replacements can loosen or fracture with time.

Referral Decisions/Red Flags

Patients with persistent pain, locking episodes, or significant loss of motion require further evaluation. Septic arthritis usually requires a combined medical and surgical approach.

SECTION 3   ELBOW

Dislocation of the Elbow

Definition

The elbow is the most commonly dislocated joint in children; in adults, it is second only to the shoulder and finger. Typically, a dislocated elbow is the result of a fall on an outstretched hand. More than 80% of elbow dislocations are posterior; posterolateral dislocations are most common (**Figure 1**). A dislocation may be complete or "perched" (subluxated, with the trochlea resting on top of the coronoid process). The lateral collateral ligament is always disrupted, and other soft-tissue restraints commonly are injured as well. Concomitant fractures of the radial head/coronoid (in adults this is referred to as the "terrible triad") (**Figure 2**) or medial epicondyle (in children) may be present. Neurovascular structures such as the brachial artery, median nerve, and ulnar nerve also may be injured.

Clinical Symptoms

Extreme pain, swelling, and inability to bend the elbow after a fall on an outstretched hand are characteristics of a dislocated elbow.

Tests

Physical Examination

Note areas of abnormal prominence and tenderness. The most important part of the examination is the neurovascular evaluation. Check the radial pulse and capillary refill. Assess motor and sensory function of the median, radial, and ulnar nerves.

Figure 1 AP (**A**) and lateral (**B**) views demonstrate posterolateral dislocation of the elbow.

Figure 2 Lateral view of an elbow demonstrates the "terrible triad" of dislocation and fractures of the radial head and coronoid.

Diagnostic Tests

AP and lateral radiographs of the elbow are adequate to make a diagnosis. Look carefully for associated fractures and bony fragments incarcerated in the joint, as these may cause widening of the joint space. In the pediatric patient, a comparison radiograph of the contralateral elbow may help secure the diagnosis.

Differential Diagnosis

- Fracture-dislocation of the elbow (same deformity, evident on radiographs)
- Fracture of the distal humerus (evident on radiographs)
- Fracture of the olecranon process of the ulna (evident on radiographs)
- Hemarthrosis (positive fat pad sign)
- Occult fractures (positive fat pad sign)
- Synovitis (normal radiographs, no deformity)

Adverse Outcomes of the Disease

Persistent loss of motion is common, especially in extension. Although most simple dislocations (ie, without fractures) are stable after reduction, persistent or recurrent instability is possible and should be specifically addressed rather than treated with prolonged immobilization. Heterotopic bone formation and the development of arthritis of the elbow joint also are possible.

Treatment

Reduction of an elbow dislocation should be performed as soon as possible after injury. Because of the possibility of occult fractures and the potential for neurovascular complications, reduction of elbow dislocations ideally should be performed by an orthopaedic surgeon unless this would result in an unacceptable delay in treatment. Reduction usually can be accomplished in the emergency department with the patient under conscious sedation (see page 25). Sedation may be supplemented by aspirating the hemarthrosis and injecting 10 mL of 1% lidocaine into the joint from a lateral approach (**Figure 3**). If muscle spasm or marked swelling precludes reduction with the patient under conscious sedation, general anesthesia may be required.

Flexing the elbow tenses the triceps attachment to the olecranon and makes the reduction more difficult. The reduction should be performed by holding the elbow relatively extended (flexed about 45°) and applying slow, steady, downward traction on the forearm in line with the long axis of the humerus and

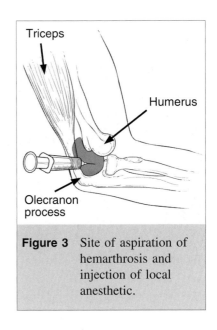

Figure 3 Site of aspiration of hemarthrosis and injection of local anesthetic.

then gently increasing flexion of the elbow. Gentle pressure over the olecranon tip as you are flexing the elbow also will help facilitate the reduction. The reduction usually is easily felt (a "clunk") and, once achieved, generally is most stable with the elbow flexed and the forearm pronated. The stability of the reduction should be tested by slowly extending the elbow until the beginning of some subluxation is felt. The arm should be splinted at 90° of flexion (but avoiding more than 100° of flexion, which may contribute to vascular compromise as swelling develops).

After reduction, the neurovascular examination must be repeated. After applying a splint, obtain AP, lateral, and oblique radiographs to confirm the reduction. Failure to obtain a perfectly concentric reduction suggests the possibility of a bony or cartilaginous intra-articular loose body or extensive soft-tissue injury, either of which may require surgical treatment.

Motion should begin 5 to 7 days after reduction and progress gradually during the next 3 to 6 weeks. A brace that blocks terminal extension is typically required during this time to maintain a concentric joint. The extension block may be removed at 3 to 4 weeks, with the aim of achieving full extension of the elbow 6 to 8 weeks after the dislocation, at which time the brace may be discontinued. At all times, radiographs must demonstrate a concentric reduction; if there is any concern, immediate referral is necessary. NSAIDs can be useful during this period and may decrease the incidence of heterotopic bone formation.

Adverse Outcomes of Treatment

Fracture and neurovascular injury are possible during the reduction maneuver. The ulnar nerve, because of its proximity, may become entrapped in the elbow joint. Subsequent vascular problems may result from compressive bandages or splinting in more than 100° of elbow flexion. Prolonged immobilization leads to elbow contracture and pain and at the same time may not correct the underlying instability. Failure to identify and address persistent instability may lead to the difficult situation of chronic instability. Chronic instability (especially chronic posterolateral rotatory instability of the elbow) is unusual; it may require surgical reconstruction.

Referral Decisions/Red Flags

Patients with associated neurovascular or bony injury (radial head/coronoid) require further evaluation, although a gentle reduction may be attempted to avoid lengthy delays. Incomplete reduction, as shown on radiographs, should never be accepted but should be referred immediately (**Figure 4**). Patients with a flexion contracture that prevents functional activities of daily living may require further evaluation.

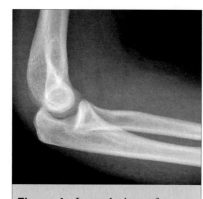

Figure 4 Lateral view of an elbow with an incomplete reduction.

Fracture of the Distal Humerus

Fracture Patterns

- Supracondylar fracture
- Transcondylar fracture
- Intercondylar fracture
- T condylar fracture
- Lateral/medial condylar fracture

Definition

Fractures of the distal humerus are relatively uncommon, accounting for only 2% of fractures in adults. Because these fractures are often comminuted and intra-articular, the potential morbidity is high. Classification schemes used for these fractures can be quite complex, but the most important factors to consider in deciding on the best course for initial treatment are whether the fracture is displaced (**Figures 1** and **2**), whether the fracture involves the joint surface, and whether the skin and neurovascular structures are involved.

ICD-9 Codes
812.0 Fracture of humerus, upper end, closed
812.1 Fracture of humerus, upper end, open
812.2 Fracture of humerus, shaft, closed
812.3 Fracture of humerus, unspecified
812.40 Fracture of humerus, lower end, closed, unspecified part
812.5 Fracture of humerus, lower end, open

Figure 1 AP radiograph of elbow demonstrates displaced supracondylar fracture. (Reproduced with permission from Beaty JH, Kasser JR: Fractures about the elbow. *Instr Course Lect* 1995;44: 199-215.)

A   B

Figure 2 **A,** Nondisplaced T condylar fracture of the distal humerus. **B,** Displaced intercondylar fracture of the distal humerus. (Adapted from Mehne DK, Jupiter JB: Fractures of the distal humerus, in Browner BD, Jupiter JB, Levine AM, et al, eds: *Skeletal Trauma: Fractures, Dislocations, Ligamentous Injuries.* Philadelphia, PA, WB Saunders, 1992, pp 1146-1176.)

SECTION 3   ELBOW

Clinical Symptoms

Marked swelling, ecchymosis, deformity, and pain about the elbow after an injury are common. Patients report increased pain with attempted flexion of the elbow.

Tests

Physical Examination

Swelling and deformity usually are clearly visible with any displaced fracture. Inspect the skin around the site to identify any open wounds. Palpation around the joint may reveal an effusion, and crepitus may be felt with gentle flexion. Palpate the radial pulse and check capillary refill. Assess median, radial, and ulnar nerve function. Any of the peripheral nerves crossing the fracture may be injured, but ulnar nerve dysfunction is most common. Brachial artery occlusion is less common but requires early diagnosis and treatment to avoid devastating complications. Check the wrist and shoulder on the affected side for associated injuries.

Diagnostic Tests

AP and lateral radiographs of the elbow, as well as other radiographic views as clinically indicated, are adequate in most patients. Without radiographic evidence of fracture, look carefully for a fat pad sign indicative of bleeding into the joint, often from an occult fracture (**Figure 3**). In the pediatric patient, comparison views may help differentiate a true fracture from a growth plate. CT may be necessary to fully define the extent of the fracture.

Differential Diagnosis

- Elbow dislocation (evident on radiographs)
- Olecranon fracture (evident on radiographs)
- Radial head fracture (evident on radiographs)
- Rupture of the distal biceps tendon (radiographs negative)

Adverse Outcomes of the Disease

Unfortunately, some degree of residual pain and stiffness is common. Other complications include deformity with malunion, nonunion, and ulnar neuropathy. Vascular injury may lead to ischemia in the forearm and hand or to compartment syndrome of the forearm muscle compartments (see page 58). Prompt treatment is required to salvage function.

Figure 3 Lateral radiograph of elbow. Note the anterior and posterior fat pad signs (arrows).

Treatment

The goal of treatment is to achieve and maintain a stable reduction that permits early motion. Stable, nondisplaced fractures may be treated with splinting for 10 days, followed by protected range of motion. Unfortunately, most distal humerus fractures are displaced to some degree, requiring open reduction and internal fixation. Other techniques, such as hinged external fixation or primary total elbow replacement, might be considered under circumstances such as severe osteoporosis and/or fracture comminution.

Adverse Outcomes of Treatment

Pain and stiffness may persist after treatment. Deformity, nonunion, arthritis, and ulnar neuropathy may develop, as well as symptoms related to the prominent implants used for internal fixation. Infection, nerve damage, or hardware failure may complicate surgery.

Referral Decisions/Red Flags

Patients with displaced or open fractures of the distal humerus need further evaluation to determine whether surgical stabilization of the fracture is necessary. Likewise, patients with associated neurovascular injury need further evaluation.

Patients treated nonsurgically require close follow-up for complications such as fracture displacement and joint stiffness. Delayed vascular compromise may occur because of progressive swelling and/or tight splinting. Failure to regain motion is also an indication for referral.

SECTION 3 ELBOW

Fracture of the Olecranon

ICD-9 Code

813.01
Fracture of olecranon process
of ulna

Definition

The olecranon is the portion of the ulna that constitutes the bony prominence of the posterior elbow. Because of its subcutaneous location, the olecranon is easily fractured as a result of a direct blow to the elbow or a fall on an outstretched hand with the elbow flexed. As with other fractures, the most important consideration is determining whether the fracture is displaced or nondisplaced. Most of these fractures are displaced and can be further classified as noncomminuted or comminuted fractures of the olecranon or fracture-dislocations of the elbow (**Figure 1**).

Clinical Symptoms

A history of trauma followed by marked swelling and ecchymosis is typical. When an associated dislocation is present, the elbow will appear deformed as well. Because of the close proximity of the ulnar nerve, the trauma itself or the resultant swelling may compress the nerve and cause numbness in the little and ring fingers.

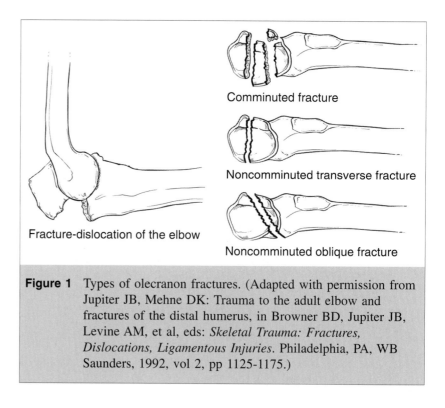

Comminuted fracture

Noncomminuted transverse fracture

Fracture-dislocation of the elbow

Noncomminuted oblique fracture

Figure 1 Types of olecranon fractures. (Adapted with permission from Jupiter JB, Mehne DK: Trauma to the adult elbow and fractures of the distal humerus, in Browner BD, Jupiter JB, Levine AM, et al, eds: *Skeletal Trauma: Fractures, Dislocations, Ligamentous Injuries.* Philadelphia, PA, WB Saunders, 1992, vol 2, pp 1125-1175.)

SECTION 3 ELBOW

Tests

Physical Examination

Examination usually reveals marked swelling of the entire elbow joint. Superficial abrasions at the site of impact are common and must be distinguished from deep wounds, which would make the injury an open fracture. Gentle palpation may reveal a defect if the fracture is displaced. Flexion of the elbow produces pain and is met with resistance. Median, radial, and ulnar nerve function should be assessed; of these, ulnar nerve injury is the most common. Radial and ulnar pulses and capillary refill should be assessed, but significant vascular injury is uncommon with this fracture.

Diagnostic Tests

AP and lateral radiographs usually are adequate to confirm the diagnosis (**Figure 2**).

Differential Diagnosis

- Dislocation of the elbow (more grotesque deformity, evident on radiographs)
- Fracture of the coronoid process of the olecranon (nearly always associated with an elbow dislocation)
- Fracture of the distal humerus (more proximal area of pain, evident on radiographs)
- Fracture of the radial head (lateral elbow pain increases with forearm rotation, fracture may be difficult to see on radiographs)

Figure 2 Lateral radiograph of an elbow demonstrates an olecranon fracture.

Adverse Outcomes of the Disease

Loss of motion and/or stability in the elbow is possible. Because the triceps inserts on the tip of the olecranon, active elbow extension may be lost with displaced fractures. Arthritis of the elbow may develop.

Treatment

Nondisplaced fractures of the olecranon may be treated with a posterior splint. To avoid excessive pull on the triceps and possible loss of reduction, splint the elbow in approximately 45° of flexion. Follow-up radiographs should be obtained 7 to 10 days after the injury to ensure that the fracture has not become displaced. To avoid significant permanent loss of motion, protected motion should begin within 2 to 3 weeks. To maintain hand strength and flexibility, instruct patients to squeeze a rubber ball or commercially available hand exerciser for 5 minutes at least twice each day.

SECTION 3 ELBOW

Most olecranon fractures are displaced and are best treated surgically. Occasionally, a displaced fracture in a debilitated elderly patient who is a poor risk for surgery may be treated with a sling and early range-of-motion exercises, as pain allows.

Adverse Outcomes of Treatment

Elbow stiffness, loss of motion, or arthritis may develop despite treatment. Nonunion or displacement of the fracture due to hardware failure is possible. After surgical treatment, irritation from the implants used to fix the fracture commonly occurs, necessitating a second procedure for implant removal.

Referral Decisions/Red Flags

Patients with displaced fractures or open fractures need further evaluation for possible surgical treatment.

Fracture of the Radial Head

Definition

Fractures of the radial head and neck result from falls on an outstretched hand. The most commonly used classification system, the modified Mason classification, separates these fractures into three types (**Figure 1**). Type I is a nondisplaced or minimally displaced fracture. Type II includes radial head fractures that are displaced more than 2 mm at the articular surface and angulated neck fractures that produce articular incongruity or a mechanical block. Type III fractures are severely comminuted fractures of the radial head and neck.

ICD-9 Codes

813.05
Fracture of head of radius

813.06
Fracture of neck of radius

Clinical Symptoms

Following a fall on the outstretched hand, pain and swelling develop over the lateral aspect of the elbow. Loss of elbow motion may be related to pain inhibition and joint effusion, but a mechanical block to full forearm pronation and supination may be present in type II and III injuries. Radial head fractures also may be present in the context of an elbow dislocation ("terrible triad" injury). Rarely, the radial head fracture may be associated with an injury of the forearm (called an Essex-Lopresti fracture), and the forearm and wrist should be assessed.

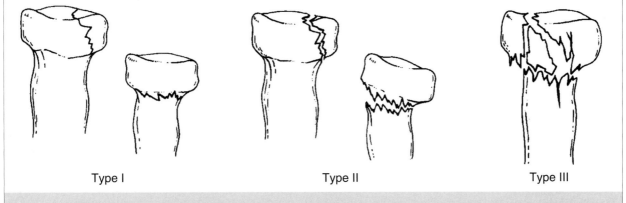

Type I   Type II   Type III

Figure 1   Modified Mason classification of radial head fractures. (Adapted with permission from Jupiter JB, Mehne DK: Trauma to the adult elbow and fractures of the distal humerus, in Browner BD, Jupiter JB, Levine AM, et al, eds: *Skeletal Trauma: Fractures, Dislocations, Ligamentous Injuries.* Philadelphia, PA, WB Saunders, 1992, vol 2, pp 1125-1175.)

SECTION 3   ELBOW

Tests

Physical Examination

Tenderness to palpation is localized to the lateral aspect of the joint, and a joint effusion can often be palpated. Passive forearm rotation is limited and may be associated with palpable crepitus. Elbow flexion and extension also may be limited by pain.

Tenderness over the forearm and/or wrist may signify a more extensive soft-tissue injury involving the radioulnar interosseous membrane and the distal radioulnar joint. Presence of this type of injury makes treatment more difficult. Medial elbow tenderness and ecchymosis also may be present, signifying a medial collateral ligament strain or tear.

Diagnostic Tests

Type I fractures may be difficult to visualize radiographically but should be suspected based on positive clinical findings. Type II and III fractures are usually obvious on AP and lateral radiographs. CT is occasionally necessary to define the extent of the fracture.

Differential Diagnosis

- Elbow dislocation (clinical deformity and diffuse pain)
- Hemarthrosis of the elbow (present with radial head fracture or with other bony or soft-tissue injury)
- Olecranon fracture (pain and tenderness over the posterior tip of the elbow)
- Supracondylar fracture of the humerus (location of pain, tenderness, and deformity)

Adverse Outcomes of the Disease

Loss of motion, especially the last 10° to 15° of extension, is common, even with type I injuries. Posttraumatic arthritis of the radiocapitellar joint also may develop.

Treatment

Type I fractures should be treated with a sling or splint for comfort and early active motion as soon as pain allows. Because early motion is the key to a successful outcome, aspiration of the associated elbow hemarthrosis may be considered.

Aspiration with local anesthetic injection is useful diagnostically in type II fractures to determine whether a mechanical block to forearm rotation is present. When the fracture involves less than 2 mm articular step-off of a partial articular segment and no block to rotation, treatment should consist of early range of motion, as in type I fractures.

Otherwise, open reduction and internal fixation is preferred. Open reduction and internal fixation of the radial head is most effective when there are three or fewer articular segments. More complex fractures are more amenable to prosthetic replacement.

Type III fractures usually are best treated by early open reduction and internal fixation of the bone fragments or radial head replacement. When associated injuries of the ulnar collateral ligament or the interosseous membrane are present, excision alone of the fragments is contraindicated, as this could lead to persistent elbow instability.

Adverse Outcomes of Treatment

Loss of motion, instability, and wrist pain caused by proximal radial migration after radial head excision can all occur. Infection, nerve damage, hardware failure, malunion, loss of motion, and arthritis are possible following surgical intervention.

Referral Decisions/Red Flags

Type II fractures that block rotation, type III fractures, and any fracture associated with elbow dislocation or instability should be referred for surgical consideration. Failure of nonsurgical treatment, manifested by persistent pain or limited motion, also indicates the need for further evaluation.

SECTION 3 ELBOW

Lateral and Medial Epicondylitis

Synonyms

Lateral epicondylitis:

    Lateral tendinosis of the elbow

    Tennis elbow

Medial epicondylitis:

    Golfer's or bowler's elbow

    Medial tendinosis of the elbow

Definition

Lateral epicondylitis and tennis elbow are the terms most commonly used to describe a condition that produces pain and tenderness at the site of origin of the extensor carpi radialis brevis muscle (lateral epicondyle of the humerus). Although the term *epicondylitis* is commonly used, the pathology and point of maximal pain are in the tendon substance just distal and slightly anterior to the epicondyle (**Figure 1**). The term *elbow tendinitis* also is inaccurate because it implies an inflammatory origin. In fact, the histologic pattern of lateral epicondylitis is one of tissue degeneration with fibroblast and microvascular hyperplasia and the absence of inflammation. The term *lateral tendinosis* of the elbow is probably the most accurate but rarely is used.

Medial epicondylitis (also called golfer's or bowler's elbow) is similar to lateral epicondylitis in etiology and pathology and occurs in the common tendinous origin of the flexor/pronator muscles just distal to the medial epicondyle. Medial epicondylitis is much less commonly encountered than lateral epicondylitis.

Figure 1   Location of pain in lateral epicondylitis.

Clinical Symptoms

The typical patient with lateral epicondylitis is between 35 and 50 years of age and reports a gradual onset of pain in the lateral elbow and forearm during activities involving gripping and wrist extension, such as lifting, turning a screwdriver, or hitting a backhand in tennis. With time, the pain may become more severe and may occur at rest or during activities as minimal as holding a cup of coffee or using a key. Less commonly, the patient may relate the onset of symptoms to an acute event, such as a direct blow to the elbow or a sudden maximal muscle contraction.

The pain of medial epicondylitis typically occurs with active wrist flexion and forearm pronation, such as takes place in a golf swing, baseball pitching, the pull-through strokes of swimming, weight lifting, bowling, and many forms of manual labor.

Tests

Physical Examination

The most consistent finding in lateral epicondylitis is localized tenderness over the common extensor origin 1 cm distal and slightly anterior to the lateral epicondyle (**Figure 2**). During the examination, it is best to have the patient's elbow flexed to 90° and the forearm pronated. Tapping lightly on the lateral epicondyle may be painful. Pain in the region also may be produced by gripping with resisted extension of the wrist when the elbow is in extension. To help differentiate lateral epicondylitis from other painful elbow conditions, ask the patient to lift a stool or chair with the palm up (using the wrist flexors) and then the palm down (using the wrist extensors). Patients with lateral epicondylitis will have pain when lifting with the palm down.

With medial epicondylitis, the area of tenderness is just distal to the medial epicondyle, and the pain is exacerbated by pronating the forearm and flexing the wrist against resistance. These patients also may have pain when lifting a chair with the palm up.

Diagnostic Tests

AP and lateral radiographs of the elbow are necessary to rule out arthritis or osteochondral loose bodies. Rarely, an area of calcification may be seen at the attachment of the extensor

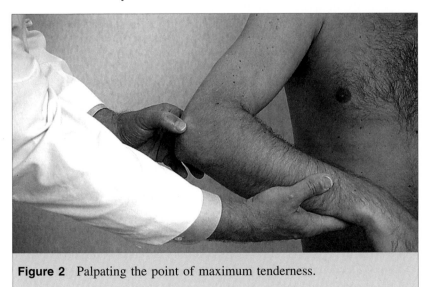

Figure 2 Palpating the point of maximum tenderness.

SECTION 3   ELBOW

muscles to the lateral epicondyle or the flexor/pronator mass to the medial epicondyle of the humerus. MRI is helpful in confirming the diagnosis and severity, but it is rarely helpful in predicting treatment outcome.

Differential Diagnosis

- Cubital tunnel syndrome (compression of the ulnar nerve, paresthesias in little and ring fingers)
- Fracture of the radial head (radiographs should differentiate; pain and tenderness over the radial head that are exacerbated by passive pronation and supination)
- Lateral plica (patient describes locking episodes and loss of elbow extension)
- Osteoarthritis of the radiocapitellar portion of the elbow joint (radiographs should differentiate; similar examination to radial head fracture but without a history of acute trauma)
- Osteochondral loose body (medial or lateral joint line pain, symptoms of locking)
- Radial tunnel syndrome (compression of the posterior interosseous nerve, tenderness typically approximately 5 cm distal to lateral epicondyle)
- Synovitis of the elbow (swelling, palpable effusion)
- Triceps tendinitis (tenderness above the olecranon)

Adverse Outcomes of the Disease

Persistent pain is the most common problem. Weakness or poor endurance with motions that involve forceful wrist flexion/extension or forearm pronation/supination, such as heavy or repetitive lifting, also is common. Inability to participate optimally in sport is common. Rupture of the flexor/pronator mass or the extensor mass from the respective epicondyle is seen occasionally.

Treatment

Modifying or eliminating the activities that cause symptoms is the most important step in treatment. In the case of tennis-related epicondylitis, this may include changing to a lighter-weight tennis racket, changing the tension of the racket strings, or overwrapping the handle to make it slightly larger or using a racket with a larger grip. For patients with severe and long-standing conditions, this activity modification may have to be permanent. NSAIDs and rub-in anti-inflammatory creams may be helpful during acute exacerbations. Use of a commercial tennis elbow strap worn just below the elbow during heavy-lifting activities may be helpful as well. Application of heat or ice may relieve pain and inflammation. Once the pain has decreased, gentle stretching and forearm strengthening exercises can be initiated and are the key to successful treatment. Referral to a rehabilitation specialist is recommended if pain persists after 3 to 4 weeks.

If symptoms persist, corticosteroid injection into the area of maximum tenderness may be helpful in lateral or medial epicondylitis (see pages 377-378). Advise patients that they might experience an increase in pain for 1 to 2 days after the injection. No more than three injections should be given. If the pain recurs and symptoms are severe, surgery (typically involving débridement of the area of tendinosis) can be considered. More than 95% of cases of lateral epicondylitis and 85% of cases of medial epicondylitis will heal with nonsurgical treatment.

Rehabilitation Prescription

Treatment of the patient with humeral epicondylitis has four stages: (1) reduction of overload, pain, and inflammation; (2) promotion of total arm strength; (3) return to limited activities (those that are pain free); and (4) maintenance.

A home exercise program includes the use of ice following early attempts at exercise or unavoidable daily activities. Early submaximal exercise is initiated as signs and symptoms allow; for example, patient tolerance to a firm handshake is a criterion for determining whether a patient is ready for early exercise. Early use of submaximal isometrics such as squeezing a ball and manual resistive exercises for the wrist flexors, extensors, pronators, and supinators is advocated. The early goal of the home program is to promote muscle endurance and improve resistance to repetitive stress. To accomplish this goal, high repetitions per set with extremely low or no resistance are used. This promotes local muscle endurance and provides a vascular response to the exercising tissues.

If the pain persists after the patient has been on the home program for 3 to 4 weeks, formal rehabilitation may be initiated. The orders should include a thorough evaluation of muscle strength, pain, and joint mobility. No single pain-relieving modality has been found to be most effective for all patients. The rehabilitation specialist should determine the most effective modality for the individual patient based on patient tolerance and response.

Adverse Outcomes of Treatment

NSAIDs may cause gastric, renal, or hepatic complications. Although surgery always carries a small risk of complications, such as wound infection or nerve injury, the most common

SECTION 3 ELBOW

adverse outcome is incomplete pain relief despite adequate surgical release. Surgical failure may result from misdiagnosis, especially in cases involving nerve entrapment syndromes (with lateral epicondylitis, the posterior interosseous nerve; with medial epicondylitis, the ulnar nerve). Returning to work activities that were related to the onset of symptoms may be unlikely because of recurrence of symptoms or issues of secondary gain.

Referral Decisions/Red Flags

Failure of nonsurgical management indicates the need for further evaluation.

Home Exercise Program for Epicondylitis and Radial Tunnel Syndrome

- Perform the exercises in the order listed.
- To prevent inflammation, apply ice, such as a bag of crushed ice or frozen peas, to the painful area of the elbow for 20 minutes after performing the exercises.
- If you are unable to add weight or perform the indicated number of repetitions because of pain, call your doctor.

Exercise Type	Muscle Group	Number of Repetitions/Sets	Number of Days per Week	Number of Weeks
Wrist flexion (stretching)	Wrist extensor muscle group	Hold for 30 seconds; repeat 3 times. Perform on both sides.	5 to 7	3 to 4
Wrist extension (stretching)	Wrist flexor muscle group	Hold for 30 seconds; repeat 3 times. Perform on both sides.	5 to 7	3 to 4
Elbow extension	Elbow extensor muscle group	Work up to 5 sets of 10 repetitions, 2 or 3 times a day	5 to 7	3 to 4
Wrist flexion and extension	Wrist flexor and extensor muscle groups	Work up to 3 sets of 10 repetitions, 1 or 2 times a day	5 to 7	3 to 4
Forearm supination and pronation	Supinator and pronator teres	Work up to 3 sets of 10 repetitions, 1 or 2 times a day	5 to 7	3 to 4

Wrist Flexion (Stretching)

- To stretch the wrist flexors, extend the arm and hand as if signaling someone to "stop."
- Use the opposite hand to apply gentle pressure across the palm and pull it as far toward the body as it will comfortably go, keeping the arm straight. Hold for 10 to 15 seconds.
- Repeat 3 times.
- Perform on both sides, 5 to 7 days per week, for 3 to 4 weeks.

Wrist Extension (Stretching)

- To stretch the wrist extensors, extend the arm and hand out and flex the wrist so that the fingers are pointing down.
- Use the opposite hand to gently pull the hand as far toward the body as it will comfortably go, keeping the arm straight. Hold for 10 to 15 seconds.
- Repeat 3 times.
- Perform on both sides, 5 to 7 days per week, for 3 to 4 weeks.

SECTION 3 ELBOW

Elbow Extension

- Perform this exercise either standing with your weight evenly distributed over both feet or sitting.
- Holding a light weight in the hand of the injured arm, raise the arm overhead while supporting the elbow with the opposite hand.
- Straighten the elbow overhead, hold for 5 seconds, and then bend the elbow and relax.
- Work up to 5 sets of 10 repetitions, 2 or 3 times per day.
- Perform the exercise 5 to 7 days per week, for 3 to 4 weeks.

Caution: If you do not have adequate triceps strength, do not raise the weight over your head. Bend at the waist with the elbow bent to 90°. Extend your arm back and hold this position for 5 seconds. Then bend the elbow and relax.

Wrist Flexion and Extension

- To exercise the wrist flexors, rest the forearm on a hard surface with the palm up.
- Flex the wrist as shown.
- Work up to 3 sets of 10 repetitions, 1 or 2 times per day.
- To exercise the wrist extensors, rest the forearm on a hard surface with the hand extending over the side.
- Extend the wrist as shown.
- Work up to 3 sets of 10 repetitions, 1 or 2 times per day.
- Perform the exercise 5 to 7 days per week, for 3 to 4 weeks.

Note: Use no weight initially; add weight in 1-pound increments to a maximum of 5 pounds. Always start with the elbow positioned in 90° of flexion to minimize pain with the exercises. Over time, as the pain subsides, the exercises may be performed with the elbow more extended.

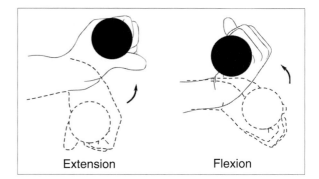

Extension   Flexion

Forearm Supination and Pronation

- Hold the forearm parallel to the ground, with the elbow bent 90°.
- To exercise the forearm supinators, pronate the forearm and then return to vertical as shown.
- Work up to 3 sets of 10 repetitions, 1 or 2 times per day.
- To exercise the forearm pronators, supinate the forearm and then return to vertical as shown.
- Work up to 3 sets of 10 repetitions, 1 or 2 times per day.
- Perform the exercise 5 to 7 days per week, for 3 to 4 weeks.

Note: Use no weight initially; add weight in 1-pound increments to a maximum of 5 pounds.

Supination   Pronation

Procedure: Tennis Elbow Injection

The classic tender spot in lateral epicondylitis of the elbow (tennis elbow) is just distal to the lateral epicondyle of the humerus with the elbow in 90° of flexion.

Note: Opinions differ regarding single- versus two-needle injection techniques. A two-needle technique is shown on the DVD.

Step 1

Wear protective gloves at all times during this procedure and use sterile technique.

Step 2

Place the patient's arm against the chest or abdomen, with the elbow flexed at least 90° and the forearm fully pronated.

Step 3

Prepare the skin with a bactericidal solution.

Step 4

Palpate just distal to the lateral epicondyle and locate the point of maximal tenderness. At this point, insert the 25-gauge needle, make a subcutaneous skin wheal with the local anesthetic, and advance through the tendon of the extensor carpi radialis brevis muscle to inject the remaining 2 to 3 mL of local anesthetic (**Figure 1**).

CPT Codes

20550
Injection(s); single tendon sheath, or ligament, aponeurosis (eg, plantar "fascia")

20551
Injection(s); single tendon origin/insertion

Current Procedural Terminology © 2010 American Medical Association. All rights reserved.

Materials

- Sterile gloves
- Bactericidal skin preparation solution
- 5-mL syringe with a 25-gauge, 1¼″ needle
- 3 to 4 mL of a 1% lidocaine solution without epinephrine
- 2-mL syringe
- 1 mL of a corticosteroid preparation
- Adhesive bandage

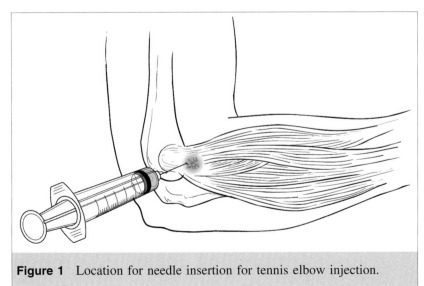

Figure 1 Location for needle insertion for tennis elbow injection.

SECTION 3 ELBOW

Step 5

Exchange syringes on the needle and inject the corticosteroid preparation. The syringe can again be exchanged and local anesthetic injected as the needle is withdrawn to avoid steroid deposition subcutaneously. This reduces the risk of depigmentation in dark-skinned patients or fat atrophy.

Step 6

Dress the puncture site with a sterile adhesive bandage.

Adverse Outcomes

Subcutaneous infiltration of the corticosteroid preparation may cause subcutaneous fat atrophy, leading to a waxy-appearing depression in the skin, and may cause depigmentation in dark-skinned patients. Although rare, infection is possible. Between 25% and 33% of patients will experience a "flare," characterized by increased pain at the injection site.

Aftercare/Patient Instructions

Advise the patient that pain may increase for 24 to 48 hours after the injection. Pain often improves with the application of ice. Acetaminophen or an NSAID also is beneficial.

SECTION 3 ELBOW

Olecranon Bursitis

Definition

Because of its superficial location on the extensor side of the elbow, the olecranon bursa is easily irritated and inflamed (**Figure 1**). Olecranon bursitis may occur secondary to trauma, inflammation, or infection. Falls or direct blows may cause an acute inflammatory bursitis. Prolonged irritation from excessive leaning on the elbow, often associated with certain occupations and avocations, may result in chronic inflammation. Olecranon bursitis also may develop in patients with chronic lung disease who lean on their elbows to aid breathing. The condition may be caused by systemic inflammatory processes, such as rheumatoid arthritis, gout, chondrocalcinosis, or hydroxyapatite crystal deposition. Infection of the olecranon bursa (septic bursitis) may occur primarily or develop as a secondary complication of aseptic bursitis.

ICD-9 Code
726.33 Olecranon bursitis

Clinical Symptoms

The swelling associated with bursitis may develop either gradually (chronic) or suddenly (infection or trauma). Pain is variable but may be intense, and it may limit motion after an acute injury or when infection is present. Such severe swelling of the bursa may occur that patients report difficulty putting on long-sleeved shirts. As the mass diminishes in size, patients may feel firm "lumps" that are tender when the elbow is bumped. These lumps or nodules are scar tissue left as the fluid recedes.

Olecranon bursitis also occurs in patients with gout or rheumatoid arthritis. Gouty tophi (masses of monosodium urate crystals) may form in the olecranon bursa as well as along the ulnar border of the forearm, in the synovium of the elbow joint, and in numerous distant locations. Tophi are found only in patients with fairly advanced gout. As with gout, rheumatoid nodules may appear in several subcutaneous locations, such as over the olecranon and the ulnar border of the forearm. With time, these nodules may spontaneously shrink or disappear.

Figure 1 Swollen olecranon bursa. (Adapted with permission from Jupiter JB, Mehne DK: Trauma to the adult elbow and fractures of the distal humerus, in Browner BD, Jupiter JB, Levine AM, et al, eds: *Skeletal Trauma: Fractures, Dislocations, Ligamentous Injuries*. Philadelphia, PA, WB Saunders, 1992, vol 2, pp 1125-1175.)

Tests

Physical Examination

Examination may reveal a large mass, up to 6 cm in diameter, over the tip of the elbow. The skin might be abraded or even lacerated if related to trauma. Redness and heat are not uncommon with acute bursitis and could indicate infection.

Exquisite tenderness usually results from an infectious or traumatic origin. Chronic, recurrent swelling usually is less tender. The dimensions of the bursa should be measured periodically to monitor progress.

Diagnostic Tests

For large, symptomatic masses, aspiration may be both diagnostic and therapeutic (see pages 382-383). After an acute injury, bloody fluid may be found. Fluid aspirated from the bursa should be analyzed for WBC count, crystals, Gram stain, and culture. The index of suspicion for infection should be high because about 20% of cases of acute bursitis have a septic cause, involving either primary or secondary infection. When the origin is traumatic, radiographs should be obtained to rule out a fracture of the olecranon process of the ulna.

Differential Diagnosis

- Fracture of the olecranon process of the ulna (evident on radiographs)
- Gouty tophus or rheumatoid nodule (a tophus or nodule generally will be smaller and more discrete than an inflamed olecranon bursa)

Adverse Outcomes of the Disease

Secondary infection, chronic recurrence or drainage, and swelling or limited motion may develop.

Treatment

If the mass is small and symptoms are mild, the bursitis should be left alone or treated symptomatically with activity modifications and possibly NSAIDs. Wearing an elbow pad and avoiding hyperflexion against hard surfaces may improve symptoms. Patients with more symptomatic bursitis should undergo aspiration of the bursa, followed by Gram stain and culture of any suspicious fluid. If there is no indication of septic bursitis, a compression bandage consisting of an 8-cm-diameter circular piece of foam and an elastic wrap should be applied. Reassess the patient in 2 to 7 days. If cultures are negative and fluid has reaccumulated in the bursa, repeat the aspiration and, if the fluid remains sterile, inject 1 mL of a corticosteroid preparation into the sac. The bursal sac may have to be aspirated two or more times. If the elbow is at risk for repeated trauma, recommend an elbow protector.

Septic olecranon bursitis requires organism-specific antibiotic coverage based on the culture and sensitivity of the aspirate (frequently involving coverage for penicillin-resistant

Staphylococcus aureus) and decompression by either surgical drainage or daily aspiration. Oral antibiotics may be administered if the septic bursitis is treated early and the patient is not immunocompromised. Hospitalization with intravenous antibiotics and surgical drainage and irrigation is indicated if the patient does not respond to oral antibiotics or if the patient has a more serious infection.

Excision of chronically inflamed aseptic bursitis is not commonly necessary and should be avoided because a chronically draining or infected sinus may develop.

Adverse Outcomes of Treatment

Secondary infection, chronic drainage, or recurrence is possible.

Referral Decisions/Red Flags

Septic bursitis or recurrence of fluid despite repeated (three or more) aspirations indicates the need for further evaluation.

SECTION 3 ELBOW

Procedure: Olecranon Bursa Aspiration

The olecranon bursa lies on the extensor aspect of the elbow, over the olecranon process of the ulna. The ulnar nerve lies adjacent to the medial face of the olecranon, behind the ulnar groove of the distal humerus. For this reason, aspiration is best done from the lateral side.

Step 1

Wear protective gloves at all times during this procedure and use sterile technique. This is important in aspirating an olecranon bursa because secondary infection may develop.

Step 2

Prepare the skin with a bactericidal solution.

Step 3

Use a 27-gauge needle to infiltrate the skin over the lateral aspect of the bursa with 1 mL of 1% lidocaine.

Step 4

Through the skin wheal, insert the 18-gauge needle attached to the 10-mL syringe into the enlarged bursa (**Figure 1**). Aspirate the contents until the bursa is flat. If there is any concern about infection, send the fluid for culture and sensitivity and do not inject the corticosteroid preparation into the cavity.

CPT Code

20605
Arthrocentesis, aspiration and/or injection; intermediate joint or bursa (eg, temporomandibular, acromioclavicular, wrist, elbow or ankle, olecranon bursa)

Current Procedural Terminology © 2010 American Medical Association. All rights reserved.

Materials

- Sterile gloves
- Bactericidal skin preparation solution
- Two 1-mL syringes
- 27-gauge, ¾" needle
- 1 mL of 1% lidocaine without epinephrine
- 10-mL syringe
- 18-gauge needle
- 1 mL of a 40 mg/mL corticosteroid preparation (optional)
- Adhesive bandage

Figure 1 Location for needle insertion for olecranon bursa aspiration.

difficult and delayed because of the vague symptoms, a lack of easily observed findings, and the frequent association with workers' compensation.

Clinical Symptoms

Symptoms vary depending on the duration and severity of the nerve compression. Early symptoms of ulnar nerve compression include aching pain at the medial aspect of the elbow and numbness and tingling in the ring and little fingers. The paresthesias occasionally radiate proximally into the shoulder and neck. Weakness of the intrinsic muscles is a late finding and can interfere with activities of daily living, such as opening jars or turning a key in a door. Visible muscle wasting implies ulnar nerve compression of several months or more.

Patients with radial tunnel syndrome present with symptoms similar to lateral epicondylitis but with pain that is 4 to 5 cm more distal than that of lateral epicondylitis. Because the posterior interosseous nerve contains only motor fibers, there is no numbness or tingling. Obvious muscular weakness is rarely encountered until late in the disease process.

Symptoms of pronator syndrome are often vague, consisting of discomfort in the forearm with occasional proximal radiation into the arm. Repetitive strenuous motions, such as industrial activities, weight training, or driving, often provoke the symptoms. Numbness may affect all or a part of the median nerve distribution. Women seem to be at greater risk than men for this syndrome, especially in the industrial setting.

Tests

Physical Examination

Inspect the elbow for deformity and measure the carrying angle. The nerve should be palpated for any masses or localized tenderness. Tapping lightly on the nerve may cause pain and paresthesias over the ulnar border of the hand and the ring and little fingers (Tinel sign).

Palpate the ulnar groove as the elbow is flexed and extended to determine if the nerve slips out of the groove. The elbow flexion test is a provocative maneuver. For this test, the patient flexes the elbow as far as possible, reporting any tingling or numbness in the hand as soon as it is felt. Record how quickly symptoms appear; if the symptoms do not develop within 60 seconds, the test is considered negative.

SECTION 3 ELBOW

Assess sensation and muscle function of the ulnar nerve. Vibration and light touch perception are the first to be affected, and the little finger and the ulnar half of the ring finger are most likely to be involved. Two-point discrimination is affected when nerve compression has progressed to axonal degeneration.

Weakness is assessed by testing abduction and adduction of the little and index fingers, the ability to cross the index and middle fingers, and thumb-to-index pinch. The ulnarly innervated extrinsic muscles are less commonly involved. Wasting of the intrinsic muscles is a late finding and produces a hollowed-out appearance between the metacarpals on the dorsal aspect of the hand.

With posterior interosseous nerve compression, the area of tenderness is directly over the radial tunnel, which lies 4 to 5 cm distal and slightly anterior to the lateral epicondyle. With radial tunnel syndrome, pain in the proximal forearm may be elicited by extending the long (middle) finger against resistance ("middle finger test").

With pronator syndrome, physical examination findings are often subtle. The most reliable test is reproduction of pain with direct pressure over the proximal portion of the pronator teres approximately 4 cm distal to the antebrachial crease while exerting moderate resistance to pronation. Resisted pronation for 60 seconds may initiate the symptoms by contracting the flexor-pronator muscle.

Diagnostic Tests

Electromyographic/nerve conduction velocity (EMG/NCV) studies provide an objective measurement of ulnar nerve compression. A reduction in velocity of 30% or more suggests significant compression of the ulnar nerve. EMG/NCV studies are usually normal in cases of radial tunnel and pronator syndromes. Plain radiographs of the elbow are indicated when previous elbow trauma has occurred.

Differential Diagnosis

- Carpal tunnel syndrome (numbness in thumb, index, and middle fingers; thenar muscle wasting)
- Herniated cervical disk or cervical radiculopathy (history, physical examination, and EMG/NCV should differentiate, although MRI may sometimes be necessary)
- Lateral epicondylitis (tenderness over lateral epicondyle/extensor attachment, no neurogenic symptoms)
- Medial epicondylitis (tenderness over the medial epicondyle; no distal weakness, paresthesias, or numbness)
- Thoracic outlet syndrome (normal NCV studies at the elbow; rarely, wasting in the hand)

■ Ulnar nerve entrapment at the wrist (strong wrist flexors and ulnar deviators, sensation intact over the dorsomedial hand and the dorsum of the little and ring fingers)

Adverse Outcomes of the Disease

Loss of strength and sensation can be progressive and permanent in long-standing cases. Pain, tenderness, and stiffness at the elbow also can persist.

Treatment

For ulnar nerve compression, modifying activities in the workplace to limit elbow flexion and direct pressure on the ulnar nerve is the most important step in treatment. At night, an elbow splint that keeps the elbow from flexing to 90° can be worn. (A towel wrapped around the elbow is sufficient if a commercial splint is not available.) A sports elbow protector can be used at work to keep from bumping the elbow. NSAIDs may be of benefit for an acute, severe episode. Corticosteroid injections are not recommended.

Surgical decompression and transposition of the ulnar nerve should be considered for patients with bothersome symptoms or mild weakness that persists despite 3 to 4 months of nonsurgical management, or for patients with significant or progressive weakness. There are several different methods of surgical decompression, but all involve inspecting the nerve and removing all sources of compression.

Decompression of the radial tunnel is indicated for patients with radial tunnel syndrome who have significant discomfort that has not responded to prolonged nonsurgical care over a period of at least 3 to 6 months.

Likewise, surgical decompression is indicated for pronator syndrome if all measures of nonsurgical treatment (including activity/job modification, anti-inflammatory medications, rehabilitation, and steroid injection) have not resulted in adequate pain relief over a period of at least 3 to 6 months.

SECTION 3 ELBOW

Adverse Outcomes of Treatment

Care should be taken that any splint applied does not have straps across the medial elbow because this could increase nerve compression. NSAIDs can cause gastric, renal, or hepatic complications. Surgery may be complicated by infection and/or nerve damage. Symptoms are not always improved after surgery. The importance of nonsurgical care and the careful selection of surgical candidates cannot be overemphasized because these nerve compression injuries are often work related and are complicated by issues of secondary gain.

Referral Decisions/Red Flags

Significant or progressive weakness or atrophy of the intrinsic muscles, increasing numbness despite nonsurgical treatment, or persistent symptoms that interfere with activities or work and have failed to respond to prolonged nonsurgical care indicate the need for further evaluation.

Rupture of the Distal Biceps Tendon

Definition

Rupture of the distal biceps brachii tendon is uncommon, accounting for less than 5% of biceps tendon ruptures, but when they do occur, complete tears of the distal biceps tendon cause significantly greater weakness than do tears of the proximal biceps tendon. If the lesion is not recognized and repaired in a timely fashion, elbow flexion and forearm supination strength is decreased by 30% to 50%. Most often, ruptures occur in men older than 40 years who have preexisting degenerative changes in the biceps tendon.

These ruptures typically are located at the insertion of the biceps tendon into the radius (radial tuberosity). The rupture may be incomplete or complete. With complete ruptures, the biceps aponeurosis may remain intact initially.

Clinical Symptoms

Patients often report a history of sudden, sharp pain in the anterior elbow following an excessive extension force on the flexed elbow. The pain typically is severe for a few hours (acute inflammatory response) and then is followed by a chronic, dull ache in the anterior elbow region that is made worse by lifting activities.

Tests

Physical Examination

Examination reveals tenderness and a defect in the antecubital fossa due to the absence of the usually prominent biceps tendon. Early on, ecchymosis will be present in the antecubital fossa and proximal forearm. With flexion of the elbow against resistance, the muscle belly retracts proximally (**Figure 1**). When the patient actively pronates and supinates the forearm with the elbow at 90°, the normal rise and fall of the biceps muscle belly is lost; this can be compared with the opposite arm.

If the rupture is incomplete, the defect will not be apparent, but the patient will exhibit pain and weakness on flexion and supination of the elbow against resistance. If the rupture is complete but the bicipital aponeurosis is intact, the defect is not as obvious; however, comparison with the opposite side helps to confirm the diagnosis.

ICD-9 Code

841.9
Sprains and strains of elbow and forearm, unspecified site

Figure 1 Clinical appearance of distal biceps tendon rupture. (Reproduced with permission from Ramsey ML: Distal biceps tendon injuries: Diagnosis and management. *J Am Acad Orthop Surg* 1999;7:199-207.)

SECTION 3 ELBOW

Diagnostic Tests

AP and lateral radiographs of the elbow usually are normal, but they may reveal an avulsion fracture of the bicipital tuberosity. MRI is usually necessary to confirm the diagnosis. MRI will also help to distinguish between an avulsion of the tendon from the radial tuberosity versus a rupture at the muscle-tendon junction (not common), which has a poorer prognosis.

Differential Diagnosis

- Bicipital tendinosis (tendon degenerative changes without rupture)
- Cubital bursitis (enlargement of the bursa between the biceps tendon and the radial tuberosity; may occur as a primary condition or secondary to other conditions)
- Entrapment of the lateral antebrachial cutaneous nerve (pain and dysesthesia at the lateral aspect of the proximal forearm)
- Pronator syndrome (no weakness or defect)

Adverse Outcomes of the Disease

Loss of elbow flexion strength is noted initially, but over time flexion strength improves; on average, only a 15% residual loss of strength is seen. Loss of forearm supination, on the other hand, is more significant and permanent, with up to a 50% loss seen. Loss of forearm supination power (eg, turning a screwdriver) is more dysfunctional for manual laborers or individuals who perform activities that require a lot of forearm twisting. With time, the muscle retracts and becomes fibrotic. In this situation, surgical repair either is not possible or the results are compromised, with less predictable return of muscle strength.

Treatment

Most patients with complete ruptures do better with surgical repair of the tendon. Partial ruptures may be managed nonsurgically with activity modification and intermittent splinting, but if this treatment fails, surgical repair is indicated. Nonsurgical management is used with older patients who are sedentary and do not require normal elbow flexor/supinator strength and endurance. Nonsurgical treatment also may be appropriate for the nondominant arm in selected patients and in cases of delayed diagnosis.

SECTION 3 ELBOW

Adverse Outcomes of Treatment

Full return of muscle strength may not occur. Injury to the radial nerve is possible. Infection, heterotopic ossification, and chronic pain may ensue.

Referral Decisions/Red Flags

Because of the adverse and progressive effect on muscle strength, rupture of the distal tendon of the biceps should be evaluated for possible surgical repair within 1 to 2 weeks of the injury. Surgical exposure and ability to repair the tendon is more difficult if referral is delayed beyond the first 2 weeks of injury.

SECTION 3 ELBOW

Ulnar Collateral Ligament Tear

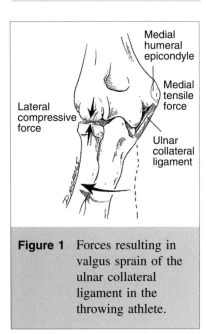

Figure 1 Forces resulting in valgus sprain of the ulnar collateral ligament in the throwing athlete.

Definition

The ulnar collateral ligament is the primary structure resisting valgus stress at the elbow. Trauma to this ligament (including strains and tears) is relatively uncommon and rarely leads to symptomatic instability or disability in the general population. The overhead throwing athlete (particularly in baseball and javelin), however, places repetitive valgus stress across the medial elbow and the ulnar collateral ligament (**Figure 1**), which can result in injury to the ligament, leading to instability and disability that may require treatment in these athletes.

Clinical Symptoms

Onset may be acute, with the athlete experiencing a "pop" while throwing, followed by medial elbow pain. Most commonly, patients have a gradual onset of symptoms with progressive medial elbow pain with throwing. Paresthesias along the ulnar nerve distribution while throwing is a common symptom. Swelling and ecchymosis are usually minimal. This injury is being seen with increasing frequency at younger ages, especially in high school athletes. A history of abuse to the arm (excessive number of pitches per game, excessive innings per year, year-round baseball, use of "breaking" pitches—curve or slider—at a young age) is common.

Tests

Physical Examination

Examination generally demonstrates tenderness over the ulnar collateral ligament, and there may be some loss of terminal extension. Swelling and ecchymosis are generally absent. There is usually pain over the ulnar collateral ligament with valgus stress testing, although gross opening of the joint is uncommon. The milking maneuver and the moving valgus stress test also are useful physical examination tests. With the milking maneuver, the patient or examiner pulls on the patient's thumb to create a valgus stress with the forearm supinated and the elbow flexed to 90°. A positive test is when the patient describes pain with this maneuver. With the moving valgus stress test, this same valgus load is applied while moving the elbow into full flexion and extension (**Figure 2**). The test is positive if more intense pain at the medial elbow is reported by the patient when the elbow is

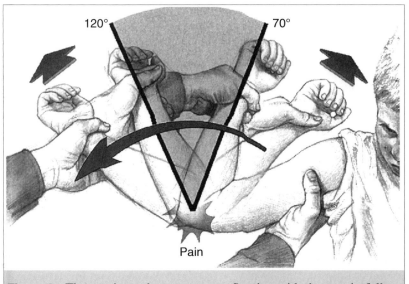

Figure 2 The moving valgus stress test. Starting with the arm in full flexion, the examiner applies a constant valgus torque to the elbow and then quickly extends the elbow. The test is positive when pain is elicited when the elbow is flexed between 70° and 120°. (Adapted with permission from the Mayo Foundation for Medical and Education Research, Rochester, MN.)

flexed between 70° and 120°. Tenderness over the ulnar nerve and a positive Tinel sign also may be present and can lead to an inaccurate diagnosis of primary ulnar neuritis.

Diagnostic Tests
AP and lateral radiographs are necessary to rule out fracture. Ossification within the ulnar collateral ligament may be seen in chronic cases. Posteromedial olecranon osteophytes, loose bodies, and marginal spurring also may be seen in chronic cases. MRI with intra-articular contrast is a reasonable diagnostic tool for diagnosing pathology of the ulnar collateral ligament.

Differential Diagnosis
- Cubital tunnel syndrome (stability examination, history; frequently coexists with ulnar collateral ligament injury)
- Medial epicondyle avulsion (evident on radiographs, adolescent age group)
- Medial epicondylitis (history and stability examination; typically, older age group)

SECTION 3 ELBOW

Adverse Outcomes of the Disease

Persistent pain and disability in throwing sports are most common. Rarely are problems encountered with activities of daily living or in nonthrowing sports. Chronic stiffness and loss of motion may be encountered.

Treatment

Nonsurgical care, including rest, NSAIDs, rehabilitation, stretching and strengthening exercises, and activity modification, is appropriate following such an injury. Corticosteroid injections in the ulnar collateral ligament may cause weakening and attenuation of the ligament and should be avoided. A very slow return to sport (involving a detailed progressive throwing program) should be stressed. If pain relief is the main goal of the patient, nonsurgical care is likely to be successful. If a return to a highly competitive level of a throwing sport is the main goal, surgery may be necessary. If symptoms in an athlete have failed to respond to an appropriate course of nonsurgical care within 3 months, surgical reconstruction (the so-called Tommy John surgery) should be considered. The patient must realize that postoperative rehabilitation is critical and lengthy, requiring approximately 12 months before return to competition. In the properly selected athlete, surgery is over 90% successful in returning the athlete to the preinjury level of competition. With the alarming trend of ulnar collateral ligament injuries in younger baseball players, emphasis should be placed on education and prevention in youth sports (ie, following pitch counts, limiting the number of innings pitched per season or per year, avoiding year-round baseball, and delaying the throwing of breaking pitches until the young athlete's body matures).

Adverse Outcomes of Treatment

Surgical risks include stiffness, nerve injury, infection, and persistent pain.

Referral Decisions/Red Flags

Failure of nonsurgical management in the high-level throwing athlete who wishes to continue to compete at this level indicates the need for further evaluation.

PAIN DIAGRAM
Hand and Wrist

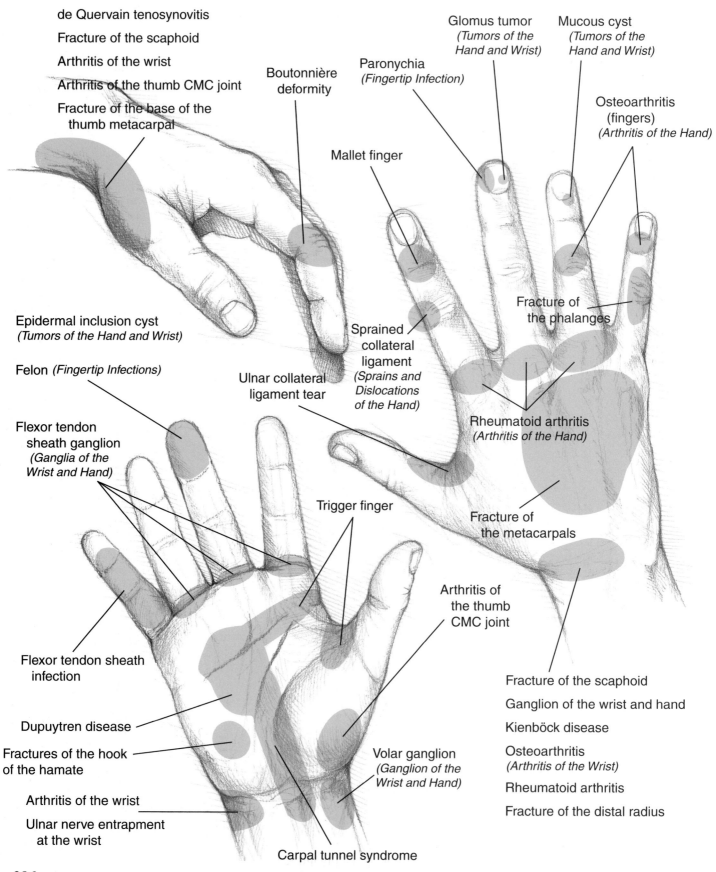

de Quervain tenosynovitis

Fracture of the scaphoid

Arthritis of the wrist

Arthritis of the thumb CMC joint

Fracture of the base of the
thumb metacarpal

Boutonnière
deformity

Glomus tumor
*(Tumors of the
Hand and Wrist)*

Mucous cyst
*(Tumors of the
Hand and Wrist)*

Paronychia
(Fingertip Infection)

Osteoarthritis
(fingers)
(Arthritis of the Hand)

Mallet finger

Epidermal inclusion cyst
(Tumors of the Hand and Wrist)

Felon *(Fingertip Infections)*

Flexor tendon
sheath ganglion
*(Ganglia of the
Wrist and Hand)*

Sprained
collateral
ligament
*(Sprains and
Dislocations
of the Hand)*

Ulnar collateral
ligament tear

Fracture of
the phalanges

Rheumatoid arthritis
(Arthritis of the Hand)

Trigger finger

Fracture of
the metacarpals

Flexor tendon sheath
infection

Arthritis of
the thumb
CMC joint

Dupuytren disease

Fractures of the hook
of the hamate

Volar ganglion
*(Ganglion of the
Wrist and Hand)*

Arthritis of the wrist

Ulnar nerve entrapment
at the wrist

Carpal tunnel syndrome

Fracture of the scaphoid

Ganglion of the wrist and hand

Kienböck disease

Osteoarthritis
(Arthritis of the Wrist)

Rheumatoid arthritis

Fracture of the distal radius

Hand and Wrist

Section Editor

John G. Seiler III, MD

Georgia Hand, Shoulder & Elbow
Atlanta, GA

Contributor

Michael Huxford, MEd, ATC, CSCS

Sports Medicine Coordinator
Rehabilitative Services
Institute for Sports Medicine
Children's Memorial Hospital
Chicago, IL

ANATOMY OF THE HAND AND WRIST

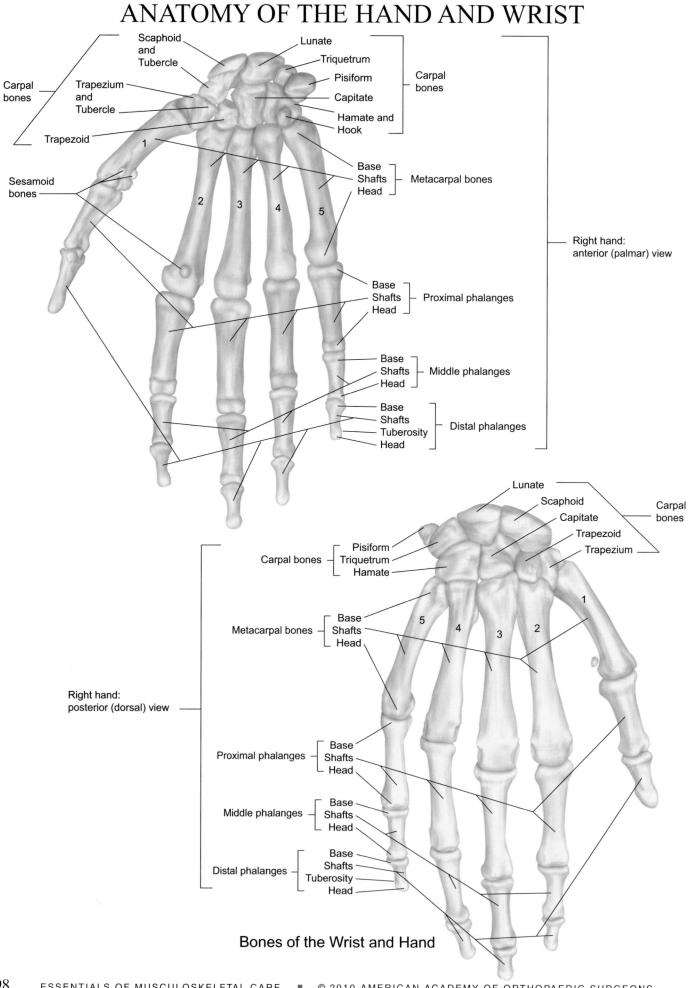

Carpal bones

Scaphoid and Tubercle

Trapezium and Tubercle

Trapezoid

Lunate

Triquetrum

Pisiform

Capitate

Hamate and Hook

Carpal bones

Sesamoid bones

1
2
3
4
5

Base
Shafts
Head — Metacarpal bones

Right hand: anterior (palmar) view

Base
Shafts
Head — Proximal phalanges

Base
Shafts
Head — Middle phalanges

Base
Shafts
Tuberosity
Head — Distal phalanges

Right hand: posterior (dorsal) view

Lunate

Scaphoid

Capitate

Trapezoid

Trapezium

Carpal bones

Carpal bones —
Pisiform
Triquetrum
Hamate

Metacarpal bones —
Base
Shafts
Head

5
4
3
2
1

Proximal phalanges —
Base
Shafts
Head

Middle phalanges —
Base
Shafts
Head

Distal phalanges —
Base
Shafts
Tuberosity
Head

Bones of the Wrist and Hand

Overview of the Hand and Wrist

Carpal tunnel syndrome, trigger finger, ganglion formation, carpometacarpal (CMC) arthritis of the thumb, and radiocarpal arthritis are among the more common hand and wrist problems that bring patients to a primary care physician. Patients with chronic hand and wrist problems typically have one or more of the following symptoms: pain, instability, stiffness, swelling, weakness, numbness, or a mass.

To begin the evaluation, obtain a history from the patient, including a statement of the chief symptom, a thorough history of the present condition, and a general medical history. The history of the present condition should include the duration of symptoms, the specific type and location of symptoms, factors that improve or worsen the symptoms, and previous treatments. After obtaining the history, a physical examination should be done. With these two pieces of information, a working diagnosis can be established in a high percentage of patients. Diagnostic testing, which often includes plain radiographs, should be done to help confirm the working hypothesis that has been synthesized from the history and physical examination. Additional diagnostic evaluation commonly used for the hand includes electrophysiologic evaluation (electromyography or nerve conduction velocity tests), Doppler ultrasonography, and MRI and CT with or without arthrogram contrast.

Location of Pain

The best method of localizing the pain is to have the patient use one finger to identify the point of maximum tenderness (see page 396). Categorize the pain as being in one of the following four areas: radial, ulnar, volar, or dorsal (**Figure 1**). This localization of pain by anatomic region will help narrow the field of probable diagnoses.

Radial Pain

Wrist pain in patients younger than 30 years most commonly results from trauma. Posttraumatic tenderness and pain over the radial aspect of the wrist may suggest a fracture of the scaphoid, which is the most commonly missed fracture in the wrist and hand. In the absence of trauma, pain associated with tenderness over the radial styloid is most likely de Quervain (wrist) tenosynovitis. Pain that is dorsal and slightly more proximal may be caused by intersection syndrome (tenosynovitis of the radial wrist extensors) or superficial radial neuritis. Pain that

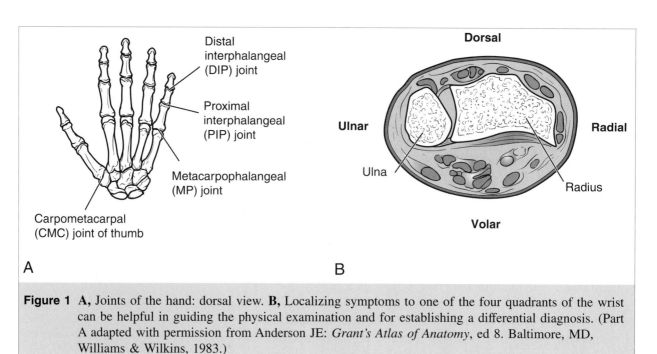

Figure 1 **A,** Joints of the hand: dorsal view. **B,** Localizing symptoms to one of the four quadrants of the wrist can be helpful in guiding the physical examination and for establishing a differential diagnosis. (Part A adapted with permission from Anderson JE: *Grant's Atlas of Anatomy*, ed 8. Baltimore, MD, Williams & Wilkins, 1983.)

occurs without numbness in patients older than 40 years is likely caused by posttraumatic arthritis or osteoarthritis. Pain at the base of the thumb in women in this age group is likely to be caused by CMC arthritis.

Dorsal Pain

Generalized dorsal wrist discomfort may be associated with radiocarpal arthritis. Pain in this region associated with a well-defined mass over the dorsoradial aspect of the wrist is usually a ganglion cyst. Pain and loss of motion in the wrist can also be caused by ligamentous injury (scapholunate ligament injury or lunotriquetral ligament injury) to the wrist or by Kienböck disease (osteonecrosis of the lunate). Plain radiographs are valuable in the initial assessment of these patients.

Ulnar Pain

Pain in this region after trauma can be caused by a tear of the triangular fibrocartilage complex, which is located distal to the ulnar styloid. Swelling and tenderness over the dorsoulnar or volar aspects of the wrist are likely to be caused by a tendinitis of the ulnar wrist extensor (extensor carpi ulnaris) or flexor (flexor carpi ulnaris) tendons.

Volar Pain

Carpal tunnel syndrome, ganglion cyst formation, and tenosynovitis are the most common causes of volar wrist pain. Carpal tunnel syndrome is commonly associated with numbness and tingling in the radial three digits (thumb plus index and long fingers) and, often, half of the ring finger. Other causes of discomfort include a volar ganglion cyst, which should be easily palpable on the volar radial aspect of the wrist, or wrist tendinitis. Swelling over the volar region suggests inflammation of the finger flexor tendons. Patients with radiocarpal arthritis might have pain over both the dorsal and volar aspects of the wrist. Volar wrist pain also can be caused by arthritis between the pisiform and the triquetrum bones.

Chronic Wrist and Finger Instability

Diagnosis of wrist instability is often complex, requiring considerable experience in history taking, physical examination, and interpretation of radiographs. Typical symptoms are sensations of slipping, snapping, or clunking with certain wrist motions after an injury. The unstable structure might be a joint (following a tear of the supporting and stabilizing ligaments that hold together the carpal bones) or a subluxating tendon (following a tear of the restraining ligaments, or retinaculum, that contain the tendon). Plain PA radiographs of the wrist might show separation between the scaphoid and the lunate (Terry Thomas sign), indicating a tear of the intrinsic ligament binding the scaphoid and the lunate (scapholunate dissociation). Chronic ligamentous instability commonly occurs in the metacarpophalangeal (MP) joint of the thumb and can occur in any of the proximal interphalangeal (PIP) joints or MP joints.

Stiffness

Morning stiffness is a common symptom of arthritis or tenosynovitis and may be associated with carpal tunnel syndrome or trigger finger. Patients with trigger finger often have pain, and they commonly (and erroneously) localize the problem to the PIP joint when it locks or "jumps" as the finger is flexed. In fact, the source of the problem is in the palm, where the thickened flexor tendon catches under the proximal (A1) tendon pulley at the distal palmar crease. Tenderness and palpable catching just distal to this crease confirm the diagnosis.

Swelling

Swelling in the joints of the hand and wrist is caused by synovitis, which can be secondary to osteoarthritis, infection, or a systemic inflammatory disease such as rheumatoid arthritis or gout. A history of penetrating trauma or immunocompromise in patients who present for evaluation of swelling should suggest infection as opposed to inflammatory disease. Plain radiographs are useful in diagnosing osteoarthritis and rheumatoid arthritis.

Swelling around the tendons can occur in association with rheumatoid arthritis and/or overuse syndromes such as de Quervain tenosynovitis. Pain and swelling around the wrist flexor or extensor tendons suggest tendinitis; plain radiographs may show a calcific deposit close to the involved tendon in patients who develop calcific tendinitis.

Weakness

Weakness in the hand may be secondary to pain, as with CMC or radiocarpal arthritis or intrinsic muscle disease. Weakness without pain suggests possible peripheral nerve entrapment or central nervous system disease. Ulnar nerve entrapment at the elbow will result in decreased grip and pinch strength in addition to loss of sensation in the little and ring fingers. Wasting of the intrinsic muscles is seen on physical examination in advanced cases.

Numbness

Dysesthesias, paresthesias, and hand-based numbness and tingling are commonly caused by entrapment neuropathy. **Figure 2** shows the typical sensory distribution of the median, ulnar, and radial nerves; however, variations from this pattern can occur. Positive provocative signs (Tinel sign, Phalen maneuver, Durkan carpal compression test) and abnormal sensory test results should be considered indicative of carpal tunnel syndrome. With carpal tunnel syndrome, the numbness characteristically occurs in the thumb, the index and long fingers, and, often, the radial half of the ring finger; some patients report that the entire hand is numb.

Loss of sensation in the little and ring fingers usually is caused by entrapment of the ulnar nerve at the elbow or the wrist. Patients with thoracic outlet syndrome often report symptoms at the ulnar side of the hand and forearm, but this condition is much less common than ulnar nerve entrapment at the elbow. Both the Tinel sign and elbow flexion tests should be negative with thoracic outlet syndrome.

Neck pain associated with a positive Spurling test and with loss of sensation in the thumb and index finger suggests a common cervical radiculopathy. Electrophysiologic testing is commonly used to confirm the clinical diagnosis in patients who present for evaluation of numbness.

Masses

The most common mass in the hand and wrist is a ganglion cyst. These cysts most often occur in four locations: the dorsoradial and volar radial aspects of the wrist, the proximal

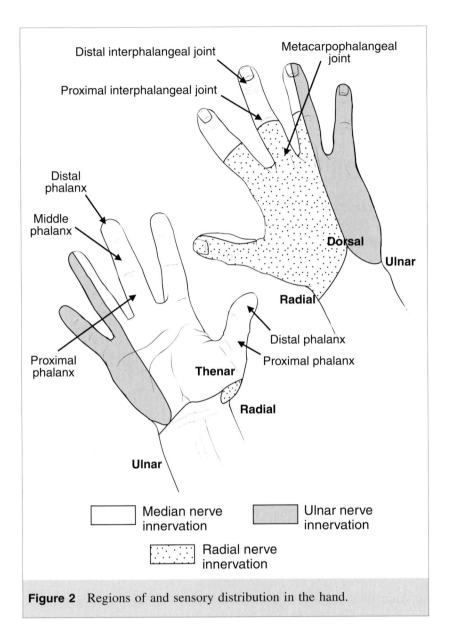

Distal interphalangeal joint

Metacarpophalangeal joint

Proximal interphalangeal joint

Distal phalanx

Middle phalanx

Dorsal

Ulnar

Proximal phalanx

Radial

Distal phalanx

Proximal phalanx

Thenar

Radial

Ulnar

Median nerve innervation

Ulnar nerve innervation

Radial nerve innervation

Figure 2 Regions of and sensory distribution in the hand.

finger flexor crease, and the distal interphalangeal joint. Multilobulated masses along the sides of the finger are most likely giant cell tumors. Nontender nodules in the palm and cords that cross both the MP and PIP joints are consistent with Dupuytren contracture. A hard mass at the dorsal base of the index metacarpal is usually a carpal boss—a bony mass consisting of spurs from the second and third metacarpals, the trapezoid, and the capitate. A serpiginous mass that follows the path of the tendon sheaths is often tenosynovitis. Masses with bluish discoloration or masses that have a pulsation are usually vascular in origin.

Physical Examination of the Hand and Wrist

Inspection/Palpation

Dorsum

Observe the alignment of the fingers. Inspect the nails for pitting and other evidence of systemic disorders. Look for swelling and synovitis of the finger and wrist joints. Note any osteophytes or bony prominences associated with degenerative arthritis. Muscle atrophy between the metacarpals is caused by weakness of the intrinsic muscles.

Palm

Look for atrophy of the thenar muscles, which are innervated by the median nerve, and the hypothenar muscles, which are innervated by the ulnar nerve. Note any thickening of the palmar fascia associated with Dupuytren contracture. Pain elicited by pressure over the thumb metacarpophalangeal joint suggests arthritis or instability of this joint. Position the patient's hands with the palms facing each other to best visualize atrophy of the thenar muscles. Swelling in the joints of the thumb also is prominent in this position.

Wrist Flexion and Extension: Zero Starting Position

To measure wrist flexion and extension, a goniometer is needed. Place the patient's forearm in pronation and the carpus aligned with the plane of the forearm. Place the goniometer on the dorsum of the wrist or on the radial side of the forearm (**A**). Aligning the goniometer on the ulnar side may falsely elevate the measurement because of the mobility of the fifth metacarpal. Wrist motion occurs at the radiocarpal and midcarpal joints. Normal wrist palmar flexion (**B**) is 75° to 80°, and normal dorsal extension (**C**) is 70° to 80°.

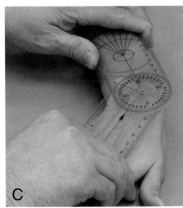

Wrist Radial and Ulnar Deviation

To measure radial and ulnar deviation, a goniometer is needed. Place the patient's forearm in pronation and the carpus aligned with the plane of the forearm. Align the goniometer with the third metacarpal and the axis of the forearm (**A**). In radial and ulnar deviation, the carpal rows move as linked segments. The buttress of the radial styloid limits radial deviation so that its arc of motion is significantly less. Normal radial deviation (**B**) is 20° to 25°, and normal ulnar deviation (**C**) is 35° to 40°.

Finger Flexion and Extension

Finger joint motion occurs primarily in the flexion-extension plane, with flexion accounting for most finger joint motion. A goniometer is needed to measure finger flexion and extension. From a functional perspective, finger flexion is a composite movement of motion of the metacarpophalangeal, proximal interphalangeal, and distal interphalangeal joints. To estimate the loss of digital flexion, have the patient maximally flex the fingertip. In young and middle-aged adults, the fingertip should touch the distal palmar crease (**A**). Flexion and extension also can be measured individually at the metacarpophalangeal, proximal interphalangeal, and distal interphalangeal joints (**B**). The wrist should be in neutral when measuring finger flexion. If the wrist is flexed, the extensor digitorum longus will be effectively tethered, thereby limiting finger flexion. Finally, active motion should be compared with passive motion.

Finger Abduction and Adduction

Abduction and adduction of the fingers occur in the plane of the palm, primarily at the metacarpophalangeal joints and centered on the long finger. Ask the patient to spread the fingers, then close them together three times. Abduction (**A**) is movement of the fingers away from the long finger; adduction (**B**) is movement of the other fingers toward the long finger.

more than 10 to 12 hours old. Sensation and tendon function should be tested in the affected hand or finger. Inspect the forearm for the presence of red streaks that indicate lymphangitis. The inner aspect of the elbow and the axilla should be palpated for the presence of enlarged lymph nodes. The patient's temperature should be checked.

Diagnostic Tests

AP and lateral radiographs of the affected part are necessary to rule out a fracture or the presence of a foreign body. These views also may reveal gas in the soft tissues. Routine laboratory studies may not show significant abnormality for wounds seen shortly after injury. If an infection is suspected, however, a swab of the wound should be sent for a Gram stain and aerobic and anaerobic cultures.

Differential Diagnosis

- Foreign body with secondary infection (foreign body apparent on radiograph, ultrasound, or CT)

Adverse Outcomes of the Disease

Any of the following conditions could develop as a result of an untreated animal bite: sepsis in the joint, deep space infection, septic tenosynovitis, osteomyelitis, or rabies. Patients also may lose sensation and motion, and possibly the affected fingers, following an animal bite. Chronic lymphedema with hand and finger stiffness is also possible.

Treatment

Débridement, wound irrigation with 500 to 1,000 mL of saline solution or an antibiotic irrigation solution, and outpatient antibiotics are appropriate for superficial wounds that do not have a nerve, tendon, or bony injury. An anesthetic block will facilitate débridement of bite wounds on the finger. When the bite wound is on the back of the hand, 3 to 10 mL of local anesthetic should be infiltrated around the wound. Oral amoxicillin-clavulanate, 875 mg twice a day for 5 days, is one standard antibiotic regimen for the treatment of early infection.

Primary suturing of animal bite wounds is controversial and can be hazardous. Suturing should be performed only when the wound is clean following débridement and usually is best completed over a passive drain (Penrose type). Because of the higher rate of infection associated with cat bites, these wounds should not be sutured. In general, it is safest to leave animal bites open.

Table 1 Summary Guide to Tetanus Prophylaxis in Routine Wound Management[a]

History of Tetanus Immunization (Doses)	Clean, Minor Wounds		All Other Wounds	
	Td[b]	TIG	Td[b]	TIG
Uncertain or <3 doses	Yes	No	Yes	Yes
3 or more doses	No[c]	No	No[d]	No

[a]Important details on the CDC Web site: http://wwwnc.cdc.gov/travel/yellowbook/2010/chapter-2/tetanus.aspx.

[b]For children <7 years old, DTaP or DTP (DT, if pertussis vaccine contraindicated) preferred to tetanus toxoid alone. For children ≥7 years of age, Td preferred to tetanus toxoid alone. For adolescents and adults to age 64, tetanus toxoid as Tdap is preferred, if the patient has not previously been vaccinated with Tdap.

[c]Yes, if more than 10 years since last dose.

[d]Yes, if more than 5 years since last dose. More frequent boosters are not needed and can accentuate side effects.

Td = tetanus and diphtheria toxoids, TIG = human tetanus immune globulin.

(Adapted with permission from the Centers for Disease Control and Prevention.)

When signs of active infection are present, the wound should be managed open and allowed to close by secondary intention. Intravenous antibiotics are indicated in this situation. Empiric therapy can be started with intravenous ampicillin-sulbactam, 1.5 to 3.0 g every 6 hours, pending culture results and sensitivities. Tetracycline can be used in patients with a penicillin allergy. Antibiotic therapy should be organism specific whenever possible. The patient may be switched to oral antibiotics in 48 hours if the wound is healing satisfactorily. Tetanus prophylaxis should be given as outlined in **Table 1**.

If the animal is suspected of being infected with rabies, contact local or state public health officials regarding the need for rabies prophylaxis.

Adverse Outcomes of Treatment

Infection secondary to primary wound closure can occur. Patients also may have allergic reactions to antibiotics.

Referral Decisions/Red Flags

Any patient with an animal bite that involves the tendon, nerve, joint capsule, or an underlying fracture requires further evaluation.

Arthritis of the Hand

Synonyms

Degenerative joint disease
Osteoarthritis
Rheumatoid arthritis

Definition

Osteoarthritis and secondary degenerative joint disease are the most common causes of arthritis of the hand and wrist. These conditions are characterized by progressive loss of articular cartilage, reactive bony changes at the joint margins, and subchondral cyst formation. The cause of primary osteoarthritis is unknown. Secondary osteoarthritis develops in joints affected by trauma, mechanical problems, or preexisting lesions.

Rheumatoid arthritis is a systemic condition that affects synovial tissue. All deformities, joint destruction, and pathologic anatomy that occur in patients with rheumatoid arthritis are a result of synovial hypertrophy and inflammation. The boggy synovium stretches the joint capsule and ligaments, causing deformity and joint instability. The articular cartilage also may be destroyed. Rheumatoid synovitis may also involve the tenosynovium and invade the flexor and extensor tendons, disrupting their motion and function.

Clinical Symptoms

In osteoarthritis, the distal interphalangeal (DIP) and proximal interphalangeal (PIP) joints are most often involved. Patients report stiffness and loss of motion in the fingers. In rheumatoid arthritis, the wrist and metacarpophalangeal (MP) joints are most often involved (**Figure 1**). Extensor or flexor tenosynovitis (inflammation of the tendon sheath) also is common, resulting in pain that is caused by activation, whereas patients with osteoarthritis have more pain with joint palpation. Patients with rheumatoid arthritis have increased pain in the morning and after extended activities.

Tests

Physical Examination

Patients with rheumatoid arthritis involving the hands have fusiform swelling of multiple joints, with some joints more swollen than others. Rheumatoid arthritis commonly involves the MP joint and the wrist joint. A boggy mass over the dorsum

Figure 1   Advanced rheumatoid arthritis. **A,** Clinical appearance. Note the severe ulnar drift of the metacarpophalangeal (MP) joint and the limited finger extension. **B,** PA radiograph demonstrating the severe ulnar drift of the MP joints (white arrows) and the destruction of the wrist (black arrow).

of the hand and crepitus with movement also are common, as is flexor tenosynovitis with crepitus at the wrist or in the fingers. Ulnar drift of the fingers may exist at the level of the MP joint. Other findings include contractures of the fingers at the PIP joints (boutonnière deformity) or hyperextension at the PIP joints with flexion at the DIP joints (swan-neck deformity).

Patients with osteoarthritis of the hand have bony nodules at the DIP joint (Heberden nodes). These nodules may be painful at first, but the pain usually resolves. Nodules also may occur at the PIP joints (Bouchard nodes). Involvement of the MP joints is much less common with osteoarthritis. When it occurs at this location, it is often the result of previous trauma.

Diagnostic Tests

PA, oblique, and lateral views with the fingers positioned in different degrees of flexion, allowing each finger to be examined in detail, are necessary. When a single digit is involved, isolated PA and true lateral views of the digit also are appropriate. Serologic studies should be ordered for patients who have the characteristic changes of inflammatory arthritis but for whom the diagnosis has not been established.

Differential Diagnosis

- Pyogenic arthritis (may resemble the swollen joints of rheumatoid arthritis) (bacteria in joint aspirate, markedly elevated white blood cell count)

Adverse Outcomes of the Disease

Rheumatoid arthritis can be slowly progressive, resulting in the typical rheumatoid hand deformity (**Figure 1**). Progressive osteoarthritis can cause joint destruction, particularly at the DIP, PIP, and wrist joints, with decreased mobility and function.

Treatment

Rheumatoid arthritis has no cure. NSAIDs and other anti-inflammatory medications should be optimized. Newer medications such as etanercept (Enbrel) or infliximab (Remicade) may be more effective in limiting symptoms but may be associated with other medical complications. Cortisone injections can be extremely helpful for a severely inflamed joint or tendon sheath (see pages 422-423). Nonsurgical treatment may include referral to an experienced occupational therapist to assist with splinting and the use of modalities. Occupational therapy and splinting can reduce deformity and limit symptoms but may not alter the natural history of the disease.

Treatment of osteoarthritis typically includes NSAIDs and, occasionally, temporary splinting of an involved joint for pain relief. Consultation with a hand therapist can be helpful to assist with hand splints and externally applied modalities such as home paraffin treatments and externally applied rub-in creams. Surgery for pain relief or stabilization may be necessary.

Adverse Outcomes of Treatment

NSAIDs may cause gastric, hepatic, and renal complications. Corticosteroids may adversely affect the immune system. Cortisone injections should be used very judiciously because tendon rupture may occur. Infection also is a risk but can be minimized with careful sterile technique.

Referral Decisions/Red Flags

When a cortisone injection for extensor tenosynovitis is not effective, surgery to excise the inflamed synovium can prevent rupture of the tendon. Patients who cannot extend their digits, especially the little finger, ring finger, or thumb, may have ruptured the extensor tendon, and immediate further evaluation is needed.

Patients with rheumatoid arthritis who report increasing deformity and increasing pain in the hand may need reconstructive surgery.

Further evaluation is required for patients with osteoarthritis pain no longer controlled with splinting and NSAIDs and who have radiographic evidence of joint destruction.

Procedure: Metacarpophalangeal or Proximal Interphalangeal Joint Injection

Note: Opinions differ regarding single- versus two-needle injection techniques. Proponents of the single-needle technique believe that one needle is less painful for the patient than two. Because the corticosteroid preparation is thicker than the local anesthetic, however, a slightly larger gauge needle is required at the outset. A two-syringe, two-needle technique is described on the DVD.

Injections are performed on the extensor aspect of either the metacarpophalangeal (MP) or the proximal interphalangeal (PIP) joint.

The entry site for the MP joint is the small sulcus just below the prominent metacarpal head that is most obvious with the finger flexed 20° (**Figure 1A**). Identify this sulcus while moving the joint through a small amount of flexion and extension. Applying axial traction to the finger can facilitate localization of the joint.

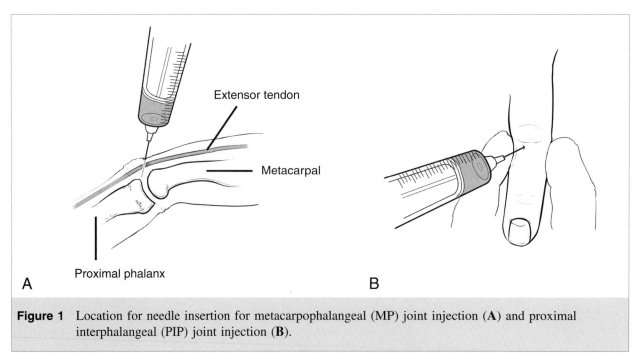

Extensor tendon

Metacarpal

Proximal phalanx

A   B

Figure 1 Location for needle insertion for metacarpophalangeal (MP) joint injection (**A**) and proximal interphalangeal (PIP) joint injection (**B**).

Identify the PIP joint in the same manner. Be aware, however, that the dorsal rim of the middle phalanx is often more easily palpated with this joint in extension (**Figure 1B**).

Step 1
Wear protective gloves at all times during this procedure and use sterile technique.

Step 2
Cleanse the skin with a bactericidal skin preparation solution.

Step 3
Insert the 25-gauge needle at the joint level on the dorsolateral side of the joint. Inject 0.5 mL of a 1% local anesthetic preparation into the joint, change syringes, and then, with the new syringe, inject 0.5 to 1.0 mL of corticosteroid preparation. Slight pressure against the syringe plunger should make the joint bulge slightly on either side.

Alternate method: Combine the local anesthetic medication with the corticosteroid solution into one syringe. Insert a 25-gauge needle at the joint level on the dorsolateral side of the joint and inject the preparation into the joint.

Step 4
Dress the puncture wound with a sterile adhesive bandage.

Materials
• Sterile gloves
• Bactericidal skin preparation solution
• Two 3-mL syringes with a 25-gauge needle
• 0.5 mL of a 1% local anesthetic solution without epinephrine
• 0.5 to 1.0 mL corticosteroid preparation
• Adhesive dressing

Adverse Outcomes

Although rare, infection is possible. Subcutaneous fat atrophy may occur if the corticosteroid preparation is injected external to the joint. This may produce a depressed area of thin, tender, and unsightly skin. Some patients experience changes in skin pigmentation following injection. Occasionally, these changes in skin coloration are permanent.

Aftercare/Patient Instructions

The joint might be sore for 24 to 48 hours after injection. Instruct the patient to return to your office if undue swelling, pain, or redness occurs. Ice massage and the use of acetaminophen or an NSAID will control local symptoms after injection.

SECTION 4 HAND AND WRIST

Arthritis of the Thumb Carpometacarpal Joint

Figure 1 Carpometacarpal (CMC) arthritis of the thumb.

Synonyms

Carpometacarpal degenerative arthritis

Degenerative arthritis of the basal joint

Definition

Idiopathic degenerative arthritis of the thumb carpometacarpal (CMC) joint (**Figure 1**) most commonly occurs in women between the ages of 40 and 70 years. The idiopathic variety is caused by anatomic factors (joint configuration and ligamentous laxity) that predispose the joint to instability, shear forces, and subsequent degenerative change.

Clinical Symptoms

The most common symptom is pain at the base of the thumb that occurs with grip and pinch activities. The pain may radiate proximally into the wrist and forearm. Decreased pinch strength is a common symptom. Patients also may note instability, "catching," or "clicking" with certain movements. Late manifestations include stiffness of the CMC joint in adduction with secondary metacarpophalangeal hyperextension.

Carpal tunnel syndrome may coexist with or mimic the symptoms of CMC arthritis.

Tests

Physical Examination

The hallmark of this condition is tenderness over the palmar and radial aspects of the joint in the region of the base of the thumb. Manipulation of the CMC joint with simultaneous longitudinal loading (compression) causes pain and often some crepitus or instability. The grind test for thumb CMC arthritis readily reproduces the pain of CMC arthritis (see page 414). With the palm facing up and the back of the hand resting on the table, the thumb is pushed down toward the table with the metacarpophalangeal and proximal interphalangeal joints extended. The CMC joint relocation test, in which dorsal pressure is placed on the thumb metacarpal and the CMC joint is relocated by applying pressure in a palmar direction, is also useful in localizing the point of maximum discomfort (see page 415).

Figure 2 Radiographic appearance of CMC arthritis of the thumb.

Diagnostic Tests

PA and lateral radiographs of the thumb show joint space narrowing, subchondral sclerosis, and varying degrees of subluxation or dislocation at the CMC joint (**Figure 2**).

Differential Diagnosis

- Arthritis of the wrist (evident on radiographs)
- Carpal tunnel syndrome (positive Phalen maneuver, decreased sensation in median nerve distribution)
- de Quervain tenosynovitis (positive Finkelstein test)
- Flexor carpi radialis tendinitis (pain with resisted wrist flexion, swelling over flexor carpi radialis tendon)
- Fracture of the scaphoid (tenderness over the anatomic snuffbox)
- Scaphoid-trapezium-trapezoid arthritis (tenderness over the scaphoid-trapezium-trapezoid joint)
- Volar radial ganglion (palpable mass over the palmar surface of the wrist)

Adverse Outcomes of the Disease

Chronic pain, loss of pinch and grip strength, adduction contracture of the thumb (thumb held against the index finger), and chronic metacarpophalangeal joint instability can occur.

Treatment

Initial treatment should consist of placing the thumb in a thumb spica splint for 3 weeks, with NSAIDs for pain relief. If symptoms recur, intermittent splinting that immobilizes the entire thumb should be continued. If splinting fails, a corticosteroid preparation may be injected into the joint (see pages 427-428). Although injections do not alter the natural history of the disease, many patients report pain relief that lasts a few months with each injection. Multiple injections may be appropriate in some cases. A hand therapist may be consulted to help fabricate splints and assist with the use of externally applied modalities, such as iontophoresis, ice, heat, or rub-in creams.

Adverse Outcomes of Treatment

NSAIDs can cause gastric, renal, or hepatic complications. Infection can develop after corticosteroid injection. Rapid progression of arthritis is possible as a result of multiple corticosteroid injections.

Referral Decisions/Red Flags

Failure of nonsurgical treatment indicates the need for further evaluation.

Procedure: Thumb Carpometacarpal Joint Injection

Note: Opinions differ regarding single- and two-needle injection techniques. Proponents of the single-needle technique believe that one needle is less painful for the patient than two. Because the corticosteroid preparation is thicker than the local anesthetic, however, a slightly larger-gauge needle is required at the outset.

Step 1

Wear protective gloves at all times during this procedure and use sterile technique.

Step 2

Before putting on the gloves, mark the level of the carpometacarpal (CMC) joint on the dorsum of the hand with your thumbnail by gently indenting the skin at the interval between the base of the thumb metacarpal and the trapezium.

Step 3

Cleanse the skin over the CMC joint at the marked site with a bactericidal skin preparation solution.

Step 4

Insert the 25-gauge needle, attached to the syringe with the anesthetic solution, at the mark on the back of the CMC joint. Inject 0.5 mL of the 1% anesthetic subcutaneously.

Step 5

Pull on the end of the thumb to open the joint space. Advance the needle into the joint and inject 0.5 to 1.0 mL of the anesthetic solution (**Figure 1**). If resistance is encountered, redirect the needle and reinsert. After the anesthetic solution is injected, leave the needle in place and change syringes.

Step 6

Inject 0.5 mL of the corticosteroid preparation through the same needle tract. The injection of fluid should meet little resistance if the needle is in the CMC joint.

Step 7

Dress the puncture site with a sterile adhesive bandage.

CPT Code

20600
Arthrocentisis, aspiration and/or injection; small joint or bursa (eg, fingers, toes)

Current Procedural Terminology © 2010 American Medical Association. All rights reserved.

Materials

- Sterile gloves
- Bactericidal skin preparation solution
- Two 3-mL syringes with a 25-gauge needle
- 0.5 mL corticosteroid preparation
- 2 mL of a 1% local anesthetic without epinephrine
- Adhesive bandage

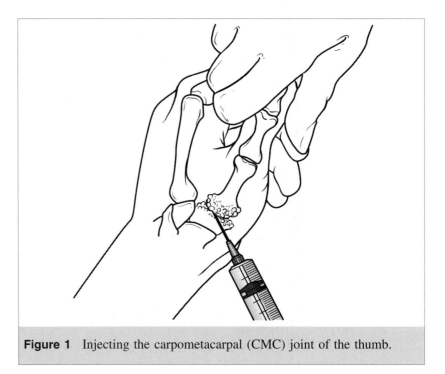

Figure 1   Injecting the carpometacarpal (CMC) joint of the thumb.

Adverse Outcomes

Depigmentation and/or fat atrophy at the site of injection, injury to sensory branches of the radial nerve, and joint space infection are possible.

Aftercare/Patient Instructions

Advise the patient that 33% of patients may experience a flare of discomfort, manifested by increased joint pain, for 1 to 2 days. Ice massage and the use of acetaminophen or an NSAID will facilitate control of local symptoms that stem from the injection. Also, the patient can wear a thumb spica splint for 2 or 3 days after the injection. The patient should experience relief within 5 to 7 days after the injection.

Arthritis of the Wrist

Synonym

Synovitis

Wrist joint arthritis

Definition

Arthritis in the wrist most commonly occurs secondary to previous trauma (eg, fractures of the distal radius) or rheumatoid arthritis. Pseudogout and primary osteoarthritis also may affect the wrist.

Clinical Symptoms

Patients with rheumatoid arthritis typically report generalized swelling, tenderness, and limited motion. Hand function is often impaired by the synovitis and resultant instability of the carpal bones. The result is radial deviation of the wrist, ulnar deviation of the fingers, inefficient wrist and finger tendon function, decreased grip strength, and pain with daily activities.

Degenerative arthritis of the wrist is associated with swelling, pain, and limited motion of the wrist.

Tests

Physical Examination

Examination reveals swelling, increased warmth, limited motion, and pain on palpation of the radiocarpal joint. Patients with rheumatoid arthritis often have associated involvement of the metacarpophalangeal joints and deformity at the wrist and fingers. The ulna may appear prominent (caput ulnae).

In posttraumatic degenerative arthritis, the finger joints usually appear normal.

Diagnostic Tests

PA and lateral radiographs are helpful in distinguishing the various types of arthritis. Generalized thinning of the bone structure (osteopenia) with erosions in the area of the joint surface is characteristic of rheumatoid arthritis. Subchondral sclerosis, joint space narrowing, spur formation, and, in some cases, erosion characterize primary or secondary osteoarthritis (**Figure 1**). Early calcification of the triangular fibrocartilage complex may indicate pseudogout, which can be confirmed by the presence of calcium pyrophosphate crystals in synovial fluid aspirate.

Laboratory studies, including erythrocyte sedimentation rate and tests for rheumatoid factor, antinuclear antibodies, and uric acid, may help confirm the diagnosis.

ICD-9 Codes
712.23 Pseudogout of the wrist
714.0 Rheumatoid arthritis
715.13 Osteoarthritis of the wrist, primary
715.23 Osteoarthritis of the wrist, secondary
715.93 Osteoarthritis of the wrist, unspecified
716.13 Traumatic arthropathy of the wrist
716.92 Traumatic arthropathy unspecified, forearm

Figure 1 PA radiograph showing osteoarthritis of the wrist. Note the subchondral sclerosis of the radius and the loss of radiocarpal joint space (black arrow). The scapholunate interval is also widened (white arrow).

Differential Diagnosis

- Septic arthritis of the wrist (acute onset, severe pain and restriction of wrist motion, systemic signs of infection)
- Tenosynovitis (normal radiographs, swelling over the involved tendon)

Adverse Outcomes of the Disease

Pain, loss of motion and/or strength, and impaired function in the wrist and fingers are possible.

Treatment

Medical management depends on the type of arthritis present. Temporary immobilization in a splint can help relieve pain and swelling. In the absence of infection, injection of a corticosteroid may provide temporary pain relief (see pages 431-432). Surgery is usually necessary when hand function decreases, when the joint becomes unstable, or when nonsurgical treatment fails to relieve pain. Surgical treatment usually focuses on improving stability and limiting discomfort.

Adverse Outcomes of Treatment

Loss of motion and persistent pain can develop. NSAIDs can cause gastric, renal, or hepatic complications.

Referral Decisions/Red Flags

Patients with a possible wrist infection require immediate evaluation. Those with radiographic evidence of advanced disease from degenerative or rheumatoid arthritis and those who do not respond to splinting and NSAIDs also are candidates for further evaluation.

Procedure: Wrist Aspiration/Injection

Step 1
Wear protective gloves at all times during this procedure and use sterile technique.

Step 2
Cleanse the area with a bactericidal skin preparation solution.

Step 3
Palpate the distal edge of the radius between the extensor carpi radialis brevis and extensor digitorum communis tendons. The depression just distal to the distal edge of the radius indicates the radiocarpal joint.

Step 4
Inject 1% local anesthetic in the subcutaneous tissue and joint capsule with the 25-gauge needle and then remove the needle.

Step 5
Insert the 22-gauge needle into the same site to aspirate the joint fluid. The joint fluid should be submitted for crystal analysis, total cell count and differential, Gram stain, and culture and sensitivity.

Step 6
If infection is not apparent, change the syringe and inject 0.5 to 1.0 mL of the corticosteroid preparation. The corticosteroid preparation may be mixed with an equal amount of 2% local anesthetic for pain relief.

Step 7
Dress the puncture wound with a sterile adhesive bandage.

Adverse Outcomes
Infection is possible. The infection may progress because corticosteroids can mask the usual signs of infection.

CPT Code

20605
Arthrocentisis, aspiration and/or injection; intermediate joint or bursa (eg, temporomandibular, acromioclavicular, wrist, elbow or ankle, olecranon bursa)

Current Procedural Terminology © 2010 American Medical Association. All rights reserved.

Materials
- Sterile gloves
- Bactericidal skin preparation solution
- 3-mL syringe with a 25-gauge needle
- 3-mL syringe with a 22-gauge needle
- 1-mL syringe
- 0.5 to 1.0 mL of 1% local anesthetic without epinephrine
- 0.5 to 1.0 mL corticosteroid preparation (optional)

SECTION 4 HAND AND WRIST

Aftercare/Patient Instructions

Instruct the patient to watch for signs of infection, such as increasing pain, swelling, heat, or redness, and to call your office if any of these signs occur. Follow-up with the patient to review the culture results is usually appropriate.

Boutonnière Deformity

Synonyms

Central slip extensor tendon injury

Jammed finger

ICD-9 Code

736.21
Boutonnière deformity

Definition

Boutonnière deformity occurs when the central portion of the extensor tendon ruptures at its insertion onto the middle phalanx (**Figure 1**), causing the proximal interphalangeal (PIP) joint to flex from the unopposed pull of the flexor tendon. The head of the proximal phalanx "buttonholes" between the lateral bands of the extensor tendon mechanism. As a result, the lateral bands are displaced below the axis of rotation of the PIP joint, causing it to flex further. More distally, the lateral bands are displaced dorsal to the axis of the distal interphalangeal (DIP) joint, causing it to extend or hyperextend.

Clinical Symptoms

Patients typically report a history of trauma. The finger is held partially flexed at the PIP joint and extended or hyperextended at the DIP joint. With a recent injury, the PIP joint is painful and tender. Initially, the boutonnière deformity may not be apparent, but it can develop over 7 to 21 days as the intact lateral bands of the extensor tendon slip inferiorly.

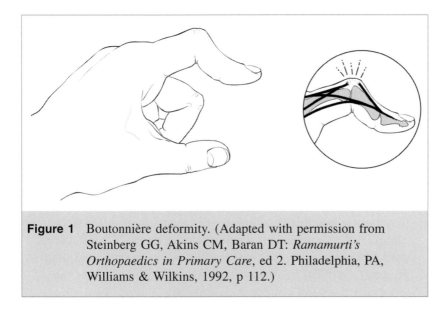

Figure 1 Boutonnière deformity. (Adapted with permission from Steinberg GG, Akins CM, Baran DT: *Ramamurti's Orthopaedics in Primary Care*, ed 2. Philadelphia, PA, Williams & Wilkins, 1992, p 112.)

Tests

Physical Examination

Ask the patient to extend the injured finger and observe the position of the PIP and DIP joints. The PIP joint will be flexed more than 30°, and the DIP joint will be extended or hyperextended. To demonstrate less severe deformities, hold the metacarpophalangeal and wrist joints in flexion and ask the patient to extend the PIP joint. A patient who lacks 15° to 20° of extension at the PIP joint probably has a rupture of the central slip of the extensor tendon.

Diagnostic Tests

AP and lateral radiographs will rule out a fracture or a pseudo-boutonnière deformity, in which the PIP joint is fixed in flexion and radiographs show calcification at the lateral aspect of the PIP joint.

Differential Diagnosis

- Dislocation of the PIP joint (painful, locked joint following surgery)
- Fracture around the PIP joint (radiographs required to confirm)
- Pseudoboutonnière deformity (PIP joint fixed in flexion, radiographs show calcification at the lateral aspect of the PIP joint)
- Rupture of the flexor tendon sheath (annular pulley) (painful flexor tendon sheath following injury)
- Sprain of the PIP joint (may be difficult to differentiate on initial examination; sprains have isolated collateral ligament tenderness and/or instability)

Adverse Outcomes of the Disease

Flexion contracture of the PIP joint and extension contracture of the DIP joint are both possible.

Treatment

Nonsurgical treatment is usually preferable. The PIP joint should be splinted in extension for 6 weeks in a young patient or for 3 weeks in an elderly patient (**Figure 2**). The DIP joint is left free. Active and passive motion should be initiated at the DIP joint.

If the injury is more than 1 or 2 weeks old at presentation, it may not be possible to achieve full extension at the first visit. The use of a dynamic extension splint (**Figure 2C**) is required until full extension is achieved, followed by a static splinting program. Surgical treatment is occasionally necessary if the deformity does not correct with splinting.

Figure 2 Static extension splint (**A**), commercial static splint (**B**), and dynamic extension splint (**C**) for the proximal interphalangeal (PIP) joint. (Reproduced from Culver JE: Office management of athletic injuries of the hand and wrist. *Instr Course Lect* 1989;38:473-486.)

Adverse Outcomes of Treatment

Failure to achieve full extension, residual PIP flexion deformity, or both are possible.

Referral Decisions/Red Flags

Failure to achieve full extension, residual deformity, or both are indications for further evaluation.

Carpal Tunnel Syndrome

ICD-9 Code

354.0
Carpal tunnel syndrome

Synonyms

Median nerve compression

Median nerve entrapment at the wrist

Definition

Carpal tunnel syndrome (entrapment of the median nerve at the wrist) is the most common compression neuropathy in the upper extremity. It most commonly affects middle-aged or pregnant women.

Any condition that reduces the size or space of the carpal tunnel (**Figure 1**) can cause compression of the median nerve, resulting in paresthesias, pain, and sometimes paralysis. Common precipitating conditions include tenosynovitis of the adjacent flexor tendons (repetitive overuse trauma or rheumatoid arthritis), tumors, and medical conditions such as pregnancy, diabetes mellitus, and thyroid dysfunction.

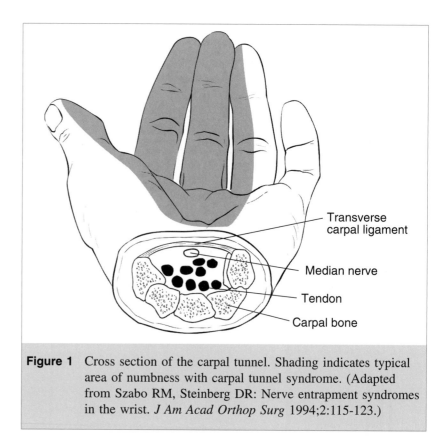

Figure 1   Cross section of the carpal tunnel. Shading indicates typical area of numbness with carpal tunnel syndrome. (Adapted from Szabo RM, Steinberg DR: Nerve entrapment syndromes in the wrist. *J Am Acad Orthop Surg* 1994;2:115-123.)

Clinical Symptoms

The symptoms most commonly reported are numbness and tingling into the radial three digits of the hand (thumb, index, and long fingers). Patients also may report a vague aching that radiates into the thenar area. Aching also may be perceived in the proximal forearm, and occasionally the pain can extend to the shoulder. The pain is typically accompanied by paresthesias or numbness in the median distribution (thumb and index finger, long finger, and radial half of the ring finger, or some combination thereof). Often the symptoms are worse at night.

Patients report that they frequently drop objects, or that they cannot open jars or twist off lids. Pain or numbness sometimes is made worse by activities that require repetitive motion of the hand, repetitive activities, or stationary tasks performed with the wrist held flexed or extended for long periods, such as driving or reading. Patients often awaken at night with pain or numbness and typically report the need to rub or shake the hand to "get the circulation back." When the compression is severe and long-standing, persistent numbness and thenar atrophy can occur (**Figure 2**).

Figure 2 Thenar atrophy.

Tests

Physical Examination

Inspect the hand for thenar atrophy. Testing thumb opposition against resistance may reveal weakness of the thenar muscles (see page 410). Evaluate the sensation in the fingers.

The Phalen maneuver is the most useful clinical test. It is performed by placing the wrists in flexion (see page 413). Avoid excessive elbow flexion when performing this test. Aching and numbness in the distribution of the median nerve within 60 seconds (often within 15 seconds or less) is a positive test for carpal tunnel syndrome. Tapping over the median nerve at the wrist may produce tingling in some or all of the digits in the median nerve distribution (see page 412). Thumb pressure (see page 412) over the median nerve at the wrist for up to 30 seconds may elicit pain or paresthesias in the median distribution.

Patients with carpal tunnel syndrome may be unable to distinguish the two points of a caliper as separate points when they are closer than 5 mm together (see page 411). Two-point discrimination of 5 mm is considered normal.

Diagnostic Tests

Radiographs of the wrist should be obtained if the patient has limited wrist motion. Most often, the diagnosis of carpal tunnel syndrome is made by clinical history and physical examination findings. Electrophysiologic testing is the most useful confirmatory test. These studies must be interpreted with caution, however. Some patients have no clinical signs or symptoms yet have abnormal nerve conduction velocity studies. Conversely, as many as 5% to 10% of patients with carpal tunnel syndrome have normal results.

Differential Diagnosis

- Arthritis of the carpometacarpal joint of the thumb (painful motion)
- Cervical radiculopathy affecting the C6 nerve (neck pain, numbness in the thumb and index fingers only)
- Diabetes mellitus with neuropathy (history)
- Flexor carpi radialis tenosynovitis (tenderness near the base of the thumb)
- Hypothyroidism (abnormal results on thyroid function tests)
- Pronator syndrome (median nerve compression at the elbow) (tenderness at the proximal forearm)
- Ulnar neuropathy (first dorsal interosseous weakness, numbness of the ring and little fingers)
- Volar radial ganglion (mass near the base of the thumb above the wrist flexion crease)
- Wrist arthritis (limited motion evident on radiographs)

Adverse Outcomes of the Disease

Permanent loss of sensation, hand strength, and fine motor skills are possible.

Treatment

For mild cases, splinting the wrist (in a neutral position wrist splint) and a short-term course of NSAIDs are suggested. The splint should be worn at night (at a minimum) and can be worn during the day if doing so does not interfere with the patient's work or daily activities. If these measures fail, consider injecting a corticosteroid into the carpal canal (see pages 441-442). Injection has diagnostic as well as therapeutic benefits, but improvement may be only temporary. Care must be taken to avoid direct injection into the median nerve, which may cause severe pain.

Work-related carpal tunnel syndrome may be improved with ergonomic modifications, such as using keyboard or forearm supports, adjusting the height of computer keyboards, and avoiding holding the wrist in a flexed position (as with dental hygienists).

Carpal tunnel syndrome that occurs during pregnancy usually resolves when the pregnancy terminates; therefore, treatment should consist of splinting and other nonsurgical measures, such as injection of a corticosteroid.

Surgical management is often necessary for patients who have fixed sensory loss or weakness of the thenar muscles and for those who have intolerable symptoms despite a course of nonsurgical treatment.

Rehabilitation Prescription

The purpose of nonsurgical management of carpal tunnel syndrome is to diminish the pressure on the median nerve at the wrist. In the early stages, the use of a night splint with the wrist in neutral position (0° of extension) is advocated. The wrist splint is worn for 3 to 4 weeks, during the day as well as at night. To reduce inflammation and pain, ice is used in the early stages. Heat is used to increase circulation and to promote tendon gliding. Exercises to promote tendon gliding are very important in the early stages of treatment (see page 440).

If the symptoms do not respond to the home program, the patient should be referred to a certified hand therapist. The therapist should evaluate range of motion, muscle strength, and sensory changes to determine the next stage of treatment. Strengthening exercises, continued use of a night splint, and ergonomic evaluation of the patient's job station should be part of the management of this condition. Other therapeutic modalities, such as iontophoresis, may be beneficial.

Adverse Outcomes of Treatment

NSAIDs can cause gastric, renal, or hepatic complications. Fluid retention, flushing of the skin, and shakiness can result from taking oral corticosteroids. Injecting corticosteroids is associated with the risk of an intraneural injection, which can have long-term adverse consequences. Prolonged nonsurgical treatment in patients with persistent sensory loss or motor weakness can result in loss of sensation and thenar atrophy.

Referral Decisions/Red Flags

Failure of nonsurgical treatment after 3 months warrants further evaluation. Persistent numbness, weakness, atrophy of the thenar muscles, or any combination of these are indications for further evaluation.

Home Physical Therapy Program for Carpal Tunnel Syndrome

- Apply heat to the hand for 15 minutes before performing the exercises, and apply ice (a bag of crushed ice or frozen peas) to the hand for 20 minutes after each exercise session to prevent inflammation.

- If numbness steadily worsens, if the exercises increase the pain, or if the pain does not improve after you have performed the exercises for 3 to 4 weeks, call your doctor.

Exercise Type	Targeted Structure	Number of Repetitions/Sets	Number of Days per Week	Number of Weeks
Nerve and tendon gliding	Median nerve	10 to 15 repetitions	6 to 7	3 to 4

Nerve and Tendon Gliding

- With the affected hand raised, make a fist with the thumb outside the fingers (1).

- Extend the fingers, keeping the thumb close to the side of the hand (2).

- Extend the hand at the wrist (bend it backward, toward the forearm), keeping the fingers straight (3).

- With the wrist straight, extend the thumb as shown (4).

- Keeping the thumb extended, extend the hand at the wrist (5).

- Reach behind your hand and grasp the thumb with the thumb and forefinger of the opposite hand. Pull the thumb downward, away from the palm of your hand (6).

- Repeat 10 to 15 times.

- Perform the exercises 6 to 7 days a week, for 3 to 4 weeks.

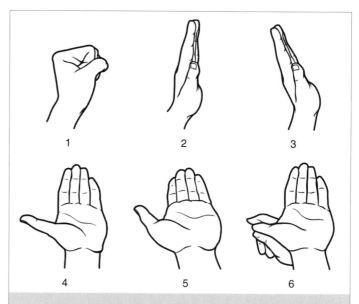

(Adapted with permission from Donatelli R, Wooden M, eds: *Orthopaedic Physical Therapy*. Philadelphia, PA, Elsevier, 2001.)

Procedure: Carpal Tunnel Injection

Note: Opinions differ regarding single- and two-needle injection techniques. Proponents of the single-needle technique believe that one needle is less painful for the patient than two. Because the corticosteroid preparation is thicker than the local anesthetic, however, a slightly larger gauge needle is required at the outset.

Step 1
Wear protective gloves at all times during this procedure and use sterile technique.

Step 2
Cleanse the volar aspect of the wrist with a bactericidal skin preparation solution.

Step 3
Insert the needle 1 cm proximal to the wrist flexion crease and in line with the ring finger metacarpal. Direct the needle toward the hand at an angle of 30° to 45° (**Figure 1**). Have the patient flex the fingers fully into the palm; then advance the needle approximately 1.0 to 1.5 cm until resistance is felt. If the patient reports paresthesias, redirect the needle.

Step 4
Instruct the patient to slightly wiggle the tips of the ring and little fingers. If this causes slight movement of the tip of the needle, the needle is safely positioned.

Step 5
Ask the patient to extend the fingers as gentle pressure is applied to the syringe. The distal excursion of the flexor tendons of the ring and little fingers will carry the point of the needle into the carpal canal.

Step 6
Ask the patient if any paresthesias occurred with the introduction of the needle. If the patient reports any tingling, then the needle is too close to the nerve and must be repositioned. Otherwise, inject 1 to 2 mL of local anesthetic into the carpal canal. If resistance is encountered on attempting to

CPT Code

20526
Injection, therapeutic (eg, local anesthetic, corticosteroid), carpal tunnel

Current Procedural Terminology
© 2010 American Medical Association. All rights reserved.

Materials
- Sterile gloves
- Bactericidal skin preparation solution
- Two 3-mL syringes with a 25-gauge needle
- 2 to 5 mL of a 1% local anesthetic without epinephrine
- 1 to 2 mL of a corticosteroid preparation
- Adhesive bandage

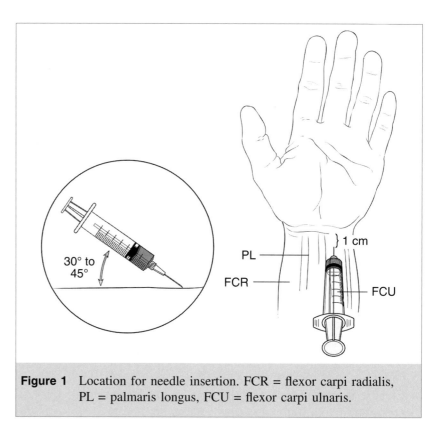

Figure 1   Location for needle insertion. FCR = flexor carpi radialis, PL = palmaris longus, FCU = flexor carpi ulnaris.

inject the local anesthetic, the tip of the needle is embedded in the flexor tendons. Maintain some pressure on the syringe while slowly withdrawing the needle, until the anesthetic flows freely. Leave the needle in place and change syringes. Inject 1 to 2 mL of corticosteroid into the carpal canal and then remove the needle.

Step 7
Dress the puncture wound with a sterile adhesive bandage.

Adverse Outcomes
Infection or intraneural injection is possible.

Aftercare/Patient Instructions
Advise the patient that mild soreness may develop, that the hand and fingers may be numb for 1 to 2 hours following the injection, and that the injection could require 24 to 48 hours to take effect.

de Quervain Tenosynovitis

Synonym

Stenosing tenosynovitis

Definition

de Quervain tenosynovitis is swelling or stenosis of the sheath that surrounds the abductor pollicis longus and extensor pollicis brevis tendons at the wrist (**Figure 1**). The inflammation thickens the tendon sheath (tenosynovium) and constricts the tendon as it glides in the sheath. This can cause pain, swelling, and a triggering phenomenon, resulting in locking or sticking of the tendon as the patient moves the thumb. The disorder is common in middle-aged women and is often precipitated by repetitive use of the thumb.

Clinical Symptoms

Patients report swelling over the radial styloid and pain that is aggravated by attempts to move the thumb or make a fist. They also may notice creaking as the tendon moves.

Tests

Physical Examination

Examination reveals swelling and tenderness over the tendons of the first dorsal compartment in the region of the distal radius. Crepitus may be palpable as the patient flexes and extends the thumb. Full flexion of the thumb into the palm, followed by ulnar deviation of the wrist (see Finkelstein Test, **Figure 2** and page 412), produces pain and is diagnostic for de Quervain tenosynovitis.

Diagnostic Tests

Even though this is largely a clinical diagnosis, PA and lateral radiographs of the wrist should be considered to rule out any bony abnormality that might be a precipitating cause, such as a deformed radial styloid process resulting from trauma. Calcification associated with tendinitis occasionally can be seen on radiographs.

ICD-9 Code

727.04
de Quervain tenosynovitis

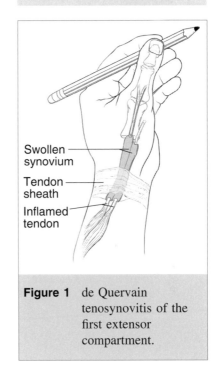

Swollen synovium

Tendon sheath

Inflamed tendon

Figure 1   de Quervain tenosynovitis of the first extensor compartment.

Figure 2 Finkelstein test. Arrow indicates location of pain when test is positive. (Adapted with permission from the American Society for Surgery of the Hand: *de Quervain's Stenosing Tenosynovitis*. Englewood, CO, 1995.)

Differential Diagnosis

- Carpometacarpal arthritis of the thumb (swelling over the joint, pain with joint compression)
- Dorsal wrist ganglion (palpable mass)
- Flexor carpi radialis tendinitis (pain and swelling over the tendon)
- Fracture of the scaphoid (tenderness over the anatomic snuffbox)
- Intersection syndrome
- Superficial radial neuritis
- Wrist arthritis (pain with movement, evident on radiographs)

Adverse Outcomes of the Disease

Chronic pain, loss of strength, and loss of thumb motion can occur; tendon rupture is possible but rare.

Treatment

Initial treatment should consist of a 2-week course of NSAIDs and a thumb spica splint that immobilizes both the wrist and thumb. If this initial treatment fails, the tendon sheath may be injected with a corticosteroid preparation, taking care not to inject the steroid into the tendon (see pages 445-446). After injection, the thumb is immobilized in a long opponens splint for 48 hours. The patient should have no more than three injections.

Surgical treatment should be considered if corticosteroid injections are not successful.

Adverse Outcomes of Treatment

NSAIDs may cause gastric, renal, or hepatic complications. The patient may experience some discomfort from wearing the splint and will stop using it. Corticosteroids can sometimes cause subcutaneous atrophy and unsightly loss of pigmentation. Infection after corticosteroid injection also is a risk, but this can be largely avoided by careful use of sterile technique. Injury to the radial sensory nerve or incomplete release is possible with surgical treatment.

Referral Decisions/Red flags

Failure to respond to splinting and corticosteroid injections indicates the need for further evaluation.

Procedure: de Quervain Tenosynovitis Injection

Note: Opinions differ regarding single- and two-needle injection techniques. Proponents of the single-needle technique believe that one needle is less painful for the patient than two. Because the corticosteroid preparation is thicker than the local anesthetic, however, a slightly larger-gauge needle is required at the outset.

Step 1

Wear protective gloves at all times during this procedure and use sterile technique.

Step 2

Cleanse the skin with a bactericidal skin preparation solution.

Step 3

Insert the 27-gauge needle at a 45° angle to the skin in line with the two tendons (**Figure 1**). If the patient reports paresthesia into the thumb, the needle has depolarized the sensory branch of the radial nerve. Reposition the needle 2 to 3 mm dorsal or volar, to a position that does not cause paresthesia.

Step 4

Create a skin wheal with 0.5 mL of 1% local anesthetic and advance the needle until it strikes one of the underlying tendons. Inject the remaining anesthetic while slowly withdrawing the needle, until the anesthetic flows freely. Leave the needle in place and change syringes.

Step 5

Inject 2 mL of corticosteroid preparation into the tendon sheath. Palpation of the tendon sheath proximal to the point of injection should reveal swelling as the corticosteroid is injected. In general, there will be some dilation of the sheath with a successful injection.

Step 6

Dress the puncture site with a sterile adhesive bandage.

CPT Code

20500
Injection(s); single tendon sheath, or ligament, aponeurosis (eg, plantar "fascia")

Current Procedural Terminology © 2010 American Medical Association. All rights reserved.

Materials

- Sterile gloves
- Bactericidal skin preparation solution
- Two 3-mL syringes with a 27-gauge, 7/8″ needle
- 2 mL of corticosteroid preparation
- 2 mL of a 1% local anesthetic without epinephrine

Figure 1   Location for needle insertion for de Quervain injection.

Adverse Outcomes

Subcutaneous fat atrophy can follow subcutaneous infiltration of the corticosteroid preparation, leading to a waxy-appearing depression in the skin. In addition, although rare, infection is possible.

Aftercare/Patient Instructions

Increased pain is not uncommon after the injection, especially in the first 24 to 48 hours. At least one third of patients will experience increased discomfort during this time.

Dupuytren Contracture

Synonyms

Dupuytren disease

Palmar fibromatosis

Viking disease

ICD-9 Code

728.6
Dupuytren contracture

Definition

Dupuytren contracture is a nodular thickening and contraction of the palmar fascia (**Figure 1**). The disease has a dominant genetic component, particularly involving people of northern European descent. Dupuytren contracture most commonly affects men older than 50 years. Associated factors include epilepsy, diabetes mellitus, pulmonary disease, alcoholism, smoking, and repetitive trauma (vibrational).

Figure 1   Dupuytren contracture of the ring finger. **A,** Drawing showing affected palmar fascial cord. **B** and **C,** Clinical appearance in an individual with bilateral Dupuytren contracture. The ring finger of the right hand, the little finger of the left hand, and both palms are affected. (Part A adapted with permission from the American Society for Surgery of the Hand: *Dupuytren's disease*. Englewood, CO, 1995.)

Clinical Symptoms

Patients initially notice one or more painless nodules near the distal palmar crease that are moderately sensitive to pressure. The nodule or nodules may gradually thicken and contract, causing the finger to flex at the metacarpophalangeal (MP) joint and, occasionally as the disease progresses, the proximal interphalangeal (PIP) joint. The ring finger is most commonly involved, followed by the little finger, the long finger, the thumb, and the index finger. Although extension is limited, finger flexion is often normal. The condition is usually painless in its later stages, but as the contractures increase, patients have trouble grasping objects, pulling on gloves, and putting the hand into a pocket. Sensation in the affected fingers usually is normal unless the patient has concomitant carpal tunnel syndrome.

Tests

Physical Examination

Examination reveals a palmar skin nodule that in the early stages may resemble a callus. As the disease progresses, the abnormal cords extend distally and sometimes proximally to the nodule. These bands may cross the PIP joint and commonly cross the MP joint, holding the finger in a contracted position. The bands are seldom tender unless the patient is in the early stages of the disease.

Diagnostic Tests

Diagnosis is made upon clinical examination. Radiographs are not needed.

Differential Diagnosis

- Flexion contracture secondary to joint or tendon injury (no cords or bands)
- Locked trigger finger (no associated nodules)

Adverse Outcomes of the Disease

Progressive flexion contracture of the fingers and limited function are possible.

Treatment

Splinting or other nonsurgical treatment is not curative, but night splints may slow the progression of the contractures. Percutaneous aponeurotomy may be appropriate in some cases for the treatment of isolated cords. Collagenase injection to the involved cord is currently under investigation as a form of treatment. Surgery involves excising the thick cords, releasing the joint contractures, and often complex skin closure. Surgery is considered when there is a 30° fixed flexion deformity of the MP joint or a 10° deformity of the PIP joint. More severe contractures are more difficult to correct, have a higher incidence of recurrent contracture, and require a longer course of postoperative occupational therapy.

Adverse Outcomes of Treatment

Patients may experience nerve injury, skin loss, and recurrence of the disease postoperatively.

Referral Decisions/Red Flags

Patients with significant contractures (greater than 30°) of the MP joints who are troubled by the lack of extension are candidates for further evaluation. Likewise, patients with involvement of the PIP joint in association with Dupuytren disease require close follow-up.

Fingertip Infections

ICD-9 Codes

054.6
Herpetic whitlow

681.01
Pulp abscess

681.02
Paronychia of finger

Synonyms

Felon
Paronychia

Definition

Infections of the fingertip typically occur in two locations: in the pulp, or palmar tip, of the finger (felon) and in the soft tissues directly surrounding the fingernail (paronychia) (**Figure 1**). *Staphylococcus aureus* is the most common causative organism in both conditions.

Felons usually are caused by a puncture wound and most commonly occur in the thumb or index finger (**Figure 2**). Herpetic whitlow, a virally mediated hand infection that is

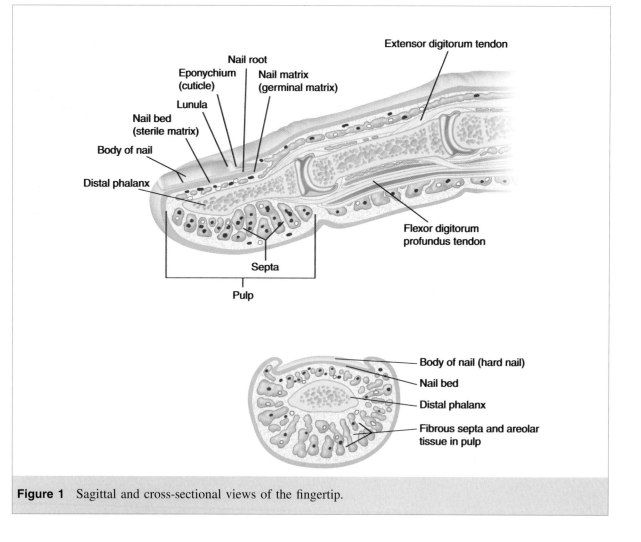

Figure 1 Sagittal and cross-sectional views of the fingertip.

characterized by the formation of vesicles filled with clear fluid, also can occur in and around the fingertip (**Figure 3**). Differentiating a felon from herpetic whitlow is important, as incision and drainage of a felon usually is indicated, whereas incision of a whitlow is contraindicated and observation is sufficient. Health care workers who are frequently exposed to the herpes simplex virus from human saliva (eg, respiratory therapists, dental hygienists) are at increased risk for herpetic whitlow. Paronychial infections often occur after a manicure or the development of a nail deformity, such as a hangnail or an ingrown nail.

Clinical Symptoms

A felon is characterized by severe pain and swelling in the pad of the fingertip. With a felon, the entire pulp of the fingertip is swollen, tense, red, and very tender. Also, a puncture wound may be visible.

Paronychial infection is characterized by swelling of the tissues about the fingernail, usually along one side and about the base of the nail. Occasionally, the swelling extends completely around the nail and is then referred to as a "run-around abscess." The pain associated with a paronychia is not as intense as that with a felon.

Swelling associated with a felon or paronychia should not extend proximal to the distal flexion crease. Any such extension suggests a deeper, more complex process, such as an infection involving the flexor tendon sheath. Significantly increased pain with passive motion also may indicate flexor tendon sheath infection.

Tests

Physical Examination

The fingertip should be examined for the location and extent of the swelling. The presence of small vesicles suggests herpetic whitlow. Tenderness, redness, and fluctuance are more characteristic of a bacterial abscess (paronychia or felon).

Diagnostic Tests

Plain radiographs show soft-tissue swelling. Late in the course of infection, osteomyelitis of the distal phalanx may occur and is evident on radiographs as partial or complete resorption of the distal tuft of the phalanx. More aggressive surgical débridement is required in these cases.

Figure 2 Felon of the index finger. (Reproduced from Stern PJ: Selected acute infections. *Instr Course Lect* 1990;39:539-546.)

Figure 3 Herpetic whitlow. (Reproduced from Stern PJ: Selected acute infections. *Instr Course Lect* 1990;39:539-546.)

Figure 4 **A,** A felon. **B,** An oblique incision. **C,** Drawing of a central volar longitudinal incision shows hemostat used to spread the wound, releasing septal fluid.

Differential Diagnosis

- Chronic fungal infection (not responsive to antibiotics)
- Epidermal inclusion cyst (dorsal swelling proximal to the nail, usually not very painful)
- Septic tenosynovitis (increased pain with active and passive motion of finger)

Adverse Outcomes of the Disease

Untreated felons (**Figure 4A**) may lead to osteomyelitis of the distal phalanx. Nail deformities and progressive infection involving the distal joint and/or the flexor tendon sheath also may develop late in the course of these infections. Untreated felons may occasionally rupture into the flexor tendon sheath and cause septic flexor tenosynovitis.

Treatment

Most felons require surgical drainage under digital block anesthesia (see pages 455-457) and tourniquet control. Either of two incisions can be used: a central volar longitudinal incision or a dorsal midaxial incision. When a puncture wound is present, the wound should be incorporated into the incision when feasible.

When a collection of pus can be seen under the skin on the pad side of the finger, use an oblique incision (**Figure 4B**) or a central longitudinal incision extending from the flexion crease to the fingertip (**Figure 4C**). Culture the drainage for aerobic and anaerobic organisms. It is most important to use a curved hemostat to break up the septae of the digital pulp to ensure that the abscess is completely evacuated. To allow drainage, keep the wound open, using a gauze packing strip, and remove it in 1 to

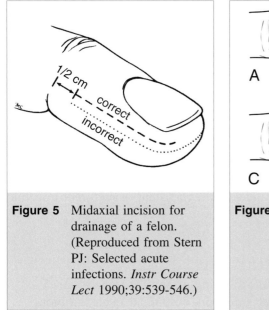

Figure 5 Midaxial incision for drainage of a felon. (Reproduced from Stern PJ: Selected acute infections. *Instr Course Lect* 1990;39:539-546.)

Figure 6 Removing a portion of a nail for paronychia. **A,** Use an elevator to separate the nail from the dorsal skin. **B,** Use an elevator to separate the nail from the underlying nail bed. **C,** With straight scissors, divide the nail itself. **D,** Remove the nail segment with a hemostat by applying gentle traction. (Adapted from the American Society for Surgery of the Hand: *Regional Review Course Manual.* Rosemont, IL, American Society for Surgery of the Hand, 1998, pp 7/8-7/9.)

2 days. Allow the wound to close by secondary intention; never suture the wound.

When no collection of pus is readily visible under the skin, use a dorsal midaxial incision (**Figure 5**). For the thumb, make the incision on the radial (noncontact) side; for the fingers, the ulnar (noncontact) side. Extend the incision to the fingertip but do not wrap it around the tip. Make the incision down to the bone where the soft-tissue attachments to the bone can be separated by blunt dissection with a small hemostat. Use open packing gauze and then remove it in 1 to 2 days.

Treatment of an early-stage paronychia is usually nonsurgical. Application of warm, moist soaks for 10 minutes four times a day, combined with an oral antibiotic for 5 days, is usually adequate. Because *S aureus* is the most likely causative organism, an oral cephalosporin such as cephalexin, 250 mg four times per day, or dicloxacillin, 250 mg four times per day, is a good initial choice. In patients at high risk for methicillin-resistant *S aureus* (MRSA), the addition of sulfamethoxazole and trimethoprim may be appropriate.

In later stages, when a purulent collection is noted at the nail bed margin or under the nail, drainage can be performed by elevating the skin fold at the margin of the nail. More severe infections require partial or complete removal of the nail (**Figure 6**). Under digital or metacarpal block anesthesia, the nail can be carefully elevated from the underlying sterile matrix using a hemostat or blunt metal probe. The nail can be completely removed by freeing the overlying cuticle, and the nail bed protected by a nonadherent gauze carefully tucked underneath the cuticle and extending to the tip of the finger. The wound should be checked in 2 to 3 days. The patient should be advised that the nail can be expected to grow out within several (up to 6) months.

Adverse Outcomes of Treatment

A painful scar may develop as a result of a misplaced incision, or a nail deformity can develop from injury to the germinal matrix. Inadequate drainage with persistent or recurrent infection may occur.

Referral Decisions/Red Flags

Persistent or progressive swelling or any evidence of an ascending hand or limb infection, despite adequate antibiotic treatment and surgical decompression, is an indication for further evaluation.

SECTION 4   HAND AND WRIST

Procedure: Digital Anesthetic Block (Hand)

Note: Two techniques are shown. The dorsal web space block is preferred by some because they believe the injection is less painful for the patient. Others prefer the volar block because they believe it is more effective.

Technique 1: Dorsal Web Space Block

Step 1
Wear protective gloves at all times during this procedure and use sterile technique.

Step 2
Cleanse all surfaces of the base of the finger with a bactericidal skin preparation solution.

Step 3
Draw 3 mL of the local anesthetic into the syringe.

Step 4
Insert the 27-gauge needle into the web space alongside the extensor tendon (**Figure 1A**). Advance the needle until it is almost at the volar skin and inject 1 mL of the local anesthetic.

CPT Code

64450
 Injection, anesthetic agent; other peripheral nerve or branch.

Current Procedural Terminology © 2010 American Medical Association. All rights reserved.

Materials

- Sterile gloves
- Bactericidal skin preparation solution
- 3-mL or 5-mL syringe with a 27-gauge needle
- 3 or 5 mL of 1% local anesthetic without epinephrine
- Sterile dressing

Figure 1 Technique 1. **A,** Dorsal location for needle insertion into the web space alongside the extensor tendon. **B,** Dorsal location for needle insertion along the top of the extensor tendon. **C,** Location for needle insertion into the web space on the opposite side of the finger.

Step 5
Withdraw the needle and insert it along the top of the extensor tendon (**Figure 1B**). Inject 1 mL of the solution.

Step 6
Repeat the procedure in the web space on the opposite side of the finger (**Figure 1C**).

Step 7
Dress the puncture site with a sterile adhesive dressing.

Technique 2: Volar Block

Step 1
Wear protective gloves at all times during this procedure and use sterile technique.

Step 2
Cleanse all surfaces of the base of the finger with a bactericidal skin preparation solution.

Step 3
Draw 5 mL of the local anesthetic into the syringe.

Step 4
Insert the 27-gauge needle into the palmar midline of the digit near the distal palmar crease. The first injection (approximately one third of the anesthetic) should be made at the midline. The needle should then be repositioned and another one third of the anesthetic injected toward the radial digital nerve. Reposition the needle again and inject the remainder of the anesthetic toward the ulnar digital nerve (**Figure 2**).

Step 5
Dress the injection site with a sterile adhesive dressing.

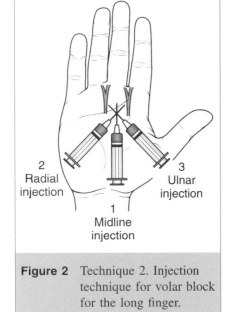

Figure 2 Technique 2. Injection technique for volar block for the long finger.

Adverse Outcomes

Although rare, infection is possible. Necrosis of a digit is possible if epinephrine is used in the anesthetic solution. Never inject circumferentially around the base of a digit, as this could cause circumferential hydrostatic pressure that can reduce circulation to the finger.

Aftercare/Patient Instructions

Advise the patient that local swelling at the site of the block should resolve in a few hours. Instruct the patient to call your office if the finger becomes dusky or completely white and to avoid touching hot surfaces or using sharp objects until all sensation has returned.

SECTION 4 HAND AND WRIST

Fingertip Injuries/ Amputations

Definition

Fingertip injuries and amputations are common. Some apparent amputations are actually crush injuries or lacerations. In addition to the soft tissue of the pulp, the distal phalanx and nail may be involved.

Clinical Symptoms

Patients report a history of a crush injury or a knife injury to the fingertip. The latter usually involves a finger in the nondominant hand.

Tests

Physical Examination

The fingertip should be inspected carefully to determine the vascularity and sensation of the skin flaps and if bone is exposed. The orientation of the amputation also should be noted (**Figure 1**) because the level and angle of amputation may determine appropriate treatment. The nail bed should be carefully examined for a painful subungual hematoma that should be drained and for lacerations of the nail bed that should be repaired. The vascularity of the tip, as well as sensation, should be noted.

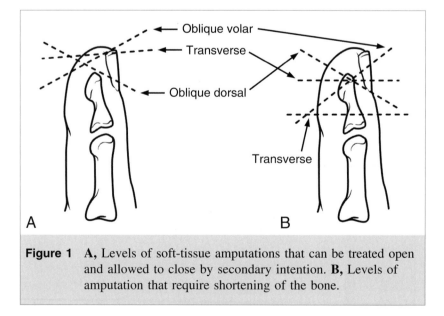

Figure 1 **A,** Levels of soft-tissue amputations that can be treated open and allowed to close by secondary intention. **B,** Levels of amputation that require shortening of the bone.

Diagnostic Tests

If bone is exposed or if the finger is markedly swollen, AP and lateral radiographs of the finger should be obtained.

Differential Diagnosis

- Amputation with injury to the nail matrix (evident on clinical examination)
- Amputation with open fracture (evident on radiographs)

Adverse Outcomes of the Disease

A painful amputation stump, dystrophic nail, loss of motion in the finger, and loss of grip and pinch strength are possible. Cold sensitivity/Raynaud phenomenon, a painful neuroma, or an epidermal inclusion cyst also can develop. Complex regional pain syndrome also is possible.

Treatment

The goals of treatment are to provide the fingertip with good soft-tissue coverage and adequate sensation, and to preserve as much length as is consistent with good function. Whether or not bone is exposed and the angle of the amputation relative to the long axis of the finger often dictate the appropriate treatment options (Figure 1).

If no bone is exposed, the physician must decide if the skin can be closed without excess tension. If not, the wound should be allowed to close by secondary intention. Fingertip wounds of 1 cm or less almost always heal well without closure. Initial treatment consists of thorough débridement and irrigation of the finger under a digital block and application of sterile dressings and a distal splint for comfort and contact protection. The initial dressings should be changed after 24 to 72 hours. Wet to dry dressings using normal saline solution twice a day are then applied. The patient should be taught how to apply these dressings and how to put on the removable splint at home. The dressing changes are continued until the tip has healed. Finger range-of-motion exercises should begin after 48 hours. Once the wound has healed, tip desensitization techniques can be started in occupational therapy. In most cases, allowing the wound to heal by secondary intention provides good function and acceptable cosmetic results and retains maximum finger length. Almost all fingertip injuries involving an area less than 1 cm square can be treated with débridement and the application of a dressing.

If bone is exposed, a decision must be made whether to shorten the bone or to provide skin coverage by a reconstructive flap procedure. As a general guide, the exposed phalanx of any of the fingers can be shortened to provide soft-tissue coverage without sacrificing function. Shortening the thumb is more controversial. Associated nail bed injuries require special attention (see page 504).

Treatment of amputation in children younger than 6 years differs somewhat from the treatment in adults. Most children heal rapidly and can be treated with local care and serial dressings. For some patients, "composite" grafting, or reapplication of the amputated fingertip as a full-thickness skin graft, is desirable. After thorough débridement and defatting, the skin of the amputated fingertip is sutured to the finger as a composite graft. Even if this graft does not survive (approximately 50% do survive), it serves as a biologic dressing until reepithelialization of the fingertip occurs. For fingertip injuries in children, always use absorbable sutures to limit the anxiety that occurs in follow-up visits.

The tetanus immunization status of the patient must be checked and updated if necessary. If the wound is grossly contaminated and/or crushed, or if the patient has diabetes mellitus, antibiotics may be used.

Replantation should be considered if the thumb is amputated at or proximal to the interphalangeal (IP) joint, if a finger is amputated proximal to the middle of the middle phalanx, or if multiple fingers are amputated. A replantation center should be contacted for specific instructions. The amputated part is wrapped in sterile gauze soaked in normal saline solution and placed in a plastic bag, and then the bag is placed on ice. The replantation team will usually make the determination if replantation is possible.

Most patients function quite well with single-finger amputations. Some patients are concerned with cosmesis, in which case a cosmetic finger prosthesis can be fitted.

Referral Decisions/Red Flags

Patients with thumb amputations proximal to the IP joint and multiple finger amputations are suitable candidates for specialty evaluation. Patients with single-finger amputations who desire replantation also should be referred to a replantation center.

Flexor Tendon Injuries

Synonyms

Jersey finger
Rugger jersey finger
Tendon laceration or rupture

Definition

The flexor tendons of the hand are vulnerable to laceration and rupture. Complete lacerations of both the flexor digitorum sublimis (FDS) and flexor digitorum profundus (FDP) cause immediate loss of flexion at the proximal interphalangeal (PIP) and distal interphalangeal (DIP) joints. Incomplete or partial lacerations can be missed on initial examination, only to present several days later as a complete rupture in the weakened tendon.

Ruptures of flexor tendons also can occur in patients with osteoarthritis, in patients with rheumatoid arthritis or other inflammatory arthritides, or as a result of trauma. Patients with rheumatoid arthritis may experience tendon rupture from direct synovial invasion of the tendon or from chronic wear over bony osteophytes. The latter type usually occurs during athletics (eg, football, wrestling, or rugby) when a player grabs another's jersey (thus the name jersey finger). When the fingers flex, the ring finger is most prominent and, therefore, the profundus tendon of the ring finger is most commonly ruptured during this activity.

Clinical Symptoms

Each finger is supplied with two flexor tendons: the FDP inserts onto the distal phalanx, and the FDS inserts onto the middle phalanx (**Figure 1**). Therefore, if the FDP is cut but the FDS is intact, patients can flex the PIP and metacarpophalangeal (MP) joints but not the DIP joint. If the FDS is cut but the FDP is intact, patients can flex the DIP, PIP, and MP joints (**Figure 2**). Because of the close proximity of the digital nerves to the flexor tendons, open injuries to the flexor tendons are commonly associated with injuries to the digital nerves as well. In this situation, patients will report numbness on one or both sides of the finger.

With traumatic rupture of the FDP, the ring finger becomes caught, as in a sports jersey (**Figure 3**), and the profundus tendon is avulsed from its insertion, possibly accompanied by a bony fragment. This injury can be missed or diagnosed late because it is often considered to be a jammed finger.

ICD-9 Codes

727.64
Rupture of flexor tendons of hand and wrist, nontraumatic

842.10
Tendon injuries of the hand, unspecified site

842.11
Tendon injuries of the hand, carpometacarpal

842.12
Tendon injuries of the hand, metacarpophalangeal

842.13
Tendon injuries of the hand, interphalangeal

842.19
Tendon injuries of the hand, midcarpal

Figure 1 Extrinsic flexor tendons of the finger. FDP = flexor digitorum profundus, FDS = flexor digitorum sublimis (Adapted with permission from Green DP, ed: *Operative Hand Surgery*, ed 2. New York, NY, Churchill Livingstone, 1988, p 1971.)

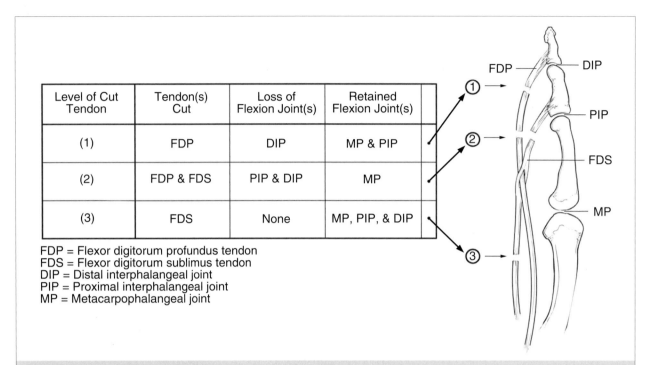

Level of Cut Tendon	Tendon(s) Cut	Loss of Flexion Joint(s)	Retained Flexion Joint(s)
(1)	FDP	DIP	MP & PIP
(2)	FDP & FDS	PIP & DIP	MP
(3)	FDS	None	MP, PIP, & DIP

FDP = Flexor digitorum profundus tendon
FDS = Flexor digitorum sublimus tendon
DIP = Distal interphalangeal joint
PIP = Proximal interphalangeal joint
MP = Metacarpophalangeal joint

Figure 2 Effects of flexor tendon injuries on flexion of the finger joint. (Adapted with permission from Green DP, ed: *Operative Hand Surgery*, ed 2. New York, NY, Churchill Livingstone, 1988, p 1971.)

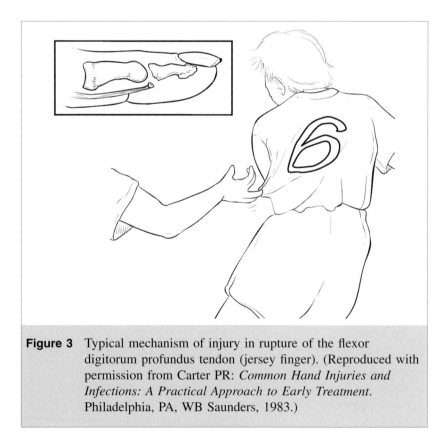

Figure 3 Typical mechanism of injury in rupture of the flexor digitorum profundus tendon (jersey finger). (Reproduced with permission from Carter PR: *Common Hand Injuries and Infections: A Practical Approach to Early Treatment.* Philadelphia, PA, WB Saunders, 1983.)

Tests

Physical Examination

First, test for active flexion; then test for strength of flexion. If the peritendinous structures are intact, the patient may retain flexion even in the presence of a complete laceration; however, flexion will be weak. Test flexion strength at both the DIP and PIP joints by asking the patient to flex the injured finger against your finger as you apply resistance.

Check flexion of the FDP by asking the patient to flex the fingertip at the DIP joint while the PIP joint is held in extension (see page 409). To test the integrity of the FDS, hold the fingers straight, then have the patient flex each finger individually at the PIP joint (see page 410). With a lacerated FDS but an intact FDP, PIP flexion will not occur when the other fingers are held extended. This is because the FDP tendons cannot function independently. This test is not reliable at the little finger because 20% to 30% of the population has a band connecting the ring and little fingers that prevents independent function of the sublimis to the little finger. In addition, in some patients, the FDP of the index finger can weakly flex the finger with the other fingers held extended.

Partial lacerations may pose a diagnostic challenge. Patients typically have full range of motion, but they have more *pain* with active flexion than would be expected. When the diagnosis is unclear, evaluation for possible surgical exploration should be considered.

Patients with a tendon rupture may have mild swelling over the flexion surface of the DIP joint and tenderness along the palmar surface of the finger. Test the strength of flexion at the DIP joint. When flexion is weak, rupture of the FDP must be considered a possibility. Patients with rheumatoid arthritis may not remember the point at which the tendon ruptured; they usually report only that the finger will not flex.

Sensation in the finger also should be evaluated because open tendon injuries are often accompanied by injuries to the nearby digital nerves. The vascular status of injured fingers should be checked and documented as well.

Diagnostic Tests

PA and lateral radiographs of the involved finger may show a small avulsed fragment from the distal phalanx in an FDP rupture. These views also may identify a fracture.

Figure 4 Flexor tendon splint.

Differential Diagnosis

- Anterior interosseous nerve paralysis (no laceration)
- Partial tendon laceration (full flexion with pain and weakness)
- Stenosing tenosynovitis ("trigger finger") with the finger locked in extension (no visible wound, tenderness over the proximal flexor pulley)

Adverse Outcomes of the Disease

Loss of flexion and loss of grip and pinch strength in the involved and adjacent fingers is possible.

Treatment

The principal goal of initial treatment is to correctly identify the condition and ensure that the patient is evaluated for surgical repair. Patients with flexor tendon injuries should be referred for consultation and surgical repair; initial treatment consists of cleaning and repairing superficial wounds and splinting the hand in the position shown in **Figure 4**. Ideally, surgical exploration and repair should be performed within 1 week after injury.

Adverse Outcomes of Treatment

Postoperative infection or failure of the repair is possible.

Referral Decisions/Red Flags

Patients with any type of suspected flexor tendon injury (rupture or laceration) require further evaluation for surgical repair.

Flexor Tendon Sheath Infections

Synonym

Septic tenosynovitis

ICD-9 Code

727.89
Abscess of bursa or tendon

Definition

The flexor tendons of the fingers and thumb are enclosed in a specialized tenosynovial sheath that extends from the distal palm to the area of the distal interphalangeal (DIP) joint (**Figure 1**). Inoculations of this space from a puncture wound can cause severe finger infections. Infections within this space can develop from a puncture wound or can spread to the sheath from more superficial infection. These bacterial infections can be progressive and require both prompt diagnosis and treatment.

Clinical Symptoms

Patients typically present with a history of a recent puncture wound to the flexor surface of the finger or thumb. Progressive swelling of the entire digit and significant pain develop 24 to 48 hours after injury (**Figure 2**).

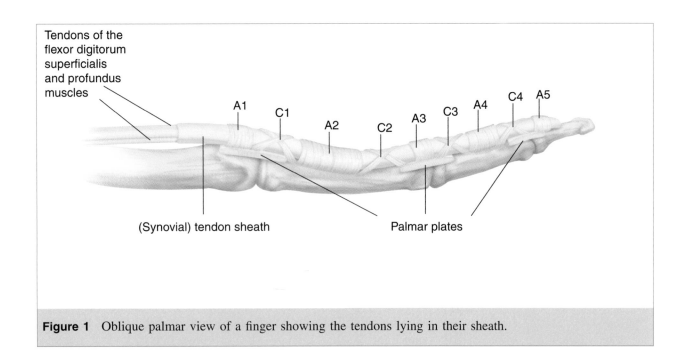

Tendons of the flexor digitorum superficialis and profundus muscles

A1 C1 A2 C2 A3 C3 A4 C4 A5

(Synovial) tendon sheath   Palmar plates

Figure 1   Oblique palmar view of a finger showing the tendons lying in their sheath.

SECTION 4 HAND AND WRIST

Figure 2 Clinical appearance of septic tenosynovitis. Septic tenosynovitis of the ring finger (**A**) and the long finger (**B**). Note the flexed position of the affected finger at rest. (Part A reproduced from Stern PJ: Selected acute infections. *Instr Course Lect* 1990;39:539-546.)

Tests

Physical Examination

Signs of a well-established septic flexor tenosynovitis are characterized by the Kanavel signs: (1) fusiform swelling of the finger, (2) significant tenderness along the course of the tendon sheath, (3) a marked increase in pain on passive extension, and (4) a flexed position of the finger at rest (**Figure 3**).

Diagnostic Tests

Radiographs may show soft-tissue swelling or, rarely, a foreign body or subcutaneous air.

Differential Diagnosis

- Aseptic flexor synovitis (negative bacterial cultures as might be seen in rheumatoid arthritis)
- Cellulitis (little or no pain with active motion of the finger)

Adverse Outcomes of the Disease

These infections progress rapidly; therefore, complications such as skin loss or loss of the entire finger are possible. Further, these infections can progress to the deep spaces of the hand and ultimately gain access to the forearm. Late problems include significant stiffness from adhesions and involvement of the bone and joint.

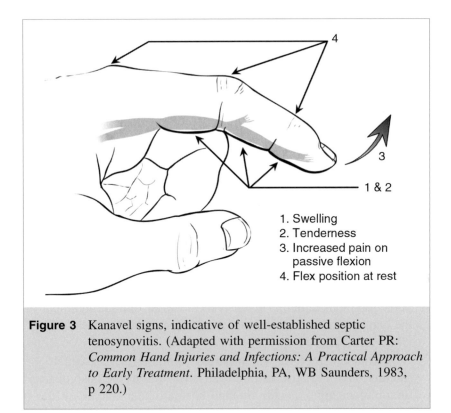

1. Swelling
2. Tenderness
3. Increased pain on passive flexion
4. Flex position at rest

Figure 3 Kanavel signs, indicative of well-established septic tenosynovitis. (Adapted with permission from Carter PR: *Common Hand Injuries and Infections: A Practical Approach to Early Treatment.* Philadelphia, PA, WB Saunders, 1983, p 220.)

Treatment

If septic tenosynovitis is suspected but the swelling is not severe, parenteral antibiotics should be initiated, and the patient should be reevaluated in 12 to 24 hours. Both *Staphylococcus* and *Streptococcus* should be covered. If the patient responds to parenteral antibiotics, these should be continued for 24 to 72 hours and then switched to oral antibiotics for an additional 7 to 14 days. If the patient has an established purulent flexor tenosynovitis or if the infection progresses or does not respond to antibiotic treatment, urgent referral for surgical drainage is indicated.

Adverse Outcomes of Treatment

Finger stiffness can persist, despite successful treatment of septic tenosynovitis.

Referral Decisions/Red Flags

Patients with well-established septic tenosynovitis and those who do not respond to antibiotic treatment require evaluation for possible surgery.

Fracture of the Base of the Thumb Metacarpal

ICD-9 Codes

815.01
Fracture of the metacarpal bone(s), base of thumb, closed

815.11
Fracture of the metacarpal bone(s), base of thumb, open

816.00
Fracture of one or more phalanges of hand, site unspecified, closed

Synonyms

Bennett fracture
Rolando fracture

Definition

A Bennett fracture is an oblique fracture of the base of the thumb metacarpal that enters the carpometacarpal (CMC) joint. This fracture has two pieces, one large and one small. The small volar fragment remains attached to the volar oblique ligament of the carpus, and the major metacarpal fragment displaces at the CMC joint (**Figure 1**).

A Rolando fracture, which is less common than a Bennett fracture, is a Y-shaped intra-articular fracture at the base of the thumb metacarpal. A comminuted intra-articular fracture at the base of the thumb metacarpal also occurs.

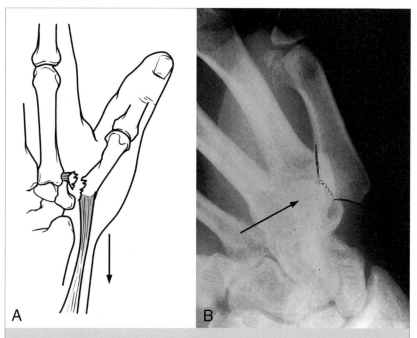

Figure 1 Fracture-subluxation of the base of the thumb metacarpal (Bennett fracture). **A,** Drawing showing the mechanism of injury. The medial fragment of the thumb metacarpal is stabilized by the intact volar oblique ligament. The arrow indicates the proximal pull of the abductor pollicis longus tendon. **B,** Radiograph showing a Bennett fracture.

Clinical Symptoms

Patients report pain and limited motion. Swelling and ecchymosis about the base of the thumb are common and are indicative of a metacarpal fracture or CMC dislocation.

Tests

Physical Examination

The thumb is painful to palpation at the base of the metacarpal. Examination also shows that, when the tip of the thumb is held into the palm, the base of the thumb metacarpal is displaced radially and posteriorly. The patient cannot move the thumb without pain.

Diagnostic Tests

AP, lateral, and oblique radiographs of the thumb will demonstrate these fractures.

Differential Diagnosis

- Arthritis of the CMC joint (narrow joint space evident on radiographs)
- Dislocation of the CMC joint (evident on radiographs)
- Fracture of the scaphoid (evident on radiographs)
- Synovitis of the CMC joint (swollen joint, normal radiographs)

Adverse Outcomes of the Disease

Posttraumatic arthritis of the CMC joint is possible, resulting in pain at the base of the thumb, along with loss of motion and pinch strength.

Treatment

The goal of treatment is to restore the axial length of the thumb and to replace the metacarpal shaft fragment against the smaller volar lip fragment. Although anatomic reduction of the fracture is the goal, even with some offset a good functional outcome is possible. A Bennett fracture almost always requires some form of surgical fixation to achieve stability in the joint.

Nondisplaced two-part fractures of the base of the thumb metacarpal can be treated in a thumb spica cast for 4 weeks.

Adverse Outcomes of Treatment

After surgery, pin tract irritation and infection can occur, as can tenderness around the surgical plates and screws. Displacement of the fracture (loss of position) and posttraumatic arthritis also are possible.

Referral Decisions/Red Flags

Intra-articular base of the thumb metacarpal fractures often require surgical treatment. These patients should be considered for early referral.

Fracture of the Hook of the Hamate

Synonyms

Fracture of the hamular process

Fracture of the hamate

ICD-9 Codes

814.08
Fracture of the hamate bone, closed

814.18
Fracture of the hamate bone, open

Definition

A fracture of the hook of the hamate involves the palmarmost aspect of the hamate bone of the wrist (**Figure 1**). Fractures of the hook of the hamate most commonly occur in players of racquet sports, golf, and baseball.

Clinical Symptoms

Patients most commonly present with a history of either repetitive trauma or direct trauma, as from grounding a golf club inadvertently or hitting a baseball, with resultant pain in the base of the ulnar side of the hand.

Figure 1   Palmar (**A**) and dorsal (**B**) views of the bones and ligaments of the wrist. P = pisiform, Tq = triquetrum, H = hamate, C = capitate, Tp = trapezoid, Tz = trapezium, S = scaphoid, L = lunate, U = ulna, R = radius. (Adapted with permission from Trumble TE, ed: *Principles of Hand Surgery and Therapy*. Phildelphia, PA, WB Saunders, 2000, pp 92 and 109.)

Figure 2 **A,** Fracture of the hook of the hamate (black arrow) seen on carpal tunnel view. Note the relationship of the pisiform (white arrow) to the hamate. **B,** CT scan demonstrates the fracture. (Part A reproduced from Johnson TR, Steinbach LS, eds: *Essentials of Musculoskeletal Imaging.* Rosemont, IL, American Academy of Orthopaedic Surgeons, 2003, p 344.)

Tests

Physical Examination

Pressure over the hook of the hamate will elicit pain, and swelling may be observed. Resisted flexion of the little finger with the wrist in ulnar deviation often increases the pain. Numbness along the ulnar nerve distribution (little finger and ulnar half of the ring finger) may be present. The hook is located 1 to 2 cm distal to and 1 to 2 cm radial to the pisiform.

Diagnostic Tests

Plain radiographs are often interpreted as normal. A carpal tunnel view may show the hook fracture (**Figure 2A**). Often a CT scan is necessary to demonstrate the fracture (**Figure 2B**).

Differential Diagnosis

- Flexor carpi ulnaris tendinitis (tenderness with wrist flexion)
- Little finger carpometacarpal joint fracture (tenderness more distal and dorsally, increases with wrist flexion)
- Pisiform fracture (tender more proximally, over the pisiform)
- Pisotriquetral arthritis (painful pisotriquetral compression)
- Ulnar artery thrombosis (abnormal Allen test)

Adverse Outcomes of the Disease

If left untreated and, often, if treated, hook of the hamate fractures go on to form a nonunion. The nonunion is usually painful and may require additional treatment. If the nonunion is long-standing, tendon rupture to the little finger may occur.

Treatment

Early, the hand should be immobilized in a neutral position with a splint or cast. Usually in the course of the process, excision of the hook of the hamate is necessary to control symptoms of wrist discomfort and reduce the risk of tendon rupture.

Adverse Outcomes of Treatment

Excision of the hook of the hamate can be associated with some loss of little finger flexion and power grip.

Referral Decisions/Red Flags

Hook of the hamate fractures should be referred for early evaluation and treatment.

Fracture of the Distal Radius

ICD-9 Codes

813.41
Colles fracture, Smith fracture

813.42
Dupuytren's fracture

813.52
Other fractures of distal end of radius (alone)

Synonyms

Barton fracture
Chauffeur's fracture
Colles fracture
Die-punch fracture
Smith fracture

Definition

Fractures involving the distal radius are among the most frequently occurring fractures in adults (**Figure 1**). The most common type is the Colles fracture (**Figure 2**), in which the distal radius fracture fragment is tilted upward, or dorsally. The articular surface of the radius may or may not be involved, and the ulnar styloid is usually fractured. A Smith fracture is the opposite of a Colles fracture: the distal fragment is tilted downward, or volarly. A Barton fracture (**Figure 3**) is an intra-articular fracture associated with subluxation of the carpus, either dorsally or volarly, along with the displaced articular fragment of the radius. A chauffeur's fracture is an oblique fracture through the base of the radial styloid. A die-punch

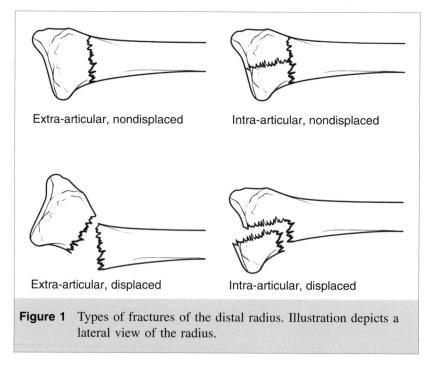

Extra-articular, nondisplaced

Intra-articular, nondisplaced

Extra-articular, displaced

Intra-articular, displaced

Figure 1   Types of fractures of the distal radius. Illustration depicts a lateral view of the radius.

Figure 2 Colles fracture. **A,** PA view shows loss of ulnar inclination (black arrow), shortening of the radius (white arrow), and the intra-articular extent of the fracture (arrowhead). **B,** Lateral view shows the radius is translated dorsally (lines) and is dorsally angulated about 30° (arrow). (Reproduced from Johnson TR, Steinbach LS, eds: *Essentials of Musculoskeletal Imaging*. Rosemont, IL, American Academy of Orthopaedic Surgeons, 2003, pp 339-340.)

Figure 3 Reverse (volar) Barton fracture. Note the volarly displaced distal radius fragment (black arrow), the increased volar angulation (line), and the volar subluxation of the carpus (arrowhead). (Reproduced from Johnson TR, Steinbach LS, eds: *Essentials of Musculoskeletal Imaging*. Rosemont, IL, American Academy of Orthopaedic Surgeons, 2003, p 340.)

fracture is a depressed fracture of the articular surface opposite the lunate or scaphoid bone. The most important concepts for classifying distal radius fractures are whether they are open or closed and whether they are displaced or nondisplaced.

Clinical Symptoms

The usual history is a fall on an outstretched hand. Patients have acute pain, tenderness, swelling, and deformity of the wrist.

Tests

Physical Examination

Look for swelling, deformity, and discoloration around the wrist and distal radius. Observe for skin injury and bleeding (usually with fat droplets in the blood) that would suggest an open fracture. Test for sensation in the hand over the median, radial, and ulnar nerve distribution. Also check the circulation to the fingertips. Examine the elbow for swelling and tenderness.

Diagnostic Tests

AP and lateral radiographs of the forearm, including the wrist, are necessary. Radiographs of the elbow should be obtained when elbow swelling and tenderness are present because some patients will have combined injuries to the distal end of the radius, the forearm, and the elbow.

Differential Diagnosis

- Carpal fracture-dislocation (evident on radiographs)
- Fracture of the scaphoid (tenderness over anatomic snuffbox, possibly evident on radiographs)
- Tenosynovitis of the wrist (normal radiographs)

Adverse Outcomes of the Disease

Malunion, loss of wrist motion, loss of finger motion, complex regional pain syndrome, decreased grip strength, posttraumatic arthritis, or (uncommonly) compartment syndrome can occur when a fracture of the distal radius is not treated.

Treatment

Open fractures require irrigation and débridement and antibiotics. Initial treatment usually focuses on reduction and splinting of the fracture. For most fractures, a sugar tong splint is appropriate. Anatomic reduction is ideal, but less-than-perfect bone alignment can be associated with a good functional outcome. Older, less active persons are more tolerant of residual deformity than are younger individuals. There is significant controversy in the orthopaedic literature as to what constitutes an acceptable reduction.

General guidelines for acceptable radiographic alignment after reduction of distal radius fractures are as follows (**Figure 4**): (1) On the lateral view, no more than 5° of dorsal angulation is acceptable. (2) On the AP view, no less than 15° of radial inclination is acceptable. (3) A step-off in the articular surface greater than 2 mm should be reduced. If these parameters are not met, early referral to an orthopaedic surgeon should be considered.

AP and lateral radiographs of the fracture should be repeated each week for several weeks after the fracture to determine if the alignment is satisfactory.

For nondisplaced and minimally displaced extra-articular fractures, a sugar tong splint should be applied for 2 to 3 weeks and a short arm cast for an additional 2 to 3 weeks. (Two weeks in a sugar tong splint plus 2 weeks in a short arm cast is adequate full-time immobilization for some older, less active

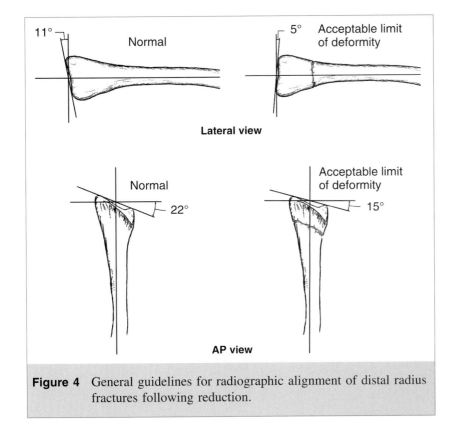

Figure 4 General guidelines for radiographic alignment of distal radius fractures following reduction.

patients.) After the short arm cast is removed, the patient should wear a removable splint for 3 weeks to allow removal for bathing and gentle exercise. The patient should be encouraged to move the shoulder and elbow of the injured arm through a full range of motion twice a day to prevent shoulder stiffness. Likewise, active and passive finger motion (five sets, four times a day) should be encouraged.

Displaced fractures often are unstable and require additional internal and/or external fixation techniques.

Adverse Outcomes of Treatment

Recurrence of deformity, malunion, loss of wrist motion (flexion, extension, pronation, and supination), posttraumatic wrist arthritis, carpal tunnel syndrome, loss of finger motion, compartment syndrome, or paresthesias of the radial sensory nerve all can result following treatment.

Referral Decisions/Red Flags

Displaced fractures that exceed the parameters outlined above and intra-articular fractures require further evaluation. Fractures that initially are nondisplaced but that show progressive collapse on radiographic follow-up require further evaluation. Clinical examination that demonstrates any neurologic dysfunction necessitates urgent referral.

Fracture of the Metacarpals and Phalanges

Synonyms

Boxer's fracture

Fighter's fracture

Definition

Metacarpal fractures are among the most common fractures in adults (**Figure 1**). The most common fracture in the hand is a boxer's fracture, an injury of the distal metaphysis of the fifth metacarpal that results when the closed fist strikes an object (**Figure 2**). In phalangeal fractures in adults, the distal phalanx is the most commonly injured (**Figure 3**), followed by the proximal and then the middle phalanx. Approximately 20% of these fractures are intra-articular.

ICD-9 Codes

815.00 - 815.19
Fracture of metacarpal bone(s), closed or open. These codes require a fifth digit. Please refer to ICD-9 for subclassification.

Continued on next page

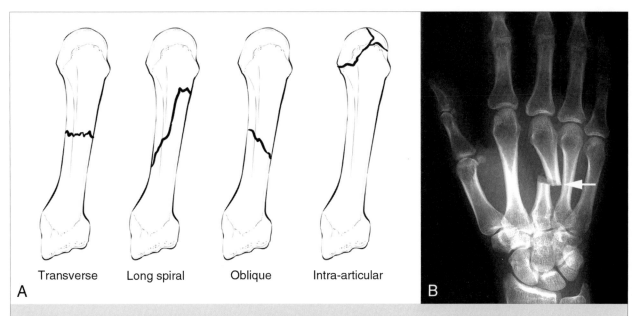

Transverse   Long spiral   Oblique   Intra-articular

A

B

Figure 1 **A,** Types of metacarpal fractures. **B,** PA view of a right hand shows a displaced transverse fracture of the middle metacarpal (arrow). (Part A adapted with permission from Dabezies EJ, Schutte JP: Fixation of metacarpal and phalangeal fractures with miniature plates and screws. *J Hand Surg* 1986;11A:283-288. Part B reproduced from Johnson TR, Steinbach LS, eds: *Essentials of Musculoskeletal Imaging.* Rosemont, IL, American Academy of Orthopaedic Surgeons, 2003, p 347.)

ICD-9 Codes (continued)

816.00 - 816.13
Fracture of one or more phalanges of hand, closed or open. These codes require a fifth digit. Please refer to ICD-9 for subclassification.

817.0
Multiple fractures of hand bones, closed

817.1
Multiple fractures of hand bones, open

Figure 2 Boxer's fracture. **A,** Drawing shows the direction of force that causes the fracture. **B,** PA view of a left hand shows an angulated fracture of the neck of the fifth metacarpal (arrow). The degree of angulation shown here is well tolerated without loss of function. (Part A adapted with permission from Green DP, ed: *Operative Hand Surgery*, ed 3. New York, NY, Churchill Livingstone, 1993. Part B reproduced from Johnson TR, Steinbach LS, eds: *Essentials of Musculoskeletal Imaging*. Rosemont, IL, American Academy of Orthopaedic Surgeons, 2003, p 347.)

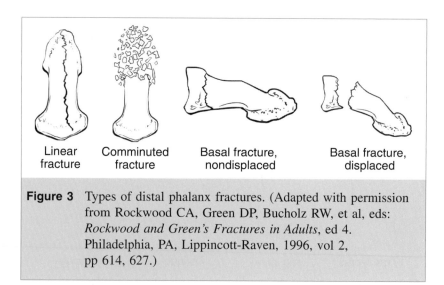

| Linear fracture | Comminuted fracture | Basal fracture, nondisplaced | Basal fracture, displaced |

Figure 3 Types of distal phalanx fractures. (Adapted with permission from Rockwood CA, Green DP, Bucholz RW, et al, eds: *Rockwood and Green's Fractures in Adults*, ed 4. Philadelphia, PA, Lippincott-Raven, 1996, vol 2, pp 614, 627.)

Phalangeal fractures are more common than metacarpal fractures in children. The most common fracture involves the physis of the little finger. Growth disturbances from physeal injuries of the phalanges are rare.

characteristic. Patients have pain on palpation of the snuffbox, and any type of wrist motion, such as gripping, is painful. Swelling about the back and radial side of the wrist also is common. If the patient reports a history of a high-energy injury, such as a car accident, ligamentous injuries and resultant carpal instability (perilunar instability) are possible in addition to the scaphoid fracture.

Tests

Physical Examination

Palpation over the anatomic snuffbox reveals marked tenderness. Likewise, pressure over the scaphoid tubercle on the underside of the wrist will produce pain. In addition, the patient may have decreased motion and grip strength. An intra-articular effusion is not uncommon for patients who present with an acute scaphoid fracture. Assess function of the median, ulnar, and radial nerves, as well as circulatory status.

Diagnostic Tests

Scaphoid fractures may not be visible on PA and lateral radiographs of the wrist obtained at the time of initial injury. Therefore, if these radiographs appear normal, obtain a PA view with the wrist in ulnar deviation and an oblique view to help visualize the fracture (**Figure 3**). If this series of initial radiographs is normal but the pain persists for 2 to 3 weeks, the PA and oblique views should be repeated. If the radiographs are still normal, an MRI should be ordered.

Differential Diagnosis

- de Quervain tenosynovitis (positive Finkelstein test)
- Fracture of the distal radius (evident on plain radiographs)
- Scapholunate dissociation (increased gap between scaphoid and lunate [**Figure 4**])
- Wrist arthritis (narrowing of joint space, evident on radiographs)

Adverse Outcomes of the Disease

Nonunion, decreased grip strength and range of motion, and osteoarthritis of the radiocarpal joint are possible.

Treatment

Patients with significant snuffbox tenderness (even with normal radiographs) should be treated initially as though they have a scaphoid fracture and placed in a thumb spica splint. Close follow-up with additional radiographs or MRIs will identify

Figure 2 The triangular area outlined on this hand is the anatomic snuffbox. EPL = extensor pollicis longus; EPB = extensor pollicis brevis.

Figure 3 PA view with the wrist in ulnar deviation demonstrating a scaphoid fracture (arrow).

SECTION 4 HAND AND WRIST

Figure 4 Clenched-fist view showing scapholunate dissociation (arrow) with increased gap between the scaphoid and the lunate.

occult scaphoid fractures. Because the interval to treatment can be important in minimizing the risk of nonunion, patients should be immobilized at the time of initial presentation until a definitive diagnosis can be reached. Once the diagnosis of an acute nondisplaced fracture of the scaphoid has been confirmed, treatment is controversial because agreement is lacking on the optimal type of immobilization for these fractures. Data are conflicting regarding the optimal position of the wrist, whether the elbow should be immobilized, and whether the thumb should be included in the cast. Immobilization for 6 weeks in a long arm-thumb spica cast with the wrist in a neutral position may be necessary. If radiographs obtained after this time show that the fracture is healing, apply a short arm-thumb spica cast. If the fracture line appears to be getting wider, however, indicating resorption at the fracture site, or if the fracture shows any displacement, then further evaluation for possible surgery is indicated.

If the patient has pain over the region of the snuffbox but the initial radiographs are normal, place the hand and wrist in a thumb spica splint for 1 to 2 weeks and then obtain repeat radiographs. If the radiographs are still normal but tenderness over the scaphoid persists, order an MRI. If the image is positive, treat the hand as for an acute nondisplaced scaphoid fracture.

It may be difficult to determine on routine radiographs whether a scaphoid fracture has healed, and immobilization may be discontinued too soon. As a general rule, the closer the fracture line is to the proximal pole, the longer the time for healing. For fractures of the distal pole, the average time for healing is 6 to 8 weeks. Fractures of the middle third require 8 to 12 weeks to heal, and fractures of the proximal pole can take 12 to 24 weeks or longer. If plain radiographs do not clearly reveal that the fracture has healed, an axial CT scan can be ordered to better visualize the fracture site.

Adverse Outcomes of Treatment

Loss of motion from prolonged immobilization and/or loss of grip strength can result.

Referral Decisions/Red Flags

All patients with displaced fractures of the scaphoid require early further evaluation for possible surgical treatment. All patients with scaphoid fractures in association with other wrist ligament injuries (perilunar instability) require urgent referral to a hand surgeon. Patients who show cystic absorption at the fracture site or displacement of the fracture after immobilization, or those with nondisplaced fractures that have not healed after 2 months of immobilization, require further evaluation for possible surgical treatment.

SECTION 4 HAND AND WRIST

Ganglion of the Wrist and Hand

ICD-9 Codes

727.41
Ganglion of joint

727.42
Ganglion of tendon sheath

727.43
Ganglion, unspecified

Figure 1 Wrist ganglion.

Synonyms

Flexor tendon sheath ganglion

Mucous cyst

Synovial cyst

Volar retinacular ganglion

Definition

A ganglion is a cystic structure that arises from the capsule of a joint or a tendon synovial sheath (**Figure 1**). The cyst contains a thick, clear, mucinous fluid identical in composition to joint fluid. Through degeneration or tearing of the joint capsule or tendon sheath, a connection to the joint or tendon sheath with a one-way valve is established. Thus, synovial fluid can enter the cyst but cannot flow freely back into the synovial cavity. Ganglions vary in size, and significant symptoms may result from increased pressure on surrounding structures.

Ganglions are the most common soft-tissue tumors of the hand, generally affecting individuals between the ages of 15 and 40 years. These benign tumors typically develop, and sometimes disappear, spontaneously. Common locations include the dorsum of the wrist, the volar radial aspect of the wrist, and the base of a finger. The latter typically arises from the proximal annular ligament (A1 pulley) of the flexor tendon sheath. These also are known as volar retinacular ganglia.

Mucous cysts are a type of ganglion that develops from an arthritic interphalangeal joint, most commonly in women between the ages of 40 and 70 years.

Clinical Symptoms

Wrist

Patients typically present with a lump, which may or may not be painful (**Figure 2**). The pain is described as aching and is aggravated by activities that require frequent movement of the wrist. Ganglia in the wrist often vary in size, with an increase in size associated with times of increased activity. A history of variation in size is a key factor to distinguish a ganglion from other soft-tissue tumors.

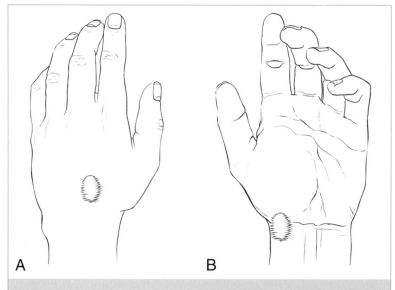

Figure 2 Clinical appearance of dorsal (**A**) and volar (**B**) wrist ganglia. (Adapted with permission from the American Society for Surgery of the Hand: *Ganglion Cysts.* Englewood, CO, 1995.)

Figure 3 Flexor tendon sheath ganglion. (Adapted with permission from the American Society for Surgery of the Hand: *Ganglion Cysts.* Englewood, CO, 1995.)

Occasionally, a ganglion will occur in an area of the wrist where it may result in compression of the median or ulnar nerve. In this situation, sensory symptoms in the fingers and/or weakness of the intrinsic muscle may develop.

Hand and Finger

Patients with flexor tendon sheath cysts report tenderness when grasping and have a bump at the base of the finger (usually at the level of the proximal flexion crease) (**Figure 3**). A tender mass in this area usually is a flexor tendon sheath ganglion.

Patients with mucous cysts have swelling on the dorsum of the finger distal to the distal interphalangeal (DIP) joint (**Figure 4**). They also may report a cycle of the cyst breaking open, draining a clear, jellylike fluid, and healing. Treatment often is sought when the cyst becomes painful, ulcerated, or infected or is cosmetically displeasing. Patients also may have furrowing of the fingernail because of pressure of the cyst on the nail matrix.

SECTION 4   HAND AND WRIST

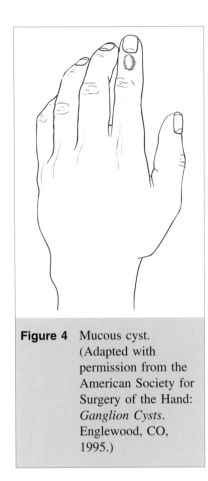

Figure 4 Mucous cyst. (Adapted with permission from the American Society for Surgery of the Hand: *Ganglion Cysts.* Englewood, CO, 1995.)

Tests

Physical Examination—Wrist

A dorsal ganglion is typically a smooth, round or multilobulated structure on the dorsoradial aspect of the wrist that becomes more prominent with flexion. It usually is positioned directly over the scapholunate joint but can occur more distally, even though its stalk usually emanates from the scapholunate joint.

A volar radial ganglion usually is a less well-defined mass situated between the flexor carpi radialis tendon and the radial styloid. It may extend underneath the radial artery and, in some cases, may adhere to the radial artery. On palpation, the ganglion may appear to pulsate and can be confused with an aneurysm. Symptoms also become more pronounced with extreme flexion or extension.

A ganglion is mildly tender with pressure. A prominent ganglion often will transilluminate when a penlight is shined through it from the side. Solid tumors will not transilluminate.

If a definite mass is not visible, the possibility of an occult ganglion, which is characterized by more subtle swelling, should be considered. Palpation must be especially thorough and careful to identify a small tender mass that is different from what is felt on the opposite wrist. MRI may be necessary to determine if an occult ganglion is present.

Physical Examination—Hand and Finger

A volar retinacular ganglion of the flexor tendon sheath is characterized by a small, firm, tender mass at the base of the finger in the area of the metacarpophalangeal flexion crease, most often at the long or ring fingers (**Figure 3**). These ganglions are sometimes difficult to detect because of their small size. They rarely affect motion and do not move with excursion of the tendon.

Mucous cysts usually lie to one side of the extensor tendon at the DIP joint (**Figure 4**). Initial clinical findings include a mass or a blister. Periarticular arthritic nodules may contain mucous cysts.

Diagnostic Tests

PA, lateral, and oblique radiographs of the hand or PA and lateral radiographs of the wrist or the involved finger should be obtained to rule out bony pathology. In most cases, ganglia are not associated with radiographic changes. With a mucous cyst, degenerative changes and a small bony spur usually are seen rising from the dorsum of the distal phalanx at the DIP joint.

Differential Diagnosis

Wrist

- Arthritis (evident on radiographs)
- Bone tumor (evident on radiographs)
- Intraosseous ganglion (evident on radiographs)
- Kienböck disease (collapse of the lunate)
- Soft-tissue tumor, benign or malignant (solid mass on palpation, rare)

Hand and Finger

- Dupuytren disease (presence of cords or bands)
- Epidermal inclusion cyst (history of laceration and repair)
- Giant cell tumors (different locations, but usually about the phalanges)
- Lipoma (larger in size, often in the palm)
- Soft-tissue tumor, benign or malignant (solid mass on palpation, rare)

Adverse Outcomes of the Disease

Wrist

Patients may experience a decrease in grip strength and painful wrist motion; they also may complain about the unsightly bump. On rare occasions, a ganglion will cause significant compression on the median nerve.

Hand and Finger

Patients often have pain in the hand and finger and an obvious deformity at the fingernail. Infection also can occur in association with a mucous cyst.

Treatment

Wrist

When the patient has significant symptoms, immobilizing the wrist will relieve symptoms and may cause the ganglion to decrease in size. However, immobilization is rarely a permanent solution. Occasionally, aspiration of a dorsal wrist ganglion will lead to resolution (see pages 493-494). Because of the proximity of the radial artery, volar wrist ganglions should be aspirated with great care.

When the patient has significant symptoms or is seriously bothered by the appearance of the wrist ganglion, then surgical excision is indicated.

Hand and Finger

Treatment of a ganglion of the tendon sheath consists of needle rupture followed by massage to disperse the contents of the cyst or injection with 1% or 2% local anesthetic until the cyst pops. Exercise caution when performing a needle rupture because of the proximity of the neurovascular bundle. Surgical management is occasionally required for painful flexor sheath ganglia.

Aspiration and/or rupture of a mucous cyst is not recommended because of the danger of introducing an infection into the DIP joint. If infection occurs, the patient should be started on a first-generation cephalosporin (unless allergic), tetanus immunization status should be updated if necessary, and a specialist should be consulted promptly.

Adverse Outcomes of Treatment

Wrist

Recurrence of wrist ganglia occurs in 5% to 10% of patients after surgical excision and in up to 90% after needle aspiration. Injury to the radial artery can occur as a result of aspiration of a volar wrist ganglion.

Hand and Finger

Recurrence of hand and finger ganglia is quite common. Skin loss is possible, as is injury to the digital nerve.

Referral Decisions/Red Flags

Wrist

Any mass with atypical findings should be evaluated with additional diagnostic tests or excisional biopsy. Recurrence after aspiration also is an indication for further evaluation.

Hand and Finger

Persistence of a painful or bothersome cyst after one or two attempts at needle rupture or aspiration indicates that surgical excision should be considered. Increased erythema and pain in a mucous cyst suggests infection that may require surgical treatment.

Procedure: Dorsal Wrist Ganglion Aspiration

Step 1
Wear protective gloves at all times during this procedure and use sterile technique.

Step 2
Cleanse the area with a bactericidal skin preparation solution.

Step 3
Use a syringe with a 27-gauge needle to infiltrate 1% local anesthetic into the area immediately proximal to and surrounding the ganglion. Remove the 27-gauge needle and change to the 18-gauge needle.

Step 4
Penetrate the ganglion with the 18-gauge needle and attempt to withdraw as much fluid as possible (**Figure 1**). With your free hand, compress the ganglion and displace the thick fluid toward the needle. As you compress the mass, you may need to move the needle to the right or left slightly to break small cavities within the ganglion. Injecting corticosteroid has not been shown to influence the recurrence rate and is not recommended.

Step 5
Apply a sterile dressing.

Adverse Outcomes
Infection and recurrence of the ganglion are possible. Injury to the radial artery also can occur following attempts to aspirate volar wrist ganglia.

Materials

- Sterile gloves
- Bactericidal skin preparation solution
- 3-mL syringe with a 27-gauge, ¾" needle
- 18-gauge needle
- 3 mL of a 1% local anesthetic without epinephrine
- Elastic bandage

SECTION 4 HAND AND WRIST

Figure 1 Location for needle insertion for dorsal wrist ganglion aspiration.

Aftercare/Patient Instructions

Instruct the patient to wear the elastic bandage for 1 week, removing it only for bathing.

Human Bite Wounds

Synonyms

Clenched-fist injury

Fight bite

Definition

Human bite wounds to the hand occur either directly, from a bite (usually to the fingers), or indirectly, when the hand strikes a tooth (clenched-fist injury). Few infections of the hand can progress more quickly or result in more significant complications. Both early recognition and appropriate treatment are important.

Human bite wounds result in greater concentrations of bacteria, especially anaerobic species, than most animal bite wounds. *Eikenella corrodens* can cause infections in human bite wounds, but the most common organisms causing these infections are α-hemolytic streptococci and *Staphylococcus aureus*.

ICD-9 Codes

882.0
Open wound of hand except finger(s) alone, without mention of complication

882.1
Open wound of hand, except fingers, complicated

882.2
Open wound of hand, except fingers, with tendon involvement

883.0
Open wound of finger(s) without mention of complication

883.1
Open wound of finger(s), complicated

883.2
Open wound of finger(s), with tendon involvement

Clinical Symptoms

The history of the injury and a laceration is diagnostic but may be difficult to elicit. Warmth, swelling, pain, and a purulent discharge are often present (**Figure 1**). Examination may reveal evidence of damage to underlying structures, including lack of extension or flexion due to tendon damage or a loss of sensation over the tip of the finger due to nerve injury.

Figure 1 **A,** Mechanism of tendon laceration and intra-articular contamination by saliva in human bite. **B,** An injury to a tendon that is cut in flexion will retract as the joint extends. (Adapted with permission from Carter PR: *Common Hand Injuries and Infections: A Practical Approach to Early Treatment.* Philadelphia, PA, WB Saunders, 1983.)

Figure 2 Possible tooth injury over the MP joint of the long finger. (Reproduced from Pollak AN, Barnes L, Ciotola JA, Gulli B, eds: *Emergency Care and Transportation of the Sick and Injured*, ed 10. Rosemont, IL, American Academy of Orthopaedic Surgeons, 2010, p. 822.)

Tests

Physical Examination

Measure and record the location of the laceration. A small laceration over the ring or little finger is a sign of a possible clenched-fist injury. Be alert for a tooth wound that is proximal to the metacarpophalangeal (MP) joint when the finger is extended but lies over the knuckle when the fist is clenched (**Figure 2**). Document the location and severity of swelling, erythema, and any purulent discharge. When the injury is on the dorsum of the hand, significant swelling may occur quickly (within 2 to 3 hours). Assess function of the flexor and extensor tendons and sensory nerves distal to the laceration. Examine the forearm for signs of ascending infection (eg, lymphangitic streaks, enlarged epitrochlear nodes).

Diagnostic Tests

PA, lateral, and oblique radiographs of the hand should be obtained to rule out an underlying fracture or the presence of a foreign body. Aerobic and anaerobic cultures should be obtained when any drainage is present. A white blood cell count can serve as a baseline for following the clinical course, but this test may be within normal limits in the early phases after injury.

Differential Diagnosis

- Laceration from a sharp object (accurate history)
- Septic joint caused by a retained foreign body (possibly evident on radiographs)

Adverse Outcomes of the Disease

Tendon rupture and/or laceration can occur as a result of the bite. An abscess involving the deep palmar space, osteomyelitis, joint sepsis, joint stiffness, and possibly septic tenosynovitis can develop with a delay in treatment.

Treatment

Bite wounds can be treated on an outpatient basis if the joint has not been penetrated, if there has been no tendon or bony injury, and when medical treatment is sought within 8 hours of the injury.

Anesthetize the wound with a 1% plain lidocaine solution and carefully examine and débride the skin edges and any underlying necrotic tissue. The extensor mechanism over the MP joints should be examined with the finger flexed to assess for damage to the tendons or penetration of the underlying joint. It is important to explore the wound with the patient's fingers both

Table 1 Guide to Tetanus Prophylaxis in Routine Wound Management[a]

History of Tetanus Immunization (Doses)	Clean, Minor Wounds		All Other Wounds	
	Td[b]	TIG	Td[b]	TIG
Uncertain or <3 doses	Yes	No	Yes	Yes
3 or more doses	No[c]	No	No[d]	No

[a]Important details on the CDC Web site: http://wwwnc.cdc.gov/travel/yellowbook/2010/chapter-2/tetanus.aspx.

[b]For children < 7 years old, DTaP or DTP (DT, if pertussis vaccine contraindicated) preferred to tetanus toxoid alone. For children ≥ 7 years of age, Td preferred to tetanus toxoid alone. For adolescents and adults to age 64, tetanus toxoid as Tdap is preferred, if the patient has not previously been vaccinated with Tdap.

[c]Yes, if more than 10 years since last dose.

[d]Yes, if more than 5 years since last dose. More frequent boosters are not needed and can accentuate side effects.

(Adapted with permission from the Centers for Disease Control and Prevention.)

flexed and extended. If the possibility of joint infection exists, an arthrotomy is necessary to irrigate the joint. Irrigate the wound with a large amount of an antibiotic irrigation solution and apply saline-soaked gauze or a nonadherent dressing. Human bites should never be closed primarily.

Immobilize the hand in a bulky dressing that incorporates a dorsal plaster splint that holds the hand in a safe position (with the MP joint at 60° to 90° of flexion and the interphalangeal joints in a resting, extended position). Appropriate tetanus prophylaxis should be given as outlined in Table 1, followed by antibiotics. Penicillin and a first-generation cephalosporin provide adequate coverage in most instances. Tetracycline can be used for patients who are allergic to penicillin. If cultures obtained from specimens taken at the time of initial wound care are positive, antibiotic type and dosage should be adjusted accordingly.

Advise patients who present soon after injury and without an established abscess to return within 24 hours for a recheck to confirm that infection has not developed. After the first 24 hours, daily whirlpool treatment or twice-daily dressing changes can be started. The wound should be allowed to close by secondary intention. For established infections, urgent surgical débridement and intravenous antibiotics are usually necessary. Early referral is necessary in these cases.

Adverse Outcomes of Treatment

Inadequate evaluation or treatment can lead to significant complications, including the need for amputation in advanced cases. Infection may develop with primary wound closure. Patients may experience sensitivity to antibiotics.

SECTION 4 HAND AND WRIST

Referral Decisions/Red Flags

Wounds that involve the joint, tendon, nerve, or bone require further evaluation. A bite wound that becomes infected despite treatment with antibiotics also requires further evaluation.

Kienböck Disease

Synonym

Osteonecrosis of the carpal lunate

Definition

Kienböck disease—osteonecrosis of the carpal lunate—most commonly affects men between the ages of 20 and 40 years (**Figure 1**). Patients may have a history of trauma, but the cause of the disrupted blood supply is frequently difficult to establish. With progression of the disease, the lunate collapses and fragments ultimately lead to end-stage arthritis of the wrist.

Clinical Symptoms

Pain, stiffness, and diffuse swelling over the dorsal-central aspect of the wrist are common. Patients often report weakness or an inability to grasp heavy objects.

Tests

Physical Examination

Examination typically reveals tenderness directly over the lunate bone (mid-dorsal wrist area, just distal to the radius). Grip strength usually is decreased. With progression of the disease, dorsal swelling and limited wrist motion are common.

Diagnostic Tests

PA and lateral radiographs of the wrist are indicated. In the early phase of Kienböck disease, radiographs show increased density (whiteness) of the lunate bone compared with the surrounding carpal bones. In later stages, the dead bone will fragment and collapse, resulting in generalized degenerative arthritis of the wrist (**Figure 2**).

Differential Diagnosis

- Fracture of the distal radius (evident on radiographs)
- Fracture of the scaphoid (evident on radiographs)
- Ganglion (discrete mass, normal radiographs)
- Scapholunate dissociation (increased distance between the scaphoid and lunate on radiographs)
- Tenosynovitis of the extensor tendon (diffuse swelling over extensor tendon extending onto the hand)

ICD-9 Codes
715.23 Osteoarthrosis of the wrist, secondary
732.3 Kienböck disease

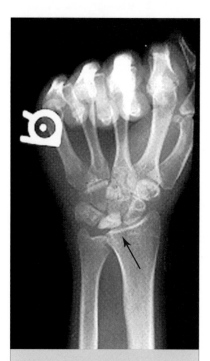

Figure 1 PA clenched-fist view of left hand of patient with Kienböck disease shows significant sclerosis of the lunate (arrow) and possible early collapse.

Figure 2   Radiographic classification of Kienböck disease according to the method of Lichtman and associates, modified by Weiss and associates. (Reproduced with permission from the American Society for Surgery of the Hand: *Hand Surgery Update*. Rosemont, IL, American Academy of Orthopaedic Surgeons, 1994, p 86.)

■ Wrist arthritis (narrowing of joint space but normal contour of lunate)

Adverse Outcomes of the Disease

Untreated Kienböck disease can result in progressive arthritis.

Treatment

If radiographs are normal, or if the lunate shows significant sclerosis, splint the wrist in a neutral position for 3 weeks. Wrist radiographs should be obtained with the shoulder abducted 90° and the elbow flexed 90° to obtain a true measure of the relationship between the radius and the ulna at the wrist (ulnar variance). NSAIDs may make the patient more comfortable. If pain persists after 3 weeks, further evaluation is indicated. In general, MRI is necessary to complete staging of the disease.

Adverse Outcomes of Treatment

Loss of motion, chronic pain, and decreased grip strength are possible.

Referral Decisions/Red Flags

If plain radiographs show any abnormality of the lunate, further evaluation is indicated. Persistent dorsal wrist pain, despite 3 weeks of immobilization, also is an indication for further evaluation.

Mallet Finger

Synonyms

Baseball finger
Terminal extensor tendon rupture

ICD-9 Code

736.1
Mallet finger

Definition

A mallet finger deformity is caused by rupture, laceration, or avulsion of the insertion of the extensor tendon at the base of the distal phalanx. Sometimes, instead of the tendon tearing, the injury avulses a fragment of the distal phalanx at the tendinous attachment (Figure 1).

Clinical Symptoms

Patients report pain and an inability to straighten the finger at the distal interphalangeal (DIP) joint. In addition to an extension lag at the DIP joint, patients may report a compensatory change of hyperextension in the proximal interphalangeal joint.

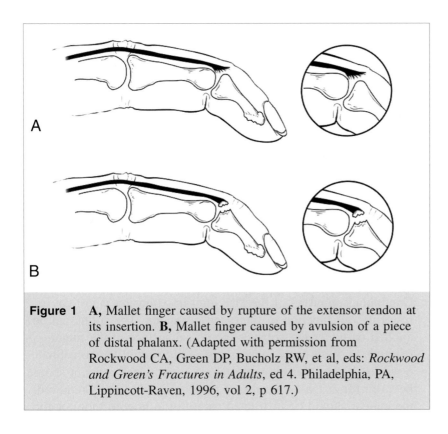

Figure 1 A, Mallet finger caused by rupture of the extensor tendon at its insertion. **B,** Mallet finger caused by avulsion of a piece of distal phalanx. (Adapted with permission from Rockwood CA, Green DP, Bucholz RW, et al, eds: *Rockwood and Green's Fractures in Adults*, ed 4. Philadelphia, PA, Lippincott-Raven, 1996, vol 2, p 617.)

Figure 2 Types of splints used in the treatment of mallet finger. **A,** Dorsal aluminum splint; **B,** Commercial splint. (Reproduced from Culver JE Jr: Office management of athletic injuries of the hand and wrist. *Instr Course Lect* 1989;38:473-482.)

Tests

Physical Examination

Examination reveals that the DIP joint is in flexion and that the patient is unable to actively extend the joint although it can be passively extended. The dorsal area of the DIP joint initially is tender and slightly swollen, but about 2 weeks after the injury occurs, the fingertip usually is not painful.

Diagnostic Tests

A lateral radiograph may reveal a small bony avulsion from the dorsal side of the distal phalanx. With large dorsal avulsion fragments, the distal phalanx may displace in a palmar direction from the unopposed pull of the flexor tendon.

Differential Diagnosis

- Fracture of the distal phalanx (evident on radiographs)
- Fracture-dislocation of the DIP joint (evident on radiographs)

Adverse Outcomes of the Disease

Permanent extensor lag of the DIP joint is possible. Persistent deformity associated with flexion of the fingertip is also possible, despite treatment.

Treatment

Continuous splinting of the DIP joint in extension is critical to restoring full function of the extensor tendon. The splint can be applied on either the volar or the dorsal surface of the finger (**Figure 2**). With acute injuries, the splint should be worn for 6 weeks. If the injury is more than 3 months old, a splint should be worn for at least 8 weeks. If prolonged splinting is required, the patient should be instructed carefully in how to monitor for skin problems, as excessive skin pressure can result in skin breakdown.

Advise patients to maintain the DIP joint in extension when the splint is removed for cleaning. If the fingertip droops at any time after the splint is applied, the healing process is disrupted and the period of splinting must be extended. Four or 5 days after the splint is applied, check the dorsal skin for maceration or pressure spots. If the joint does not come into full extension by the second visit, the patient should be evaluated for possible surgical pinning.

Visits every 2 to 3 weeks are helpful to monitor progress and usually lead to a better outcome than if the splint is applied and the patient is not seen again until 6 to 8 weeks later. At the end of the splinting period, if no extensor lag is evident, guarded active flexion is started, with splinting continued at night for 2 to 4 weeks.

Certain occupations (eg, cooking, dishwashing, typing) make splint wear difficult, and patients whose lifestyle requires doing these tasks repeatedly should be evaluated for possible surgical pinning.

Adverse Outcomes of Treatment

Prolonged splinting can result in skin breakdown.

Referral Decisions/Red Flags

Patients with volar subluxation of the distal phalanx and/or an avulsed bony fragment that involves more than one third of the joint surface require further evaluation.

Nail Bed Injuries

ICD-9 Codes

883.0
Open wound of finger(s) without mention of complication

883.1
Open wound of finger(s), complicated

883.2
Open wound of finger(s), with tendon involvement

Synonyms

Smashed finger
Subungual hematoma

Definition

Many injuries to the fingertip are crushing in nature, resulting in various degrees of injury to the fingernail, nail bed, and distal phalanx (**Figure 1**). The types of nail bed injuries include simple lacerations, stellate lacerations, severe crush injuries, and avulsions. Approximately 50% are associated with fractures of the distal phalanx.

Clinical Symptoms

Patients usually have pain and obvious injury to the fingertip.

Tests

Physical Examination

Determine the extent of the injury, noting any subungual hematoma and its extent, avulsion or laceration of the nail, and whether an associated fracture of the distal phalanx is displaced or nondisplaced. When the fingernail is avulsed, note the extent of injury to the nail bed (both germinal and sterile matrices). Examine the fingernail for attached remnants of the nail bed. An avulsion of the fingernail in a child or infant may be associated with a physeal injury, in which case referral to a specialist is indicated.

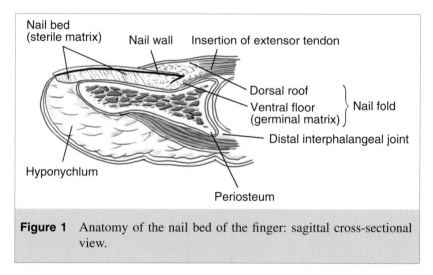

Figure 1 Anatomy of the nail bed of the finger: sagittal cross-sectional view.

Diagnostic Tests
PA and lateral radiographs of the finger are necessary when a fracture of the distal phalanx is suspected.

Differential Diagnosis

- Mallet finger (unable to fully extend the distal interphalangeal joint)

Adverse Outcomes of the Disease

If the patient has sustained damage to the nail bed, particularly the germinal matrix, a permanent nail deformity may result.

Treatment

Subungual Hematomas
Painful subungual hematomas can be treated with decompression. After scrubbing the finger and applying a disinfectant, create a hole in the fingernail over the hematoma, using battery-operated microcautery, if available, or a heated paper clip or 18-gauge needle. The hole must be large enough to allow continued drainage. Penetrate only through the nail and avoid perforating too deeply into the nail bed, as this is extremely painful and may result in scarring of the nail bed.

Nail Bed Lacerations
For lacerations of the nail bed with injury to the nail plate, the nail plate should be removed and the nail bed repaired. This should be performed with adequate anesthesia (see pages 455-457), with sterile preparation of the finger, and the use of a finger tourniquet. Elevate all or part of the nail plate using a small scissors. The entire nail can be removed or just enough to allow visualization of the laceration and suture placement. Irrigate the wound, remove the hematoma, and meticulously suture the nail bed using No. 6-0 or 7-0 bioabsorbable gut suture. After repair, stent the nail fold open by placing some xeroform gauze or a piece of a red rubber catheter into the nail fold. This gauze can be left in place because it will grow out with the new nail. An associated minimally displaced or nondisplaced fracture usually will be stabilized with the repair.

Nail Avulsions
The proximal portion of the nail bed (germinal matrix) may be avulsed and lying on top of the nail fold (**Figure 2**). This must be replaced underneath the nail fold and sutured in place. The sutures should be placed through the proximal fold to pull the nail bed into the fold. If the nail avulsion is associated with a fracture, the distal phalanx may need to be stabilized. Any nail

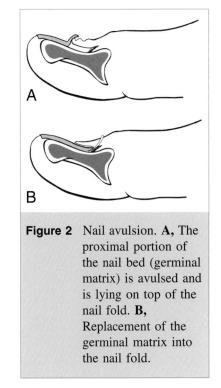

Figure 2 Nail avulsion. **A,** The proximal portion of the nail bed (germinal matrix) is avulsed and is lying on top of the nail fold. **B,** Replacement of the germinal matrix into the nail fold.

bed tissue adherent to the fingernail should be gently removed with a scalpel and sewn in place in the nail bed defect using small bioabsorbable suture. A large fragment of nail or the whole nail itself, when it has a large amount of nail bed still attached to it, should not have the tissue removed; rather, sew the entire fragment anatomically in place. Any injuries to the nail fold should be repaired with No. 5-0 gut, nylon, or monofilament suture. Injuries in children should be repaired with bioabsorbable sutures.

Wound Care

The finger should be dressed with antibacterial ointment, nonadherent gauze, sterile gauze, and an outer wrap. The finger should be splinted for protection.

Adverse Outcomes of Treatment

Abnormal growth and subsequent deformity of the nail can occur.

Referral Decisions/Red Flags

Nail bed injuries with complex lacerations or loss of tissue or injury to the germinal matrix may require more involved surgical treatment. Associated open fractures of the distal phalanx require further evaluation.

Procedure: Fishhook Removal

Retrograde extraction of a fishhook is difficult because of the barb (**Figure 1**). Most fishhook injuries involve the skin and subcutaneous tissues only. Although many techniques of fishhook removal have been described, only two are discussed here (**Figures 2** and **3**). Remember to wear protective gloves at all times during this procedure and use sterile technique.

Technique 1

Step 1
Cleanse the skin with a bactericidal skin preparation solution.

Step 2
Use a 27-gauge needle to infiltrate the skin with 2 to 3 mL of 1% local anesthetic.

Step 3
Grasp the exposed end of the hook (shank) with the thumb and index finger and rotate the hook to force the barb out through the skin.

Step 4
Cut the barbed end of the hook with a wire cutter.

Step 5
Remove the rest of the hook retrograde. It will back out easily once the barb is gone.

Step 6
Apply a topical antibiotic and a sterile bandage to the wound.

Technique 2

Step 1
Cleanse the skin with a bactericidal skin preparation solution.

Step 2
Inject 2 to 3 mL of 1% local anesthetic about the hook.

Step 3
Using a hemostat, grasp the belly of the hook at the point where it penetrates the skin.

CPT Code

Appropriate E/M CPT Code (if no incision is used to remove fishhook)

10120
Incision and removal of foreign body, subcutaneous tissues; simple (if incision is used to remove fishhook)

Current Procedural Terminology
© 2010 American Medical Association. All rights reserved.

Materials

- Sterile gloves
- Bactericidal skin preparation solution
- 3-mL syringe with a 27-gauge needle
- 3 mL of a 1% local anesthetic without epinephrine
- Wire cutter
- Hemostat
- #15 blade

Figure 1 Embedded fishhook with parts labeled.

Treatment

Initial treatment may involve a short course of NSAIDs or injection of corticosteroid into the tendon sheath (see pages 519-520). Care must be exercised to avoid injecting the tendon, as corticosteroid injected into a tendon may predispose it to rupture. If symptoms persist, a second injection in 3 to 4 weeks is indicated. However, because patients with rheumatoid disease are already at increased risk for tendon rupture, only one injection is indicated for these patients before surgical release should be considered. If two injections fail to resolve the trigger finger, surgical release should be considered.

Adverse Outcomes of Treatment

NSAIDs can cause gastric, renal, or hepatic complications. Repeated corticosteroid injections might lead to rupture of the flexor tendon and also may injure the digital sensory nerve. Infection also is a risk. In patients with diabetes mellitus, steroid injections may increase blood glucose levels. Rarely, injury to the distal nerve may occur at surgery.

Referral Decisions/Red Flags

Failure of nonsurgical treatment, development of contractures in the PIP joint, and/or a locked finger (in flexion or extension) indicate a need for further evaluation. Patients with rheumatoid arthritis in whom the problem does not resolve after a single injection also need additional evaluation. Patients with type 1 diabetes mellitus who cannot tolerate steroid injection require specialty evaluation.

Procedure: Trigger Finger Injection

The flexor tendons pass beneath a pulley situated just distal to the distal palmar crease. Palpating this area as the patient flexes and extends the finger reveals a click or snapping sensation as the enlarged tendon passes beneath the pulley.

Note: Opinions differ regarding single- and two-needle injection techniques. Proponents of the single-needle technique believe that one needle is less painful for the patient than two. Because the corticosteroid preparation is thicker than the local anesthetic, however, a slightly larger gauge needle is required at the outset. The DVD shows a two-needle, two-syringe technique.

Step 1

Wear protective gloves at all times during this procedure and use sterile technique.

Step 2

Cleanse the palm with a bactericidal skin preparation solution.

Step 3

Identify the lump on the tendon. Infiltrate the skin at the distal palmar crease, which directly overlies the tendon, and inject the anesthetic at that level.

Step 4

Inject 0.5 mL of a 1% anesthetic solution into the subcutaneous tissue and then advance the needle into the tendon sheath and inject the rest of the anesthetic (**Figure 1**). Continue to insert the needle as the patient moves the affected finger through a small arc of flexion and extension. When the needle touches the moving tendon, the patient will experience a scratchy sensation. If the needle moves, it has penetrated the tendon and should be partially withdrawn until the scratchy sensation occurs. At this point, the needle tip is inside the tendon sheath but external to the tendon.

Step 5

Leave the needle in place, change syringes, and then inject the corticosteroid preparation.

CPT Code

20550
Injection(s); single tendon sheath, or ligament, aponeurosis (eg, plantar "fascia")

Current Procedural Terminology © 2010 American Medical Association. All rights reserved.

Materials

- Sterile gloves
- Bactericidal skin preparation solution
- 2 to 3 mL of a 1% local anesthetic without epinephrine
- Two 3-mL syringes with a 25-gauge needle
- 1 mL of a corticosteroid preparation
- Adhesive dressing

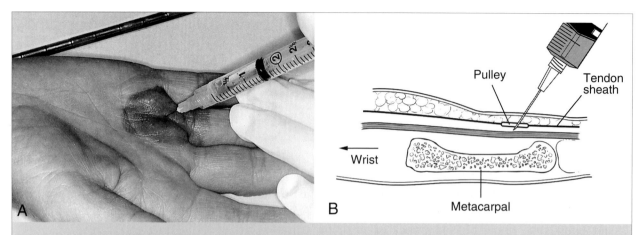

Figure 1 **A,** Location for needle insertion for trigger finger injection. **B,** Proper positioning of the needle, through the pulley and into the tendon sheath.

Step 6
Check the finger for filling of the tendon sheath with the solution.

Step 7
Dress the puncture site with a sterile adhesive bandage.

Adverse Outcomes

Injection of a corticosteroid into the subcutaneous tissues may lead to depigmentation and/or local fat atrophy, resulting in a tender, unsightly depression beneath the skin.

Aftercare/Patient Instructions

Advise the patient of possible significant discomfort for 1 to 2 days following any injection of a corticosteroid. Also, the finger may be numb for 1 to 2 hours until the local anesthetic wears off. Instruct the patient to return to your office if swelling, redness, or inordinate pain occurs. The patient should be able to use the finger in a normal fashion after the injection.

Tumors of the Hand and Wrist

Definition

Most tumors in the hand and wrist are benign, with primary malignant tumors and skeletal metastases accounting for less than 1% of these neoplasms. Ganglia are the most common benign soft-tissue tumors, followed by giant cell tumors and epidermal inclusion cysts. Enchondromas are the most common benign neoplasm of the bones of the hand, accounting for 90% of all cases. Squamous cell carcinomas are the most common malignant neoplasm of the hand, and chondrosarcomas are the most common primary malignant bone tumor in the hand. Malignant melanomas are frequently seen in the upper extremity because of exposure of the arm to the sun.

ICD-9 Codes
195.4 Malignant neoplasm, upper limb
213.5 Benign neoplasms of short bones of upper limb
229.8 Benign neoplasms of other and unspecified sites

Clinical Symptoms

Many tumors of the hand are painless. The exception is a glomus tumor, which characteristically is extremely painful and sensitive to cold. Enchondromas present with pain after a patient sustains a pathologic fracture through the weakened bone. Lipomas can cause pain and numbness in the fingers if the lesion is compressing an adjacent nerve. Masses located near joints can cause loss of motion.

Tests

Physical Examination

Note the position, size, and characteristics of the mass (**Figures 1** and **2**). These factors help to narrow the diagnostic possibilities.

A ganglion cyst is characterized as a mass located over the dorsal or volar radial aspect of the wrist, over the flexion crease of the finger at the level of the web space, or over the top of the distal interphalangeal joint of a finger.

Epidermal inclusion cysts typically occur around the end of a digit or at the end of an amputation stump. Pressing a small flashlight against an inclusion cyst will not transilluminate the mass, but this same maneuver will transilluminate a ganglion cyst.

A giant cell tumor is characterized by a multinodular, firm, nontender mass located around an interphalangeal joint, usually of the thumb or the index or long finger.

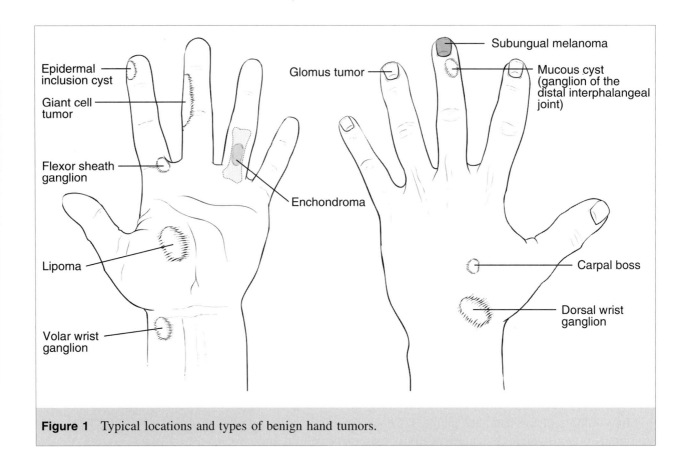

Figure 1 Typical locations and types of benign hand tumors.

A blue or red area visible under the fingernail could be a glomus tumor, subungual hematoma, or foreign body. However, subungual discoloration in the absence of trauma should raise a suspicion of melanoma. Likewise, a mole (nevus) that changes shape or color can indicate a malignant melanoma.

Lipomas typically are superficial, soft, reasonably well defined, and nontender on palpation. A frequent location in the hand is the thenar eminence. When lipomas are located on the palmar surface of the wrist, compression of the median or ulnar nerve may occur.

Recurrent paronychia infections and chronic nail deformities can be caused by underlying squamous cell carcinoma. A diagnosis of Kaposi sarcoma should be suspected in a patient with AIDS who develops skin nodules or red-brown plaques.

A symptomatic enchondroma is characterized by tenderness and swelling over the involved phalanx (usually the proximal). A pathologic fracture may be present.

A carpal boss is a dorsal prominence at the base of the third metacarpal or second metacarpal. These dorsal osteophytes may be confused with a neoplasm. A ganglion is sometimes associated with a carpal boss.

Figure 2 Clinical appearance of various hand tumors. **A,** Ganglion (mucous) cyst. **B,** Epidermoid cyst. **C,** Giant cell tumor. **D,** Glomus tumor. **E,** Melanoma. **F,** Lipoma. **G,** Squamous cell carcinoma. **H,** Enchondroma. (Reproduced from Evers B, Klammer HL: Tumors and tumorlike lesions of the hand. *Arch Am Acad Orthop Surg* 1997;1:37-42.)

Diagnostic Tests

PA and lateral radiographs of the involved finger or PA, lateral, and oblique views of the hand should be obtained.

Differential Diagnosis

See **Table 1** and **Figure 1** for a complete listing.

Adverse Outcomes of the Disease

Ganglions can result in limited joint motion. Nail changes, skin atrophy, and infection can develop as a result of a mucoid cyst. Drainage is a problem associated with epidermal mucoid cysts. Patients with giant cell tumors may have limited tendon function because of peritendinous adhesions. Nerve compression can develop as a result of lipoma. With an enchondroma, fracture can occur. Squamous cell carcinomas and malignant melanoma can metastasize and result in death.

Table 1 Common Benign Tumors of the Hand and Wrist

Type of Tumor*	Common Location(s)	Patient Age and Sex	Signs and Symptoms	Radiographic Findings
Ganglion cyst (see Ganglia of the Wrist and Hand, p 488)				
Epidermal inclusion cyst	Fingertip or anywhere from penetrating injury	Teens to middle age; more common in men	Painless, slow growing; does not transilluminate	Round soft-tissue mass, also in distal phalanx
Giant cell tumor of tendon sheath	Digits on palmar surface	> 30 years; ratio of men to women, 2:3	Slowly enlarging painless mass	20% show cortical erosion
Glomus tumor	50% occur under fingernail	30 to 50 years; ratio of women to men, 2:1	Triad of symptoms: marked pain, cold intolerance, very tender; blue discoloration of nail	Some show erosion on lateral view
Lipoma	Thenar area in palm and first web space	30 to 60 years; slight predominance in women	Painless, slow growing; might cause nerve entrapment	No bony involvement, soft-tissue mass
Enchondroma	In proximal phalanges or metacarpals	10 to 60 years; affects men and women equally	Might become painful after trauma because of fracture	Radiolucent expansive lesion, cortex thin, fracture and areas of calcification possibly visible

* See **Figure 1**.

Treatment

Treatment is based on the diagnosis. For some tumors, MRI will add significant additional information regarding the nature of the mass. Surgical excision and histologic examination are required for most expanding or symptomatic masses.

Adverse Outcomes of Treatment

Ganglions recur at the same site in 5% to 10% of patients. The recurrence rate of giant cell tumors is relatively high after surgical excision. Joint stiffness can develop after treatment of pathologic fractures caused by enchondromas.

Referral Decisions/Red Flags

Patients with a painful or expanding mass, one that interferes with function, or one believed to be malignant require further evaluation. Pigmented subungual lesions should be referred for evaluation.

Ulnar Nerve Entrapment at the Wrist

Synonym

Ulnar tunnel syndrome

ICD-9 Code

354.2
Lesion of ulnar nerve

Definition

Entrapment of the ulnar nerve at the wrist usually is caused by a space-occupying lesion such as a lipoma, ganglion, ulnar artery aneurysm, or muscle anomaly (**Figure 1**). Repetitive trauma, such as operating a jackhammer or using the base of the hand as a hammer, also may cause ulnar neuropathy at the wrist. Ulnar nerve entrapment at the wrist is less common than ulnar nerve entrapment at the elbow.

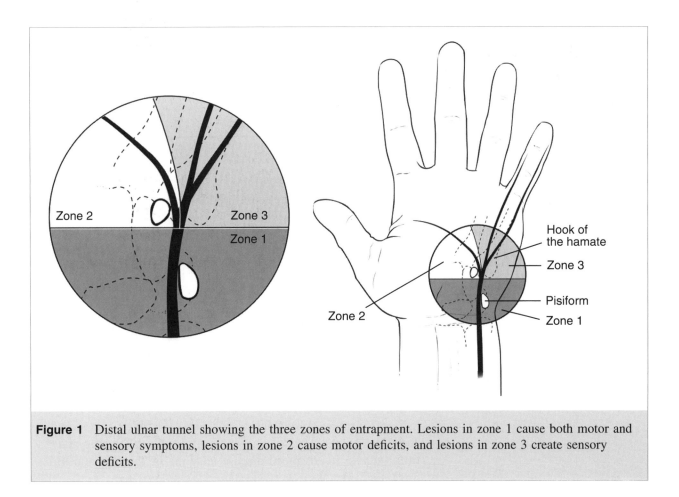

Figure 1   Distal ulnar tunnel showing the three zones of entrapment. Lesions in zone 1 cause both motor and sensory symptoms, lesions in zone 2 cause motor deficits, and lesions in zone 3 create sensory deficits.

Figure 2 Intrinsic muscle wasting indicative of ulnar nerve entrapment at the wrist.

Clinical Symptoms

Patients may or may not have pain, but they often report weakness and numbness.

Tests

Physical Examination

Inspect the hypothenar eminence for atrophy. Assess sensory and motor function of the ulnar nerve. In some patients, only the motor branch of the ulnar nerve may be affected, sparing the sensory branches; however, with sensory involvement, tapping over the ulnar nerve in the hypothenar region will produce tingling in the ring and little fingers (Tinel sign). Sensation over the dorsal and ulnar aspects of the hand is normal. When the ulnar nerve is involved at the elbow, almost all patients will have both sensory and motor involvement, with numbness over the dorsal and ulnar sides of the hand. Motor weakness is detected by atrophy of the hypothenar and intrinsic muscles or weakness of the intrinsic muscles (muscles that spread the finger) (**Figure 2**).

Diagnostic Tests

Results of electrophysiologic studies may be abnormal and may differentiate ulnar entrapment at the wrist from the more common entrapment at the elbow.

Differential Diagnosis

- Carpal tunnel syndrome (usually involves the thumb and the index, long, and ring fingers)
- Cervical (C7-C8) radiculopathy (more proximal muscle involvement, numbness on the dorsum of the hand)
- Peripheral neuropathy (from diabetes, alcoholism, or hypothyroidism; more generalized numbness)
- Thoracic outlet syndrome (symptoms more diffuse)
- Ulnar artery thrombosis in the hand (positive Allen test, firm cord on the ulnar side of the hand)
- Ulnar neuropathy at the elbow or cubital tunnel syndrome (sensory changes on the dorsum of the hand)
- Wrist arthritis (pain, limited motion, evident on radiographs)

Adverse Outcomes of the Disease

Loss of intrinsic muscle function causes decreased grip strength and pinch. Sensory loss, when present, involves the ring and little fingers. In advanced disease, clawing of the ring and little fingers can develop.

Treatment

Because the usual cause of ulnar entrapment at the wrist is extrinsic compression (because of a lipoma, ganglion, or tumor, for example), treatment is usually surgical. When the obvious cause is external pressure, such as resting the hypothenar area on a keyboard or desk, then the use of padding or a change in position could help.

Adverse Outcomes of Treatment

Postoperative infection, persistent symptoms, or both are possible.

Referral Decisions/Red Flags

Patients with ulnar weakness and neuropathy need further evaluation.

PAIN DIAGRAM
Hip and Thigh

Snapping hip

Trochanteric bursitis

Dislocation of the hip

Fracture of the pelvis

Hip fracture
  (Fracture of the Proximal Femur)

Hip impingement

Inflammatory arthritis
  and other conditions

Osteoarthritis of the hip

Osteonecrosis of the hip

Strains of the hip

Transient osteoporosis of the hip

Trochanteric
bursitis

Lateral femoral cutaneous
nerve syndrome

Fracture of the femoral shaft

Strains of the thigh

ESSENTIALS OF MUSCULOSKELETAL CARE   ■   © 2010 AMERICAN ACADEMY OF ORTHOPAEDIC SURGEONS

Hip and Thigh

Section Editors

Craig J. Della Valle, MD
Associate Professor
Department of Orthopaedic Surgery
Rush University Medical Center
Chicago, IL

Kathleen Weber, MD, MS
Assistant Professor
Department of Orthopaedic and Internal Medicine
Rush University Medical Center
Chicago, IL

Michael Huxford, MEd, ATC, CSCS
Sports Medicine Coordinator
Rehabilitative Services
Institute for Sports Medicine
Children's Memorial Hospital
Chicago, IL

Shane J. Nho, MD, MS
Assistant Professor
Section of Sports Medicine
Department of Orthopaedic Surgery
Rush University Medical Center
Chicago, IL

ANATOMY OF THE HIP AND THIGH

12th rib

Quadratus lumborum muscle

Transversus abdominis muscle (cut)

Iliohypogastric nerve

Ilioinguinal nerve

Psoas minor muscle

Psoas major muscle

Genitofemoral nerve

Lateral cutaneous nerve of thigh

Iliacus muscle

Femoral nerve

Superior pubic ramus

Greater trochanter of femur

Iliopsoas muscle passes backward to insertion on lesser trochanter

Shaft (body) of femur

T12
L1
L2
L3
L4
L5

Origin of psoas major muscle from vertebral bodies, transverse processes, and intervertebral disks (T12-L4) and origin of psoas minor muscle from vertebral bodies (T12, L1)

Lumbar plexus

Lumbosacral trunk

Iliac crest

Anterior superior iliac spine

Iliopectineal bursa

Iliofemoral ligament of hip joint (Y ligament of Bigelow)

Anterior Muscles of the Pelvis

Anterior superior iliac spine
Iliacus muscle

Psoas major muscle
Gluteus medius muscle
Inguinal ligament

Pubic tubercle
Iliopsoas muscle
Tensor fasciae latae muscle
Pectineus muscle

Adductor longus muscle

Gracilis muscle
Sartorius muscle
Rectus femoris muscle
Vastus lateralis muscle
Vastus intermedius muscle
Vastus medialis muscle

Iliotibial tract
Rectus femoris tendon (becoming part of quadriceps femoris tendon)
Lateral patellar retinaculum
Patella
Medial patellar retinaculum
Patellar ligament
Sartorius tendon
Gracilis tendon
Semitendinosus tendon
Tibial tuberosity

Iliac crest
Gluteal aponeurosis over gluteus medius muscle

Gluteus maximus muscle

Greater trochanter

Semitendinosus muscle

Biceps femoris muscle (long head)
Adductor minimus part of adductor magnus muscle

Semimembranosus muscle
Iliotibial tract
Gracilis muscle
Biceps femoris muscle
Short head
Long head
Semimembranosus muscle
Semitendinosus muscle
Popliteal vessels and tibial nerve
Common fibular (peroneal) nerve
Plantaris muscle
Gastrocnemius muscle
Medial head
Lateral head
Sartorius muscle

Muscles of the Anterior Thigh

Muscles of the Posterior Thigh and Gluteus

Overview of the Hip and Thigh

Hip or proximal thigh pain generally comes from one of the following sources: (1) the hip joint itself, (2) the soft tissues around the hip and pelvis, (3) the pelvic bones, or (4) referred pain from the lumbar spine. Diagnosing pathology involving the hip joint and pelvis is often possible with a careful history and physical examination combined with plain radiographs; in some cases, however, advanced imaging studies such as MRI, CT, or nuclear medicine scans may be required.

The hip joint, consisting of the articulation between the cartilaginous surfaces of the femoral head and the pelvic acetabulum, is a diarthroidal, synovial ball-and-socket joint (**Figure 1**). The acetabulum is formed by the confluence of the ilium, the ischium, and the pubis, and the articular surface that is created is horseshoe shaped. The proximal femur consists of the femoral head and neck and the greater and lesser trochanters. The greater trochanter is a large bony prominence found at the lateral base of the femoral neck; it serves as the attachment site for the abductor musculature (the gluteus medius and minimus). The lesser trochanter is a smaller bony prominence located on the medial aspect of the proximal femur;

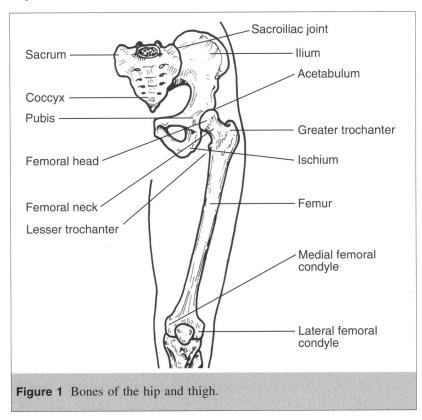

Figure 1 Bones of the hip and thigh.

it serves as the attachment site for the iliopsoas tendon (a powerful hip flexor).

Radiographic examination of the hip should include an AP radiograph of the pelvis and either a frog-lateral view of the pelvis or AP and lateral radiographs of the involved hip. Radiographs should be evaluated carefully for displaced or nondisplaced fractures, degenerative changes of the hip joint (including joint space narrowing), hip dysplasia, and changes in bony architecture, such as lytic or blastic lesions that could suggest a primary or metastatic tumor.

Type of Pain

Pain arising from the hip joint may be secondary to osteoarthritis, osteonecrosis, inflammatory conditions such as rheumatoid arthritis, septic arthritis, fractures of the proximal femur or pelvis, or dislocations of the femoral head. Patients with these conditions usually report pain in the groin or the anterior aspect of the proximal thigh, but pain may be present in the buttock or lateral aspect of the thigh or may be referred to the supracondylar region of the knee. Hip joint pathology is often associated with a decrease in range of motion that in degenerative conditions is associated with difficulty in activities such as putting on shoes. A limp also may be present, and patients with traumatic injuries (such as proximal femoral or pelvic fractures) are typically unable to bear weight on the extremity and are unable to perform a straight-leg raise.

Problems involving the bony pelvis include traumatic high-energy fractures, insufficiency fractures associated with osteoporosis, avulsion fractures from attached tendons, and primary or metastatic tumors. Problems involving both the hip joint and bony pelvis often manifest as pain in the groin, buttock, or lateral thigh.

Conditions that affect the soft tissues around the hip, such as trochanteric bursitis, lateral femoral cutaneous nerve impingement, and snapping hip syndrome, typically cause pain on the lateral or anterolateral aspect of the proximal thigh. Patients with an injury of the adductor muscles will note pain in the groin; hamstring injuries are associated with pain in the buttock or posterior aspect of the thigh.

The sacroiliac (SI) joint is relatively immobile. Some individuals have been found to experience more SI mobility than others and may experience SI pain. High-energy injuries such as high-energy pelvic ring disruption can lead to significant SI pain. Other conditions that involve the SI joint, such as seronegative arthritides or traumatic arthritis, can cause buttock and posterior thigh pain but are unlikely to restrict function.

Pathology in the lumbar spine may present as referred pain to the buttock and posterior thigh or as pain that radiates down the ipsilateral extremity in a radicular pattern. Patients with degenerative problems of the lumbar spine or strains of the lumbar musculature may have pain limited to the buttock, whereas disorders that cause entrapment of the spinal nerves (such as disk herniations) will cause pain that radiates in a dermatomal pattern. With these conditions, patients typically do not have symptoms referable to the groin, significant discomfort with rotation of the hip, or limited range of motion of the hip joint, although they often present with what they describe as "pain in the hip."

Nonmusculoskeletal pathology may present as groin or hip pain, and if the source of pain is obviously not the hip joint, these etiologies must be explored. Constitutional symptoms such as fever, chills, and weight loss should be explored to rule out malignancy or infection. Inguinal or abdominal hernias and rectus abdominus strains may present with pain in the groin or anterior thigh and may be difficult for the patient to distinguish from hip pathology. Gastrointestinal disorders such as inflammatory bowel disease, diverticulosis, diverticulitis, or appendicitis may mimic hip pain. Pain from abdominal aortic aneurysms may mimic groin pain. Urinary tract infections or nephrolithiasis also may cause pain referred to the hip region.

Pathology of the reproductive system also may present as pain in the groin or hip area. Prostatitis, epididymitis, hydroceles, varicoceles, testicular torsions, and testicular neoplasms all have been known to cause groin pain in men. Ectopic pregnancy, dysmenorrhea, endometriosis, and pelvic inflammatory disease may cause pain in this location in women. Pelvic floor muscles that are weak or too tight can produce hip, buttock, or groin pain. If any of these disorders are suspected, a referral should be made to the appropriate specialists.

Gait

A brief examination of the patient's gait can be very helpful in making a diagnosis. Ask the patient to walk briskly up and down the hall several times at a brisk pace. An abductor or gluteus medius lurch is manifested by a lateral shift of the body to the weight-bearing side with ambulation. This type of gait often occurs in patients who have intra-articular hip pathology (osteoarthritis, inflammatory arthritis, or osteonecrosis of the hip). Pain associated with a limp suggests pathology around the pelvis or hip and requires further investigation.

Musculoskeletal Conditioning of the Hip

A conditioning program consists of three basic phases: stretching exercises, to improve range of motion; strengthening, to improve muscle power; and proprioception, to enhance balance and

SECTION 5 HIP

agility. In addition, the exercise session should begin with an active warm-up, and plyometric exercises may be added for power after basic strength and flexibility have been achieved. Patient handouts are provided here for the stretching and strengthening exercises. Advanced proprioceptive exercises and plyometric exercises should be done under the supervision of a rehabilitation specialist or other exercise professional.

The goal of a conditioning program is to enable people to live a more fit and healthy lifestyle by being more active. A well-structured conditioning program also will prepare the individual for participation in sports and recreational activities. The greater the intensity of the activity that the individual wishes to engage in, the greater the intensity of the conditioning that will be required. If the individual participates in a supervised rehabilitation program that provides instruction in a conditioning routine—instead of using only an exercise handout such as provided here—the focus should be on developing and committing to a home exercise fitness program. A conditioning program for the body as a whole that includes exercises for the shoulder, knee, foot, and spine as well as the hip is described in Musculoskeletal Conditioning: Helping Patients Prevent Injury and Stay Fit, beginning on page 183.

The muscles of the hip and pelvis are important in walking and running activities. Both the shoulder and the hip are ball-and-socket joints, but because of its anatomy, the hip is more stable than the shoulder. An exercise program for conditioning of the hip should include an active warm-up; stretching, strengthening, and proprioceptive exercises; and, once basic stretching and strengthening have been achieved, plyometrics for power.

Active Warm-Up

The hip muscle groups are large and require an adequate warm-up, such as riding on a stationary bicycle or jogging for 10 minutes to raise the core body temperature. In addition, dynamic stretching exercises such as leg swings can be used to warm up the synovial fluid in the hip joint and actively stretch the muscles before activity.

Strengthening Exercises

Exercises that isolate muscle contraction and do not stimulate co-contractions are important for strengthening the hip muscles. In general, weight-bearing exercises produce co-contractions, and non–weight-bearing exercises do not. Co-contractions are important for stabilizing the joint that is being strengthened. Strengthening of the large hip muscle groups requires heavier weights and few (6 to 12) repetitions. After beginning with a weight that allows the patient to perform 6 to 8 repetitions initially, working up to 12 repetitions should be the goal of the strengthening phase. The exercises described below isolate the gluteus medius (posterior fibers), the gluteus maximus, and the internal and external rotators, which often are weak and therefore contribute to hip pathology.

Static Stretching Exercises

Static stretching should be done to increase the flexibility of the muscles surrounding the hip. A static stretch is performed at the end of the available range of painless motion of the muscle and joint.

Proprioceptive Conditioning and Plyometrics

In addition to strength, the athlete requires balance and power. Neuromuscular training, which improves communication between the muscles and the proprioceptors, includes balance and perturbation exercises as well as plyometrics. Balance involves the visual, vestibular, and proprioceptive systems. With balance training, the athlete consciously attempts to hold a posture for 30 to 60 seconds. These exercises might include balancing on one leg or balancing on one leg while touching the other foot to different points on the ground within reach. With perturbation training, the athlete stands on an unstable surface such as a balance board while it is being perturbed by an outside force. Jumping exercises, such as jumping forward and backward over a barrier, are a basic form of plyometrics. These should be attempted only by individuals with full range of motion and adequate strength in the hip, pelvic and abdominal, and back muscles. These types of plyometric and proprioceptive exercises should be supervised by a rehabilitation specialist or other exercise professional.

SECTION 5 HIP

Home Exercise Program for Hip Conditioning

■ Before beginning the conditioning program, warm up the muscles and the hip joint by riding a stationary bicycle or jogging for 10 minutes and performing leg swings as follows: While standing, swing one leg forward and backward 10 times and then side-to-side 10 times. Repeat with the opposite leg. Place one hand against a wall for balance if needed.

■ When performing the stretching exercises, you should stretch slowly to the limit of motion, taking care to avoid pain. If you experience pain with the exercises, call your doctor.

■ After performing the active warm-up and strengthening exercises, static stretching exercises should be performed to maintaining or increase flexibility.

Exercise	Muscle Group	Number of Repetitions/Sets	Number of Days per Week
Strengthening			
Hip extension (prone)	Gluteus maximus	6 to 8 repetitions, progressing to 12 repetitions	2 to 3
Side-lying hip abduction	Gluteus medius	6 to 8 repetitions, progressing to 12 repetitions	2 to 3
Internal hip rotation	Medial hamstrings	6 to 8 repetitions, progressing to 12 repetitions	2 to 3
External hip rotation	Piriformis	6 to 8 repetitions, progressing to 12 repetitions	2 to 3
Stretching			
Seat side straddle	Adductor muscles Medial hamstrings Semitendinosus Semimembranosus	4 repetitions/2 to 3 sets	Daily
Modified seat side straddle	Hamstrings Adductor muscles	4 repetitions/2 to 3 sets	Daily
Leg stretch	Hamstrings	4 repetitions/2 to 3 sets	Daily
Sitting rotation stretch	Piriformis External rotators Internal rotators	4 repetitions/2 to 3 sets	Daily
Knee to chest	Posterior hip muscles	4 repetitions/2 to 3 sets	Daily
Leg crossover	Hamstrings	4 repetitions/2 to 3 sets	Daily
Cross overstand	Hamstrings	4 repetitions/2 to 3 sets	Daily
Iliotibial band stretch	Tensor fascia	4 repetitions/2 to 3 sets	Daily
Quadriceps stretch (prone)	Quadriceps	4 repetitions/2 to 3 sets	Daily

Strengthening Exercises

Hip Extension (Prone)

- Lie face down with a pillow under your hips and one knee bent 90°. Elevate the leg off the floor, lifting the leg straight up with the knee bent.
- Lower the leg to the floor slowly, to a count of 5. Ankle weights should be used. Start with weight light enough to allow 6 to 8 repetitions and work up to 12 repetitions.
- Repeat on the other side.
- Perform the exercise 2 to 3 days per week.
- Once you have worked up to 12 repetitions, add as much weight as can be lifted only 8 times, working up to 12 repetitions again. Continue this cycle of adding weight and increasing repetitions.

Side-Lying Hip Abduction

- Lie on your side while cradling your head in your arm. Bend the bottom leg for support.
- Slowly move the top leg up and back to 45°, keeping the knee straight. Lower the leg slowly, to a count of 5, and relax it for 2 seconds. Ankle weights should be used, starting with weight light enough to allow 6 to 8 repetitions, working up to 12 repetitions.
- Repeat on the other side.
- Perform the exercise 2 to 3 days per week.
- Once you have worked up to 12 repetitions, add as much weight as can be lifted only 8 times, working up to 12 repetitions again. Continue this cycle of adding weight and increasing repetitions.

Internal Hip Rotation

- Lie on your side on a table with a pillow between your thighs. Bend the top leg 90° at the hip and 90° at the knee.
- Start with the foot of the top leg below the level of the top of the table; lift to the finish position, which is rotated as high as possible.
- Lower the leg slowly, to a count of 5. Ankle weights should be used, starting with weight light enough to allow 6 to 8 repetitions, working up to 12 repetitions.
- Repeat on the other side.
- Perform the exercise 2 to 3 days per week.
- Once you have worked up to 12 repetitions, add as much weight as can be lifted only 8 times, working up to 12 repetitions again. Continue this cycle of adding weight and increasing repetitions.

Start

Finish

External Hip Rotation

- Lie on your side on a table with the bottom leg bent 90° at the hip and 90° at the knee.
- Start with the foot below the level of the top of the table; lift to the finish position, which is rotated as high as possible.
- Lower the leg slowly, to a count of 5. Ankle weights should be used, starting with weight light enough to allow 6 to 8 repetitions, working up to 12 repetitions.
- Repeat on the other side.
- Perform the exercise 2 to 3 days per week.
- Once you have worked up to 12 repetitions, add as much weight as can be lifted only 8 times, working up to 12 repetitions again. Continue this cycle of adding weight and increasing repetitions.

Stretching Exercises

Seat Side Straddle

- Sit on the floor with your legs spread apart.
- Place both hands on the same ankle and bring your chin as close to your knee as possible. Hold the stretch for 30 seconds and then relax for 30 seconds.
- Repeat on the other side.
- Repeat the sequence 4 times, performing 2 to 3 sets daily.

Modified Seat Side Straddle

- Sit on the floor with one leg extended to the side and the other leg bent as shown.
- Place both hands on the ankle of the extended leg and bring your chin as close to your knee as possible. Hold the stretch for 30 seconds and then relax for 30 seconds.
- Reverse leg positions and repeat on the other side.
- Repeat the sequence 4 times, performing 2 to 3 sets daily.

Leg Stretch

- Sit on the floor with your legs straight and your hands grasping the calf of one leg.
- Slowly lift and pull the leg toward your ear, keeping your back straight and the other leg flat on the floor or bent slightly if necessary for comfort. Hold the stretch for 30 seconds and then relax for 30 seconds
- Repeat with the other leg.
- Repeat the sequence 4 times.
- Perform 2 to 3 sets daily.

Sitting Rotation Stretch

- Sit on the floor with both legs straight out in front of you.
- Cross one leg over the other, place the elbow of the opposite arm on the outside of the thigh, and support yourself with your other arm behind you.
- Rotate your head and body in the direction of the supporting arm. Hold the stretch for 30 seconds and then relax for 30 seconds.
- Reverse positions and repeat the stretch on the other side.
- Repeat the sequence 4 times.
- Perform 2 to 3 sets daily.

Knee to Chest

- Lie on your back on the floor with your knees bent and your heels flat on the floor.
- Grasp one knee and slowly bring it toward your chest as far as it will go. Hold the stretch for 30 seconds and then relax for 30 seconds.
- Repeat with the other leg; then do both legs together.
- Repeat the sequence 4 times.
- Perform 2 to 3 sets daily.

Leg Crossover

- Lie on the floor with your legs spread and your arms at your sides.
- Keeping the leg straight, bring your right toe to your left hand.
- Try to keep the other leg flat on the floor, but you may bend it slightly if needed for comfort. Hold the stretch for 30 seconds and then relax for 30 seconds.
- Repeat with the left leg and the right hand.
- Repeat the sequence 4 times. Perform 2 to 3 sets daily.

Crossover Stand

- Stand with your legs crossed, with your feet close together and your legs straight.
- Slowly bend forward and try to touch your toes. Hold the stretch for 30 seconds and then relax for 30 seconds.
- Repeat with the position of the legs reversed.
- Repeat the sequence 4 times.
- Perform 2 to 3 sets daily.

SECTION 5 HIP

Iliotibial Band Stretch

- Stand next to a wall for support.
- Begin with your weight distributed evenly over both feet, and then cross one leg behind the other.
- Lean the hip of the crossed-over leg toward the wall until you feel a stretch on the outside of the leg. Hold the stretch for 30 seconds and then relax for 30 seconds.
- Repeat on the opposite side.
- Repeat the sequence 4 times.
- Perform 2 to 3 sets daily.

Quadriceps Stretch (Prone)

- Lie on your stomach with your arms at your sides and your legs straight.
- Bend one knee up toward your buttocks and grasp the ankle with the hand on the same side.
- Pull on the ankle. Hold the stretch for 30 seconds and then relax for 30 seconds.
- Repeat on the opposite side.
- Repeat the sequence 4 times.
- Perform 2 to 3 sets daily.

SECTION 5   HIP

Physical Examination of the Hip and Thigh

Inspection/Palpation

Anterior View

With the patient standing, look for atrophy of the anterior thigh musculature and note the overall alignment of the hip, knee, and ankle.

Posterior View

With the patient standing, look for atrophy of the buttock and posterior thigh musculature. Note any pelvic obliquity (one iliac crest lower than the opposite side). Limb-length discrepancy will cause one iliac crest to be lower than the other, but this apparent obliquity can be corrected by placing blocks under the shorter limb. Fixed pelvic obliquity from a spinal deformity cannot be corrected by this maneuver. Palpate the iliac crests, the posterior iliac spine (deep to the dimples of Venus), and the greater trochanter. A Trendelenburg test can be conducted at this time to determine gluteus medius weakness. For the Trendelenburg test, the patient is instructed to stand first on one leg and then the other for comparison. With normal hip abductor strength, the pelvis will stay level or the side opposite the stance leg will elevate slightly. With abnormal abductor strength in the stance leg, the contralateral iliac crest will drop. This is a positive Trendelenburg test (see page 548).

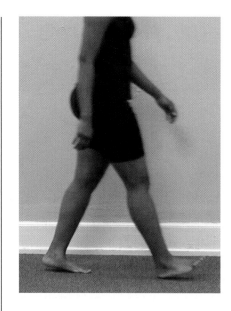

Gait

To assess gait, observe the patient walk across the room. Hip deformities often cause a limp that can range in severity from barely detectable to a marked swaying of the trunk and slowing of gait. Patients with a painful hip joint may have an antalgic gait; that is, they shorten the stance phase on the affected side to avoid placing weight across the painful joint. A Trendelenburg gait, characterized by a lateral shift of the body weight, is seen in patients with weakness of the abductor musculature; this is sometimes primary but is more often secondary to a degenerative disorder of the hip. As the hip joint degenerates and friction within the hip joint increases, it becomes more difficult for the abductor musculature to level the pelvis during gait.

Anterior View, Supine

With the patient supine, palpate to identify any masses, abnormal adenopathy, or tenderness in the region of the anterior superior iliac spine (ASIS) or greater trochanter. (The examiner is palpating the ASIS in the photograph.) Patients with avulsion of the sartorius or rectus femoris will report tenderness at or directly inferior to the ASIS. Patients with meralgia paresthetica (entrapment of the lateral femoral cutaneous nerve) will report tenderness immediately medial to the ASIS and hypoesthesia over the distal lateral thigh.

Patients who report a popping sensation in the hip while ambulating most likely have a thickened iliotibial band that snaps over the greater trochanter as the hip moves into flexion and internal rotation. Have the patient re-create the snapping and palpate the iliotibial band as it snaps over the greater trochanter. This may be visible (and at times can be seen from across the room).

Lateral View, Side-Lying

Place the patient in a side-lying position on the unaffected side to facilitate the examination. Structures in the region of the greater trochanter may be palpated with the patient in the supine position, but examination of this area is easier with the patient lying on the unaffected side. Tenderness to palpation directly over the greater trochanter reproduces pain with greater trochanteric bursitis. Tenderness at the proximal tip of the trochanter may indicate gluteus medius tendinitis. Tenderness at the posterior margin of the trochanter may indicate external rotator tendinitis.

Range of Motion

Flexion: Zero Starting Position

To evaluate hip flexion, the patient is supine on a firm, flat surface with the hip not being examined held in enough flexion to flatten the lumbar spine. Flattening the lumbar spine prevents excessive lordosis, which may camouflage a hip flexion contracture. Avoid positioning the opposite hip in excessive flexion, as this will rock the pelvis into abnormal posterior inclination, thereby creating a false-positive hip flexion contracture. Instead, flex the opposite hip to a position where the lumbar spine just starts to flatten or, more precisely, to a position where the inclination of the pelvis is similar to that of a normal standing posture (ie, the anterior superior iliac spine is inferior to the posterior iliac spine by only 2° to 3°).

Maximum Flexion

Maximum hip flexion is the point at which the pelvis begins to rotate. Normal hip flexion in adults is 110° to 130°.

Hip Flexion Contracture—Thomas Test

The Thomas test is used to evaluate for hip flexion contracture or psoas tightness. Begin with the patient sitting at the end of the examination table with the legs extending far enough that when the patient lies supine, the table edge will not contact the posterior aspect of the calves. Have the patient then assume a supine position, with the legs hanging off the end of the table. Instruct the patient to pull one hip into maximum flexion. Observe the contralateral hip to see if it also flexes off the surface of the table. A normal hip will remain on the table or flex very slightly. Greater flexion indicates psoas tightness or a flexion contracture.

Abduction and Adduction: Zero Starting Position

The Zero Starting Position is with the pelvis level and the limbs at a 90° angle to a transverse line across the anterior superior iliac spines.

SECTION 5   HIP

Abduction

To assess hip abduction, a goniometer is needed. Start with the patient supine and the limbs at a 90° angle to a transverse line across the anterior superior iliac spines. Abduct the leg until maximum abduction is reached, which is when the pelvis begins to tilt, a movement that you can detect by keeping your hand on the patient's opposite anterior superior iliac spine when moving the leg. Normal hip abduction in adults is 35° to 50°.

Adduction

To measure adduction, a goniometer is needed. Start with the patient supine. Flex the opposite extremity to allow adduction of the affected extremity (**A**). Maximum adduction is reached when the pelvis starts to rotate. If flexing the opposite extremity is impractical, measure adduction by moving the affected extremity over the top of the opposite limb (**B**). Normal hip adduction in adults is 25° to 35°.

Internal-External Rotation in Flexion

In adults, it is more practical to measure hip rotation with the hips in flexion; however, this technique should not be used in children or when assessment of femoral torsion or a more precise measurement of hip rotation in a "walking" position is required.

To evaluate hip rotation in flexion, with the patient supine, flex the hip and knee to 90°, with the thigh held perpendicular to the transverse line across the anterior superior iliac spines. Measure internal rotation by rotating the tibia away from the midline of the trunk, thus producing inward rotation of the hip **(A)**. Measure external rotation by rotating the tibia toward the midline of the trunk, thus producing external rotation at the hip **(B)** (see page 1105).

Muscle Testing

Hip Flexors

To assess the hip flexor muscles, ask the seated patient to flex the hip upward as you resist the effort with your hand by pushing down on the distal thigh just above the knee.

Hip Extensors

To assess the hip extensor muscles, with the patient prone, place the knee in approximately 90° of flexion and ask the patient to extend the hip as you resist the effort with your hand by pushing against the distal thigh.

Hip Abductors

To assess the hip abductors, have the patient lie on the unaffected side. Ask the patient to abduct the hip as you resist the effort with your hand on the lateral aspect of the thigh. Note that hip abductor strength also can be assessed by using the Trendelenburg test.

Hip Adductors

To assess the hip adductors, with the patient supine, place your hand on the medial aspect of the distal thigh and ask the patient to adduct the hip as you resist the effort.

SECTION 5 HIP

Special Tests

Trendelenburg Test

The Trendelenburg test is used to evaluate hip abductor strength, primarily the gluteus medius. Stand behind the patient to observe the level of the pelvis. Ask the patient to stand on one leg. With normal hip abductor strength, the pelvis will remain level. If hip abductor strength is inadequate on the stance limb side, the pelvis will drop below level on the opposite side, indicating a positive test.

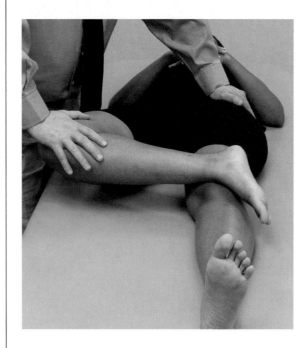

FABER Test

The FABER (flexion-abduction-external rotation) test, sometimes called the figure-of-4 test, Patrick test, or Jansen test, is a stress maneuver to detect hip and sacroiliac pathology. With the patient supine, place the affected hip in flexion, abduction, and external rotation with the patient's foot on the opposite knee. Stabilize the pelvis with your hand on the contralateral anterior superior iliac spine and press down on the thigh of the affected side. If the maneuver is painful, the hip or sacroiliac region may be affected. Increased pain with this test also may be a nonorganic finding (see page 165).

Log Roll Test

With the patient supine, internally and externally rotate the relaxed lower extremity. Pain in the anterior hip or groin, particularly with internal rotation, is considered a positive result. A positive test may indicate acetabular or femoral neck pathology, such as in osteoarthritis or femoral head osteonecrosis.

Piriformis Test

With the patient lying on the unaffected side and the hip and knee flexed to approximately 90°, stabilize the pelvis with one hand and use your other hand to apply flexion, adduction, and internal rotation pressure at the knee, pushing it to the examination table. If a tight piriformis is impinging on the sciatic nerve, pain may be produced in the buttock and even down the leg.

SECTION 5 HIP

Scouring Test

With the patient supine and the hip flexed and adducted, use the patient's knee and thigh to apply a posterolateral force through the hip as the femur is rotated in the acetabulum. Passively flex, adduct, and internally rotate the hip while longitudinally compressing to scour the inner aspect of the joint (**A**). To scour the outer aspect, abduct and externally rotate the hip while maintaining flexion during longitudinal compression (**B**). Pain or a grating sound or sensation is a positive result and may indicate labral pathology, a loose body, or other internal derangement.

Hamstring Flexibility

With the patient supine and the contralateral hip and knee maintained in full extension, instruct the patient to flex the hip to 90° and then, while maintaining this position, actively extend the knee fully. Patients unable to obtain within 10° of full knee extension are considered to have hamstring tightness.

SECTION 5   HIP

Dislocation of the Hip (Acute, Traumatic)

Definition

Dislocation of the hip occurs when the femoral head is displaced from the acetabulum. Because of its strong capsule and deep acetabulum, the hip is rarely dislocated in adults. The causative injury usually is high-energy trauma, such as a motor vehicle accident or a fall from a height. Posterior dislocations (femoral head posterior to the acetabulum) are far more common than anterior dislocations, accounting for more than 90% of these injuries.

Clinical Symptoms

Dislocation of the hip is a severe injury. Patients have pain and are typically unable to move the lower extremity. Patients often have other associated musculoskeletal injuries, and there is a high prevalence of associated head, intra-abdominal, and chest injuries.

Tests

Physical Examination

A posterior dislocation results in the affected limb being short, with the hip fixed in a position of flexion, adduction, and internal rotation (**Figure 1**). Assess the status of distal pulses

ICD-9 Codes	
831.01	Posterior dislocation, closed
831.02	Obdurator dislocation, closed
831.03	Other anterior dislocation, closed
831.11	Posterior dislocation, open
831.12	Obdurator dislocation, open
831.13	Other anterior dislocation, open

SECTION 5 HIP

Figure 1 The clinical appearance of an individual with a posterior dislocation of the right hip. (Reproduced with permission from Pollak AN, Barnes L, Cioltola JA, Gulli B, eds: *Emergency Care and Transportation of the Sick and Injured*, ed 10. Rosemont, IL, American Academy of Orthopaedic Surgeons, 2010, p 1042.)

and the function of the sciatic and femoral nerves. Sciatic nerve palsies are common (8% to 20% incidence), with the peroneal division of the sciatic nerve most commonly affected.

With an anterior dislocation, the hip assumes a position of mild flexion, abduction, and external rotation. Femoral nerve palsy may be present, but nerve injuries are less frequent with anterior dislocations.

Inspect the extremity for abrasions about the anterior aspect of the knee or for a knee effusion. Significant knee ligament injuries are commonly associated with hip dislocations because most hip dislocations typically occur from a direct blow to the flexed hip and knee. An associated fracture of the ipsilateral femur or acetabulum may be present.

Diagnostic Tests

Radiographs should include an AP view of the pelvis and AP and lateral views of the femur, including the knee. In the normal pelvis, the size of the femoral heads and joint spaces will be symmetric on AP radiographs. With a posterior hip dislocation (**Figure 2**), the affected femoral head appears smaller than the contralateral, normal femoral head; with an anterior hip dislocation (**Figure 3**), the affected femoral head appears larger. Associated fractures of the acetabulum (particularly fractures of the posterior wall) are common; in these cases, a CT scan should be obtained to fully define the fracture pattern (**Figure 4**). Following reduction of the dislocation, it is imperative to ensure that the reduction is completely concentric without interposition of associated bony fragments or residual subluxation; if there are any questions regarding these parameters, a CT scan should be obtained.

Figure 2 Posterior dislocation of the left hip with an associated fracture of the femoral head (arrow).

Figure 3 AP radiograph of the pelvis demonstrates an anterior dislocation of the left hip (arrow).

Figure 4 CT scan of the pelvis shows a displaced fracture of the posterior wall of the acetabulum (arrow).

Differential Diagnosis

- Fracture of the acetabulum or pelvis (pain in the groin and/or buttock)
- Fracture of the hip or shaft of the femur (pain in the groin, buttock, and thigh)

Adverse Outcomes of the Disease

Osteonecrosis of the femoral head is the most common early complication and occurs in approximately 10% of patients. Dislocation of the hip joint tears the hip capsule and disrupts the blood supply to the femoral head; a delay in reduction or incomplete reduction increases the risk of osteonecrosis. Osteonecrosis may not be apparent for as long as 2 or 3 years after the injury, and thus these patients require follow-up over several years. Posttraumatic arthritis (secondary to the severe impact to the cartilaginous surfaces), sciatic or femoral nerve injury, and chronic pain may occur.

Treatment

An acute traumatic hip dislocation is an emergency. A reduction should be performed as soon as possible to decrease the risk of osteonecrosis. The reduction should be performed in an atraumatic fashion to avoid damage to the articular cartilage or fracture of the femoral head or acetabulum. Associated fractures of the femoral head or intra-articular loose bodies should be ruled out before the reduction is performed. Repeat radiographs and, frequently, a postreduction CT are necessary to identify unrecognized intra-articular bony fragments and to confirm a perfectly concentric reduction; if bony fragments are identified within the joint, they must be surgically removed. Nerve and vascular function should be carefully evaluated and documented both before and after the reduction. Postreduction treatment of an uncomplicated dislocated hip is early crutch-assisted ambulation with weight bearing as tolerated until the patient is free of pain, usually 2 to 4 weeks after the injury. Patients should then begin hip abduction and extension exercises and use a walking aid in the hand opposite the involved hip until they can walk without a limp. Associated fractures of the acetabulum often require surgical treatment to ensure that adequate stability has been restored to the joint; small retained bony fragments can often be removed arthroscopically.

Adverse Outcomes of Treatment

Despite a rapid closed reduction, osteonecrosis may still occur. The impact of the injury itself may cause severe damage to the cartilaginous surfaces of the femoral head or the acetabulum, resulting in posttraumatic arthritis. A delay in time to reduction or incomplete reduction increases the risk of osteonecrosis of the femoral head. Even when a rapid, closed complete reduction is performed, osteonecrosis may occur. Articular cartilage damage or femoral head and acetabulum fractures may occur during reduction.

Referral Decisions/Red Flags

All traumatic dislocations of the hip are serious injuries requiring immediate attention.

Fracture of the Femoral Shaft

Definition

The shaft, or diaphysis, of the femur is defined as the portion of the femur from the subtrochanteric region to the supracondylar area (**Figure 1**). In most adults, fractures of the femoral shaft are caused by high-energy trauma, such as a motor vehicle accident. As such, this injury is severe and is potentially associated with life-threatening pulmonary, intra-abdominal, and head injuries. Pathologic fractures of the femoral shaft are less common, occur in bone weakened by osteopenia or tumors, result from low-energy injuries such as a simple fall, and have a much lower incidence of associated complications.

Clinical Symptoms

Patients with femoral shaft fractures present with severe pain in the thigh along with an obvious deformity and are typically unable to move, let alone bear weight on the extremity. Patients who have sustained the injury as a result of high-energy trauma are likely to have multisystem injuries and may not be alert or able to respond to questioning.

Tests

Physical Examination

Inspect for deformity, swelling, and open injuries. It is important to recognize that a femoral shaft fracture can act as a distracting injury, causing the examiner to overlook other associated musculoskeletal injuries; thus, a thorough examination of the entire extremity is mandatory to rule out associated injuries. Ligamentous injuries of the ipsilateral knee are common; however, often the knee cannot be examined until the patient is anesthetized for surgical treatment. Evaluate and document the vascular status of the limb distal to the fracture. Assess function of the femoral, peroneal, and posterior tibial nerves. In the presence of deformity and vascular compromise, simple manual longitudinal traction should be applied to determine whether the deformity is the cause of the ischemia. As these are typically high-energy injuries, standard advanced trauma life support (ATLS) protocols should be applied to evaluate for and potentially treat associated life-threatening injuries.

ICD-9 Codes
821.01 Fracture of the femoral shaft, closed
821.1 Fracture of the femoral shaft, open

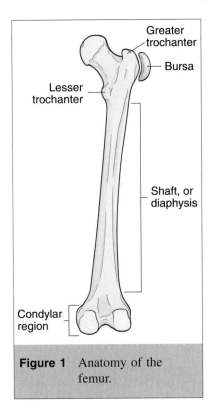

Figure 1 Anatomy of the femur.

Greater trochanter

Bursa

Lesser trochanter

Shaft, or diaphysis

Condylar region

Figure 2 Lateral radiograph shows a femoral shaft fracture.

Figure 3 AP radiograph shows a femoral neck fracture (arrows) in a patient with a femoral shaft fracture in the same extremity caused by high-energy trauma.

Diagnostic Tests

The fracture is confirmed by AP and lateral radiographs of the femur (**Figure 2**). High-energy trauma can disrupt adjacent joints; therefore, radiographs of the hip, knee, and pelvis must be obtained. It is particularly important to identify an ipsilateral fracture of the femoral neck because treatment options differ and failure to identify a concomitant femoral neck fracture can lead to nonunion of the femoral neck fracture or osteonecrosis of the femoral head (**Figure 3**). If vascular compromise is identified, arterial studies are required.

Differential Diagnosis

- Fracture of the pelvis, acetabulum, or proximal femur (evident on radiographs)
- Malignant or metastatic lesion of the femur (pain in the thigh with activity or at rest, evident on radiographs)
- Osteomyelitis with bone destruction (pain in the thigh, evident on radiographs)
- Soft-tissue injury without fracture (pain, swelling, ecchymosis of the thigh, pain with hip and/or knee motion)
- Stress fracture of the femur (pain in the thigh that increases with weight bearing; may be evident on plain radiographs, but MRI may be needed to confirm the diagnosis)

Adverse Outcomes of the Disease

The most significant adverse outcomes are those associated with violent trauma or long-bone fractures, such as fat embolism, adult respiratory distress syndrome, and multisystem organ failure. An acute arterial injury may be life threatening and requires immediate recognition and treatment. Complications of open fractures, such as infection, may result in chronic osteomyelitis. Even if uneventful healing occurs, the high energy associated with these injuries may have long-lasting effects on associated soft tissues. Persistent pain, limp, and difficulty returning to jobs that require manual labor are not uncommon.

Treatment

Immediate, temporary splinting may be applied for comfort and to provide stabilization during transfers, followed by the application of skeletal traction until surgical intervention is undertaken. Skeletal traction pins can be applied to the distal femur or the proximal tibia. These provide patient comfort and prevent shortening of the extremity, which can be difficult to overcome once the fracture is treated surgically. Surgical treatment is indicated for the vast majority of patients to lessen the risk of pulmonary and other systemic complications related to recumbency. Patients with open fractures should receive appropriate tetanus prophylaxis along with immediate systemic antibiotic treatment, followed by emergent surgical débridement of the soft-tissue injury as soon as the patient is medically stabilized.

Adverse Outcomes of Treatment

Nonunion, malunion, and infection are potential problems with any fracture treated surgically.

Referral Decisions/Red Flags

Femoral shaft fractures are markers of a high-energy traumatic injury and thus require appropriate evaluation and treatment of associated musculoskeletal, head, thoracic, and intra-abdominal injuries. Open injuries require special attention to ensure that appropriate tetanus prophylaxis and intravenous antibiotics are administered, along with prompt surgical débridement and fracture fixation.

SECTION 5 | HIP

Fracture of the Pelvis

Definition

Pelvic fractures include fractures of the pelvic ring and the acetabulum. Pelvic injuries range in severity from stable, low-energy fractures (typically seen in older patients) that heal readily when treated nonsurgically to unstable, high-energy fractures that are associated with massive blood loss and resultant hemodynamic instability that can lead to death if not stabilized emergently. Stable pelvic ring fractures generally involve only one side of the pelvic ring. For example, a unilateral fracture of the superior and inferior pubic ramus is a stable injury. Unstable pelvic ring fractures disrupt the ring at two sites. For example, a fracture of a superior and inferior pubic ramus combined with a fracture of the sacrum or ilium is considered an unstable pelvic fracture. Another unstable pattern is disruption of the symphysis pubis combined with a fracture of the sacrum or disruption of one or both sacroiliac ligaments (**Figure 1**). Acetabular fractures are by definition intra-articular injuries that can lead to posttraumatic arthritis if displaced. Acetabular fractures usually are high-energy injuries.

Figure 1 AP view of the pelvis reveals an unstable pelvic fracture with disruption of the symphysis pubis (arrow) and sacroiliac joint (arrowhead).

Clinical Symptoms

Low-energy pelvic fractures are often seen in elderly patients. Presenting symptoms are similar to those in patients with a fracture of the proximal part of the femur, including pain in the groin with attempts at weight bearing or an inability to bear weight on the extremity. Pain is typically localized to the groin, the lateral hip, or the buttock area. Most pelvic and acetabular fractures are high-energy injuries and are associated with other musculoskeletal injuries as well as traumatic injuries to the head, chest, and abdomen.

Tests

Physical Examination

Low-energy pelvic fractures are associated with pain on attempted range of motion of the hip and on attempted straight-leg raising. Patients who are able to ambulate have an antalgic gait pattern.

Patients with high-energy pelvic fractures require treatment in a trauma center with the application of standard trauma protocols, including an initial evaluation of the airway, breathing, and circulatory status of the patient. The cervical spine should be examined to ensure that there is no pain with attempted range of motion. Inspect the pelvic area for swelling, ecchymosis, and obvious deformity as well as for lacerations, which may represent an open fracture of the pelvis. Palpation and gentle compression of the pelvis often will localize the area of injury. The neurovascular status of the lower extremities should be evaluated carefully because peripheral nerve injuries are not uncommon and pelvic fractures that involve the sacrum can directly damage the spinal nerve roots. Unstable fractures also may be associated with genitourinary injuries of the prostate and bladder. If blood is present in the perineal area, a urologic consultation should be obtained before placing a Foley catheter.

A thorough history should be obtained, with special attention paid to any history of chest pain, palpitation, syncope, loss of consciousness, or shortness of breath that may have resulted in a fall. Appropriate referral is indicated if there is concern for associated medical conditions.

Diagnostic Tests

Standard trauma protocols include an AP radiograph of the chest, a lateral view of the cervical spine, and an AP view of the pelvis. The AP pelvis view typically identifies most pelvic fractures. If a pelvic fracture is seen on this view, pelvic inlet and outlet views (**Figure 2**) should be obtained to assist with identification of the injury pattern. If an acetabular fracture is demonstrated, oblique views of the pelvis are required to fully

SECTION 5   HIP

Figure 2 Pelvic inlet (**A**) and outlet (**B**) views are useful for determining rotational and vertical displacement of the pelvis. Note the displacement and rotation of the left pubic ramus.

Figure 3 CT scan of the pelvis shows an unstable fracture of the left side of the sacrum (arrow).

define the extent of the fracture. CT scans are often needed to define these complex injuries and plan for appropriate surgical intervention (**Figure 3**).

Differential Diagnosis

- Hip arthritis (pain in the groin or buttock, limited hip motion, evident on radiographs)
- Hip fracture (pain in the groin or buttock, shortened and externally rotated leg)
- Hip strain (pain in the groin or buttock)
- Stress fracture of the pelvis or sacrum (MRI imaging may be necessary for diagnosis)
- Tumors involving the bony pelvis or sacrum (pain in the low back, groin, rectum, and/or buttock; evident on radiographs)

Adverse Outcomes of the Disease

High-energy injuries are associated with a significant prevalence of associated musculoskeletal, head, chest, and abdominal trauma. These injuries may result in serious sequelae, including death. Associated genitourinary injuries are common and can lead to pain and/or sexual dysfunction. Neurologic injuries may be permanent, leading to abnormal motor and/or sensory dysfunction of the ipsilateral lower extremity. Although nonunion of these fractures is uncommon, malunion of the pelvis sometimes occurs and may lead to deformity of the pelvis and/or limb-length discrepancy with persistent pain. Acetabular fractures, classified as intra-articular injuries, can result in posttraumatic arthritis secondary to chondral injury that occurs when the femoral head strikes the acetabulum. This may occur even if the fracture is fixed anatomically with rigid internal fixation. Patients with pelvic ring and acetabular fractures are at substantial risk for thromboembolic complications. Even if these injuries proceed to uneventful bony union, the psychosocial implications of these injuries are substantial because many patients have persistent pain that may result in an occupation change.

Treatment

The treatment of pelvic fractures is determined by the degree of pelvic instability and the presence of associated injuries. Pelvic fractures associated with minor injuries, such as falls in the elderly patient, are common and typically have a stable pattern. Treatment of these low-energy stable fractures consists of analgesics, relative rest, and gait training for protected weight bearing with a walker. It is important to monitor the patient and implement prophylactic measures to help prevent potential complications related to immobility, such as venous thromboembolism and skin breakdown. Most patients require protected weight bearing for about 6 weeks, until the pain has subsided and the fracture demonstrates early healing. These patients should also undergo evaluation and treatment of osteoporosis to prevent the occurrence of future fragility fractures.

High-energy pelvic fractures often are life threatening. Initial treatment focuses on hemodynamic resuscitation along with identification and treatment of associated injuries. As a temporizing measure, a sheet can be tautly and carefully applied around the patient's pelvis to decrease pelvic volume and effect a temporary reduction, thereby potentially reducing pelvic bleeding. Skeletal traction may be used once the patient has been deemed to be hemodynamically stable until definitive surgical treatment is performed for patient comfort and to effect a temporary reduction of the fracture.

Adverse Outcomes of Treatment

Degenerative arthritis of the sacroiliac joint or the hip joint, heterotopic ossification, malunion, nonunion, or neurovascular injury may occur. Sexual dysfunction is a known sequela of these injuries, along with problems associated with concomitant musculoskeletal injuries.

SECTION 5 HIP

Referral Decisions/Red Flags

High-energy displaced pelvic fractures and open pelvic fractures are best managed at a level I trauma center, where a multidisciplinary approach can be used to optimize patient survival. Fractures involving the acetabulum or the sacroiliac joint require evaluation for possible surgical reduction and fixation.

Fracture of the Proximal Femur

Synonym

Hip fracture

Definition

Hip fractures (proximal femur fractures) are a common injury in elderly individuals with osteoporosis. These fractures generally involve either the femoral neck or the intertrochanteric region. Both types occur with approximately the same frequency and affect a similar patient population; however, surgical treatment of the two injuries differs. Femoral neck fractures also are known as intracapsular hip fractures and thus by definition occur in the region of the proximal femur that is within the hip capsule itself (**Figure 1**). Intracapsular hip fractures often lead to a disruption of the blood supply to the femoral head, and thus nonunion and osteonecrosis are common complications of this injury. Intertrochanteric hip fractures are extracapsular, occurring in the region of the proximal femur between the base of the femoral neck and the distal aspect of the lesser trochanter (**Figure 2**), and they require more robust fixation than do femoral neck fractures. They are associated with lower rates of osteonecrosis or nonunion, as the blood supply to the femoral head is not typically disrupted; however, implant failure is a much more common problem with these injuries.

ICD-9 Codes
820.0 Femoral neck (transcervical) fracture, closed
820.00 Femoral neck (intracapsular) fracture, closed
820.01 Femoral neck (epiphysis) fracture, closed
820.02 Femoral neck (midcervical) fracture, closed
820.03 Femoral neck (base of neck) fracture, closed
820.09 Femoral neck (head of femur, subcapital) fracture, closed
820.1 Femoral neck (transcervical) fracture, open
820.10 Femoral neck (intracapsular) fracture, open
820.11 Femoral neck (epiphysis) fracture, open
820.12 Femoral neck (midcervical) fracture, open
820.13 Femoral neck (base of neck) fracture, open
820.19 Femoral neck (other) fracture, open
820.21 Intertrochanteric femur fracture, closed
820.22 Subtrochanteric fracture, closed
820.31 Intertrochanteric fracture, open
820.32 Subtrochanteric fracture, open

Figure 1 AP view shows a displaced femoral neck fracture (arrow).

Figure 2 AP view shows an intertrochanteric fracture of the hip (arrow).

SECTION 5   HIP

Advanced age is the most important risk factor for a proximal femur fracture. The frequency of hip fractures generally doubles with each decade beyond age 50 years. There are several reasons for this. Decreased proprioceptive function and loss of protective responses increase the likelihood that elderly individuals will fall. Also, because elderly individuals walk slowly, when they fall they tend to fall to the side as opposed to forward, so the lateral thigh and hip region often strikes the ground first. Dizziness, stroke, syncope, peripheral neuropathies, and medications are other factors that can compromise balance and predispose elderly patients to hip fractures.

White women are two to three times more likely to sustain a hip fracture than African American or Hispanic women. Other risk factors include sedentary lifestyle, smoking, alcoholism, use of psychotropic medication, dementia, osteoporosis, and living in an urban area.

Clinical Symptoms

Most patients report a fall followed by pain in the groin and the inability to bear weight on the extremity or ambulate. A few patients will be able to walk with crutches, a cane, or a walker but have groin or buttock pain on weight bearing that worsens with ambulation. Occasionally, patients report pain referred to the supracondylar region of the knee. Elderly patients with hip pain after a fall should be treated as if they have a hip fracture until proven otherwise.

Tests

Physical Examination

A patient with a displaced femoral neck or intertrochanteric fracture, when supine, lies with the limb externally rotated, abducted, and if the fracture is displaced, the leg will also be shortened. A patient with a stress fracture or a nondisplaced fracture of the femoral neck may have no obvious deformity. Attempts by the examiner to gently rotate the limb while the hip is extended elicit pain, and the patient will be unable to perform a straight-leg raise (lift the heel on the affected side off the bed while keeping the knee straight).

Diagnostic Tests

An AP view of the pelvis and cross-table lateral views of the involved hip reveal most fractures of the proximal femur. It is important to avoid a frog-lateral radiograph in a patient with a suspected proximal femur fracture, as this will cause severe pain and may cause displacement of a nondisplaced fracture. An MRI should be obtained if the history and physical examination are suggestive of a fracture but plain radiographs are negative (**Figure 3**).

Figure 3   T1-weighted MRI shows a nondisplaced intertrochanteric hip fracture (arrow).

Differential Diagnosis

- Pathologic fracture (underlying or associated tumor, benign or malignant)
- Pelvic fracture (normal hip joint motion, pain on external rotation)
- Stress fracture of the femoral neck or pelvis (normal but painful hip motion)

Adverse Outcomes of the Disease

Proximal femur fractures are generally markers of poor health, and medical complications frequently accompany these injuries, including thromboembolic events, pneumonia, decubitus ulcers, and urinary tract infections. One-year mortality following proximal femur fractures in elderly patients has been reported at 10% to 30%, and patients often lose both ambulatory capacity and functional independence. Complications directly related to the fracture include nonunion and osteonecrosis.

Treatment

Most proximal femur fractures are treated surgically because the risks of nonsurgical treatment (primarily related to the extended period of bed rest required, with the associated risk of thromboembolic events, pneumonia, decubitus ulcers, and general deconditioning) generally outweigh the risks of surgical treatment of all except the most medically unstable patients and nonambulatory and/or demented patients who have minimal pain associated with transfers.

Patients diagnosed with a proximal femur fracture should be evaluated by an orthopaedic surgeon, an internist, and an anesthesiologist in a timely manner to expedite surgical treatment. Patients should undergo a thorough evaluation to determine if medical comorbidities are present that can be optimized preoperatively to decrease the risk of perioperative morbidity and mortality. Thromboembolic prophylaxis of some form (mechanical, pharmacologic, or both in combination) should be instituted immediately because these patients are at extraordinarily high risk for thromboembolic events. Numerous studies have suggested that a delay of more than 48 hours from the time of injury to surgical intervention is associated with increased mortality. Therefore, surgical intervention should not be delayed longer than 48 hours unless some other intervention will substantially decrease the patient's perioperative risk from surgical treatment. Although skin traction has been commonly used in the past to relieve preoperative discomfort, recent prospective randomized studies have shown that it is less effective than a pillow placed beneath the patient's knee.

SECTION 5 HIP

The form of surgical treatment selected is determined primarily by fracture location (femoral neck versus intertrochanteric), displacement, and patient activity level. Intertrochanteric fractures are treated with either a screw and side plate (**Figure 4A**) or an intramedullary nail (**Figure 4B**). Nondisplaced or valgus impacted femoral neck fractures are treated by percutaneous fixation with multiple (typically three) screws (**Figure 4C**). Displaced fractures in elderly patients are typically treated with prosthetic replacement (arthroplasty) (**Figure 4D**), (either hemiarthroplasty for minimal ambulators or nonambulators or total hip arthroplasty for patients who are able to ambulate before surgery) because the risks of nonunion and osteonecrosis approach 50% if fracture fixation is performed. Femoral neck fractures in patients younger than 60 years are typically associated with high-energy trauma and constitute a surgical emergency because anatomic surgical fixation in a timely manner is required for optimal outcomes. Bone mineral density measurement should be part of the evaluation of patients who present with fractures of the femoral neck or intertrochanteric area of the femur. If low bone mineral density is found, appropriate treatment should be instituted.

Adverse Outcomes of Treatment

Femoral neck fractures treated with internal fixation are associated with osteonecrosis of the femoral head and fracture nonunion. In hips treated with either hemiarthroplasty or total hip arthroplasty, prosthetic dislocation can occur. The most common complications of surgical treatment of an intertrochanteric fracture are posttraumatic arthritis and/or failure of fixation with nonunion (**Figure 5**). All patients with proximal

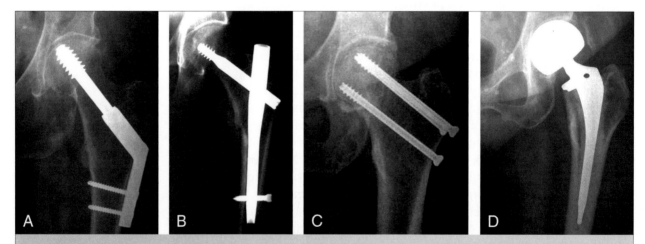

Figure 4   Postoperative AP radiographs. **A,** Intertrochanteric hip fracture treated with a screw and side plate. **B,** Intertrochanteric hip fracture treated with an intramedullary nail. **C,** Nondisplaced femoral neck fracture treated with three cannulated screws. **D,** Displaced femoral neck fracture treated with cemented arthroplasty of the hip.

femur fractures should undergo evaluation for osteoporosis and treatment as appropriate because they are at substantial risk for fracture of the contralateral hip and other fragility fractures, such as distal radius and vertebral compression fractures.

Referral Decisions/Red Flags

A femoral neck fracture in a patient younger than 60 years constitutes a surgical emergency because the risk of osteonecrosis and fracture nonunion is substantial. Prompt surgical fixation and an anatomic reduction decrease the risk of these complications. In a patient with a history and physical examination suggestive of a fracture but with negative plain radiographs, an MRI should be obtained to definitively diagnose or rule out a proximal femur fracture. All proximal femur fractures should be considered for surgical treatment given the high risk of complications associated with nonsurgical treatment.

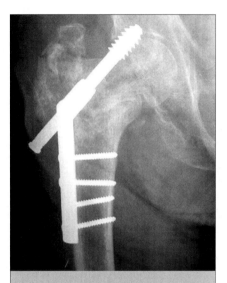

Figure 5 AP radiograph shows a failed fixation following an intertrochanteric hip fracture.

SECTION 5 HIP

Hip Impingement

Synonyms

Femoral acetabular impingement (FAI)

Definition

Hip impingement, or femoral acetabular impingement (FAI), occurs when areas of osseous deformities on the acetabular rim, the femoral head–neck junction, or both abut at extremes of hip motion and cause injury to the acetabular labrum and cartilage. Studies have demonstrated that most labral tears occur after repetitive microtrauma as a result of these subtle structural deformities.

Clinical Symptoms

Patients with hip impingement can range in age from teenagers to middle-aged weekend athletes. Pain secondary to hip impingement may occur after an acute event, but more often the patient reports an insidious onset of pain that becomes more severe with time. The location of the pain is important because intra-articular hip pathology is classically associated with groin pain. With hip impingement, patients may place a hand over the side of the hip and report that they feel a deep pain located between their fingers and thumb; this is known as the "C sign." Some patients also may report pain on the lateral aspect of the hip over the greater trochanter, with associated hip abductor weakness. Associated catching, locking, or clicking also may be present. Many patients describe worsening pain with prolonged sitting or pain with stair climbing, getting in and out of a car, putting on shoes or socks, or activities that require rotational movement.

Tests

Physical Examination

Decreased hip flexion and internal rotation compared with the opposite extremity may be observed in patients with hip impingement. The classic provocative maneuver is to place the hip in maximum flexion, adduction, and internal rotation (FADDIR); pain with this maneuver is a positive impingement sign (**Figure 1**).

Diagnostic Tests

AP and lateral radiographs of the hip are indicated for patients with pain and limited internal rotation of the hip. The classic radiographic features are a loss of femoral head–neck offset on either the AP or lateral view (cam impingement), a crossover sign (pincer impingement), or both, in the setting of normal joint space (**Figure 2**).

Figure 1   The FADDIR (flexion, adduction, internal rotation) maneuver.

Figure 2   Radiographs of patient with hip impingement. **A**, AP view of the left hip demonstrates a preserved joint space with a cam deformity (arrow) of the femur and crossover sign (*) on the acetabulum. The solid line indicates the anterior wall; the dashed line indicates the posterior wall. **B**, Cross-table lateral view also demonstrates the loss of femoral head concavity (arrow).

Figure 3 T2-weighted coronal MR arthrogram of a right hip demonstrates a labral tear (arrow).

In pure femoral cam impingement, the anterior femoral neck loses its normal concave anatomy and instead has a "bump" that impinges on the anterosuperior labrum with flexion, causing labral tears and delamination of the adjacent cartilage.

In pincer impingement, the acetabulum is involved. The morphology of a normal acetabulum is anteverted, in that the posterior rim is more lateral than the anterior rim. Pincer acetabular impingement arises when the anterior acetabular rim is prominent relative to the posterior rim, resulting in a radiographic appearance in which the anterior wall is more lateral than the posterior wall. This is known as the crossover sign. Either MRI or CT with three-dimensional constructions can provide further information about the three-dimensional anatomy of the hip. MRI may be falsely negative for evidence of labral tears or articular cartilage injury because of variable technique or interpretation. MR arthrography of the hip has been shown to be the most accurate modality for demonstrating associated labral tears and osseous abnormalities (**Figure 3**).

Differential Diagnosis

- Athletic pubalgia/sports hernia (pain over rectus insertion and adductor tendons)
- Developmental dysplasia of the hip (evident on radiographs)
- Femoral cutaneous nerve entrapment (sensory changes, burning pain, normal hip range of motion)
- Groin strains (normal radiographs)
- Osteoarthritis (narrow joint space on radiographs with associated osteophytes, subchondral sclerosis and cystic changes)
- Osteonecrosis of the femoral head (evident on plain radiographs or MRI)
- Psoas impingement or snapping psoas tendon (audible snap in groin reproducible with flexion, circumduction, and extension)
- Trochanteric bursitis (local tenderness of the greater trochanter, pain with resisted hip abduction, normal motion)
- Tumor of the pelvis or spine (back pain, night pain, normal hip range of motion)

Adverse Outcomes of the Disease

Hip impingement and other hip deformities may be the etiology for 60% to 80% of cases of osteoarthritis of the hip. The assertion that hip impingement can potentially cause osteoarthritis has not been scientifically proved, but long-term prospective natural history studies may provide strong support for this idea. If hip impingement is a major contributor to hip osteoarthritis, it is thought that surgical intervention for hip pain secondary to hip impingement may delay the onset or potentially even prevent hip osteoarthritis.

Treatment

The initial treatment of all patients is nonsurgical and consists of a combination of acetaminophen, NSAIDs, and activity modification. A rehabilitation specialist familiar with nonarthroplasty hip joint dysfunction should be consulted for hip range of motion and strength training, with the goal of restoring muscular balance to the hip. Modalities such as deep tissue massage or active release therapy may be helpful in patients with associated tendinitis or stiffness around the hip secondary to long-standing hip impingement. Fluoroscopically guided intra-articular hip injections with a combination of a local anesthetic and a corticosteroid are both diagnostic and therapeutic, and complete pain relief is the most accurate test to determine an intra-articular etiology for hip pain. Many patients have relief of their hip pain after a course of nonsurgical treatment.

Patients with hip impingement that has been refractory to nonoperative treatment are candidates for surgical intervention. Hip impingement was originally treated with open surgical hip dislocation to safely provide exposure to the femoral head–neck junction and the acetabular rim. More recently, arthroscopic techniques have been developed to perform surgery for hip impingement. Early postoperative mobilization and range of motion with a continuous passive motion machine and a stationary bicycle are important for motion recovery. Postoperative rehabilitation is important for restoration of motion and the return to functional as well as sporting activities.

Adverse Outcomes of Treatment

Adverse outcomes of nonsurgical treatment include complications related to the chronic use of NSAIDs, such as gastric, renal, or hepatic problems. Extended treatment with acetaminophen in large doses can lead to hepatic toxicity. Postoperative complications associated with hip arthroscopy can include temporary numbness in the groin or the dorsal aspect of the foot secondary to nerve palsy. A small number of patients have long-standing numbness over the lateral thigh secondary to surgery near the lateral femoral cutaneous nerve. Other potential postoperative complications with either open or arthroscopic surgery include heterotopic ossification, deep vein thrombosis, and stiffness. In rare cases, postoperative femoral neck fracture and joint instability can occur. The long-term result of untreated hip impingement is the development of early osteoarthritis.

SECTION 5 HIP

Referral Decisions/Red Flags

Patients who have persistent hip or groin pain, especially with flexion and internal rotation of the hip, that is refractory to nonsurgical treatment should be referred for further evaluation and potential surgical intervention. Hip pain in a young patient can be difficult to diagnose, and early referral is appropriate.

Inflammatory Arthritis

Synonym

Synovitis of the hip

Definition

Most inflammatory conditions that involve the hip are local manifestations of systemic disorders; however, these conditions may first present with hip symptoms. Although any of the inflammatory arthritides listed in the differential diagnosis may involve the hip, the prevalence of hip involvement is highest in rheumatoid arthritis and ankylosing spondylitis. End-stage arthritis of the hip also is commonly observed in patients with systemic lupus erythematosus, but this is often secondary to osteonecrosis.

With few exceptions, the pathophysiology of inflammatory arthropathies results from an immunologic host response to antigenic challenge. The exact cause remains unclear, but epidemiologic and genetic evidence supports a genetic component to many inflammatory arthritides.

ICD-9 Codes

714.0
Rheumatoid arthritis

716.65
Monoarthritis, unspecified, pelvic region or thigh

716.95
Arthropathy, unspecified, pelvic region or thigh

Clinical Symptoms

Inflammatory arthritis of the hip is characterized by a dull, aching pain in the groin, lateral thigh, or buttock region. The pain is often episodic, with patients experiencing morning stiffness, improvement with moderate activity, and increased pain and stiffness following vigorous activity. Patients often will note a progressive limp as well as limited range of motion, which may manifest as difficulty with dressing or putting on shoes. With increasing time and disease progression, symptoms are indistinguishable from osteoarthritis of the hip.

Tests

Physical Examination

Gait abnormalities such as an antalgic gait (short stance phase on the affected side) are common in the earlier phases of the disease, whereas a Trendelenburg gait develops with progressive loss of articular cartilage. Hip range of motion is often restricted, with a loss of internal rotation the most sensitive finding in adults with hip joint disease. Synovial inflammation can be detected by placing the patient in a prone position with the knee flexed and applying gentle rotation to the extremity (as if rolling a rolling pin), moving the hip only. If synovial inflammation is present, this maneuver will cause pain.

SECTION 5 HIP

Figure 1 AP view of the hip shows inflammatory arthritis of the hip with concentric joint space narrowing (arrow), minimal osteophytes, and generalized osteopenia.

Diagnostic Tests

An AP view of the pelvis as well as AP and frog-lateral radiographs of the involved hip are obtained. In the early stages of inflammatory conditions, radiographs may show subtle osteopenia and/or a joint effusion. In later stages of inflammatory arthritis, symmetric joint space loss and periarticular bone erosions are typical (**Figure 1**).

For a patient with a history and physical examination consistent with acute synovitis of the hip, laboratory studies should include complete blood count, acute phase reactants (erythrocyte sedimentation rate or C-reactive protein), rheumatoid factor, and antinuclear antibody tests. When an effusion is present, aspiration performed under fluoroscopic guidance can be considered. The aspirate should be sent for culture, cell count with differential analysis, and inspection for crystalline deposits.

Differential Diagnosis

- Ankylosing spondylitis (stiffness of the spine and hips, low back pain, evident on radiographs)
- Calcium pyrophosphate deposition disease (uncommon in the hip)
- Gout (rare in hip, previous diagnosis of gout most probable, pain in the groin or buttock)
- Hemophilic arthropathy (previous diagnosis of hemophilia, pain with motion, evident on radiographs)
- Infection (acute onset, pain in the groin, fever, marked restriction of motion)
- Inflammatory bowel disease (previous diagnosis of bowel disease most probable, groin and buttock discomfort)
- Osteoarthritis of the hip (pain in the groin or buttock, limited range of motion)
- Osteonecrosis (dull ache in the groin or buttock, evident on radiographs and/or MRI)
- Reiter syndrome (arthritis, conjunctivitis, pain in the hip, urethritis)
- Rheumatoid arthritis (pain in the groin or buttock, decreased range of motion, evident on radiographs, other joint involvement, evidence of synovitis)
- Stress fracture (pain in the groin or buttock with activity, evident on MRI)
- Systemic lupus erythematosus (pain in the groin or buttock, limited range of motion, other joint involvement)
- Trochanteric bursitis (pain in the lateral aspect of the thigh)

Adverse Outcomes of the Disease

Adverse outcomes of the disease include persistent pain, progressive gait abnormalities, and joint contractures, which may lead to decreased ambulatory capacity and loss of functional independence.

Treatment

For noninfectious inflammatory arthritis, a nonsurgical treatment plan administered in conjunction with a rheumatologist may include NSAIDs, disease-modifying agents, acetaminophen or other analgesics, the use of an assistive device held in the hand contralateral to the affected hip; and activity modification. Intra-articular corticosteroid injections can be considered, but they generally require fluoroscopic guidance for accurate placement. A rehabilitation program emphasizing range-of-motion exercises and pain-free strengthening can be helpful but may exacerbate the patient's symptoms. Total hip arthroplasty is the treatment of choice for patients with advanced symptoms that have failed to respond to nonsurgical treatment.

Adverse Outcomes of Treatment

Adverse outcomes of nonsurgical treatment include complications related to the chronic use of NSAIDs, such as gastric, renal, or hepatic problems. Extended treatment with acetaminophen in large doses can lead to hepatic toxicity. Corticosteroids are often used as part of the treatment algorithm and can lead to osteonecrosis of the femoral head. The most common short-term complications related to total hip arthroplasty include neurovascular injury, thromboembolic events, infection, leg-length inequality, and prosthetic dislocation. Wear-related complications are unusual because this patient population is typically inactive; however, prosthetic loosening requiring revision surgery may still occur.

Referral Decisions/Red Flags

For noninfectious arthritis, symptoms recalcitrant to nonsurgical treatment that lead to persistent pain and functional disability indicate the need for further evaluation.

SECTION 5   HIP

Lateral Femoral Cutaneous Nerve Syndrome

Synonym

Meralgia paresthetica

Definition

Compression or entrapment of the lateral femoral cutaneous nerve is characterized by pain, burning (dysesthesia), or hypoesthesia over the lateral thigh. Motor nerve dysfunction does not occur, because the lateral femoral cutaneous nerve is a sensory nerve. The nerve is most susceptible to compression where it exits the pelvis just medial to the anterosuperior iliac spine. This syndrome can be caused by several factors, including obesity, compression from tight clothing or straps around the waist (eg, tool belt or backpack), scar tissue from previous operations, significant trauma (especially involving hip extension), or mild repetitive trauma over the course of the nerve. The nerve also can be injured during anterior surgical approaches to the hip, pelvis, or acetabulum. Rarely, pathologic intrapelvic or abdominal processes (cecal tumors) cause compression of the lateral femoral cutaneous nerve.

Clinical Symptoms

Symptoms associated with this condition include pain and dysesthesia in the anterolateral or lateral thigh that sometimes extends to the lateral knee. Uncommonly, patients report aching in the groin area and, if the condition is acute, pain radiating to the sacroiliac joint area. Joggers describe the pain as an "electric jab" each time the affected hip extends, usually after running a short distance.

Tests

Physical Examination

Hypoesthesia or dysesthesia in the distribution of the lateral femoral cutaneous nerve is typical, with the most reproducible spot of hypoesthesia above and lateral to the knee (**Figure 1**). Burning is most consistent in this area. Pressure or tapping over the nerve where it exits the pelvis just medial to or directly over the anterosuperior iliac spine can produce tenderness or

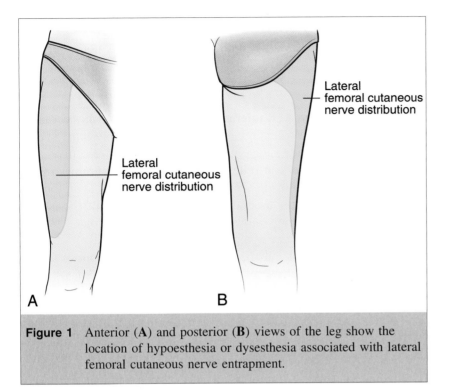

Figure 1 Anterior (**A**) and posterior (**B**) views of the leg show the location of hypoesthesia or dysesthesia associated with lateral femoral cutaneous nerve entrapment.

reproduce paresthesias along the distribution of the nerve. Muscle weakness and reflex changes are absent. Abdominal and pelvic examinations are needed to exclude intra-abdominal pathology.

Diagnostic Tests

An AP radiograph of the pelvis will rule out any bony abnormality, and AP and lateral radiographs of the hip may be appropriate when the patient has restricted internal rotation of the hip and groin pain. CT or MRI is appropriate to investigate a suspected intrapelvic mass.

Differential Diagnosis

- Diabetes mellitus or other causes of peripheral neuropathy (numbness in the feet)
- Hip arthritis (limited internal rotation, limp)
- Intra-abdominal tumor (pelvic or abdominal mass, hematochezia, weight loss)
- Lumbar disk herniation (L1 through L4 motor and sensory changes, positive prone rectus femoris stretch test)
- Trochanteric bursitis (tenderness over trochanter, stiffness when rising)

SECTION 5   HIP

Adverse Outcomes of the Disease

Pain and dysesthesia will continue if the patient is not treated.

Treatment

Numbness is often well tolerated, but burning dysesthesia can become intolerable. Removing the source of compression, such as a tight waistband, a weight-lifting belt, or mild repetitive trauma to the nerve, can relieve the symptoms of burning. In obese patients, significant weight loss often relieves symptoms. Infiltration of the area around the nerve where it exits the pelvis near the anterosuperior iliac spine with a corticosteroid preparation may reduce symptoms. Neuropathic pain medications, such as gabapentin, may be useful in appropriate patients. Surgical release of the nerve is rarely required; its most common indication is in patients with persistent burning dysesthesia.

Adverse Outcomes of Treatment

In some instances, symptoms persist despite treatment.

Referral Decisions/Red Flags

A suspected pelvic or abdominal mass signals the need for immediate further evaluation. The presence of intolerable symptoms that have failed to respond to nonsurgical treatment also indicates the need for further evaluation.

Osteoarthritis of the Hip

Synonyms

Degenerative arthritis of the hip

Osteoarthrosis of the hip

Definition

Osteoarthritis of the hip is characterized by a loss of articular cartilage in the hip joint. The osteoarthrosis may be primary (idiopathic) or secondary to hip diseases during childhood, trauma, osteonecrosis, previous joint infection, or other conditions.

Clinical Symptoms

The classic presentation is a gradual onset of anterior thigh or groin pain. Some patients have pain in the buttock or the lateral aspect of the thigh. The pain may be referred to the distal thigh (knee) and may be perceived only in the knee. Initially, pain occurs only with activity, but gradually the frequency and intensity of the pain increase to the point that pain occurs at rest and at night. As osteoarthritis progresses, patients develop decreased range of motion, which may manifest as a limp and difficulty putting on trousers or shoes. Ambulatory capacity gradually decreases as pain increases. Occasionally, patients will have a severe limp and stiffness but little pain.

Careful questioning may reveal a history of hip problems as an infant or toddler (indicative of developmental dysplasia of the hip), as a small child (indicative of Legg-Calvé-Perthes disease), or as an adolescent (suggestive of slipped capital femoral epiphysis). Patients with osteoarthritis of the hip may have other coexisting conditions, as listed in the differential diagnosis.

Tests

Physical Examination

The earliest sign of osteoarthritis of the hip is a loss of internal rotation as determined by range-of-motion testing. Gradually, global decreases in range of motion occur, and many patients develop a fixed external rotation and flexion contracture. Flexion contractures are particularly problematic because they greatly affect gait patterns, as the patient must compensate by increasing lumbar spine extension to afford hip extension. In addition, an antalgic gait (short stance on the painful leg) and an abductor lurch (swaying the trunk far over the affected hip) develop as the body tries to compensate for the pain and secondary weakness in the hip abductor muscles.

ICD-9 Codes

715.05
Osteoarthritis of the hip, generalized

715.15
Primary (idiopathic) osteoarthritis of the hip, localized

715.25
Secondary osteoarthritis of the hip (eg, Legg-Calvé-Perthes disease)

715.35
Primary or secondary osteoarthritis of the hip, localized

716.15
Traumatic arthritis of the hip

SECTION 5 HIP

Figure 1 AP radiograph showing degenerative joint disease of the hip with joint space narrowing (black arrow), osteophyte formation (white arrow), subchondral cyst formation (black arrowhead), and subchondral sclerosis (white arrowhead).

Diagnostic Tests

AP and lateral radiographs of the hip are indicated for patients with pain and limited internal rotation of the hip. The classic radiographic features of osteoarthritis of the hip are joint space narrowing, osteophyte formation, subchondral cyst formation, and subchondral sclerosis (**Figure 1**).

Differential Diagnosis

- Degenerative lumbar disk disease (normal hip motion)
- Femoral cutaneous nerve entrapment (sensory changes, burning, normal motion)
- Herniated lumbar disk (diminished knee reflex, sensory changes)
- Inflammatory arthritis of the hip (rheumatoid arthritis, systemic lupus erythematosus, ankylosing spondylitis)
- Osteonecrosis of the femoral head (evident on radiographs)
- Trochanteric bursitis (local tenderness, normal motion)
- Tumor of the pelvis or spine (back pain, night pain, normal motion)

Adverse Outcomes of the Disease

Osteoarthritis of the hip is a progressive condition with a natural history of increasing pain and a subsequent decrease in function associated with progressive gait abnormality. In the end stages of the disease, pain is severe, occurring at night and at rest and severely limiting ambulation, and large fixed contractures of the hip develop secondarily. Progressive bone loss of the femoral head or the acetabulum may occur but is uncommon.

Treatment

Initial treatment of all patients is nonsurgical and consists of a combination of acetaminophen, NSAIDs, activity modification, and the use of an assistive device held in the hand contralateral to the affected hip. Non–weight-bearing exercise (such as the use of a stationary bicycle or swimming) and hip strengthening are occasionally helpful but may exacerbate symptoms. Intra-articular injections with corticosteroids are used occasionally; they generally require fluoroscopic guidance for accurate placement.

Vigorous, young patients in whom nonsurgical treatment fails and who have a biomechanical derangement of the hip may be candidates for a realignment osteotomy of the proximal femur or the acetabulum. Hip fusion is a potential surgical option for a young patient who either must return to work as a manual laborer or who leads a vigorous lifestyle. The vast majority of patients in whom nonsurgical treatment fails, however, are most appropriately treated with total hip replacement surgery (**Figure 2**). Total hip replacement is associated with dramatic decreases in pain as well as increases in function and is among the most cost-effective medical interventions available when quality-adjusted years of life are considered. Metal-on-metal hip resurfacing (**Figure 3**), which uses a cap on the femoral head as opposed to the stemmed femoral component used in a conventional total hip arthroplasty, may be an appropriate alternative for young, active patients. It has the potential benefits of preserving proximal femoral bone stock (should revision surgery be required in the future) and allowing the return to higher level activities, such as running sports, that are not typically recommended following conventional total hip arthroplasty with a stemmed femoral component.

Adverse Outcomes of Treatment

Adverse outcomes of nonsurgical treatment include complications related to the chronic use of NSAIDs, such as gastric, renal, or hepatic problems. Extended treatment with acetaminophen in large doses can lead to hepatic toxicity. The most common short-term complications related to total hip arthroplasty include neurovascular injury, thromboembolic events, infection, leg-length inequality, and prosthetic dislocation. Long-term complications of total hip arthroplasty are more common in young, active patients and relate primarily to wear of the bearing surface and loosening of the components that may require revision surgery. Patients who are treated with osteotomy or hip fusion may require further surgical intervention in the form of total hip arthroplasty if the surgery is unsuccessful, subsequent arthritis develops, or pain relief is incomplete.

Referral Decisions/Red Flags

Patients who have persistent pain despite nonsurgical treatment including acetaminophen, multiple different NSAIDs, activity modification, and/or the use of an assistive device require appropriate referral for further evaluation of potential surgical intervention. Young patients may be referred earlier to determine if an alternative to conventional total hip arthroplasty (such as redirectional osteotomy, hip fusion, or hip resurfacing) is appropriate.

Figure 2 AP radiograph of the hip of a patient with osteoarthritis following total hip arthroplasty.

Figure 3 AP radiograph of a hip following metal-on-metal hip resurfacing.

SECTION 5 HIP

Osteonecrosis of the Hip

ICD-9 Code

733.42
Aseptic necrosis of femoral
head and neck

Synonyms

Aseptic necrosis of the hip
Osteonecrosis of the hip

Definition

Osteonecrosis of the hip results from the death of varying amounts of bone in the femoral head. The causative event may be traumatic disruption of the vascular supply to the femoral head or deficient circulation from other causes (eg, microvascular thrombosis in patients with sickle cell anemia). Initially, only the osteocytes and other cells are affected, but with time the bone structure fragments and collapses. As a result, the overlying articular surface collapses and progressive arthritis develops.

Osteonecrosis affects 10,000 to 20,000 new patients per year in the United States, occurs with greater frequency in the third through fifth decades of life, and often is bilateral. Risk factors include trauma (hip dislocation or femoral neck fracture), history of corticosteroid use, alcohol abuse, sickle cell disease, rheumatoid arthritis, and systemic lupus erythematosus. Of note, the association with corticosteroids generally is related to the amount and duration of medication; however, osteonecrosis sometimes develops after only one or two exposures to corticosteroids.

Clinical Symptoms

Patients usually report the indolent onset of a dull ache or a throbbing pain in the groin, lateral hip, or buttock area. Patients may report severe pain during the initial phases of the disease when bone death occurs. Secondary arthritis develops with progressive collapse of the femoral head, and symptoms may be indistinguishable from osteoarthritis. Limited range of motion may occur, and patients often report a progressive limp. The history should focus on the following risk factors for the disease:

Tests
Physical Examination

- Alcohol abuse
- Caisson disease (scuba diving)
- Chronic pancreatitis
- Corticosteroid use

- Crohn disease
- Gaucher disease
- HIV infection
- Myeloproliferative disorders
- Radiation treatment
- Rheumatoid arthritis
- Trauma
- Sickle cell disease
- Smoking
- Systemic lupus erythematosus

Patients have pain with attempted straight-leg raising (lifting the heel of the affected extremity off the examination table with the knee held straight) as well as with range of motion of the hip. Range of motion may be decreased (particularly internal rotation) in addition to being painful. Patients often have an antalgic gait (short stance phase) but may develop a Trendelenburg gait once secondary arthritis develops.

Diagnostic Tests

An AP view of the pelvis and AP and frog-lateral radiographs of the hip should be obtained. In the earliest stages of the disease, plain radiographs may be normal. With time, patchy areas of sclerosis and lucency may be present. With disease progression, a "crescent sign" appears, which is a well-defined sclerotic area just beneath the articular surface that represents a subchondral fracture. The femoral head typically becomes progressively more aspherical with time, leading to secondary degenerative changes of the acetabulum, which may appear indistinguishable from degenerative arthritis (**Figure 1**).

In patients in whom osteonecrosis is suspected but radiographic findings are normal or equivocal, MRI is indicated (**Figure 2**). Patients with unilateral atraumatic osteonecrosis may benefit from an MRI of the contralateral hip to diagnose asymptomatic disease on that side that may benefit from surgical treatment to prevent disease progression.

Differential Diagnosis

- Fracture of the femoral neck (evident on radiographs and MRI)
- Lumbar disk disease (back pain, reflex changes, radiation below knee)
- Muscle strain or groin pull (normal radiographs, intermittent limp)
- Osteoarthritis of the hip (no risk factors, absence of sclerosis within the femoral heads on radiographs)
- Septic arthritis of the hip (fever, constitutional symptoms)

Figure 1 AP view of the hip showing osteonecrosis of the femoral head with collapse (arrow).

Figure 2 Coronal T1-weighted MRI of the hip shows areas of low signal intensity consistent with osteonecrosis of the femoral heads (arrows). (Reproduced with permission from Johnson TR, Steinbach LS, eds: *Essentials of Musculoskeletal Imaging.* Rosemont, IL, American Academy of Orthopaedic Surgeons, 2004, p 470.)

SECTION 5 HIP

- Transient osteoporosis of the hip (disabling pain without previous trauma, osteopenia, patient a woman in the third trimester of pregnancy or a middle-aged man)

Adverse Outcomes of the Disease

The natural history of osteonecrosis is not well understood. In general, in patients with smaller lesions in non–weight-bearing areas and limited exposure to vascular insult, symptoms tend to resolve without femoral head collapse and arthritis developing. In patients with larger lesions and/or sustained insult to the vascular supply of the femoral head, however, femoral head collapse and secondary degenerative arthritis develop. End-stage degenerative changes also develop in these patients, including progressive pain, decreased range of motion, decreased ambulatory capacity, and limp.

Treatment

Treatment options before collapse are controversial. A myriad of different treatment options have been attempted, including protected weight bearing, pulsed magnetic electrical fields, and surgical interventions, but few studies have adequate randomization or statistical power to provide guidance with regard to selecting among these options. Surgical choices for the patient without collapse aimed at maintaining the native femoral head include core decompression (removing a core of bone from the femoral head and neck to decrease bone marrow pressure and encourage blood flow) with or without bone grafting, vascularized fibular grafting (harvesting a portion of the ipsilateral fibula with a vascular pedicle and transplanting it to the femoral head and neck to stimulate revascularization), and fresh osteochondral allografting of the femoral head. The former two options aim to relieve pressure in the femoral head that may be causing pain and stimulate healing of the lesion. Once femoral head collapse has occurred, most recommend replacement arthroplasty, although some have advocated core decompression for short-term pain relief.

Adverse Outcomes of Treatment

If attempts to preserve the femoral head fail, degenerative arthritis may develop subsequently, requiring further surgical intervention in the form of total hip arthroplasty. A unique complication of core decompression is a fracture of the femoral shaft if the core biopsy tract is placed below the level of the lesser trochanter. The results of total hip arthroplasty in this patient population are often inferior because patients may be young and vigorous and bone metabolism may be altered, placing higher demands on the prosthesis and increasing the risk of prosthetic loosening.

Referral Decisions/Red Flags

Plain radiographic evidence of or clinical suspicion for osteonecrosis requires further evaluation to determine if surgical intervention to preserve the femoral head is indicated.

SECTION 5 HIP

Snapping Hip

Definition

Snapping hip is characterized by a snapping or popping sensation that occurs as tendons around the hip move over bony prominences. The most common cause is the iliotibial band snapping over the greater trochanter. Snapping also can occur when the iliopsoas tendon slides over the pectineal eminence of the pelvis or from intra-articular tears of the acetabular labrum (the fibrocartilage rim at the periphery of the acetabulum).

Clinical Symptoms

Iliotibial band subluxation usually occurs with walking or rotation of the hip. When asked to localize their symptoms, patients will point to the trochanteric area (**Figure 1**). Some patients notice the snapping when they lie on their side with the affected side up and rotate the leg. If a trochanteric bursitis subsequently develops, patients will report increased pain when first rising in the morning, pain at night, and difficulty lying on the affected side.

Snapping caused by subluxation of the iliopsoas tendon usually is felt in the groin as the hip extends from a flexed position, as when rising from a chair. Many patients feel the snapping but have no disability. In a few patients, the snapping is either annoying or painful.

Snapping from intra-articular causes is more disabling and more likely to cause patients to reach for support.

Tests
Physical Examination

Iliotibial band subluxation can be re-created by having the patient stand and then rotate the hip while holding it in an adducted position. A snap can be palpated as the iliotibial band slides over the greater trochanter. Snapping of the iliopsoas tendon may be palpated as the hip extends from a flexed position and the tendon moves over the pectineal eminence of the pelvis. Restricted internal rotation of the involved hip, a limp, or shortening of the limb suggests problems within the hip joint. The Ober test (see page 639) is used to evaluate the tightness of the iliotibial band. For this test, the patient lies on the uninvolved side. The examiner flexes the patient's knee to 90°, then abducts the involved hip about 40° and extends it to its limit. While the hip extension and knee flexion are maintained and the pelvis is stabilized, the hip is allowed to

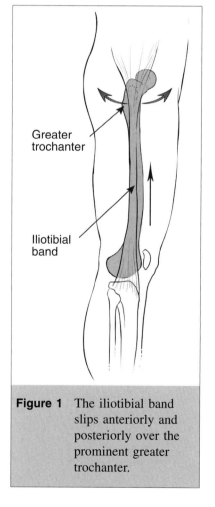

Figure 1 The iliotibial band slips anteriorly and posteriorly over the prominent greater trochanter.

Greater trochanter

Iliotibial band

adduct passively. If the hip fails to adduct to at least the midline of the body or the patient experiences pain along the iliotibial band, the test is positive.

Diagnostic Tests

AP radiographs of the pelvis and lateral hip can exclude bony pathology or intra-articular hip disease. Radiographs typically are normal for patients with a snapping hip. A CT arthrogram may be necessary to rule out intra-articular loose bodies. MRI with gadolinium may be necessary to rule out a tear of the acetabular labrum. A diagnostic, fluoroscopically guided anesthetic injection may be useful to distinguish between intra-articular and extra-articular sources of symptoms.

Differential Diagnosis

- Osteoarthritis of the hip (limited internal rotation)
- Osteochondral loose body (fragment of bone and cartilage within the joint, pain with hip motion)
- Osteonecrosis of the femoral head (compromised blood supply to the femoral head, groin pain)
- Tear of the acetabular labrum (pain, catching, or instability with hip motion)

Adverse Outcomes of the Disease

Pain and annoyance are commonly reported.

Treatment

Snapping hip is often painless, and once the diagnosis is made with certainty, patients often require only an explanation of the source of the symptoms for reassurance. Patients who are significantly bothered by the symptoms should be advised to avoid provocative maneuvers and activities so that the symptoms can subside. Treatment consists of exercises to stretch and strengthen the iliotibial band, hip abductors, hip adductors, and hip flexors. A short course of NSAIDs may reduce the discomfort associated with tendon snapping and secondary bursitis. Corticosteroid injection into the greater trochanteric bursa (for snapping iliotibial band) or into the psoas tendon sheath (for snapping iliopsoas tendon) may reduce pain.

Surgery is reserved for the uncommon cases that are disabling and fail to resolve with nonsurgical management.

SECTION 5 HIP

Rehabilitation Prescription

The functional goal of rehabilitation for a patient with a snapping hip is to reduce pain and increase the ability of the patient to return to functional activities, such as walking and running. Stretching exercises for tight muscles around the hip should be performed in conjunction with strengthening exercises. Weakness of the hip abductors is very commonly associated with tightness of the iliotibial band.

The home exercise program for snapping hip (see page 589) should include stretching and strengthening exercises. If the pain does not diminish within 2 or 3 weeks on a home program, formal rehabilitation may be ordered. The prescription should include a complete evaluation of hip strength and the flexibility of the soft-tissue structures, including the iliotibial band, the hamstrings, and the hip flexors. Increasing the endurance of the trunk muscles should be part of the rehabilitation prescription.

Adverse Outcomes of Treatment

NSAIDs can cause gastric, renal, or hepatic complications. Postoperative infection or persistent pain is possible if surgical intervention is undertaken.

Referral Decisions/Red Flags

Unclear diagnosis, intra-articular pathology, or failure of nonsurgical measures indicates the need for further evaluation.

Home Exercise Program for Snapping Hip

- Perform the exercises in the order listed.

- Apply dry or moist heat to the hip for 5 to 10 minutes before exercising to prepare the tissues. Alternatively, riding a stationary bicycle for 10 minutes will also prepare the tissues for stretching.

- Apply a bag of crushed ice or frozen peas to the hip for 20 minutes after exercising to help reduce inflammation.

- If you experience pain in the hip during or after exercising, discontinue the exercises and call your doctor.

Exercise Type	Muscle Group	Number of Repetitions/Sets	Number of Days per Week	Number of Weeks
Piriformis stretch	Piriformis	4 repetitions/2 to 3 sets	5 to 7	2 to 3
Iliotibial band stretch	Tensor fascia latae	4 repetitions/2 to 3 sets	5 to 7	2 to 3
Hip abduction	Gluteus medius	8 repetitions/2 sets, progressing to 15 repetitions/3 sets	3	2 to 3

Piriformis Stretch

- Lie on your back and bend both knees so that your feet are flat on the floor.

- Place the ankle of the affected leg on the opposite knee and clasp your hands behind the thigh as shown.

- Pull the thigh toward you until you feel a stretch in the hip.

- Hold the stretch for 30 seconds and then relax for 30 seconds.

- Perform 2 to 3 sets of 4 repetitions 5 to 7 days per week, continuing for 2 to 3 weeks.

- Perform the stretch on both sides.

Iliotibial Band Stretch

- Stand approximately 2 feet away from a wall with the affected side to the wall.
- Fully extend your arm and place your hand on the wall for support.
- Cross the uninjured leg (the leg farther from the wall) over the opposite leg.
- Lean your hips toward the wall until you feel a stretch on the outside of the injured leg.
- Hold the maximum stretch for 30 seconds and then relax for 10 seconds.
- Repeat the sequence 4 times on each side.
- Perform 2 to 3 sets of 4 repetitions 5 to 7 days per week, continuing for 2 to 3 weeks.
- Perform the stretch on both sides.

Hip Abduction

- Lie on your side with the affected hip on top. Cradle your head in your arm and bend your bottom leg to provide support.
- Slowly move the top leg up and back to 45°, keeping the knee straight. Hold this position for 5 seconds.
- Slowly lower the leg to a count of 5 and relax it for 2 seconds.
- Ankle weights should be used, starting with light enough weights to allow 2 sets of 8 repetitions and progressing to 3 sets of 15 repetitions.
- Then return to 2 sets of 8 repetitions and add weight in 2- to 3-pound increments, progressing each time to 3 sets of 15 repetitions.
- Perform the exercise 3 times per week, continuing for 2 to 3 weeks.

Strains of the Hip

Definition

Hip strain is a general term applied to injuries of the muscle-tendon units around the hip. Several muscles, including the abdominals, the hip flexors (iliopsoas, sartorius, and rectus femoris), and the hip adductors, should be considered when a patient has pain around the hip after an acute or overuse injury (**Figure 1**). Vigorous muscular contraction while the muscle is on stretch frequently causes the injury. For example, forceful hip flexion can strain the iliopsoas muscle, as when a soccer player forcibly flexes the hip to kick a ball and the leg is blocked or forcefully extended by an opponent. Overuse injuries are a common cause of hip strains.

ICD-9 Codes
843.0 Sprains and strains of hip and thigh, iliofemoral
843.1 Sprains and strains of hip and thigh, ischiocapsular
843.8 Sprains and strains of hip and thigh, other specified sites
843.9 Sprains and strains of hip and thigh, unspecified site

Clinical Symptoms

The most common presenting symptom is pain over the injured muscle that is exacerbated when that area continues to be used during strenuous activities.

Tests

Physical Examination

The deep location of the hip muscles compromises the examination, and precise localization of the injured muscle is not always possible. A strain of the hip adductors is identified

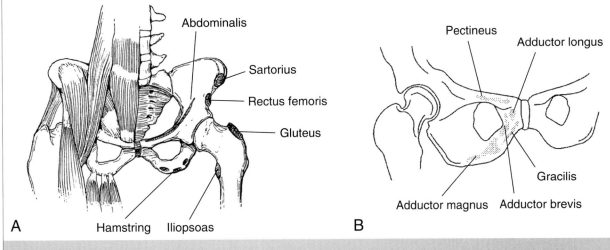

Figure 1   **A,** Anterior view of pelvis: muscle origins and insertions. **B,** Anterior view of pelvis: adductor muscle insertions. (Part A reproduced with permission from Delee JC, Drez D Jr, eds: *Orthopaedic Sports Medicine: Principles and Practice.* Philadelphia, PA, WB Saunders, 1994, vol 2, pp 1063-1085.)

Figure 2 Coronal short tau inversion recovery (STIR) sequence MRI of the pelvis demonstrates high signal intensity, indicating edema, at the origin and proximal muscle belly of several of the adductor muscles. This is consistent with a muscle strain.

by tenderness in the groin and increased pain with passive abduction. Additionally, resistive strength testing of the muscle typically elicits pain. Injury to the abdominal muscles is identified by increased pain when the patient flexes the trunk. When a hip flexor is injured, the pain is worse with flexion of the hip against resistance or with passive extension of the hip. Strain of the rectus femoris is delineated by increased pain when putting the rectus femoris on stretch. Injury to the iliopsoas typically causes pain in the deep groin or inner thigh, whereas pain from a proximal sartorius strain is more superficial and lateral.

Diagnostic Tests

AP radiographs of the pelvis and a frog-lateral view of the involved hip can rule out a fracture or other bony lesion. A bone scan or MRI can contribute useful information to help the physician arrive at the correct diagnosis, but these studies are rarely necessary except in the elite athlete (**Figure 2**).

Differential Diagnosis

- Hip avulsion fractures (may be seen with strains of the sartorius [avulsion fracture of the anterior superior iliac spine] or rectus femoris [avulsion fracture of the anterior inferior iliac spine])
- Osteonecrosis of the hip (chronic dull ache in the groin, inner thigh, or buttock; evident on radiographs, MRI)
- Pelvic or proximal femoral tumors (pain at rest or at night, increased pain with weight bearing)

Adverse Outcomes of the Disease

Chronic injury can be debilitating and threaten athletic performance. If pain persists, the patient's gait may be altered, resulting in secondary injuries.

Treatment

Rehabilitation enhances full recovery and should be initiated after confirmation of the injury. For most patients, activity modification, followed by a home exercise program, is sufficient. Elite athletes usually are treated with a more aggressive and costly regimen (**Table 1**). Rehabilitation can be divided into five phases that generally are completed within approximately 6 weeks. Phase I (48 to 72 hours) includes rest, ice, compression, and protected weight bearing with crutches if needed. Phase II (72 hours up to 1 week) includes passive range-of-motion exercises, accompanied by heat, electrical stimulation, or ultrasound. The final three phases include different isometric exercises and sport-specific training.

Table 1 Rehabilitation Guidelines for Muscle Injuries in Elite Athletes

Phase	Goals	Treatment	Time Frame
I	Reduce pain, inflammation, and bleeding	Rest, ice, and compression; crutches if needed	48 to 72 h
II	Regain range of motion	Passive range of motion, heat, ultrasound, electrical muscle stimulation	72 h to 1 week
III	Increase strength, flexibility, and endurance	Isometrics, well-leg cycling	Weeks 1 to 3
IV	Increase strength and coordination	Isotonic and isokinetic exercises	Weeks 3 to 4
V	Return to competition	Sport-specific training	Weeks 4 to 6

(Reproduced with permission from Delee JC, Drez D Jr, eds: *Orthopaedic Sports Medicine: Principles and Practice.* Philadelphia, PA, WB Saunders, 1994, vol 2, pp 1063-1085.)

The purpose of the final phases is to increase strength and flexibility and focus on returning the patient to the preinjury level of activity. If pain is exacerbated during the rehabilitation process, the patient should return to the phase of treatment that preceded the recurrence of symptoms. NSAIDs can be a useful adjunct to a rehabilitation program to reduce pain and inflammation.

Rehabilitation Prescription

Strains of the hip are usually secondary to overuse and/or muscle imbalances. For example, running long distances can result in muscle fatigue. The hip abductors, extensors, and internal and external rotators are among the weakest muscle groups in the hip, so a home exercise program that attempts to strengthen these muscles is appropriate, provided there is no pain with the exercise (see page 595).

If pain persists after the patient has been on a home program for 3 to 4 weeks, formal rehabilitation may be ordered. The prescription should include an evaluation of the trunk and hip muscles, including testing of the quadratus lumborum, abdominals, and back extensors. Once the deficits are determined, an extensive strengthening program should be initiated.

SECTION 5 HIP

Adverse Outcomes of Treatment

Recalcitrant pain may indicate a more serious injury or tendinous disruption that requires further evaluation. Recurrent injuries also are possible and are more likely to occur in competitive or weekend athletes who fail to maintain flexibility of the affected muscle. NSAIDs can cause gastric, renal, or hepatic complications.

Referral Decisions/Red Flags

Symptoms that do not respond to treatment require further evaluation to ensure that a more serious injury has not occurred and that a malignancy or osteonecrosis of the hip is not responsible for the symptoms.

Home Exercise Program for Strains of the Hip

- Perform the exercises in the order listed.
- After each set of exercises, apply a bag of crushed ice or a bag of frozen peas to the hip for 20 minutes.
- If pain in the hip is aggravated by exercising or does not go away within 3 to 4 weeks, call your doctor.

Exercise type	Muscle Group	Number of Repetitions/Sets	Number of Days per Week	Number of Weeks
Hip abduction	Gluteus medius	8 repetitions/2 sets, progressing to 12 repetitions/3 sets	3	3 to 4
Hip adduction	Adductors	8 repetitions/2 sets, progressing to 12 repetitions/3 sets	3	3 to 4
Straight-leg raises	Quadriceps	8 repetitions/2 sets, progressing to 12 repetitions/3 sets	3	3 to 4
Hip extension	Gluteus maximus	8 repetitions/2 sets, progressing to 12 repetitions/3 sets	3	3 to 4
Hip rotations	*External*: Piriformis *Internal*: Medial hamstring	8 repetitions/2 sets, progressing to 12 repetitions/3 sets	3	3 to 4

Hip Abduction

- Lie on your side with the affected hip on top. Cradle your head in your arm and bend your bottom leg to provide support.
- Slowly move the top leg up and back to 45°, keeping the knee straight.
- Hold this position for 5 seconds.
- Slowly lower the leg and relax it for 2 seconds.
- Ankle weights should be used, starting with light enough weight to allow 2 sets of 8 repetitions, progressing to 3 sets of 12 repetitions. Then return to 2 sets of 8 repetitions and add weight.
- Perform the exercise 3 days per week, continuing for 3 to 4 weeks.

Hip Adduction

- Lie on the floor on the side of the injured leg with both legs straight.
- Cross the uninjured leg in front of the injured one.
- Raised the injured (bottom) leg 6″ to 8″ off the floor.
- Hold this position for 5 seconds.
- Lower the leg and rest for 2 seconds.
- Work up to 3 sets of 10 repetitions.

Straight-Leg Raises

- Lie on the floor with the injured leg straight and the uninjured leg bent.
- Tighten the thigh muscle of the straight leg and slowly raise it 6″ to 10″ off the floor.
- Hold this position for 5 seconds.
- Work up to 3 sets of 10 repetitions.

Hip Extension

- Lie face down with a pillow under your hips and the knee on the affected side bent 90°.
- Elevate the leg off the floor to a count of 5, lifting the leg straight up with the knee bent.
- Ankle weights should be used, starting with light enough weights to allow 2 sets of 8 repetitions, progressing to 3 sets of 12 repetitions. Then return to 2 sets of 8 repetitions and add weight.
- Perform the exercise 3 days per week, continuing for 3 to 4 weeks.

Hip Rotations

- Lie face down with a pillow under your hips and the knee on the affected side bent 90°.
- Rotating from the hip, move the ankle slowly from side to side, attempting to touch the floor.
- Ankle weights should be used, starting with light enough weights to allow 2 sets of 8 repetitions, progressing to 3 sets of 12 repetitions. Then return to 2 sets of 8 repetitions and add weight.
- Perform the exercise 3 days per week, continuing for 3 to 4 weeks.

Strains of the Thigh

Definition

Injury to the thigh muscles can be temporarily painful and devastating to the avid elite or weekend athlete. The posterior thigh muscles (hamstring muscles) are injured more often than the anterior thigh muscles (quadriceps). Most hamstring strains occur when one of these muscles (biceps femoris, semimembranosus, or semitendinosus) is put on stretch during an active contraction. The strain or tear usually occurs at the musculotendinous junction. The quadriceps may sustain a similar injury; however, the quadriceps is more often injured by a direct blow.

Clinical Symptoms

A patient with a hamstring strain typically reports a sudden onset of posterior thigh pain that occurred while running, water skiing, or some other rapid movement. A "pop" may have been perceived at the onset of pain. Quadriceps contusions are associated with a direct blow during contact sports.

Tests

Physical Examination

Physical examination reveals local tenderness at the site of the injured muscle. With time, the inflammation spreads and the tenderness can become less localized. Muscle injury and associated hemorrhage may be evident by ecchymosis located in the region of the affected muscle. The hamstrings span two joints, originating above the hip on the ischial tuberosity and inserting below the knee on the tibia and fibula. Placing the hamstring on stretch to confirm the diagnosis requires flexion of the hip followed by extension of the knee. Three components of the quadriceps muscle (vastus medialis, vastus intermedius, and vastus lateralis) span only one joint. Therefore, pain associated with strain or contusion of this part of the quadriceps muscle is exacerbated by flexion of the knee and is not related to the position of the hip. The fourth component of the quadriceps muscle, the rectus femoris, spans two joints—the hip and the knee. To put this muscle on stretch, perform the prone rectus femoris test by flexing the knee with the hip in extension.

SECTION 5 HIP

Figure 1 **A,** Axial MRI of the pelvis of a 39-year-old woman who sustained an acute injury while water skiing. Area of signal change (arrow) indicates an acute hamstring injury. **B,** Sagittal MRI of the hip and thigh of the same patient also demonstrates the hamstring injury (arrow).

Figure 2 Radiograph demonstrates myositis ossificans of the thigh.

Diagnostic Tests

Radiographs or other specialized imaging studies usually are not needed in patients with a typical history and physical examination. If there is a suspicion of a fracture or bony avulsion injury, plain radiographs can be obtained. MRI can confirm a strain of the thigh (**Figure 1**), but this is rarely indicated because the history and physical examination can adequately provide a correct diagnosis.

Differential Diagnosis

- Adductor injuries (pain in the groin and inner thigh, ecchymosis, occasional sharp, stabbing pain)
- Iliopsoas strains (pain in the groin with hip flexion)
- Muscle strain of other pelvic/hip muscles (pain with ambulation)
- Pelvic avulsion fractures (pain and ecchymosis over the anterosuperior iliac spine, evident on radiographs)
- Proximal femoral tumor (pain in the groin or thigh at rest or at night, pain with weight bearing, evident on radiographs)

Adverse Outcomes of the Disease

Chronic hamstring injuries are debilitating and can end an elite athlete's career. Contusion (hemorrhage) in the quadriceps muscle may progress to myositis ossificans (**Figure 2**), with a resulting restriction of knee flexion and a possible diagnostic dilemma because the clinical appearance may simulate a malignant tumor.

Treatment

Initial treatment includes the prevention of further swelling and hemorrhage by having the patient rest and elevate the limb while applying ice and compressive wraps as needed. As time passes, the patient should begin a program of rehabilitation with stretching and strengthening of the injured muscle. The degree of rehabilitation necessary depends on the patient's general activity level and the severity of the injury. Most patients can be treated with a home exercise program. Elite athletes usually are treated with a more aggressive and costly regimen. The long-term results are generally similar. If myositis ossificans develops in the quadriceps muscle, the rehabilitation process is typically longer, but surgical excision of the ossific mass is rarely needed. NSAIDs may be used as an adjunct to a rehabilitation program to reduce pain and inflammation.

Rehabilitation Prescription

The hamstrings, adductors, and quadriceps muscle groups of the thigh are commonly injured. Sometimes a muscle imbalance of the hip and trunk is responsible for strains of these muscle groups. Early treatment consists of rest, ice, compression, and elevation (RICE) of the affected limb. In addition to RICE treatment, quadriceps injuries should be initially treated with active pain-free stretching, not passive stretching, in an attempt to prevent the development of myositis ossificans.

Depending on the severity of the injury, 1 to 3 weeks of rest may be required. Following the period of rest, early mobilization of the muscle is important to the healing process. Gentle stretching of the involved muscle group is important to regain flexibility, and strengthening is important to prevent a recurrence of the injury. An early home exercise program (see page 601) might include gentle stretching of the hamstrings and strengthening of the hip muscles, especially the abductors.

If pain and stiffness persist, formal rehabilitation may be ordered. The prescription should include a detailed assessment of the trunk and hip muscle strength, a flexibility assessment of the involved muscle, and pain-relieving modalities to promote healing of the muscle.

SECTION 5 HIP

Adverse Outcomes of Treatment

NSAIDs can cause gastric, renal, or hepatic complications. Failure to rehabilitate the injury adequately can result in chronic problems.

Referral Decisions/Red Flags

Patients with symptoms that fail to respond to appropriate rehabilitation require further evaluation.

SECTION 5   HIP

Home Exercise Program for Strains of the Thigh

- Perform the exercises in the order listed.
- Apply dry or moist heat to the thigh for 5 to 10 minutes before exercising to prepare the tissues.
- Apply a bag of crushed ice or frozen peas for 20 minutes after exercising to prevent inflammation.
- If exercising increases pain or the pain does not go away after adhering to the program for 3 to 4 weeks, call your doctor.

Exercise Type	Muscle Group	Number of Repetitions/Sets	Number of Days per Week	Number of Weeks
2-person hamstring stretch *or* 1-person hamstring stretch	Hamstrings	4 repetitions/2 to 3 sets	Daily	3 to 4
Hip abduction	Gluteus medius	8 to 12 repetitions/2 to 3 sets	3	3 to 4
Hamstring curls (standing)	Hamstrings	20 repetitions/3 sets	4 to 5	3 to 4
Straight-leg raises	Quadriceps	20 repetitions/3 sets	4 to 5	3 to 4
Straight-leg raises (prone)	Gluteus maximus	20 repetitions/3 sets	4 to 5	3 to 4
Wall slides	Quadriceps Hamstrings	20 repetitions/3 sets	4 to 5	3 to 4

2-Person Hamstring Stretch

- Lie on the floor with your legs straight or with one leg bent slightly at the knee if that is more comfortable.
- Your partner raises one of your legs just to the point of tightness and applies resistance for 30 seconds while you try to lower the leg.
- Do the same with the other leg.
- Repeat the cycle 4 times.
- Perform 2 to 3 sets of 4 repetitions daily, continuing for 3 to 4 weeks.

1-Person Hamstring Stretch

- Sit on the floor with your legs straight.
- Grasp the calf of one leg and slowly pull the leg toward your ear, keeping your back straight.
- Hold for 5 seconds.
- Do the same with the other leg.
- Repeat the cycle 4 times.
- Perform 2 to 3 sets of 4 repetitions daily, continuing for 3 to 4 weeks.

Hip Abduction

- Lie on your side with the affected hip on top. Cradle your head in your arm and bend your bottom leg to provide support.
- Slowly raise the top leg up and back to 45°, keeping the knee straight.
- Slowly lower the leg to a count of 5 and relax it for 2 seconds.
- Ankle weights should be used, starting with a weight that allows 2 sets of 8 repetitions and progressing to 3 sets of 12 repetitions.
- Then return to 2 sets of 8 repetitions and add weight in 2- to 3-pound increments, progressing each time to 3 sets of 12 repetitions.
- Perform the exercise 3 days per week for 3 to 4 weeks.

Hamstring Curls

- Stand on a flat surface with your weight evenly distributed on both feet.
- Hold onto the back of a chair or the wall for balance.
- Bend the injured knee, raising the heel of the affected leg toward the ceiling as far as you can without pain.
- Hold this position for 5 seconds and then relax.
- Perform 3 sets of 20 repetitions, 4 to 5 days per week, continuing for 3 to 4 weeks.

Straight-Leg Raises

- Lie on the floor, supporting your torso with your elbows as shown.
- Keep the injured leg straight and bend the other leg at the knee so that the foot is flat on the floor.
- Tighten the thigh muscle of the injured leg and slowly raise it 6 to 10 inches off the floor.
- Hold this position for 5 seconds and then relax.
- Perform 3 sets of 20 repetitions, 4 to 5 days per week, continuing for 3 to 4 weeks.

Straight-Leg Raises (Prone)

- Lie on the floor on your stomach with your legs straight.
- Tighten the hamstrings of the injured leg and raise the leg toward the ceiling as far as you can.
- Hold the position for 5 seconds.
- Lower the leg and rest it for 2 seconds.
- Perform 3 sets of 20 repetitions, 4 to 5 days per week, continuing for 3 to 4 weeks.

Wall Slides

- Lie on your back with the uninjured leg extending through a doorway and the injured leg extending against the wall.
- Let the foot gently slide down the wall.
- Hold the position for a maximum flexion of 5 seconds and then slowly straighten the leg.
- Perform 3 sets of 20 repetitions, 4 to 5 days per week, continuing for 3 to 4 weeks.

SECTION 5 HIP

Stress Fracture of the Femoral Neck

Synonym

Stress fracture of the hip

Definition

Femoral neck stress fractures are often misdiagnosed or missed. A failure to identify this injury may be catastrophic. Stress fractures are usually the result of a dynamic, continuing process rather than a single acute, traumatic event. Stress fractures of the femoral neck occur most commonly in military recruits and athletes, especially runners. These fractures may be classified based on the anatomic location of the fracture. Tension stress fractures, which tend to occur in older patients, are usually transverse and occur on the superior aspect of the proximal femoral neck. These injuries have a high tendency to displace. Fractures on the inferior medial side of the femur (compression side) occur more commonly in younger athletes and usually do not displace.

Clinical Symptoms

Patients usually present with vague pain in the groin, anterior thigh, or knee that is associated with activity or weight bearing and usually subsides after cessation of activity. Athletes usually report an increase in exercise intensity or activity level in the few weeks preceding symptoms.

Tests

Physical Examination

Examination of the hip may reveal pain at extreme range of motion or a limited range of motion, most significantly in internal rotation. Occasionally, the patient will walk with an antalgic gait. Tenderness at the proximal thigh or groin may be present, related to soft-tissue irritation in the area. A resisted straight-leg raising maneuver (lifting the heel of the affected side off the examination table with the knee held straight) may reproduce the groin or thigh pain.

Diagnostic Tests

Although plain radiographs are the first diagnostic test ordered, they are not diagnostic in most patients. Classic radiographic

Figure 1 Stress fracture at the base of the femoral neck. **A,** Initial AP radiograph demonstrates no apparent sign of fracture. **B,** Bone scan shows markedly increased uptake at site of femoral neck fracture (arrow). **C,** AP radiograph following a period of rest from impact activities shows increased osseous density at the site of fracture healing (arrow).

signs of stress fracture, including radiolucent lines, sclerosis, or periosteal new bone formation, usually are not apparent until 2 to 4 weeks after the onset of symptoms. Bone scans, however, can detect stress fractures as soon as 24 to 48 hours after the injury (**Figure 1**). MRI is extremely sensitive for identifying stress fractures of the femoral neck (and useful for differentiating compression-side from tension-side involvement) and should be considered in all patients with clinical evidence of a stress fracture but negative radiographs (**Figure 2**).

Figure 2 Coronal T1-weighted MRI reveals a linear stress fracture along the medial left femoral neck (white arrow) surrounded by reactive edema (black arrows). (Reproduced from Johnson TR, Steinbach LS, eds: *Essentials of Musculoskeletal Imaging*. Rosemont, IL, American Academy of Orthopaedic Surgeons, 2003, p 451.)

Differential Diagnosis

- Acute fracture of the femoral neck (evident on radiographs and MRI, history of trauma)
- Muscle strain or groin pull (normal radiographs, intermittent limp)
- Osteoarthritis of the hip (no risk factors, absence of sclerosis within the femoral heads on radiographs)
- Osteonecrosis (dull ache in groin or buttock, evident on radiographs and/or MRI)
- Pathologic fracture (underlying or associated benign or malignant tumor; evident on bone scan, MRI, or radiographs)
- Pelvic fracture (normal hip joint motion, pain on external rotation)
- Tear of the acetabular labrum (pain or instability with hip motion)

SECTION 5 HIP

Adverse Outcomes of the Disease

Unlike patients with acute femoral neck fractures, patients with stress fractures are usually healthy and active. Adverse outcomes are associated with fracture displacement and include nonunion, osteonecrosis, and progressive varus deformity.

Treatment

The treatment of stress fractures is usually guided by the type and the presence of fracture displacement. Displaced fractures in the young patient are treated as a surgical emergency, and immediate anatomic reduction and internal fixation is mandatory.

Nondisplaced compression-side (medial-side) stress fractures are treated with cessation of activity and no weight bearing with crutches until the fracture is healed. Healing usually takes 6 to 8 weeks. During this time period, serial radiographs are essential to monitor for fracture displacement or widening. Internal fixation may be necessary if the fracture progresses or the symptoms persist despite appropriate nonsurgical treatment.

All tension-side stress fractures are treated surgically whether the fracture is displaced or nondisplaced. These injuries have a high tendency to displace, and an aggressive approach is necessary. Internal fixation is the treatment of choice in these patients.

Adverse Outcomes of Treatment

Osteonecrosis of the femoral head and fracture nonunion are potential complications of internal fixation of femoral neck stress fractures.

Referral Decisions/Red Flags

A displaced femoral neck fracture in a patient younger than 60 years constitutes a surgical emergency because the risks of osteonecrosis and fracture nonunion are significant, and prompt surgical fixation decreases the risk of these complications. All stress fractures require consideration for surgical treatment given the high risk of displacement of tension-side fractures.

Femoral stress fractures may be associated with osteopenia or osteoporosis. Consider evaluation for bone density deficits in these patients.

Transient Osteoporosis of the Hip

Synonym

Bone marrow edema syndrome

ICD-9 Code

733.09
Osteoporosis not elsewhere classified or drug-induced

Definition

Transient osteoporosis of the hip is an uncommon idiopathic condition characterized by spontaneous onset of hip pain associated with radiographic osteoporosis of the femoral head and neck. The condition is most common in middle-aged men and in women during the third trimester of pregnancy. Resolution is spontaneous, usually within 6 to 12 months.

Clinical Symptoms

Patients typically have spontaneous onset of pain in the anterior thigh (groin), the lateral hip, or the buttock. Pain is usually worse with weight bearing and better at rest. Symptoms typically worsen for the first several months and then gradually abate.

Tests

Physical Examination

Patients usually have an antalgic gait and pain at the limits of hip motion.

Diagnostic Tests

Plain radiographs of the hip typically demonstrate diffuse osteoporosis of the femoral head and neck, although signs may not be evident in the early phase of the disease. MRI is helpful to rule out other diagnoses and help confirm the diagnosis of transient osteoporosis. The typical MRI findings include bone marrow edema of the femoral neck with diffuse decreased signal intensity on T1-weighted images and diffuse increased signal intensity on T2-weighted images. The signal change usually extends into the intertrochanteric region (**Figure 1**).

Figure 1 Coronal T1-weighted MRI of the pelvis shows diffuse decreased signal intensity (arrow) indicating transient osteoporosis of the hip.

SECTION 5 HIP

Differential Diagnosis

- Infections involving the proximal femur or hip joint (pain, constitutional symptoms)
- Osteonecrosis of the femoral head (pain in the groin or buttock, sclerosis on radiographs)
- Pigmented villonodular synovitis of the hip (pain in the groin or buttock, evident on MRI and biopsy)
- Stress fracture of the femoral neck (pain in the groin or buttock, evident on radiographs or MRI)
- Tumors involving the proximal femur (pain in the groin, buttock, or thigh; evident on radiographs or MRI)

Adverse Outcomes of the Disease

Fracture of the femoral neck can occur during the time the bone is weakened by osteoporosis. Pregnant women with the disease appear to be at higher risk for femoral neck fracture.

Treatment

The disease is a self-limited process that typically resolves spontaneously within 6 to 12 months after the onset of symptoms. After other diseases have been excluded and a firm diagnosis is established (usually by the characteristic MRI appearance), supportive treatment is begun. Patients are provided with mild analgesics and placed on crutches to limit weight bearing until symptoms resolve and radiographs demonstrate reconstitution of normal bone density.

Referral Decisions/Red Flags

The diagnosis may be difficult to make with certainty. In pregnant women, decisions regarding imaging studies and the choice of analgesics should be made in consultation with the patient's obstetrician. Pregnant women with the disease appear to be at greater risk for femoral neck fracture.

Trochanteric Bursitis

Synonym

Greater trochanteric bursitis

ICD-9 Code

726.5
Enthesopathy of hip region

Definition

Inflammation and hypertrophy of the greater trochanteric bursa may develop without apparent cause or in association with lumbar spine disease, intra-articular hip pathology, significant limb-length inequalities, inflammatory arthritis, or previous surgery around the hip (particularly when internal fixation devices are placed in or near the greater trochanter) (**Figure 1**).

Clinical Symptoms

Patients usually have pain and tenderness over the greater trochanter. The pain may radiate distally to the knee or ankle (but not to the foot) or proximally into the buttock. The pain is worse when the patient first rises from a seated or recumbent position, lessens somewhat after a few steps, and recurs after walking for half an hour or more. Patients report night pain and are unable to lie on the affected side. Inflammation (tendinitis) of the gluteal tendons may cause a similar pain pattern.

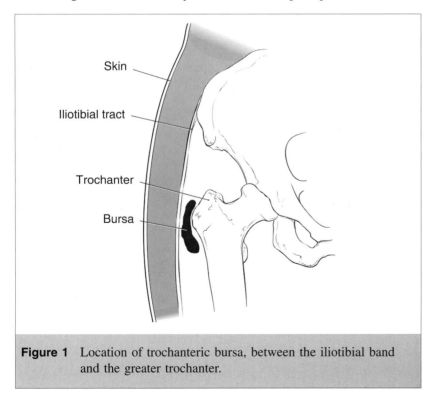

Skin

Iliotibial tract

Trochanter

Bursa

Figure 1 Location of trochanteric bursa, between the iliotibial band and the greater trochanter.

SECTION 5 HIP

Tests

Physical Examination

With the patient in the lateral decubitus position, palpate the greater trochanter (**Figure 2**). Point tenderness over the lateral greater trochanter is the essential finding. Pain is often exacerbated with active hip abduction. Tenderness above the trochanter suggests tendinitis of the gluteus medius tendon. Patients report increased discomfort with adduction of the hip or adduction combined with internal rotation.

Diagnostic Tests

AP radiographs of the pelvis and lateral radiographs of the hip are necessary to rule out bony abnormalities and intra-articular hip pathology. Occasionally, rounded or irregular calcific deposits may be seen above the trochanter at the attachment of the gluteus medius. Bone scans and MRI rarely are needed to make the diagnosis but occasionally may be helpful to rule out uncommon conditions such as occult fractures, tumors, or osteonecrosis of the femoral head.

Differential Diagnosis

- Metastatic tumor (evident on radiographs, weight loss, constitutional symptoms)
- Osteoarthritis of the hip (painful internal rotation, evident on radiographs)
- Sciatica (pain posteriorly, pain radiating to the foot, motor and sensory changes, reflex changes)

Figure 2 Palpation with the patient in the lateral decubitus position. With trochanteric bursitis, there is point tenderness over the lateral greater trochanter.

- Septic arthritis of the hip (fever, severe pain with motion)
- Snapping hip (obvious snap of the iliotibial band)
- Trochanteric fracture (evident on radiographs, persistent limp when walking, positive Trendelenburg sign)

Adverse Outcomes of the Disease

Chronic pain, a limp, or sleep disturbances are possible.

Treatment

NSAIDs, activity modifications, iliotibial band stretching, ice, and short-term use of a cane are sufficient for most patients. It is important to incorporate hip abduction strengthening as part of a comprehensive program. Injection of a local anesthetic and corticosteroid preparation into the greater trochanteric bursa (see page 614) can be helpful in relieving symptoms. Occasionally, repeat injections are required for symptomatic relief. Surgery is indicated only rarely, for refractory cases.

Rehabilitation Prescription

The pathology underlying trochanteric bursitis can be difficult to identify. Regardless, the muscles surrounding the hip joint can play an important role in the management of pain and flexibility with this condition. Regular stretching of the piriformis and tensor fascia latae may reduce pain over the greater trochanter. A home exercise program that attempts to stretch these muscles is appropriate provided the physician has identified no contraindications (see page 612).

Adverse Outcomes of Treatment

NSAIDs can cause gastric, renal, or hepatic complications. In some patients, pain may persist. Rarely, infection from the injection can develop, but this can be largely avoided by the careful use of sterile technique.

Referral Decisions/Red Flags

Failure of treatment, diagnostic uncertainty, and/or suspected fracture are indications for further evaluation.

SECTION 5 HIP

Home Exercise Program for Trochanteric Bursitis

- Perform the exercises in the order listed.
- Apply dry or moist heat to the hip for 5 to 10 minutes before exercising to prepare the tissues.
- Alternatively, riding a stationary bicycle for 10 minutes will also prepare the tissues for stretching.
- Apply a bag of crushed ice or frozen peas to the hip for 20 minutes after exercising to help reduce inflammation.
- If you experience pain in the hip during or after exercising, discontinue the exercises and call your doctor.

Exercise Type	Muscle Group	Number of Repetitions/Sets	Number of Days per Week	Number of Weeks
Piriformis stretch	Piriformis	4 repetitions/2 to 3 sets	5 to 7	2 to 3
Iliotibial band stretch	Tensor fascia latae	4 repetitions/2 to 3 sets	5 to 7	2 to 3
Hip abduction	Gluteus medius	8 repetitions/2 sets, progressing to 15 repetitions/3 sets	3	2 to 3

Piriformis Stretch

- Lie on your back and bend both knees so that your feet are flat on the floor.
- Place the ankle of the affected leg on the opposite knee and clasp your hands behind the thigh as shown.
- Pull the thigh toward you until you feel a stretch in the hip.
- Hold the stretch for 30 seconds and then relax for 30 seconds.
- Perform 2 to 3 sets of 4 repetitions 5 to 7 days per week, continuing for 2 to 3 weeks.
- Perform the stretch on both sides.

Iliotibial Band Stretch

- Stand approximately 2 feet away from a wall with the affected side to the wall.
- Fully extend your arm and place your hand on the wall for support.
- Cross the injured leg (the leg farther from the wall) over the opposite leg.
- Lean your hips toward the wall until you feel a stretch on the outside of the injured leg.
- Hold the maximum stretch for 30 seconds and then relax for 10 seconds.
- Repeat the sequence 4 times on each side.
- Perform 2 to 3 sets of 4 repetitions 5 to 7 days per week, continuing for 2 to 3 weeks.
- Perform the stretch on both sides.

Hip Abduction

- Lie on your side with the affected hip on top. Cradle your head in your arm and bend your bottom leg to provide support.
- Slowly move the top leg up and back to 45°, keeping the knee straight. Hold this position for 5 seconds.
- Slowly lower the leg to a count of 5 and relax it for 2 seconds.
- Ankle weights should be used, starting with light enough weights to allow 2 sets of 8 repetitions and progressing to 3 sets of 15 repetitions.
- Then return to 2 sets of 8 repetitions and add weight in 2- to 3-pound increments, progressing each time to 3 sets of 15 repetitions.
- Perform the exercise 3 times per week, continuing for 2 to 3 weeks.

Procedure: Trochanteric Bursitis Injection

CPT Code

20610
Arthrocentesis, aspiration and/or injection; major joint or bursa (eg, shoulder, hip, knee joint, subacromial bursa)

Current Procedural Terminology © 2010 American Medical Association. All rights reserved.

MATERIALS

- Sterile gloves
- Bactericidal skin preparation solution
- 10-mL syringe
- 20-gauge or 22-gauge 1½″ needle (use a spinal needle in larger patients)
- 3 to 5 mL of 1% lidocaine
- 40 to 80 mg of a corticosteroid preparation
- Sterile adhesive sponge
- Adhesive dressing

Note: Opinions differ regarding single- versus two-needle injection techniques. Proponents of the single-needle technique believe that one needle is less painful for the patient than two. Because the corticosteroid preparation is thicker than the local anesthetic, however, a slightly larger gauge needle is required at the outset. Physicians who prefer the two-needle technique point out that the smaller gauge needle is easier for patients to tolerate and that the pain of the second injection is dulled by the anesthetic. A two-syringe, two-needle technique is described on the DVD.

Step 1
Wear protective gloves at all times during the procedure and use sterile technique.

Step 2
Ask the patient to lie in the lateral decubitus position with the affected hip upward. Place a pillow between the patient's knees to relax the iliotibial band and reduce the pressure required to inject the solution.

Step 3
Cleanse the skin with a bactericidal skin preparation.

Step 4
Draw lidocaine into a 10-mL syringe.

Step 5
Draw the chosen dose of corticosteroid preparation into the same syringe and mix the two solutions.

Step 6
Palpate the greater trochanter and identify the point of maximum tenderness.

Step 7

Insert the needle until it contacts bone, then withdraw it 1 or 2 mm so that the tip is in the bursa and not in the bone (**Figure 1**). Usually, a 1½″ needle is sufficient, but for larger patients a spinal needle might be needed to reach the trochanteric bursa. Do not withdraw the needle too far or it will be outside the trochanteric bursa.

Step 8

Aspirate to ensure that the needle is not in an intravascular position; then inject one 1- to 2-mL aliquot of the corticosteroid preparation/local anesthetic mixture.

Step 9

Partially withdraw the needle; then reinsert it and inject another 1- to 2-mL aliquot. Continue this to infiltrate the entire bursa, an area of several square centimeters around the point of maximum tenderness.

Step 10

Withdraw the needle completely and apply gentle pressure over the injection site with a sterile dressing sponge.

Step 11

Dress the puncture wound with a sterile adhesive bandage.

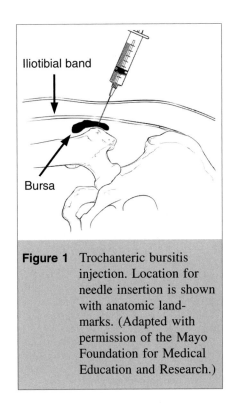

Figure 1 Trochanteric bursitis injection. Location for needle insertion is shown with anatomic landmarks. (Adapted with permission of the Mayo Foundation for Medical Education and Research.)

Adverse Outcomes

Although rare, infection or allergic reactions to the local anesthetic or corticosteroid preparation are possible. Always query the patient about medication allergies before the procedure. In some patients with diabetes mellitus, poor control of blood glucose levels may occur, but this is usually temporary. Deposition of the corticosteroid subcutaneously may cause fat atrophy or depigmentation at the injection site. A minority of patients will require a series of injections to achieve lasting pain relief; however, repeated injections with corticosteroids should be avoided.

Aftercare/Patient Instructions

Advise the patient that as the local anesthetic wears off, pain often persists or becomes worse for a few days until the corticosteroid takes effect. Instruct the patient to attempt weight bearing as tolerated and contact you if symptoms recur or if redness, fever, immobilizing pain, or any other evidence of a local problem related to the injection occurs.

SECTION 5 HIP

PAIN DIAGRAM
Knee and Lower Leg

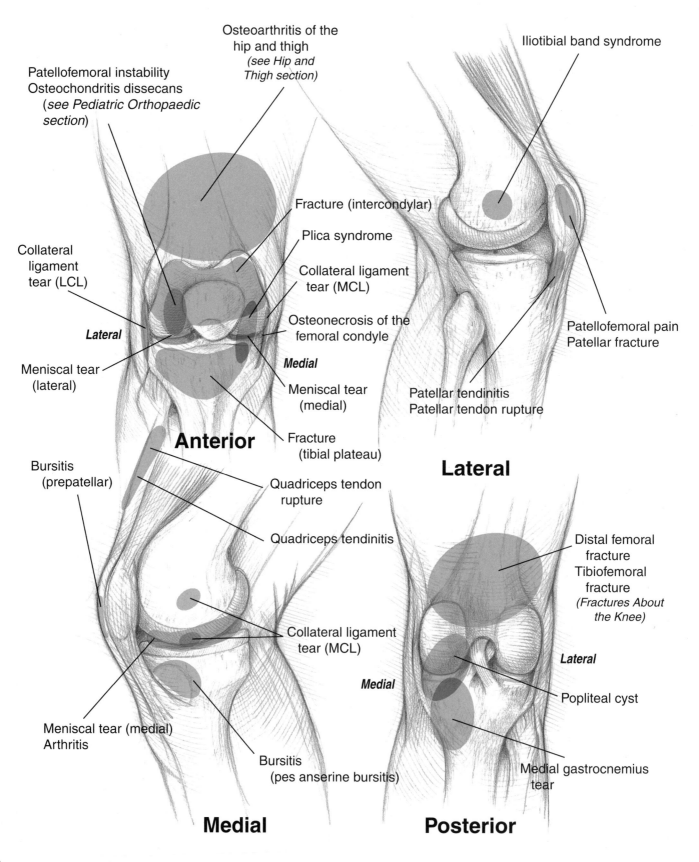

Osteoarthritis of the
hip and thigh
*(see Hip and
Thigh section)*

Patellofemoral instability
Osteochondritis dissecans
*(see Pediatric Orthopaedic
section)*

Iliotibial band syndrome

Collateral
ligament
tear (LCL)

Fracture (intercondylar)

Plica syndrome

Collateral ligament
tear (MCL)

Osteonecrosis of the
femoral condyle

Lateral

Medial

Meniscal tear
(lateral)

Meniscal tear
(medial)

Patellofemoral pain
Patellar fracture

Patellar tendinitis
Patellar tendon rupture

Anterior

Fracture
(tibial plateau)

Lateral

Bursitis
(prepatellar)

Quadriceps tendon
rupture

Quadriceps tendinitis

Distal femoral
fracture
Tibiofemoral
fracture
*(Fractures About
the Knee)*

Collateral ligament
tear (MCL)

Medial

Lateral

Popliteal cyst

Meniscal tear (medial)
Arthritis

Bursitis
(pes anserine bursitis)

Medial gastrocnemius
tear

Medial

Posterior

Knee and Lower Leg

Section Editor

Jason L. Koh, MD

Vice-Chairman
Department of Orthopaedic Surgery
NorthShore University Health System
University of Chicago
Evanston, IL

Contributor

Michael Huxford, MEd, ATC, CSCS

Sports Medicine Coordinator
Rehabilitative Services
Institute for Sports Medicine
Children's Memorial Hospital
Chicago, IL

ANATOMY OF THE KNEE AND LOWER LEG

**Knee: Cruciate and Collateral Ligaments
(Anterior View, Right Knee in Flexion)**

Anterior cruciate ligament
Lateral condyle of femur (articular surface)
Popliteus tendon
Fibular collateral ligament
Lateral meniscus
Transverse ligament of knee
Head of fibula
Gerdy tubercle

Posterior cruciate ligament
Medial condyle of femur (articular surface)
Medial meniscus
Tibial collateral ligament
Medial condyle of tibia
Tibial tuberosity

**Muscles of Leg
(Superficial Dissection)
Anterior View**

Vastus lateralis muscle
Rectus femoris tendon (becoming quadriceps femoris tendon)
Iliotibial tract
Superior lateral genicular artery
Lateral patellar retinaculum
Biceps femoris tendon
Inferior lateral genicular artery
Common fibular (peroneal) nerve
Head of fibula
Fibularis (peroneus) longus muscle
Tibialis anterior muscle
Extensor digitorum longus muscle
Fibularis (peroneus) brevis muscle
Fibula
Superior extensor retinaculum
Lateral malleolus
Inferior extensor retinaculum
Extensor digitorum longus tendons
Fibularis (peroneus) tertius tendon
Extensor digitorum brevis tendons
Dorsal digital nerves

Vastus medialis muscle
Patella
Superior medial genicular artery
Tibial collateral ligament
Medial patellar retinaculum
Inferior medial genicular artery
Infrapatellar branch (cut) of Saphenous nerve (cut)
Joint capsule
Patellar ligament
Insertion of sartorius muscle
Tibial tuberosity
Tibia
Gastrocnemius muscle
Soleus muscle
Extensor hallucis longus muscle
Medial malleolus
Tibialis anterior tendon
Medial branch of deep fibular (peroneal) nerve
Extensor hallucis longus tendon
Extensor hallucis brevis tendon
Dorsal digital branches of deep fibular (peroneal) nerve

Muscles of Leg (Superficial Dissection): Posterior View

Semitendinosus muscle
Semimembranosus muscle
Gracilis muscle
Popliteal artery and vein
Sartorius muscle
Superior medial genicular artery
Gastrocnemius muscle (medial head)
Nerve to soleus muscle
Small saphenous vein
Gastrocnemius muscle
Soleus muscle
Plantaris tendon
Flexor digitorum longus tendon
Tibialis posterior tendon
Posterior tibial artery and vein
Tibial nerve
Medial malleolus
Flexor hallucis longus tendon
Flexor retinaculum
Calcaneal branch of posterior tibial artery

Iliotibial tract
Biceps femoris muscle
Tibial nerve
Common fibular (peroneal) nerve
Plantaris muscle
Superior lateral genicular artery
Gastrocnemius muscle (lateral head)
Lateral sural cutaneous nerve (cut)
Medial sural cutaneous nerve (cut)
Soleus muscle
Fibularis (peroneus) longus tendon
Fibularis (peroneus) brevis tendon
Calcaneal (Achilles) tendon
Lateral malleolus
Superior fibular (peroneal) retinaculum
Fibular (peroneal) artery
Calcaneal branches of fibular (peroneal) artery
Calcaneal tuberosity

Overview of the Knee and Lower Leg

Knee and lower leg problems are diagnosed by obtaining an appropriate medical history, performing a physical examination, and obtaining appropriate imaging studies. Radiographs are the initial imaging study of choice. Patients with knee problems report pain, instability, stiffness, swelling, locking, or weakness. These findings may occur in or around any aspect of the knee. Careful localization of the pain and tenderness will significantly narrow the differential diagnosis. Examination of patients with knee problems also includes a screening evaluation of the hip, spine, and back because some patients with problems intrinsic to the hip present with distal thigh pain and other symptoms that mimic knee disorders, and lumbar radiculopathy may result in thigh, knee, or leg pain.

Radiographic examination of the knee includes AP, 30° weight-bearing, lateral, and axial patellofemoral (eg, Merchant or sunrise) views (**Figure 1**). If the patient is able to stand, obtain weight-bearing AP radiographs of both knees to allow comparison of the injured knee with the opposite, uninjured knee. A 30° weight-bearing view will often demonstrate arthritis or joint space loss more readily than the AP view. An axial patellofemoral view is helpful to assess the patellofemoral joint.

Figure 1 A 30° weight-bearing view shows joint space narrowing in the medial compartment of the left knee (black arrows). Note the more subtle joint space narrowing in the medial compartment of the right knee (white arrows) with less obvious degenerative change. (Reproduced from Johnson TR, Steinbach LS, eds: *Essentials of Musculoskeletal Imaging*, Rosemont, IL, American Academy of Orthopaedic Surgeons, 2004, p 532.)

Radiographs should be evaluated for changes in bony architecture, including lytic and blastic lesions, radiolucencies, and increased density.

AP radiographs are best used to evaluate medial and lateral compartment arthritis, fractures of the distal femur and proximal tibia, and alignment of the femur with the tibia. Lateral radiographs are helpful in assessing the patella for fractures and malposition (patella alta and patella baja) and in analyzing the bony architecture of the distal femur and proximal tibia. Axial patellofemoral views are best used to assess subluxation of the patella and arthritis of the patellofemoral joint.

MRI is rarely needed in the initial diagnostic workup, but it sometimes plays an important role as an advanced diagnostic tool or in surgical planning.

Acute Pain

Acute leg and knee pain usually occurs secondary to an injury. Possible diagnoses fall into several categories, any of which can be associated with acute pain (**Table 1**).

Prompt diagnosis is critical. Unreduced fractures, unreduced dislocations, or acute compartment syndrome may rapidly result in permanent residual sequelae, including significant loss of limb function.

Fractures may involve the distal femur, the patella, the proximal tibia, or the fibula. Inspect for swelling and deformity, palpate for tenderness on the bone itself, and obtain appropriate radiographs. Patellar fractures may result from direct or indirect forces, such as falls, but fractures of the tibia and femur at the knee typically result from major trauma. Knee dislocations are rare. They may occur as a result of low- or high-energy trauma and may reduce spontaneously. They may be associated with vascular injury. Patellar dislocations are often reduced at the scene when a patient or helper extends the knee. Compartment syndromes result from fractures or crush injuries and are surgical emergencies. Clinically, the predominant finding is excessive pain as the pressure increases in the tight fascial

Table 1 Possible Causes of Acute Leg and Knee Pain

Musculotendinous sprains/strains or contusions

Fractures

Dislocations

Compartment syndrome

Ligamentous injuries

Extensor mechanism injuries (quadriceps or patellar tendon rupture)

Meniscal injuries

compartment. Palpation often will not demonstrate any abnormal firmness because the subcutaneous tissue is not affected. Compartment and pressure measurements are the definitive method to establish a diagnosis. Fasciotomies should not be delayed.

Patients with ligamentous injuries often report that a "pop" occurred at the time of injury, and they present with acute pain, significant swelling, and instability. Patients with injuries to the extensor mechanism (such as quadriceps or patellar tendon rupture) report sudden weakness or collapse of the knee. A history of the mechanism of injury is crucial in diagnosing meniscal tears. A history of a twisting injury sustained with the foot planted on the ground and locking (inability to extend the knee completely) with localized pain and tenderness along the joint line are indicative of meniscal pathology. Some patients report that manipulating or pushing on the knee enabled them to "unlock" it. Contusions result from direct blows and cause localized pain and tenderness. Musculotendinous strains also can cause pain and swelling, but most do not result in instability, although there may be weakness.

Acute pain without obvious injury may be the result of infection or crystal arthropathy. Septic arthritis in the knee joint is rare in adults; when present, it is more commonly located in the prepatellar bursa. Inspection and palpation of the involved area easily determine the location of the infection. Infection in the prepatellar bursa causes swelling over the patella. With sepsis in the knee joint, a significant effusion of the knee joint occurs but not directly over the patella. Infection must be distinguished from an acute crystal arthropathy such as gout. Diagnosis is made by knee aspiration for cell count, crystal, Gram stain, and culture.

Chronic Pain

Conditions that cause chronic knee pain include osteoarthritis, overuse syndromes, tumors (including bursitis/tendinitis and anterior knee pain), and meniscal tears. Inflammatory or crystal arthropathy (such as gout) can sometimes present with an acute flare, effusions, and minimal radiographic changes. Chronic leg pain is defined as pain that has been present for more than 2 or 3 weeks. The etiology includes a spectrum of disorders. In addition to the unique conditions discussed in this chapter, chronic pain in the calf region also can be secondary to infection (osteomyelitis or pyomyositis), tumors (soft-tissue or bone), and other general disorders.

Osteoarthritis is characterized by symptoms localized to the joint line and is associated with loss of motion and radiographic changes. Degenerative meniscal tears may cause chronic pain and swelling without changes on radiographs.

Bursitis/tendinitis, anterior knee pain, and chondral injuries have similar characteristics: they are chronic, secondary to overuse, and often bilateral. The pain typically is worse with rising or walking after sitting, at night, and with prolonged exercise or use.

Primary bone or joint tumors are uncommon. Tumors are characterized by night pain (relentless pain in which the patient is unable to sleep) and often can be identified on radiographs. The most common malignant tumors are osteosarcoma (in adolescents) and chondrosarcoma (in adults). The most common benign tumor is giant cell tumor, which typically occurs in individuals aged 20 to 30 years. Metastatic disease in the knee region is uncommon.

Location of Pain

Anterior Knee Pain

Anterior knee pain is common. It often indicates chondromalacia patella. Specific tenderness at the upper pole of the patella indicates tendinitis or a partial tear of the quadriceps insertion on the patella. Tendinitis or overuse injury of the patellar tendon (also called the patellar ligament) produces pain at the inferior pole of the patella or at the tibial tubercle.

Medial Knee Pain

Pain at the medial joint line, midway between the front and back of the knee, is common with a torn meniscus, especially with degenerative tears that occur as the result of minor trauma such as twisting or rising from a squat. When the meniscal tear is sufficiently large or loose, patients also might report catching or locking. Tenderness in this area also is common with arthritis that affects the medial compartment of the knee. Pain proximal to and/or at the medial joint line, with localized swelling and a history of recent injury, usually indicates a sprain or tear of the medial collateral ligament either at its origin on the medial femoral epicondyle or in the midsubstance of the ligament.

Distal to the medial joint line lie the superficial portion of the medial collateral ligament and the pes anserinus. The latter is composed of the insertion of the sartorius, gracilis, and semitendinosus tendons and is so named because it resembles the foot of a goose. Pain in this area in the absence of trauma suggests a bursitis under the pes anserine tendons. This condition often is associated with osteoarthritis of the medial knee joint.

Lateral Knee Pain

Pain over the lateral femoral epicondyle suggests iliotibial band syndrome, usually associated with overuse. Pain over the lateral joint line usually indicates a disorder of the lateral meniscus or osteoarthritis of the lateral joint, which is more common in women.

Posterior Knee Pain

Pain at the posteromedial corner of the knee may indicate a tear of the medial meniscus (at the joint line), a popliteal (Baker) cyst, or both. Popliteal aneurysms also may be painful in the popliteal area. Patients with knee effusions may perceive popliteal pain from the distention of the joint capsule.

Instability

The knee joint is described by orthopaedic surgeons as having three compartments: two between the tibia and the femur (medial and lateral; tibiofemoral joint) and one between the patella and the femur (patellofemoral joint). The articulation between the tibia and fibula (tibiofibular joint) is rarely the source of knee symptoms. True instability means that one bony component moves on another in an abnormal fashion, such as the patella sliding laterally on the femur in recurrent subluxation of the patella, or the tibia moving anteriorly on the femur in the anterior cruciate ligament–deficient knee. Patients often use the terms "giving way," "slippage," or "buckling," which can refer to true instability or to collapse of the knee (often secondary to pain causing reflex inhibition of the quadriceps mechanism). It is important to differentiate between the two by careful history and physical examination.

Tibiofemoral Instability

Identifying the specific ligament injury that is responsible for instability can be difficult in a painful, traumatized knee because of muscle guarding. During examination, four ligament complexes should be gently assessed with the patient as relaxed as possible: the anterior cruciate ligament, the posterior cruciate ligament, the medial collateral ligament, and the lateral collateral ligament.

Chronic instability of the knee also occurs with severe arthritis because, with the loss of articular cartilage and bone height from the arthritis, the ligaments are not at full tension. In these instances, the knee may have "increased play" (greater-than-normal laxity) when the ligament is tested, but there will be a definite end point when the intact ligament finally tightens.

Patellofemoral Instability

Instability in the extensor mechanism is usually caused by a lateral dislocation or subluxation of the patella. The diagnosis is made by physical examination and radiographs. When the patella remains dislocated, the patient's knee often will be locked in approximately 45° of flexion with an obvious deformity present. Following an acute subluxation or dislocation that has reduced spontaneously, the patient usually exhibits dramatic apprehension when an attempt is made to displace the patella laterally.

SECTION 6   KNEE AND LOWER LEG

Stiffness

Stiffness of the knee is the most common symptom that accompanies an effusion. The distention of the knee joint capsule prevents full flexion, and the patient feels that the knee is "stiff" but might not notice that it is also swollen.

Arthritis is the other common cause of stiffness. Patients with arthritis often report that the knee sticks or locks momentarily as they walk. This occurs because the articular surfaces are rough and incongruous and act like two pieces of sandpaper rubbing together.

Stiffness also may result from any inflammatory condition at the knee, including arthritis, overuse syndromes, or traumatic effusion.

Swelling

With an intra-articular effusion, distention occurs around and above the patella in the suprapatellar pouch. Patients notice this as stiffness; they cannot fully flex the knee because the knee cavity is filled with synovial fluid or blood and therefore cannot be compressed.

Patients also may report knee swelling when they see soft-tissue puffiness in the infrapatellar bursa. This bursa is located behind and to either side of the patellar tendon (infrapatellar tendon).

Locking

Locking of the knee occurs when a fragment—whether torn meniscus or loose body— prevents the knee from extending fully. The knee usually can flex from the locked position, although the range of flexion also is typically limited. Often patients are able to "unlock" the knee by forcefully flexing, extending, or twisting, or making a "trick" movement.

Pseudolocking occurs with arthritis of the patellofemoral joint or between the femur and tibia, when the adjacent rough surfaces stick momentarily as they glide onto one another. This is common when the knee has been immobile, such as rising after prolonged sitting. It also can occur with minor knee conditions such as a medial synovial plica, when the synovial tissue becomes momentarily stuck under the patella as the knee extends.

Weakness

Weakness of the muscles around the knee may occur acutely or gradually. Acute catastrophic weakness usually occurs as a result of one of three types of disruption of the extensor mechanism: (1) a tear of the patellar tendon below the patella, (2) a tear of the quadriceps tendon above the patella, or (3) a fracture through the patella. With partial ruptures, the extensor mechanism might continue to function, but without proper protection, the tear may become complete. Weakness of knee flexion may be related to a hamstring strain. Weakness also can be due to reflex inhibition from knee pain or the presence of as little as 30 mL of effusion.

Musculoskeletal Conditioning of the Knee

A conditioning program consists of three basic phases: stretching exercises, to improve range of motion; strengthening, to improve muscle power; and proprioception (joint position sense) exercises, to enhance balance and agility. In addition, the exercise session should begin with an active warm-up. Plyometric exercises (high-intensity explosive exercises) may be added for power only after basic strength and flexibility have been achieved. Patient handouts are provided here for the stretching and strengthening exercises. Advanced proprioceptive exercises and plyometric exercises should be done under the supervision of a rehabilitation specialist or other exercise professional.

The goal of a conditioning program is to enable people to live a more fit and healthy lifestyle by being more active. A well-structured conditioning program also will prepare the individual for participation in sports and recreational activities. The greater the intensity of the activity that the individual wishes to engage in, the greater the intensity of the conditioning that will be required. If the individual participates in a supervised rehabilitation program that provides instruction in a conditioning routine—instead of using only an exercise handout such as provided here—the focus should be on developing and committing to a home exercise fitness program. A conditioning program for the body as a whole that includes exercises for the shoulder, hip, foot, and spine as well as the knee is described in the chapter Musculoskeletal Conditioning: Helping Patients Prevent Injury and Stay Fit, page 183.

The knee has both dynamic and static stabilizers. Muscles provide dynamic stability to the knee joint and the patellofemoral articulation. Strengthening the quadriceps and hamstrings muscle groups provides dynamic stability to the knee. In addition, the hip muscles, such as the gluteus maximus, the gluteus medius, and the internal and external rotators, help to control the movements of the femur and the position of the patellofemoral articulation. Conditioning of the knee should focus on three phases: strengthening, stretching, and neuromuscular (proprioceptive) training. Plyometrics (power training) would be added for the competitive athlete after basic

SECTION 6 KNEE AND LOWER LEG

strength and flexibility have been achieved. Advanced proprioceptive exercises and plyometric exercises should be done under the supervision of a rehabilitation specialist or other exercise professional.

Strengthening Exercises

Exercises to strengthen the quadriceps and hamstrings can be performed conveniently with progressively heavier ankle weights. The resistance training must be progressive so that the muscle is constantly stimulated to grow. Forward lunges (for the quadriceps), hamstring curls, side-lying hip abductions, and hip extensions are good strengthening exercises. The patient should begin with a weight that allows 6 to 8 repetitions and should work up to 12 repetitions. After reaching 12 repetitions with a given weight, the patient should add weight and drop back to 6 to 8 repetitions.

Stretching Exercises

The effectiveness of strengthening exercises for the quadriceps muscle group may be compromised if the range of motion of the knee is limited. Stretching the soft tissues to gain range of motion, especially after trauma or periods of immobilization, can be very effective in gaining range of motion. Hamstring stretching exercises such as leg crossovers and crossover standing increase the range of motion at the knee and hip during functional activities such as walking and running.

Once the patient has achieved normal range of motion and strength, sport-specific or work-specific training should begin. The knee musculature needs to be strong and powerful, and protective reflexes need to be optimized to reduce the risk of injury during sporting maneuvers such as sudden changes in direction while running.

Proprioceptive Training

Proprioceptive training is important for balance. Balance, or postural control, is the result of the integration of visual, vestibular, and proprioceptive afferent inputs. The goal of proprioceptive training is to enhance the activity of the proprioceptors, thereby improving their ability to protect ligaments of the knee. Several commercial devices, such as tiltboards and proprioceptive disks, are available for proprioceptive training. Advanced balance training should be performed under the supervision of a physical therapist, athletic trainer, or other exercise specialist.

Plyometric Exercises

Explosive power of the lower leg is necessary for a high level of athletic performance. Plyometrics and explosive weight training facilitate the development of power in the quadriceps, hamstrings, and gluteal muscles. Examples of plyometric exercises are jumping rope and jumping from side to side over a 6-inch-high barrier. More advanced exercises should be performed under the supervision of a physical therapist, athletic trainer, or other trained professional.

SECTION 6 | KNEE AND LOWER LEG

Home Exercise Program for Knee Conditioning

- Before beginning the conditioning program, warm up the muscles by riding a stationary bicycle or jogging for 10 minutes.
- After the active warm-up and the strengthening exercises, stretching exercises should be performed to maintaining or increase flexibility. When performing the stretching exercises, you should stretch slowly to the limit of motion, taking care to avoid pain.
- If you experience pain with exercising, call your doctor.

Strengthening and Stretching Exercises for the Knee

Exercise	Muscle Group	Number of Repetitions/Sets	Number of Days per Week
Strengthening			
Forward lunge	Quadriceps	Work up to 3 sets of 10 repetitions	3
Hamstring curl	Hamstrings	10 repetitions/5 sets/3 times per day	3
Side-lying hip abduction	Gluteus medius	6 to 8 repetitions, progressing to 12 repetitions	3
Hip extension (prone)	Gluteus maximus	6 to 8 repetitions, progressing to 12 repetitions	3
Stretching			
Leg stretch	Hamstrings	3 to 6 repetitions/3 sets	Daily
Leg crossover	Hamstrings	3 to 6 repetitions/3 sets	Daily
Crossover stand	Hamstrings	3 to 6 repetitions/3 sets	Daily
Straight-leg raise	Quadriceps	Work up to 3 sets of 10 repetitions	Daily
Straight-leg raise (prone)	Gluteus maximus	Work up to 3 sets of 10 repetitions	Daily
Wall slide	Quadriceps, hamstrings	Work up to 3 sets of 10 repetitions	Daily

Strengthening Exercises

Forward Lunges

- Stand up with the feet about 3 to 4 feet apart and with the forward foot pointing forward and the back foot angled to provide support.
- Lunge forward, bending the forward knee and keeping the back and the back leg straight. You should feel a slight stretch in the left groin area. Do not let the forward lunging knee pass beyond the toes.
- Hold the stretch for 5 seconds.
- Repeat with the opposite leg.
- Work up to 3 sets of 10 repetitions, 3 days per week.

Hamstring Curls

- Stand on a flat surface with your weight evenly distributed over both feet. Hold onto the back of a chair or the wall for balance.
- Raise the heel of one leg toward the ceiling. Hold this position for 5 seconds and then relax.
- Perform 5 sets of 10 repetitions, 3 times per day.

Side-Lying Hip Abduction

- Lie on your side, cradling your head in your arm. Bend the bottom leg for support.
- Slowly move the top leg up and back to 45°, keeping the knee straight. Hold this position for 5 seconds.
- Slowly lower the leg and relax it for 2 seconds.
- Ankle weights should be used, starting with light enough weight to allow 6 to 8 repetitions, progressing to 12 repetitions. Then return to 6 to 8 repetitions and add weight.
- Repeat on the opposite leg.
- Perform the exercise 3 times per week.

SECTION 6 KNEE AND LOWER LEG

Hip Extension (Prone)

- Lie face down with a pillow under your hips and one knee bent 90°.
- Elevate the leg off the floor to a count of 5, lifting the leg straight up with the knee bent.
- Ankle weights should be used, starting with light enough weight to allow 6 to 8 repetitions, working up to 12 repetitions. Then return to 6 to 8 repetitions and add weight.
- Repeat on the opposite leg.
- Perform the exercise 3 times per week.

Stretching Exercises

Leg Stretch

- Sit on the floor with your legs straight in front of you and place your hands on the backs of your calves. For comfort, you may slightly bend the leg not being stretched.
- Slowly lift and pull one leg toward your ear, keeping your back straight. Hold the stretch for 5 seconds.
- Alternate from side to side.
- Repeat the exercise with each leg 3 to 6 times.
- Perform the exercise daily.

Leg Crossover

- Lie on the floor with your legs spread and your arms out to the sides.
- Bring your right toe to your left hand, keeping the leg straight.
- Hold the stretch for 5 seconds.
- Alternate from side to side.
- Repeat the exercise with each leg 3 to 6 times. For comfort, you may slightly bend the leg not being stretched.
- Perform the exercise daily.

Crossover Stand

- Stand with your legs crossed.
- Keeping your feet close together and your legs straight, slowly bend forward toward your toes. Hold the stretch for 5 seconds.
- Repeat with the opposite leg crossed in front.
- Perform 3 sets of 3 to 6 repetitions daily

Straight-Leg Raise

- Lie on the floor with one leg straight and the other leg bent.
- Tighten the thigh muscle of the straight leg and slowly raise it 6 to 10 inches off the floor. Hold this position for 5 seconds. Repeat with the opposite leg.
- Work up to 3 sets of 10 repetitions.
- Perform the exercise daily.

Straight-Leg Raise (Prone)

- Lie on the floor on your stomach with your legs straight.
- Keeping the leg straight, tighten the hamstrings of one leg and raise the leg as high as you can. Hold this position for 5 seconds.
- Repeat with the opposite leg.
- Work up to 3 sets of 10 repetitions.
- Perform the exercise daily.

Wall Slides

- Stand with your back against a wall and your feet about 1 foot from the wall.
- Tuck your pelvis under so that your lower back is flat against the wall.
- Stop when your knees are bent 90°. The knees should not pass beyond the toes.
- Hold for 5 seconds and then relax. Work up to 3 sets of 10 repetitions.
- Perform the exercise daily.

SECTION 6 KNEE AND LOWER LEG

Anterior Cruciate Ligament Tear

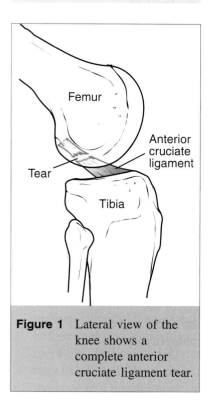

Figure 1 Lateral view of the knee shows a complete anterior cruciate ligament tear.

Synonyms

ACL tear

Anterior cruciate insufficiency

Cruciate ligament tear

Internal derangement of knee

Torn cruciate

Definition

The anterior cruciate ligament (ACL) is a primary stabilizer of the knee against anterior translation (**Figure 1**). A tear of the ACL results from a rotational (twisting) or hyperextension force applied to the knee joint that overcomes the strength of the ligament. Although partial tears can occur, injuries involving the ACL more often result in complete tears. Most ACL tears are noncontact injuries. An ACL tear is often accompanied by a significant meniscal tear. An ACL tear also can occur in association with a tear of the medial collateral ligament or, more rarely, with tears of the lateral ligaments or the posterior cruciate ligament. Uncommonly, knee injuries that disrupt multiple ligaments and result in knee instability also injure the popliteal artery; this is a limb-threatening emergency.

Clinical Symptoms

Patients with ACL tears usually report sudden pain and giving way of the knee from a twisting or hyperextension-type injury. One third of patients report an audible pop as the ligament tears. A patient who sustains an ACL tear during athletic activity usually is unable to continue participating because of pain and/or instability. The pain increases because an effusion caused by bleeding into the joint (hemarthrosis) develops rapidly.

As the swelling resolves, the patient temporarily may have no trouble moving the knee; however, if the tear is left untreated, recurrent instability develops, particularly with attempts to return to agility sports involving pivoting, running, or jumping. Chronic knee instability from an untreated ACL tear can lead to further meniscal and articular cartilage damage, with resulting degenerative arthritis.

Figure 2 Lachman test. **A,** The knee is flexed approximately 30°. The examiner gently pulls the tibia forward with the medial hand while stabilizing the distal femur with the lateral hand. In a relaxed patient, increased anterior translation of the tibia (in comparison to the uninjured knee) with a soft end point constitutes a positive test. **B,** Diagram showing movement of the tibia relative to the femur.

Tests

Physical Examination

The most sensitive test for ACL insufficiency is the Lachman test, in which the knee is flexed to 30° and the tibia is gently pulled forward while the femur is stabilized (**Figure 2**). It is critical that the patient's leg, especially the hamstrings, be relaxed. Otherwise, an accurate examination cannot be performed. Because of the subcutaneous location of the medial tibia, it is easier to grasp the tibia on the medial side (right hand for right knee, left hand for left knee) while stabilizing the femur from the lateral side with the opposite hand. If the thigh is large, the examiner may find it difficult to support the thigh in one hand. In this situation, the examiner may place his or her knee under the patient's thigh. The examiner uses one hand to stabilize the patient's thigh in this position. The examiner's other hand gently elevates the tibia from the supported femur. Increased motion of the tibia with no solid end point indicates a tear of the ACL. The anterior drawer test, performed with the knee flexed to 90°, is negative in 50% of acute ACL tears and thus is less helpful.

Diagnostic Tests

AP, lateral, and tunnel views of the knee should be ordered for every patient with a suspected ACL tear. Usually these radiographs are positive only for an effusion and possibly an avulsion fracture of the lateral capsular margin of the tibia (lateral capsular sign or Segond fracture); however, radiographs are helpful in ruling out other pathology.

MRI is sensitive for detecting ACL tears. It also is extremely useful for evaluating a knee with an acute effusion.

SECTION 6 KNEE AND LOWER LEG

Differential Diagnosis

- Fracture (tenderness over the bone, evident on radiographs)
- Meniscal tear (continued tenderness along the joint line, pain or trapping with circumduction) (may occur with ACL tear)
- Patellar dislocation/subluxation (positive apprehension sign when displacing the patella laterally)
- Patellar tendon or quadriceps rupture (inability to perform straight-leg raise)
- Posterior cruciate ligament tear (positive posterior drawer test, firm end point on Lachman test)

Adverse Outcomes of the Disease

If left untreated, the recurring instability resulting from an ACL tear may cause subsequent meniscal tears and degenerative disease. The instability also makes successful return to participation in agility sports such as soccer, football, or basketball unlikely.

Treatment

Initial treatment of an acute ACL injury includes rest, ice, and the use of crutches until the patient is able to ambulate without a limp. If the knee effusion (hemarthrosis) is tense, aspiration may be indicated to relieve symptoms (see page 647). A knee immobilizer or range-of-motion brace may be used for comfort when necessary until acute pain subsides.

Early range-of-motion exercises are important. With the patient sitting, the injured knee should be actively extended and flexed as comfort allows. Exercises should be performed repeatedly for several minutes four or five times daily. Full extension and flexion should be regained as soon as pain and swelling permit.

Definitive treatment of an ACL injury depends on the patient's age and desired activity level and any associated injuries. For young, active patients, ACL reconstruction offers the best chance for a successful return to agility sports. Older or less active individuals may be treated with physical therapy aimed at controlling the instability. ACL functional bracing also may be helpful with older or less active patients, but it usually does not provide sufficient stability for most younger patients to return to sports.

Rehabilitation Prescription

The goal of initial treatment of a torn ACL is to control the inflammation and pain with rest, ice, compression, and elevation (RICE) of the leg. In addition, maintaining the range of motion and regaining muscle strength are important to rehabilitation. Strengthening of the quadriceps and particularly the hamstring muscle group, as in balance training, is critical for knee stability following an ACL injury. Excessive anterior shearing forces during knee extension from 60° to 0°, especially from 30° to 10°, can cause damage, as can varus and valgus stress in full knee extension. Therefore, exercises that protect the ACL injury by avoiding these ranges of motion and positions, such as hamstring curls to strengthen the hamstring muscle group and isometric quadriceps contraction and straight-leg raises to strengthen the quadriceps, are used initially.

If instability, pain, and inflammation continue after 2 to 3 weeks, a formal rehabilitation program may be ordered. The prescription should include an assessment of the strength of the hip and trunk muscles, especially the hip external rotators and abductors, as well as the knee, hamstring, and quadriceps muscles. Outpatient rehabilitation for an ACL-deficient knee should emphasize strengthening of these muscle groups as well as neuromuscular training such as plyometrics and perturbation training. In addition, the rehabilitation specialist's evaluation might include structural deviations that sometimes contribute to ACL injury, such as a large Q angle, excessive foot pronation, hip anteversion, and genu recurvatum and valgum, to help determine the appropriate treatment.

Adverse Outcomes of Treatment

Nonsurgical treatment carries the risk of recurrent instability, meniscal tears, and degenerative joint disease. Scarring of the knee joint (arthrofibrosis) with loss of motion can occur after ACL injury or postoperatively after ACL reconstruction. Surgical reconstruction carries several risks: the usual risks of surgery (infection, phlebitis, pulmonary emboli, neurovascular insult, scarring, etc); the possibility that the ACL can tear again; or failure of the ACL graft to incorporate or successfully remodel, resulting in recurrence of laxity. Fracture of the tibial or patellar graft site also may occur after ACL reconstruction when a portion of the patellar tendon is used for the ACL graft.

Referral Decisions/Red Flags

Patients with suspected ACL tears and/or posttraumatic knee effusions require further evaluation and treatment. Even patients who are not candidates for ACL reconstruction can benefit from regular monitoring of the ACL tear.

SECTION 6 KNEE AND LOWER LEG

Home Exercise Program for ACL Tear

- Perform all five exercises in the order listed.

- After each exercise session, apply ice (eg, a bag of crushed ice or a bag of frozen peas) to the knee for 20 minutes or until numb, keep the leg elevated, and apply a compression bandage to the knee.

- If pain or swelling increases at any time or if it does not improve after you have adhered to the program for 3 to 4 weeks, call your doctor.

Exercise Type	Muscle Group	Number of Repetitions/Sets	Number of Days per Week	Number of Weeks
Hamstring curls (standing)	Hamstrings	20 repetitions/3 sets	4 to 5	3 to 4
Straight-leg raises	Quadriceps	20 repetitions/3 sets	4 to 5	3 to 4
Hip abduction	Gluteus medius	20 repetitions/3 sets	4 to 5	3 to 4
Hip adduction	Adductor group	20 repetitions/3 sets	4 to 5	3 to 4
Straight-leg raises (prone)	Gluteus maximus	20 repetitions/3 sets	4 to 5	3 to 4
Wall slides	Quadriceps, hamstrings	20 repetitions/3 sets	4 to 5	3 to 4

Hamstring Curls

- Stand on a flat surface with your weight evenly distributed on both feet.

- Hold onto the back of a chair or the wall for balance.

- Bend the injured knee, raising the heel of the affected leg toward the ceiling as far as possible without pain.

- Hold this position for 5 seconds and then relax.

- Perform 3 sets of 20 repetitions, 4 to 5 days a week, continuing for 3 to 4 weeks.

Straight-Leg Raises

- Lie on the floor, supporting your torso with your elbows as shown.
- Keep the injured leg straight and bend the other leg at the knee so that the foot is flat on the floor.
- Tighten the thigh muscle of the injured leg and slowly raise it 6 to 10 inches off the floor.
- Hold this position for 5 seconds and then relax.
- Perform 3 sets of 20 repetitions, 4 to 5 days a week, continuing for 3 to 4 weeks.

Hip Abduction

- Lie on your side with the injured side on top and with the bottom leg bent to provide support.
- Slowly raise the top leg to 45°, keeping the knee straight.
- Hold this position for 5 seconds.
- Slowly lower the leg and relax it for 2 seconds.
- Perform 3 sets of 20 repetitions, 4 to 5 days a week, continuing for 3 to 4 weeks.

Hip Adduction

- Lie down on the floor on the side of your injured leg with both legs straight.
- Cross the uninjured leg in front of the injured leg.
- Raise the injured leg 6" to 8" off the floor.
- Hold this position for 5 seconds.
- Lower the leg and rest for 2 seconds.
- Perform 3 sets of 20 repetitions, 4 to 5 days a week, continuing for 3 to 4 weeks.

SECTION 6 KNEE AND LOWER LEG

Straight-Leg Raises (Prone)

- Lie on the floor on your stomach with your legs straight.
- Tighten the hamstrings of the injured leg and raise the leg toward the ceiling as far as you can.
- Hold this position for 5 seconds.
- Lower the leg and rest it for 2 seconds.
- Perform 3 sets of 20 repetitions, 4 to 5 days a week, continuing for 3 to 4 weeks.

Wall Slides

- Lie on your back with the uninjured leg extending through a doorway and the injured leg extended against the wall.
- Let the foot gently slide down the wall.
- Hold this position of maximum flexion for 5 seconds and then slowly straighten the leg.
- Perform 3 sets of 20 repetitions, 4 to 5 days a week, continuing for 3 to 4 weeks.

Procedure: Knee Joint Aspiration/Injection

Aspiration of the knee joint can serve both diagnostic and therapeutic purposes. Traumatic injuries such as single- or multiple-ligament injuries, chondral or osteochondral injuries, or other fractures may produce large effusions around the knee. Pain can be relieved by draining a tense hemarthrosis. Aspiration also can help identify the etiology of an effusion. Gram stain, culture, and crystal analysis help differentiate infectious from inflammatory processes. With an injury, fat droplets from the bone marrow will accumulate on the surface of bloody aspirate placed in a small cup if an intra-articular fracture (distal femur, patella, or tibial plateau) is present.

Injection into the knee joint is the method commonly used to administer corticosteroids or other medications to an inflamed joint. Patients with an arthritic condition of the knee may obtain improvement of symptoms for significant periods with the appropriate administration of a corticosteroid or viscosupplement preparation (hyaluronic acid).

Step 1

Wear protective gloves at all times during this procedure and use sterile technique.

Step 2

With the patient supine on the examination table and with the abdominal and lower extremity muscles as relaxed as possible, maintain the knee extended.

Step 3

With a marking pen, outline the landmarks for entry into the joint. Understand that the knee joint will extend almost one handwidth above the superior aspect of the patella, especially when a joint effusion is present. Typical entry will occur from the lateral aspect of the knee 1 cm superior and 1 cm lateral to the superolateral aspect of the patella (**Figure 1**).

Step 4

Prepare the skin with a bactericidal solution.

Step 5

Use the 25-gauge needle to infiltrate the skin with 3 to 5 mL of local anesthetic at the point of entry.

CPT code

20610
Arthrocentesis, aspiration and/or injection; major joint or bursa (eg, shoulder, hip, knee joint, subacromial bursa)

Current Procedural Terminology © 2010 American Medical Association. All rights reserved.

Materials

- Sterile gloves
- Bactericidal skin preparation solution
- 25-gauge needle
- 30-mL or 60-mL syringe with an 18-gauge, 1.5″ needle
- 5 mL of a local anesthetic
- Corticosteroid or viscosupplement preparation (optional)
- Adhesive dressing

SECTION 6   KNEE AND LOWER LEG

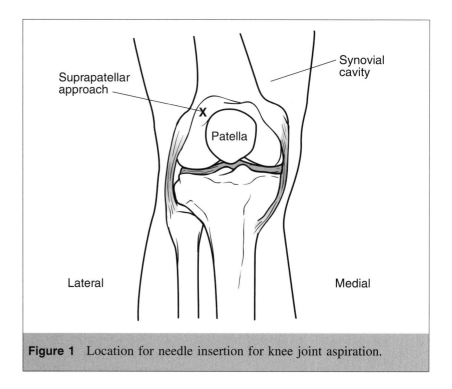

Figure 1 Location for needle insertion for knee joint aspiration.

Step 6

Using an 18-gauge, 1.5″ needle attached to a 30- or 60-mL syringe, enter the knee joint at the anesthetized site. Penetration of the joint capsule will be felt as a give or "pop." Withdraw the plunger of the syringe to aspirate the fluid; in a large effusion, the flow should be easy. If establishing flow is difficult, try changing the path of the needle slightly; the needle might be within a fat pad or thick synovium. Manual pressure can be applied to the suprapatellar region to milk more fluid out of the knee. As fluid is withdrawn, the needle may become blocked with synovium; again, a slight change in direction, with the application of forward pressure to the plunger, will usually free the needle tip and allow flow to continue.

Step 7

Once the aspiration is complete, inject medication or local anesthetic into the joint, if indicated. The aspirating syringe may be removed from the needle while maintaining the needle within the knee, and a syringe with the solution to be injected can be attached.

Step 8

When the aspiration and/or injection is complete, apply a sterile dressing.

Adverse Outcomes

As with any invasive procedure, extreme care should be taken to use sterile technique. Infection, although not common, may be introduced into the knee. Be sure that the needle path to the knee joint does not pass through any area of the skin that appears to be compromised or potentially colonized.

Aftercare/Patient Instructions

After removing a large effusion, apply a compressive wrap to minimize reaccumulation of fluid. In addition, rest and elevation of the lower extremity are recommended. Instruct the patient to notify you immediately at any sign of infection, rapid reaccumulation of fluid, or severe pain.

SECTION 6 KNEE AND LOWER LEG

Arthritis of the Knee

ICD-9 Codes

274.0
Gouty arthropathy

710.05
Systemic lupus erythematosus

712.96
Unspecified crystal arthropathy, lower leg

714.06
Rheumatoid arthritis, lower leg

715.09
Osteoarthrosis, generalized, multiple sites

715.16
Osteoarthrosis, localized, primary, lower leg

715.26
Osteoarthrosis, localized, secondary, lower leg

715.89
Osteoarthrosis involving, or with mention of more than one site, but not specified as generalized, multiple sites

716.16
Traumatic arthropathy, lower leg

716.86
Other specified arthropathy, lower leg

716.96
Arthropathy, unspecified, lower leg

Synonyms

- Degenerative joint disease
- Osteoarthritis
- Rheumatoid arthritis
- "Wear and tear" arthritis

Definition

Osteoarthritis (OA) is the most common form of knee arthritis. It can involve each of the three compartments of the knee—individually or in combination. The knee can be divided into the medial compartment, including the medial tibial plateau and the medial femoral condyle; the lateral compartment, including the lateral tibial plateau and lateral femoral condyle; and the patellofemoral joint, including the patella and the femoral trochlear groove. The medial compartment of the knee is the area most frequently involved in OA, resulting in a bowleg (genu varum) deformity. Knock-knees (genu valgum) occurs when the destructive arthritic process primarily involves the lateral compartment. Isolated patellofemoral OA can exist, especially in patients with subluxation or patella alta or baja; however, it is most frequently associated with concomitant tibiofemoral OA.

Secondary knee arthropathy usually occurs in individuals with a history of trauma, including fractures, meniscal tears, and meniscectomy, or with chronic ligament insufficiencies, such as anterior cruciate ligament–deficient knees. OA of the knee also may occur secondary to intra-articular fractures (posttraumatic) and inflammatory arthritides such as rheumatoid arthritis. Rheumatoid (inflammatory) arthritis is less common. It typically involves the joint symmetrically. Crystal arthropathies typically involve a single joint at a time and are caused by uric acid crystals (gout) or calcium pyrophosphate crystals (pseudogout) that irritate the joint.

Clinical Symptoms

OA most commonly affects patients older than 55 years, particularly those who are obese and genetically predisposed to the condition. Insidious onset of pain is common. As OA progresses, the patient will have pain on weight bearing, regardless of the initial cause. Common symptoms include buckling or giving way, which is caused by reflex quadriceps inhibition or laxity from joint erosion. The patient usually reports a history of difficulty climbing and descending stairs. Stiffness and intermittent joint swelling can limit motion at the extremes of flexion and extension. Symptoms of locking or catching, often mimicking a meniscal tear, can result from the impingement or sticking of rough joint surfaces and reflexive dysfunction of the quadriceps muscle or the impingement of inflamed synovial tissue between the joint surfaces. With severe OA, pain can occur when the patient is resting or even sleeping. With the crystal arthropathies, the symptoms typically wax and wane.

Tests

Physical Examination

Examination commonly reveals an angular (varus or valgus) deformity of the knee, which can be confirmed by a weight-bearing examination. Sometimes the opposite knee can be used for comparison; however, it is not uncommon for a patient to have windswept deformities (one knee valgus, one knee varus). The osteoarthritic knee often will have a mild effusion, with diffuse tenderness along the joint lines that at times extends into the medial hamstring tendon insertion on the anteromedial tibia. Careful palpation may reveal thickening and osteophytes along the articular margin of the femur. Crepitus around the patellofemoral joint is often present. Loss of range of motion often parallels progression of the arthritis.

Diagnostic Tests

Weight-bearing AP radiographs of both knees in full extension will show narrowing of the joint space (**Figure 1**). Radiographic findings of degenerative arthritis include asymmetric joint narrowing, bone sclerosis, periarticular cysts, and osteophytes. Radiographic findings of inflammatory arthritis include symmetric joint narrowing, disuse osteopenia, and bony erosions at the articular margins. The overall condition of the patellofemoral and tibiofemoral joints may be further assessed with lateral and axial patellofemoral views. In addition, weight-bearing AP radiographs with the knee in approximately 40° of flexion can help identify narrowing of the articular surface because these views profile different weight-bearing areas of the tibia and femur. These weight-bearing views are more sensitive for arthritis. The tunnel view (also called the intercondylar notch view) often reveals osteophytes, as well as osteochondral loose bodies.

Differential Diagnosis

- Herniated L3 or L4 disk with radiculopathy (diminished knee reflex, numbness)

SECTION 6   KNEE AND LOWER LEG

Figure 1 Weight-bearing AP radiograph of both knees shows substantial collapse of the medial joint space (black arrows) and subchondral sclerosis (white arrows).

- Meniscal tear (history of trauma and/or locking and catching) (may be concomitant)
- Osteonecrosis of the femur or tibia (patient older than 50 years, female, history of steroid use, blood dyscrasia)
- Pigmented villonodular synovitis (unexplained recurring hemarthrosis)
- Primary hip pathology (dermatomal referred pain to the knee, limited range of hip motion)
- Septic arthritis (fever, malaise, abnormal joint fluid)
- Tendinitis/bursitis (tenderness directly over a tendon or bursa)

Adverse Outcomes of the Disease

Chronic pain may ensue, with substantial loss of knee function. Walking and other weight-bearing activities may produce significant discomfort. The overall physical condition of the patient declines because a high level of activity cannot be maintained. Weight gain also often occurs.

Treatment

Nonsurgical management includes NSAIDs and perhaps the use of intra-articular injections (corticosteroids or viscosupplementation). Concomitant use of acetaminophen is often helpful. Treatment options including ice, heat, and liniments also may temporarily relieve stiffness and aching. Mechanical aids such as knee sleeves and elastic bandages can help control swelling that occurs with activity and have been shown to improve gait. Shock-absorbing shoe insoles or heels decrease impact on the knee with heel strike. Physical therapy to improve leg strength, flexibility, gait, and balance have been demonstrated to be as effective as NSAIDs for improved pain relief and function. Nonimpact exercises such as water aerobics and recumbent cycling help maintain muscle tone. Progressive resistance exercises (weight training) in pain-free arcs of motion help diminish muscle atrophy and improve muscle endurance. Using a cane or a single crutch on the side opposite the painful limb (so that the limb can be protected during the heel-strike phase) may help decrease pain while ambulating. A patient with poor balance or a history of falling should use an ambulatory assistive device, such as a walker, and may be a candidate for therapy. Severe functional limitations and pain at rest or at night indicate the failure of nonsurgical management and the need for surgical treatment. Surgical management of advanced cases often entails total knee replacement.

Rehabilitation Prescription

Rest and ice can control acute inflammation in the arthritic knee. In more chronic cases, a home exercise program of active flexion and extension range-of-motion exercises for the knee and isometric exercises for the quadriceps muscle may be useful (see Home Exercise Program for Arthritis, page 654). If a formal rehabilitation program is necessary, the prescription should include an evaluation of gait, hip and knee strength, range of motion, and balance. Weak muscles should be targeted.

Adverse Outcomes of Treatment

NSAIDs may cause gastric, renal, or hepatic complications. This is true even for cyclooxygenase-2 (COX-2)–specific NSAIDs. Chronic acetaminophen use can lead to hepatic and renal dysfunction. Repeated intra-articular injections of corticosteroids typically provide only temporary relief and may result in iatrogenic sepsis and/or accelerated destruction of cartilage.

Referral Decisions/Red Flags

Any patient with pain at rest, decreased range of motion, or significant functional limitations requires further evaluation.

SECTION 6 KNEE AND LOWER LEG

Home Exercise Program for Arthritis

Perform all five exercises, in the order listed.

- After each exercise session, apply ice (such as a bag of crushed ice or a bag of frozen peas) to the knee for 20 minutes or until numb, keep the leg elevated, and apply a compression bandage to the knee.

- If pain or swelling increases at any time or if it does not improve after you have adhered to the program for 3 to 4 weeks, call your doctor.

Exercise Type	Muscle Group	Number of Repetitions/Sets	Number of Days per Week	Number of Weeks
Hamstring curls (standing)	Hamstrings	20 repetitions/3 sets	4 to 5	3 to 4
Straight-leg raises	Quadriceps	20 repetitions/3 sets	4 to 5	3 to 4
Hip abduction	Gluteus medius	20 repetitions/3 sets	4 to 5	3 to 4
Hip adduction	Adductor group	20 repetitions/3 sets	4 to 5	3 to 4
Straight-leg raises (prone)	Gluteus maximus	20 repetitions/3 sets	4 to 5	3 to 4
Wall slides	Quadriceps, hamstrings	20 repetitions/3 sets	4 to 5	3 to 4

Hamstring Curls

- Stand on a flat surface with your weight evenly distributed on both feet.
- Hold onto the back of a chair or the wall for balance.
- Bend the injured knee, raising the heel of the affected leg toward the ceiling as far as possible without pain.
- Hold this position for 5 seconds and then relax.
- Perform 3 sets of 20 repetitions, 4 to 5 days a week, continuing for 3 to 4 weeks.

Straight-Leg Raises

- Lie on the floor, supporting your torso with your elbows as shown.
- Keep the injured leg straight and bend the other leg at the knee so that the foot is flat on the floor.
- Tighten the thigh muscle of the injured leg and slowly raise it 6 to 10 inches off the floor.
- Hold this position for 5 seconds and then relax.
- Perform 3 sets of 20 repetitions, 4 to 5 days a week, continuing for 3 to 4 weeks.

Hip Abduction

- Lie on your side with the injured side on top and with the bottom leg bent to provide support.
- Slowly raise the top leg to 45°, keeping the knee straight.
- Hold this position for 5 seconds.
- Slowly lower the leg and relax it for 2 seconds.
- Perform 3 sets of 20 repetitions, 4 to 5 days a week, continuing for 3 to 4 weeks.

Hip Adduction

- Lie down on the floor on the side of your injured leg with both legs straight.
- Cross the uninjured leg in front of the injured leg.
- Raise the injured leg 6" to 8" off the floor.
- Hold this position for 5 seconds.
- Lower the leg and rest for 2 seconds.
- Perform 3 sets of 20 repetitions, 4 to 5 days a week, continuing for 3 to 4 weeks.

SECTION 6 KNEE AND LOWER LEG

Straight-Leg Raises (Prone)

- Lie on the floor on your stomach with your legs straight.
- Tighten the hamstrings of the injured leg and raise the leg toward the ceiling as far as you can.
- Hold this position for 5 seconds.
- Lower the leg and rest it for 2 seconds.
- Perform 3 sets of 20 repetitions, 4 to 5 days a week, continuing for 3 to 4 weeks.

Wall Slides

- Lie on your back with the uninjured leg extending through a doorway and the injured leg extended against the wall.
- Let the foot gently slide down the wall.
- Hold this position of maximum flexion for 5 seconds and then slowly straighten the leg.
- Perform 3 sets of 20 repetitions, 4 to 5 days a week, continuing for 3 to 4 weeks.

Bursitis of the Knee

Synonyms

Pes anserine bursitis

Prepatellar bursitis

Definition

Bursae are sacs located between the skin and bony prominences or between tendons, ligaments, and bone. Bursae are lined with synovial tissue, which produces a small amount of fluid to decrease friction between adjacent structures. Chronic pressure or friction (overuse) causes thickening of this synovial lining and subsequent excessive fluid formation, leading to localized swelling and pain.

The prepatellar bursa on the anterior aspect of the knee is superficial and lies between the skin and the bony patella. This bursa can become inflamed (bursitis) or infected (septic bursitis) as a result of trauma to the anterior knee, such as a direct blow, or from chronic irritation from activities that require extensive kneeling, such as wrestling or carpet installation (housemaid's knee). Bacterial infections typically result from direct penetration, which may be an unrecognized event in patients who kneel extensively. *Staphylococcus aureus* and *Streptococcus* species are the most common infecting organisms.

The pes anserinus bursa lies under the insertion site of the sartorius, gracilis, and semitendinosus muscles on the medial flare of the tibia just below the tibial plateau. Although pes anserine bursitis may result from overuse, it more commonly occurs in patients with early osteoarthritis in the medial compartment of the knee.

Clinical Symptoms

At first, pain is present only with activity or direct pressure. The pain often is more severe after the patient has been sedentary for some time, and patients may notice a limp when first arising from a chair. Patients also note localized swelling over the involved structure. This swelling is most marked with prepatellar bursitis, as this bursa forms a dome-shaped swelling over the anterior aspect of the knee when it becomes inflamed and filled with fluid. Pes anserine bursitis also can be confused with medial meniscal pathology because the bursitis pain is located along the anteromedial aspect of the proximal tibia (**Figure 1**). Unlike meniscal pain, however, pes anserine bursitis pain is below the joint line.

ICD-9 Codes
726.60 Enthesopathy of knee, unspecified
726.61 Pes anserinus tendinitis or bursitis
726.65 Prepatellar bursitis

SECTION 6 KNEE AND LOWER LEG

Figure 1 Medial view of region of pes anserine tenderness.

These symptoms must be differentiated from those of arthritis. The patient with septic knee arthritis usually demonstrates intense joint pain, a large effusion, erythema, guarding of the limb, and a low-grade fever.

Tests

Physical Examination

Inspect the knee for areas of swelling and palpate structures for localized tenderness. Compression of the saphenous nerve and its infrapatellar branch by swelling of the pes anserinus bursa may cause numbness below the patella. Measure range of knee motion and then watch the patient walk. Patients with acute prepatellar bursitis typically have swelling superficial to the patella such that the patella may not be palpable in its subcutaneous position.

A patient with septic bursitis may have increased pain, warmth, and erythematous changes over the patella. With noninfectious traumatic bursitis, the area may be warm but is typically not painful or erythematous. Systemic signs (fever, elevated white blood cell count, etc) usually are not as dramatic with an infected prepatellar bursa as they are with septic arthritis of the knee; however, the clinical appearance of infectious and noninfectious bursitis may be the same. Therefore, aspiration of the bursa should be performed in all patients.

Diagnostic Tests

AP and lateral radiographs should be obtained in patients with chronic pain to rule out bony conditions. Radiographs will be normal with the exception of anterior soft-tissue swelling. With prepatellar bursitis, aspiration should be performed to rule out infection if significant erythema or warmth is present. Septic bursitis may demonstrate purulent or seropurulent material. This aspiration should be performed in a manner that does not seed the knee joint or bursa. The fluid should be sent for Gram stain and culture, cell count, crystal analysis, and synovial fluid analysis.

Differential Diagnosis

- Inflammatory arthritis (multiple joint involvement, abnormal laboratory studies)
- Medial meniscal tear (catching, locking, effusions)
- Osgood-Schlatter syndrome (preadolescent patients)
- Osteoarthritis of the knee (intra-articular effusion, osteophytes)
- Patellar fracture (intra-articular hemarthrosis, history of trauma)
- Patellar tendinitis (jumper's knee) (tenderness at the inferior pole of the patella)
- Saphenous nerve entrapment (numbness over the medial shin, dysesthesia)
- Septic arthritis of the knee (effusion of the joint but the patella can be palpated in its subcutaneous position, knee held in more flexion)
- Septic knee (flexion contracture, pain with knee motion, intra-articular swelling)
- Tumor (pain, mass)

Adverse Outcomes of the Disease

Chronic bursitis may lead to continued pain and thickening of the bursal wall. Pressure from continued swelling may cause weakening of overlying ligaments and/or tendons. Progression of a septic bursitis may result in chronic drainage or spread to the knee joint.

Treatment

Most patients with noninfected bursitis respond to nonsurgical treatment, including a short-term course of NSAIDs, ice, and activity modifications. Therapeutic modalities such as ultrasound and phonophoresis may help. Patients with identifiable tightness should perform quadriceps, hamstring, or iliotibial band stretching/flexibility exercises to prevent atrophy and maintain strength. Injection of a corticosteroid preparation is appropriate in recalcitrant cases. Surgical treatment for bursitis of the knee is the exception rather than the rule. Early-onset, mild septic bursitis can be treated with oral antibiotics. More severe infections require initial treatment with intravenous antibiotics. Repeat aspiration may help in decompressing the bursa. Surgical drainage may be necessary but is not often required.

SECTION 6 KNEE AND LOWER LEG

Adverse Outcomes of Treatment

NSAIDs may cause gastric, renal, or hepatic complications. Infection from corticosteroid injection is possible. Tendon or ligament weakening as a result of corticosteroid injection may lead to spontaneous rupture. Chronic or recurrent infection, septic arthritis, or the emergence of resistant organisms may occur.

Referral Decisions/Red Flags

Any patient whose symptoms do not respond to nonsurgical treatment or who has signs of ligament or tendon insufficiency requires further evaluation. Associated osteoarthritis in recurrent pes anserine bursitis requires evaluation. Prepatellar bursa infections may require surgical treatment when they cannot be aspirated, do not respond to antibiotics, or become recurrent.

Claudication

Definition

Claudication is activity-associated discomfort in the legs with a neurogenic or vascular etiology. Neurogenic claudication is associated with spinal stenosis. Ischemia to the cauda equina is the underlying pathology, induced by postures that mechanically compress the nerve roots with resultant paresthesias and dysesthesias. Vascular claudication is secondary to peripheral vascular disease and compromised blood flow with walking activities. It can result in a similar type of leg pain.

Clinical Symptoms

Patients with neurogenic claudication experience vague pain that begins in the buttocks and spreads to the legs while walking. Walking down inclines significantly increases symptoms secondary to the associated increased lordotic posture. Symptoms typically resolve when the patient sits or lies down. In general, the pain of neurogenic claudication tends to progress from proximal to distal in the lower extremity, whereas the pain of vascular claudication tends to start distally and radiate proximally. Claudication may lead to paresthesias and dysesthesias. Pain and paresthesias do not resolve immediately on cessation of walking in patients with neurogenic claudication. This differs from the pain associated with vascular claudication, which typically subsides when walking stops.

Tests

Physical Examination

Patients with neurogenic claudication may have no abnormal physical findings at rest, but weakness and reflex changes may develop after activities that provoke leg pain. Patients with vascular claudication have diminished or absent pulses below the waist, along with redness and pallor changes with elevation.

Diagnostic Tests

AP and lateral radiographs of the spine in patients with neurogenic claudication show degenerative changes. MRI and CT results can help define the pathology, although neither imaging study is necessary as a primary screening tool. A measure of vascular insufficiency is the ankle-brachial index (ABI). This is a vascular flow study that measures the ratio of systolic pressure at the ankle to systolic pressure in the arm; a ratio of less than 0.9 is abnormal. Doppler ultrasonographic studies and arteriography will demonstrate vascular disease in patients with vascular claudication.

ICD-9 Codes
440.21 Artherosclerosis of the extremities with intermittent claudication
440.4 Vascular claudication
721.42 Thoracic or lumbar spondylosis with myelopathy
724.02 Lumbar spinal stenosis
728.9 Unspecified disorder of muscle, ligament, and fascia

Differential Diagnosis

- Chronic compartment syndrome (athlete, pain following or during exercise)
- Herniated L3 or L4 disk with radiculopathy (diminished knee reflex, numbness)
- Meniscal tear (history of trauma and/or locking and catching)
- Osteonecrosis of the femur or tibia (patient older than 50 years, women affected more often than men, history of steroid use, blood dyscrasia)

Adverse Outcomes of the Disease

Patients with either vascular or neurogenic claudication may experience significant compromise in quality of life because of their inability to walk.

Treatment

Patients with neurogenic claudication can be treated with over-the-counter analgesic medications, intermittent NSAIDs, epidural corticosteroid injections, flexion exercises for the lumbar spine, and surgical decompression. Therapeutic options for vascular claudication include supportive measures, pharmacologic treatment, nonsurgical interventions, and surgery. Supportive measures include meticulous foot care, well-fitting and protective shoes, and the avoidance of elastic support hose.

Adverse Outcomes of Treatment

NSAIDs may lead to concomitant gastric, renal, or hepatic complications.

Referral Decisions/Red Flags

Any patient with neurogenic claudication whose symptoms do not respond to nonsurgical treatment requires further evaluation. Patients with vascular claudication require evaluation by a vascular surgeon.

Collateral Ligament Tear

Definition

The shape of the knee provides limited inherent stability. Stability of the knee joint is largely dependent on its ligaments and periarticular muscles. Therefore, injuries to knee ligaments are common. Four ligaments provide primary stabilization of the knee. The medial collateral ligament (MCL) and lateral collateral ligament (LCL) are outside the joint and stabilize the knee against valgus and varus stresses (**Figure 1**). The anterior cruciate ligament (ACL) and posterior cruciate ligament (PCL) are inside the joint and stabilize the knee against anterior and posterior stresses.

The mechanism of injury in an MCL tear (or sprain) is commonly a valgus (abduction) force without rotation, such as a clipping injury in football. The less common LCL tear is the result of a pure varus (adduction) force to the knee. Variable external rotation stress frequently occurs with MCL sprains. Injuries to the collateral ligaments can occur alone or in association with a meniscal tear or an ACL or PCL tear.

Clinical Symptoms

Many patients are able to ambulate after an acute collateral ligament injury and may be able to return to play for the remainder of the game. Patients report localized swelling or stiffness and medial or lateral pain and tenderness, but instability and mechanical symptoms, such as locking or popping, are infrequent after an isolated collateral ligament injury. Within 24 to 48 hours, localized ecchymosis and a small effusion develop. Pain may increase and motion may become limited over the first 6 to 8 hours following injury.

Tests

Physical Examination

The uninjured knee should be examined first. This helps the examiner understand what is normal for the patient and also reduces the patient's fears about the examination of the painful limb. Swelling in and around the injured ligament is common, but the presence of a significant knee effusion might indicate an associated intra-articular injury.

The MCL may be tender along its entire course, from the medial femoral condyle to its tibial insertion. Isolated tenderness at the most proximal or distal extent of the MCL may signify an avulsion-type injury. The LCL may be tender anywhere along its

Figure 1 Medial and lateral knee structures.

SECTION 6 KNEE AND LOWER LEG

Figure 2 The figure-of-4 position.

course, from the lateral femoral epicondyle to its insertion on the fibular head. The MCL is best palpated with the knee in slight flexion, but the LCL is best examined with the leg in the figure-of-4 position (**Figure 2**).

Apply a varus and then a valgus stress with the knee first in full extension and then at 30° of flexion (to relax the cruciate ligaments and posterior capsule). Laxity in full extension indicates a more extensive injury that includes the ACL and PCL plus the posterior capsule, rather than just the MCL or LCL. These injuries are knee dislocations with spontaneous reduction in which there may be a major neurovascular injury.

Increased joint space opening of less than 5 mm compared with the normal knee is considered a grade I (interstitial) tear, whereas increased opening of more than 10 mm is considered a grade III (complete) tear. A grade II (partial) tear falls between these extremes. The degree of instability may be masked in a patient with significant pain and involuntary muscle contraction. Be alert for possible false-negative results from an examination for laxity because of muscle guarding.

Diagnostic Tests

AP and lateral radiographs, although usually negative, may reveal an avulsion fracture at the femoral origin of the MCL or the fibular insertion of the LCL. MRI is sensitive for collateral ligament injuries and can be helpful in identifying other pathology.

Differential Diagnosis

- ACL tear (moderate to marked knee effusion, positive Lachman test)
- Epiphyseal fracture of the distal femur (tenderness at epiphyseal plate, evident on radiographs)
- Meniscal tear (mild to moderate knee effusion, joint line tenderness)
- Osteochondral fracture (radiographic evidence of loose osteochondral fragment)
- Patellar subluxation or dislocation with spontaneous reduction (positive apprehension sign)
- PCL tear (positive posterior drawer test)
- Tibial plateau fracture (bony tenderness, radiographic evidence of fracture)

Adverse Outcomes of the Disease

Although instability of the knee is rare, it may occur in association with disruption of the ACL and/or PCL. Lateral instability may occur after isolated LCL tears, especially in patients with varus alignment.

Treatment

Treatment of isolated MCL tears, even complete tears, is nonsurgical. Grade I sprains with no effusion usually resolve within a couple of weeks. Rest, ice, compression, and elevation (RICE), coupled with a short-term course of crutches and NSAIDs, are adequate. With grade II sprains, use of a hinged brace and weight bearing as tolerated are appropriate. For grade III injuries, use of a hinged brace with gradual return to full weight bearing over the course of 4 to 6 weeks is indicated. Rehabilitation includes early range-of-motion exercises (including bicycling) and quadriceps and hamstring progressive resistance exercises. Grade III injuries frequently require 3 to 4 months of protective bracing before the patient can return to unrestricted activity.

Although grade I and II LCL tears also should be treated nonsurgically, grade III LCL tears invariably involve a tear of the posterolateral capsular complex and are best treated surgically to avoid late instability, especially in varus knees.

Rehabilitation Prescription

Mild to moderate collateral ligament tears are initially treated with RICE to control inflammation and pain. In mild to moderate cases, early protected movement (7 days postinjury) that avoids varus or valgus stress is very important in reestablishing tensile strength and mobility of the ligament. Healing of the collateral ligament is enhanced with movement and delayed with immobilization. A hinged knee brace may provide protection to the healing ligament. A home exercise program should consist of active flexion and passive extension range-of-motion exercises for the knee and isometric exercises for the quadriceps muscle (see page 667).

If pain and inflammation continue after 3 to 4 weeks, formal physical therapy may be ordered. The prescription should include an evaluation of hip and knee muscle strength, followed by exercises targeting the weak muscles. If the range of motion of the knee joint is limited, mobilization is indicated.

Adverse Outcomes of Treatment

Instability is very uncommon after an isolated collateral ligament injury, but chronic pain and recurrence are possible. Patients are vulnerable to recurrence for 6 months; therefore, bracing for high-risk activities (contact sports) is recommended. Missed associated diagnoses, such as of meniscal and ACL tears, which can cause persistent pain or swelling or a persistent sense of instability, can complicate the course of nonsurgical treatment, and patients may ultimately require surgical intervention.

SECTION 6 KNEE AND LOWER LEG

Referral Decisions/Red Flags

Patients with hemarthrosis, significant joint effusion, or instability require further evaluation. Failure to respond to nonsurgical treatment might mean a missed diagnosis, such as an associated cruciate or posterior capsule rupture or a meniscal tear.

Home Exercise Program for Collateral Ligament Tear

- Perform the exercises in the order listed.
- These exercises should be performed with the knee braced for a grade II or III injury, as informed by your doctor using criteria in tests.
- Follow your doctor's instructions as to whether the knee should be in a brace while performing these exercises.
- Dry or moist heat may be applied to the back of the knee during the passive knee extension.
- To prevent additional inflammation, apply a bag of crushed ice or frozen peas to the injured side of the knee for 20 minutes or until numb after completing the exercises.
- If pain increases at any time or does not improve after performing these exercises for 3 to 4 weeks, call your doctor.

Exercise Type	Muscle Group	Number of Repetitions/Sets	Number of Days per Week	Number of Weeks
Hamstring curls	Hamstrings	25 to 45 repetitions/3 sets	5 to 6	3 to 4
Passive knee extension (prone)	Hamstrings	1 repetition/2 to 3 sets	5 to 6	3 to 4
Passive knee extension (seated)	Quadriceps	25 to 50 repetitions/3 sets	5 to 6	3 to 4
Quadriceps strengthening	Quadriceps	10 to 20 repetitions/2 to 3 sets	5 to 6	3 to 4

Hamstring Curls

- Stand on a flat surface with your weight evenly distributed on both feet.
- Hold onto the back of a chair or the wall for balance.
- Bend the injured knee, raising the heel of the affected leg toward the ceiling as far as possible without pain.
- Hold this position for 5 seconds and then relax.
- Perform 3 sets of 25 to 45 repetitions, 5 to 6 days a week, continuing for 3 to 4 weeks.

Seated version
- Sit on a chair with your feet flat on the floor.
- Slide the foot on the injured side back and hold the position for 5 seconds.

SECTION 6 KNEE AND LOWER LEG

Passive Knee Extension (Prone)

- Lie face down on a table or bed with your thighs supported just above the knee.
- Relax your legs and let gravity pull the knees down (into extension).
- Stay in this position for 5 to 10 minutes.
- Repeat this 2 to 3 times per day, 5 to 6 days a week, continuing for 3 to 4 weeks.

Passive Knee Extension (Seated)

- Sit in a chair with your injured leg propped up on another chair of equal height, as shown.
- Relax your leg and let gravity pull the knee down (into extension).
- Hold this position for 10 seconds.
- Perform 3 sets of 25 to 50 repetitions, 5 to 6 days a week, continuing for 3 to 4 weeks.

Quadriceps Strengthening

- Lie on the floor with the injured leg straight out and the other bent.
- Squeeze your thigh muscle for 10 seconds and then release it.
- Perform 10 to 20 repetitions, 2 to 3 sets, 5 to 6 days, continuing for 4 to 5 weeks.

Compartment Syndrome

Definition

The muscles of the leg are divided by fibrous septae into four compartments: anterior, lateral, superficial posterior, and deep posterior (**Figure 1**). Compartment syndromes are characterized by an elevation of intracompartmental pressure to a degree that compromises blood flow to the involved muscles and nerves. Although acute compartment syndromes are most common after fractures of the tibia, any condition that has the potential to cause significant swelling, such as contusions, muscle strains, or crush injuries, also can result in this limb-threatening condition. Acute compartment syndrome is an emergency requiring a fasciotomy. Compartment syndrome of the leg may affect one or more of the four compartments. The anterior compartment is the most frequently involved.

Exertional compartment syndrome of the leg, sometimes called chronic compartment syndrome, is an exercise-induced pathologic increase in tissue pressure (typically greater than 40 mm Hg) in one or more of the four muscle compartments. The result is leg pain and occasionally paresthesias radiating into the foot.

ICD-9 Codes

729.72
Nontraumatic compartment syndrome of lower extremity

958.92
Traumatic compartment syndrome of lower extremity

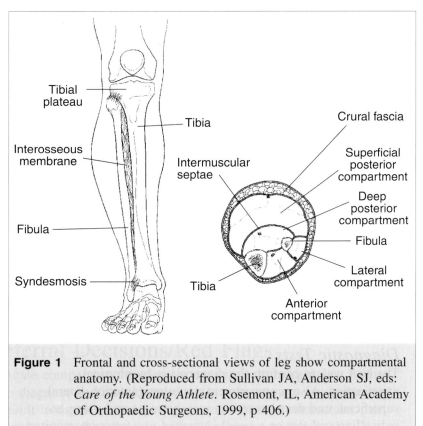

Figure 1   Frontal and cross-sectional views of leg show compartmental anatomy. (Reproduced from Sullivan JA, Anderson SJ, eds: *Care of the Young Athlete*. Rosemont, IL, American Academy of Orthopaedic Surgeons, 1999, p 406.)

Iliotibial Band Syndrome

ICD-9 Code

728.89
Iliotibial band friction syndrome

Synonyms

Iliotibial band tendinitis

Runner's knee

Definition

The iliotibial band (ITB) is a dense, fibrous band of tissue that originates from the anterior superior iliac spine region, extends down the lateral portion of the thigh, and inserts on the lateral tibia at the Gerdy tubercle. When the knee is extended, the ITB sits anterior to the lateral femoral epicondyle. When the knee is flexed past 30°, the ITB moves posterior to the lateral femoral epicondyle (**Figure 1**). ITB syndrome develops when the distal portion of the ITB rubs against the lateral femoral epicondyle, causing irritation and subsequent inflammation of the ITB. Occurring with repetitive flexion and extension of the knee, ITB syndrome is seen most commonly in long-distance runners and cyclists, but any athlete, especially those with predisposing factors for ITB tightness, such as genu varum, internal tibial rotation, and excessive foot pronation, may develop this syndrome.

Figure 1 Movement of the ITB over the prominence of the lateral femoral epicondyle with flexion and extension of the knee.

Clinical Symptoms

Patients with ITB syndrome usually describe pain at the anterolateral aspect of the knee that worsens with running, especially downhill, or cycling. This pain is usually most intense at heel strike. Also, patients may report an audible popping in the knee with walking or running. The patient is usually asymptomatic at rest before activity but may have some residual discomfort after activity.

Tests

Physical Examination

Tenderness to direct palpation is most evident directly over the lateral femoral epicondyle, 2 to 3 cm proximal to the lateral joint line. The Ober test (see page 639) may help to confirm the diagnosis. Functional testing, such as eliciting lateral knee pain when the patient hops with a flexed knee, also confirms ITB syndrome.

Diagnostic Tests

AP and lateral radiographs are usually negative with ITB syndrome, but they should be ordered to exclude other pathology presenting as lateral knee pain.

Differential Diagnosis

- Hamstring strain
- Lateral collateral ligament sprain (opening with varus stress)
- Meniscal injury (joint line tenderness, mechanical symptoms, positive McMurray test)

Adverse Outcomes of the Disease

Continued lateral knee pain may lead to decreased activity and associated lowered fitness level.

Treatment

Most patients respond to nonsurgical treatment, including physical therapy, a short-term course of NSAIDs, ice, and activity modifications. Physical therapy interventions must address the entire lower limb. A program to improve hamstring and ITB flexibility and hip abductor weakness should be initiated. ITB, tensor fasciae latae, and hip external rotator flexibility also must be addressed. Acute management may include modalities to decrease inflammation, such as phonophoresis or iontophoresis and cryotherapy. NSAIDs are also effective to help control the acute inflammatory process.

Following the initial period of inflammation control, alterations in training may be helpful for long-term prevention. Runners may alter their duration or pace of training, adjust their stride length, or reverse direction if they run on a circular track. Cyclists may adjust their seat height or foot position on the pedals. Runners with excessive pronation or excessive lateral wear may need special orthoses.

Local injection with corticosteroids may be administered only when the symptoms do not respond to stretching, physical therapy, and exercise modification. Surgery is exceedingly uncommon.

Adverse Outcomes of Treatment

NSAIDs may lead to concomitant gastric, renal, or hepatic complications. Infection, ITB weakening, and subcutaneous fat or skin atrophy may occur from corticosteroid injection.

Referral Decisions/Red Flags

Symptoms that do not respond to nonsurgical treatment require further evaluation. Further evaluation also is indicated if signs of ligament or tendon insufficiency are present.

SECTION 6 KNEE AND LOWER LEG

Gastrocnemius Tear

ICD-9 Code

844.9
Sprains and strains of knee
and leg, unspecified

Synonym

Tennis leg

Definition

Acute strains or ruptures of the medial head of the gastrocnemius muscle usually occur at the muscle-tendon junction. The injury often occurs while playing tennis, running on a hill, or jumping. These injuries are most common in athletes older than 30 years.

Clinical Symptoms

The patient typically feels a pulling or tearing sensation in the calf. Most of the pain is located proximally and medially. This injury can result in diffuse calf pain, swelling, and tenderness.

Tests

Physical Examination

The patient typically has tenderness and swelling over the medial gastrocnemius. The patient holds the ankle in plantar flexion to avoid placing tension on the injured muscle and typically ambulates with the ankle in a plantar flexed position. The patient is unable to perform a single-leg toe raise. Ecchymosis can develop in the calf over 24 hours. The patient has a negative Thompson test (see page 754), which would be positive with an Achilles tendon rupture.

Diagnostic Tests

No specific diagnostic tests are necessary to evaluate a medial gastrocnemius tear.

Differential Diagnosis

- Achilles tendinitis (more distal localization)
- Achilles tendon rupture (positive Thompson test)
- Popliteal cyst rupture (no trauma, no plantar flexion)

Adverse Outcomes of the Disease

Scar tissue may form, resulting in chronic pain, dysfunction, or reinjury due to shortening of the muscle-tendon unit. Another potential complication of a medial gastrocnemius tear is deep vein thrombosis formation due to inactivity and trauma.

Treatment

Medial gastrocnemius tears are treated nonsurgically initially with such measures as NSAIDs, rest, ice, elevation, a 0.5-inch heel lift, a calf sleeve or compression hose, and crutches. These are followed by isometric calf contractions in plantar flexion and gentle range-of-motion stretching and strengthening exercises (bilateral heel raises, heel raises with weights, single-leg heel raises).

Rehabilitation Prescription

The initial treatment goal is to control the pain and inflammation with the use of rest, ice, compression, and elevation (RICE). A home exercise program (see page 682) should include early movement: Within 7 to 21 days postinjury, gentle active and passive range-of-motion exercises should be initiated. The passive exercises should include gentle stretching of the gastrocnemius muscle group, and the active exercises should include calf raises.

If pain and limited function continue for more than 3 to 4 weeks, formal rehabilitation may be ordered. The prescription should include an evaluation of the extent of gastrocnemius and soleus muscle tightness and weakness of the gastrocnemius, and the rehabilitation specialist should design a program to increase the range of motion and improve muscle strength.

Adverse Outcomes of Treatment

NSAIDs can lead to concomitant gastric, renal, or hepatic complications. Loss of dorsiflexion may occur if range-of-motion exercises are not encouraged.

Referral Decisions/Red Flags

Persistent symptoms indicate the need for further evaluation.

SECTION 6 KNEE AND LOWER LEG

Home Exercise Program for Medial Gastrocnemius Tear

- Perform the exercises in the order listed.
- Apply moist or dry heat to the injured area before and during the heel cord stretch.
- Progress gently to the calf raises.
- To prevent further inflammation, apply a bag of crushed ice or frozen peas to the injured area for 20 minutes or until numb after performing the calf raises.
- If the exercises increase the pain or if the pain does not improve after you have performed the exercises for 3 to 4 weeks, call your doctor.

Exercise Type	Muscle Group	Number of Repetitions/Sets	Number of Days per Week	Number of Weeks
Heel cord stretch	Gastrocnemius/soleus	4 repetitions/2 to 3 sets	Daily	3 to 4
Calf raises	Gastrocnemius/soleus	10 repetitions/3 sets	3 to 4	3 to 4

Heel Cord Stretch

- Stand facing the wall with the affected leg straight and the knee of the unaffected leg bent, as shown.
- The foot of the affected leg should be turned in, and the heel should not come off the ground.
- Hold the stretch for 30 seconds with the knee straight and then relax for 30 seconds.
- Perform 2 to 3 sets of 4 repetitions daily, continuing for 3 to 4 weeks.

Calf Raises

- Stand on a flat surface with your weight evenly distributed on both feet.

- Hold onto the back of a chair or the wall for balance and lift the foot on the uninjured side.

- Keeping the knee of the injured leg straight, raise the heel off the floor as high as you can, using your body weight as resistance. (If this causes pain or discomfort, perform the exercise keeping the toes of both feet on the floor at first.)

- Work up to 3 sets of 10 repetitions, 3 to 4 days a week, continuing for 3 to 4 weeks

SECTION 6 KNEE AND LOWER LEG

Meniscal Tear

Synonyms

Internal derangement of knee

Locked knee

Torn cartilage

Definition

The medial and lateral menisci are fibrocartilaginous pads that function as shock absorbers between the femoral condyles and tibial plateaus. Meniscal tears occur alone or in association with ligament injuries such as anterior cruciate ligament tears. Meniscal tears disrupt the mechanics of the knee, leading to varying degrees of symptoms and predisposing the knee to degenerative arthritis (**Figure 1**, **Table 1**).

Clinical Symptoms

Patients with traumatic tears typically report a significant twisting injury to the knee. Older patients with degenerative tears may have a history of minimal or no trauma, with the injury occurring during an activity such as simply rising from a squatting position. Patients usually can ambulate after an acute injury and frequently are able to continue to participate in athletics.

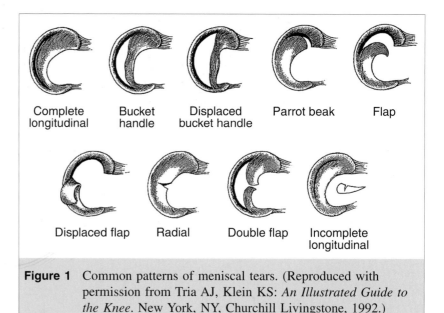

Complete longitudinal   Bucket handle   Displaced bucket handle   Parrot beak   Flap

Displaced flap   Radial   Double flap   Incomplete longitudinal

Figure 1   Common patterns of meniscal tears. (Reproduced with permission from Tria AJ, Klein KS: *An Illustrated Guide to the Knee*. New York, NY, Churchill Livingstone, 1992.)

Table 1 Classification of Meniscal Tears

Tear Type	Characteristics
Vertical longitudinal	Common, especially in the setting of anterior cruciate ligament tears; can be repaired if located in the peripheral third of the meniscus
Bucket handle	A vertical longitudinal tear displaced into the notch
Radial	Starts centrally and proceeds peripherally; not repairable because of loss of circumferential fiber integrity
Flap	Begins as a radial tear and proceeds circumferentially; may cause mechanical locking systems
Horizontal cleavage	Occurs more frequently in the older population and may be associated with meniscal cysts
Complex	A combination of tear types; more common in the older population

(Reproduced from Lieberman JR, ed: *Comprehensive Orthopaedic Review*, Vol 2. Rosemont, IL, American Academy of Orthopaedic Surgeons, 2009, p 1133.)

Traumatic tears are typically followed by the insidious onset of knee swelling and stiffness over 2 to 3 days. Mechanical symptoms such as locking, catching, and popping may then develop. Patients usually experience pain on the medial or lateral side of the knee, particularly with twisting or squatting activities. In some cases, large, unstable fragments of meniscal tissue become incarcerated in the knee joint, leading to a "locked knee." More frequently, motion is limited by a feeling of tightness in the knee secondary to the effusion. The mechanical symptoms and degree of pain tend to wax and wane.

Tests

Physical Examination

The most common finding on physical examination is tenderness over the medial or lateral joint line. Young patients who have traumatic tears that disrupt the peripheral blood supply typically present with a large effusion or hemarthrosis. In degenerative tears or tears that involve the avascular central body of the meniscus, effusions are typically small or absent. Knee motion may be limited secondary to pain or an effusion. During provocative testing, forced flexion and circumduction (internal and external rotation of the foot) frequently elicit pain on the side of the knee with the meniscal tear. The McMurray test is positive when the flexion-circumduction maneuver is associated with a painful click.

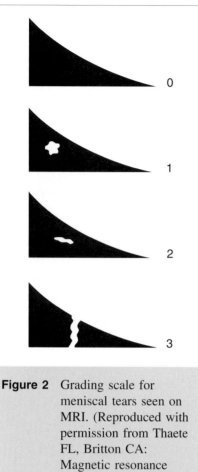

Figure 2 Grading scale for meniscal tears seen on MRI. (Reproduced with permission from Thaete FL, Britton CA: Magnetic resonance imaging, in Fu FH, Harner CD, Vince KG, Miller MD, eds: *Knee Surgery*, Philadephaia, PA, Williams & Wilkins, 1994, pp 325-352.)

Diagnostic Tests

MRI is specific and sensitive for meniscal pathology. AP, lateral, and axial patellofemoral views are indicated for patients with a history of trauma or an effusion. For patients with chronic conditions, the AP and lateral views should be weight bearing. A weight-bearing AP view with the knees flexed 45° is sensitive for early osteoarthritis and is recommended in older patients (**Figure 2**). Knee aspiration is indicated when a diagnosis of infection or crystal arthropathy is considered.

Differential Diagnosis

- Anterior cruciate ligament tear (hemarthrosis, positive Lachman test)
- Crystal disease (crystals in aspirate)
- Loose body (fragment may be evident on radiographs, but purely cartilaginous loose body may not)
- Medial collateral ligament tear (pain and instability with valgus stress)
- Osteoarthritis (joint space narrowing may be evident on weight-bearing radiographs)
- Osteochondritis dissecans (evident on radiographs, especially medial femoral condyle)
- Osteonecrosis of the femoral condyle (patient older than 50 years, pain, evident on radiographs or MRIs)
- Patellar subluxation or dislocation (tender medial patella, apprehension sign)
- Pes anserine bursitis (tender distal to medial joint line)
- Saphenous neuritis (tender to palpation along the course of the saphenous nerve)
- Tibial plateau fracture (bony tenderness, evident on radiographs)

Adverse Outcomes of the Disease

Recurrent episodes of locking and damage to the adjacent articular cartilage with subsequent osteoarthritis are possible, particularly with a delay in definitive treatment. With the exception of the outer rim, the blood supply to the meniscus is poor. Although small peripheral tears can heal, most tears are more central and cannot heal. Patients with recurrent stiffness, locking, or pain have a mechanically significant tear, which suggests ongoing internal damage. Failure to recognize and treat a traumatic tear may lead to progressive damage and a lost opportunity for surgical repair.

Treatment

A locked knee with loss of range of motion should be treated promptly with surgery. In the absence of mechanical symptoms and particularly when a degenerative tear is present, initial treatment should consist of rest, ice, compression, and elevation (RICE). A short course of oral analgesics, such as acetaminophen or ibuprofen, may facilitate return to normal activity. Traumatic tears in younger patients should be evaluated and treated aggressively. Sports activity should be restricted until MRI evaluation is performed or symptoms resolve. Arthroscopic surgical débridement or repair is indicated in younger patients with significant tears, in patients with a locked knee, and in older patients whose symptoms do not respond to nonsurgical treatment.

Rehabilitation Prescription

Initial treatment should consist of RICE to control soft-tissue edema, joint effusion, and pain. Early controlled movement is generally effective in improving mobility and reducing pain. The type of meniscal injury called a bucket-handle tear, in which the posterior fragment flips anteriorly, is beyond the scope of rehabilitation.

A home exercise program should include early, pain-free movement such as knee bends and straight-leg raises (see page 688). In addition, using a stationary bicycle may help reduce pain and increase range of motion. If the pain continues for more than 3 to 4 weeks, formal rehabilitation is an option. The prescription should include a thorough evaluation of quadriceps and hamstring strength and of the trunk and hip to determine core muscle deficits. In addition, exercises to promote healing should be initiated.

Adverse Outcomes of Treatment

NSAIDs may cause gastric, renal, or hepatic complications. Meniscal repair has a 10% to 30% failure rate, sometimes necessitating subsequent re-repair or partial meniscectomy. Persistent pain after a partial meniscectomy may occur secondary to concomitant pathology, such as osteoarthritis or saphenous neuritis. Traumatic osteoarthritis may be a late complication in the involved compartment following partial meniscectomy. Postoperative infection is rare.

Referral Decisions/Red Flags

A patient with a traumatic effusion, mechanical symptoms, or ligamentous instability requires further evaluation. Patients who do not respond to nonsurgical treatment and have persistent joint line tenderness or effusions also may require further evaluation.

SECTION 6 KNEE AND LOWER LEG

Home Exercise Program for Meniscal Tear

- Perform the exercises in the order listed.

- To prevent inflammation, apply a bag of crushed ice or frozen peas to the injured side of the knee after completing the exercises for 20 minutes or until numb.

- If the exercises increase the pain in your knee or if the pain does not improve after performing the exercises for 3 to 4 weeks, call your doctor.

Exercise Type	Muscle Group	Number of Repetitions/Sets	Number of Days per Week	Number of Weeks
Hamstring curls	Hamstrings	25 repetitions/3 sets	4 to 5	3 to 4
Straight-leg raises	Quadriceps	10 repetitions/3 sets	4 to 5	3 to 4

Hamstring Curls

- Stand on a flat surface with your weight evenly distributed on both feet.

- Hold onto the back of a chair or the wall for balance.

- Bend the injured knee, raising the heel toward the ceiling as far as possible without pain.

- Hold this position for 5 seconds and then relax.

- Perform 3 sets of 25 repetitions 4 to 5 days a week, continuing for 3 to 4 weeks.

Seated version

- Sit on a chair with your feet flat on the floor.

- Slide the foot on the injured side back and hold the position for 5 seconds.

Straight-Leg Raises

- Lie on the floor, supporting your torso with your elbows as shown.

- Keep the injured leg straight and bend the other leg at the knee so that the foot is flat on the floor.

- Tighten the thigh muscle of the injured leg and slowly raise it 6 to 10 inches off the floor.

- Hold this position for 5 seconds and then relax.

- Perform 3 sets of 10 repetitions 4 to 5 days a week, continuing for 3 to 4 weeks.

Osteonecrosis of the Femoral Condyle

Synonym

Avascular necrosis

ICD-9 Code

733.43
Aseptic necrosis of bone, medial femoral condyle

Definition

Osteonecrosis literally means "bone death." It occurs in the femoral condyle when a segment of bone loses its blood supply. The etiology is unknown, but it may begin as a stress fracture and probably involves some combination of trauma and altered blood flow. A portion of the weight-bearing surface of the medial femoral condyle is most often involved. The typical patient is a woman (female-to-male ratio 3:1) who is older than 60 years.

Osteonecrosis of the femoral condyle may be idiopathic or associated with chronic steroid therapy, renal transplantation, systemic lupus erythematosus, sickle cell anemia, and Gaucher disease. Microfracture of the subchondral bone occurs along with segmental collapse. Ultimately, progression to osteoarthritis is likely.

Clinical Symptoms

Patients typically describe a sudden, sharp pain localized to the medial compartment without obvious trauma. This pain probably develops when a shear force causes a subchondral fracture or disruption of the articular surface. An effusion may be present, and the patient may limit motion secondary to pain. Bilateral symptoms occur in less than 20% of patients.

Tests

Physical Examination

Physical examination will reveal an effusion, some loss of motion, and often a flexion contracture when the condition has gone unrecognized. Pain to palpation over the medial femoral condyle also is common.

Diagnostic Tests

Radiographically, osteonecrosis of the medial femoral condyle has been divided into stages to better define the extent of the pathology and outline appropriate care. These signs begin with flattening of the convexity of the condyle and progress through joint space narrowing, sclerosis, and osteophyte formation. The two determinants for accurate diagnosis are the area of the lesion and the percentage of involvement of the condyle. MRI or a bone scan can be helpful in making the diagnosis and determining the extent of involvement (**Figures 1** and **2**).

Differential Diagnosis

- Meniscal tears (evident on MRI)
- Osteoarthritis (tricompartmental involvement)
- Osteochondritis dissecans (sex and age predilection, location)
- Pes anserine bursitis (location)

Adverse Outcomes of the Disease

Unrecognized or untreated symptomatic osteonecrosis will progress to osteoarthritis. Current treatment seeks to slow this progression.

Figure 1 AP radiograph shows subchondral sclerosis in the medial femoral condyle with subchondral lucency (arrows), suggestive of spontaneous osteonecrosis. (Reproduced from Johnson TR, Steinbach LS, eds: *Essentials of Musculoskeletal Imaging.* Rosemont, IL, American Academy of Orthopaedic Surgeons, 2004, p 544.)

Figure 2 Coronal T2-weighted, fat-suppressed MRI shows extensive edema in the medial femoral condyle (arrows) characteristic of spontaneous osteonecrosis. (Reproduced from Johnson TR, Steinbach LS, eds: *Essentials of Musculoskeletal Imaging.* Rosemont, IL, American Academy of Orthopaedic Surgeons, 2004, p 545.)

Treatment

Nonsurgical management includes limiting weight bearing, use of an unloading brace, NSAIDs, pain medication, and a conditioning program to restore quadriceps strength and endurance with modifications as necessary to avoid knee pain when exercising. Water exercise is an excellent option. Surgical intervention, which is indicated when symptoms persist despite a course of nonsurgical treatment, can include débridement and drilling, procedures to alter the weight-bearing axis and unload the medial compartment, and, for advanced cases, total knee replacement.

Adverse Outcomes of Treatment

NSAIDs may cause gastric, renal, or hepatic complications. Surgical complications may occur. The results of procedures that alter the weight-bearing axis are mixed: risk to neurovascular structures and overcorrection are the two main concerns. Total knee replacement provides excellent pain relief and improved function but carries the possible need for future revision.

Referral Decisions/Red Flags

Failure to improve with nonsurgical treatment warrants consideration of surgical intervention. Disproportionate pain, which can indicate complex regional pain syndrome, also indicates the need for further evaluation.

SECTION 6 KNEE AND LOWER LEG

Patellar/Quadriceps Tendinitis

Synonyms

Extensor mechanism tendinitis

Jumper's knee

Definition

Extensor mechanism tendinitis is an overuse or overload syndrome involving either the quadriceps tendon at its insertion on the superior pole of the patella or the patellar tendon at the inferior pole of the patella or at its insertion at the tibial tubercle. Younger adults (younger than 40 years) with this condition often engage in jumping or kicking sports (jumper's knee) or have erratic exercise habits. Patellar or quadriceps tendinitis also sometimes develops in older patients after a lifting strain or a significant change in exercise level. Weight gain is sometimes a factor.

Clinical Symptoms

Anterior knee pain is the hallmark symptom. Patients often point to a tender spot where symptoms concentrate. The pain is often noted immediately at the end of exercise or following sitting that has been preceded by exercise. Pain may be reported with prolonged sitting, squatting, or kneeling. Climbing or descending stairs, running, jumping, or squatting often increases the pain.

Tests

Physical Examination

Palpate for tenderness at the bony attachment of the quadriceps tendon or the infrapatellar tendon. Increased heat, mild swelling, and soft-tissue crepitus also may be evident in the tender region. Examination in the area of the infrapatellar bursa (below the patella and behind the infrapatellar tendon) often reveals puffiness (**Figure 1**). Knee motion is normal but frequently is painful with resisted full extension. Pain is exacerbated by hyperflexion of the knee, which increases the stresses on the extensor mechanism. When the condition is long-standing, quadriceps atrophy may be evident. Other general knee examination tests are negative in isolated cases of tendinitis.

Inferior pole

Figure 1 Palpation of the infrapatellar bursa.

Diagnostic Tests

AP and lateral radiographs of the knee typically are negative, but lateral views may show small osteophytes or heterotopic ossification at the upper or lower pole of the patella. MRI is reserved for recalcitrant cases for which surgical treatment is being considered or for cases in which partial rupture is possible (significant weakness in extension but no palpable defect).

Differential Diagnosis

- Anterior or posterior cruciate ligament injury (positive Lachman or posterior drawer test)
- Inflammatory conditions (multisystem findings, elevated erythrocyte sedimentation rate)
- Partial rupture of the extensor mechanism (weakness, palpable defect, difficulty with straight-leg raising test)
- Patellofemoral syndrome (anterior knee pain, other abnormal patellofemoral signs but not superior or inferior pole tenderness)
- Septic arthritis of the knee (fever, warmth, painful motion, elevated erythrocyte sedimentation rate)

Adverse Outcomes of the Disease

Pain and, rarely, spontaneous rupture of the quadriceps or infrapatellar tendon may occur.

Treatment

Treatment is directed primarily at relieving symptoms and involves three critical aspects. First is a period of relative rest from aggravating activities. Depending on the severity of the condition, this period can vary from 3 to 5 days to as long as 3 to 6 weeks or more. In some instances, patients may need to use a knee immobilizer intermittently. NSAIDs may help control symptoms, but local injections of corticosteroids should be avoided because these injections significantly increase the risk of rupture of the extensor mechanism. Analgesic creams, ice after activity, and heat before activity may be helpful.

The second phase of treatment focuses on regaining pain-free range of motion, flexibility of the quadriceps and hamstrings, and strength. Exercises focusing on pain-free quadriceps strengthening and flexibility should be initiated, including eccentric loading exercises, often in conjunction with ultrasound and phonophoresis or other rehabilitation modalities. Using a

SECTION 6 KNEE AND LOWER LEG

knee sleeve with a patellar window or a compression strap at the level of the patellar tendon (infrapatellar strap) is sometimes helpful. If improvement does not occur, surgical débridement of the knee may be indicated.

The third phase of treatment is gradual resumption of the activities that caused the symptoms while continuing the exercises that have restored strength and flexibility. Using heat before activity and ice after is often helpful.

Rehabilitation Prescription

The early rehabilitation of patellar tendinitis includes rest, ice, and compression of the patellar tendon area. The home exercise program (see page 695) should include pain-free activities that promote range of motion, provide gentle stretching, return normal muscle strength to the quadriceps, and reduce any muscle weakness in the hip. Straight-leg raises, knee flexion, and stretching the quadriceps are important to early rehabilitation. If pain persists after 3 to 4 weeks, formal rehabilitation may be ordered. The prescription should include assessment of the hip and trunk muscles and patellar mobility, as well as further strengthening of the quadriceps and hamstring muscle groups. Gradual resumption of eccentric loading has been demonstrated to be effective in treating patellar tendinitis.

Adverse Outcomes of Treatment

NSAIDs may cause gastric, renal, or hepatic complications. Pain is possible, and occasionally spontaneous rupture of the tendon occurs. Persistent functional impairment is the most common disability.

Referral Decisions/Red Flags

Patients with a possible rupture of the extensor mechanism require further evaluation as soon as possible. Cases recalcitrant to nonsurgical management also require further evaluation.

Home Exercise Program for Patellar/Quadriceps Tendinitis

- Perform the exercises in the order listed.
- To prevent inflammation, apply a bag of crushed ice or frozen peas just below the kneecap after completing all the exercises.
- If the pain continues or gets worse, call your doctor.

Exercise Type	Muscle Group	Number of Repetitions/Sets	Number of Days per Week	Number of Weeks
Straight-leg raises	Quadriceps	10 repetitions/3 sets	Daily	3 to 4
Knee flexion	Hamstrings	25 repetitions/3 sets, progressing to 45 repetitions/3 sets	4 to 5	3 to 4
Prone quadriceps stretch	Quadriceps	4 repetitions/2 to 3 sets	5 to 6	3 to 4

Straight-Leg Raises

- Lie on the floor, supporting your torso with your elbows as shown.
- Keep the affected leg straight and bend the other leg at the knee so that the foot is flat on the floor.
- Tighten the thigh muscle of the affected leg and slowly raise it 6 to 10 inches off the floor.
- Hold this position for 5 seconds and then relax.
- Perform 3 sets of 10 repetitions daily, continuing for 3 to 4 weeks.

Knee Flexion

- Lie face down on a flat surface with your legs together.
- Slowly flex the affected knee (bend it up toward your buttocks) as far as possible without pain and then lower it. To add resistance, use rubber tubing while doing the exercise.
- Perform 3 sets of 25 repetitions, progressing to 3 sets of 45 repetitions.
- Perform the exercise 4 to 5 days a week, continuing for 3 to 4 weeks.

SECTION 6 KNEE AND LOWER LEG

Prone Quadriceps Stretch

- Lie face down on a flat surface with your arms at your sides and your legs straight.
- Bend the affected knee and grasp the ankle with your hand (or use a towel or rubber tubing).
- Keeping your thigh flat on the surface, pull gently and hold for 30 seconds; then relax for 30 seconds.
- Perform 2 to 3 sets of 4 repetitions 5 to 6 days a week, continuing for 3 to 4 weeks.

Patellar/Quadriceps Tendon Ruptures

Definition

A rupture of the quadriceps or patellar tendon, as well as a patellar fracture, will disrupt the extensor mechanism of the knee. Quadriceps and patellar tendon disruptions typically occur with a fall on a knee that is partially flexed. When the quadriceps muscle forcibly contracts to break the impact of the fall, the quadriceps or patellar tendon may be overwhelmed. Fractures of the patella more often result from a direct blow from a motor vehicle accident but also may occur by the indirect mechanism of a fall.

Most patients with ruptures of the quadriceps or patellar tendon are between the ages of 30 and 60 years. A history of previous quadriceps or patellar tendinitis is surprisingly uncommon.

Clinical Symptoms

Patients report significant pain and swelling after an acute injury. Walking may be possible, especially in subtotal ruptures, but patients note a sense of instability or "giving way" with ambulation.

Tests

Physical Examination

A large effusion is usually present. Palpate the knee for defects indicating the area of rupture (**Figure 1**). Fractures of the patella are usually obvious, but ruptures of the quadriceps or patellar tendon may be missed. The key to diagnosis is the patient's inability to extend the knee against gravity or perform a straight-leg raise.

Diagnostic Tests

Radiographs are appropriate to rule out a patellar fracture. The lateral view may show that the patella is higher than usual (rupture of the patellar tendon) or slightly lower than usual (rupture of the quadriceps tendon). MRI will confirm rupture of a tendon but is rarely necessary in the presence of the strong clinical findings.

ICD-9 Codes
822.0 Fracture of patella, closed
822.1 Fracture of patella, open
844.8 Sprains and strains of knee and leg, other specified sites
959.7 Injury, other and unspecified, knee, leg, ankle, and foot

SECTION 6 KNEE AND LOWER LEG

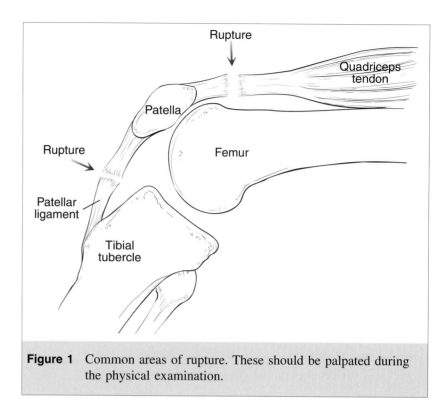

Figure 1   Common areas of rupture. These should be palpated during the physical examination.

Differential Diagnosis

- Collateral ligament tear (varus or valgus injury, medial or lateral tenderness and instability)
- Cruciate ligament disruption (effusion may be similar, but the patient is able to extend the knee)
- Meniscal tear (effusion relatively small, joint line tenderness, circumduction pain)

Adverse Outcomes of the Disease

Marked disability will develop secondary to the deficient extensor mechanism unless the rupture is surgically repaired. Delay in treatment significantly increases the difficulty of surgery and may compromise the outcome.

Treatment

Surgical repair is the treatment of choice for a complete rupture of the quadriceps or patellar tendon and for a displaced fracture of the patella. Partial tears of the tendons and nondisplaced fractures, which are uncommon, can be treated by immobilization.

Adverse Outcomes of Treatment

Postoperative infection, pain, and weakness of the extensor mechanism are possible.

Referral Decisions/Red Flags

All patients with a history and physical examination that suggest extensor mechanism rupture require further evaluation for surgery.

SECTION 6   KNEE AND LOWER LEG

Patellofemoral Instability and Malalignment

Figure 1 Acute lateral patellar dislocation of right knee. (Reproduced from Crosby LA, Lewallen DG, eds: *Emergency Care and Transportation of the Sick and Injured,* ed 10. Rosemont, IL, American Academy of Orthopaedic Surgeons, 2010, p 1045.)

Synonyms

Miserable malalignment syndrome
Patellar dislocation
Patellar subluxation

Definition

Patellofemoral instability and malalignment encompass a spectrum of pathologic conditions that include abnormal motion of the patella as it glides over the distal femur, recurrent subluxation of the patella, and recurrent dislocation of the patella. Patellofemoral instability usually occurs in a lateral direction (**Figure 1**). Medial patellar instability is rare. The term patellofemoral malalignment indicates that the patella is tilted laterally or predisposed to lateral subluxation, usually because of one or more anatomic factors. Patellar subluxation and dislocation may occur with minimal trauma (eg, a minor twist with a foot planted) in individuals with one or more anatomic predisposing factors such as patella alta, a shallow trochlear groove, a relatively flat patellar undersurface, a laterally tipped patella, ligamentous laxity, and hypermobility of the patella. In individuals with normal patellofemoral mechanics, subluxation or dislocation may be caused by direct trauma or, more frequently, by an indirect mechanism of injury. A common history is that of a right-handed softball player who dislocates the right patella while swinging the baseball bat. When the right foot is planted firmly on the ground as the torso rotates to the left, the patella lags behind, resulting in a lateral dislocation.

Clinical Symptoms

Patients usually describe severe pain, sometimes report hearing a pop, and occasionally see a deformity of the knee. Patients frequently think that the kneecap has dislocated medially because of the unusual prominence of the medial femoral condyle, which is no longer covered by the patella. The knee is usually maintained in a flexed position. The patella often reduces spontaneously, although sometimes a manual reduction is required.

Subluxation or dislocation of the patella causes tearing of the restraining medial retinacular tissue and the medial patellofemoral ligament, leading to pain, hemarthrosis, and loss of knee motion. Patients who have sustained one episode of instability are likely to sustain additional episodes, particularly when the medial soft tissues have healed in a stretched-out position and anatomic predisposing factors are present. Recurrent episodes of instability tend to be less traumatic than the initial episode, with patients experiencing milder symptoms.

In contrast to patients with patellar instability, the primary symptom in patients with symptomatic malalignment is retropatellar pain. This type of anterior knee pain usually is exacerbated when the patient uses stairs, especially when descending. Patients also may report pain with prolonged sitting (movie theater sign) or during squatting. With long-standing maltracking, progressive degenerative changes may occur, leading to patellofemoral arthrosis.

Tests

Physical Examination

Patients with acute patellar instability show apprehension at attempts to manipulate the patella, demonstrating fear and anxiety (apprehension sign) when the patella is translated laterally. Range of motion may be limited in extension and flexion because of pain or fluid in the joint. If the retinaculum is torn, there will be tenderness along the medial edge of the patella. If the medial patellofemoral ligament is torn at its origin, there will be tenderness just proximal to the medial femoral epicondyle. Patients with chronic instability exhibit the apprehension sign but may not have tenderness.

The signs of malalignment are more subtle. During gait, the patellae may tend to point inward (femoral anteversion, tibial torsion) or assume a knock-knee alignment (genu valgum). Genu valgum may be increased, and the distal portion of the vastus medialis may be dysplastic or atrophied. Increased patellar mobility also is common (lateral translation greater than one half the width of the patella), along with tightness of the lateral retinaculum (inability to elevate the lateral edge of the patella to a horizontal position). A high-riding patella (patella alta) and abnormal tracking (positive J sign) also may be observed.

Diagnostic Tests

AP, lateral, and axial patellofemoral views are necessary. An axial patellofemoral view, such as the Merchant or Laurin view, shows the relationship of the patella to the femoral trochlea. Normally, the patella is centered in the trochlea. In patients with malalignment or previous episodes of instability, radiographs may demonstrate lateral tilt or subluxation of the patella

SECTION 6 KNEE AND LOWER LEG

Figure 2 Axial patellofemoral view (Laurin view) of the knee shows patellar tilt and subluxation.

(**Figure 2**). A shallow trochlear groove with a relatively flat patellar undersurface or a patella with an acutely slanted lateral facet may be evident. In patients with excessive lateral pressure syndrome that has progressed to frank patellofemoral arthrosis, radiographs reveal joint space narrowing and other degenerative changes, especially in the lateral articulation. Axial CT may be useful in better delineating the exact nature of the patellar and trochlear relationship, particularly when surgical treatment is considered.

Differential Diagnosis

- Anterior cruciate ligament tear (increased anterior laxity with Lachman test)
- Medial collateral ligament tear (pain and laxity with valgus testing)
- Medial meniscal tear (medial joint line tenderness)
- Patellofemoral pain syndrome (pain without malalignment or instability)

Adverse Outcomes of the Disease

Anterior knee pain secondary to patellar instability or maltracking may lead to secondary quadriceps weakness, further compromising stability and exacerbating the underlying problem. Recurrent episodes of patellar instability and prolonged maltracking may limit activities of daily living and sports activities and also lead to patellofemoral arthrosis.

Treatment

The initial treatment of an acute patellar subluxation or dislocation includes application of a compressive dressing and protective splint with the knee in extension. These measures approximate the torn medial supporting structures. Aspiration of the knee should be considered in patients who have a significant effusion. Adjunctive measures include the use of oral analgesics, frequent application of ice in the first 24 to 48 hours, and modified weight bearing. The patient is instructed in isometric exercises of the quadriceps that are performed initially with the splint on. The patient is reevaluated every 2 weeks. When tenderness has resolved over the medial structures, range-of-motion and more vigorous strengthening exercises are started. The total duration of immobilization varies, depending on symptoms, but should not exceed 6 weeks, and quadriceps exercises may be begun even during this early stage of immobilization. Loose bodies seen on radiographs after patellar reduction may need to be removed.

Initial treatment of patients with chronic recurrent maltracking or instability should include exercises emphasizing quadriceps strengthening and flexibility. An elastic brace with a lateral buttress can facilitate the return to occupational or recreational activities. Occasionally, physical therapy modalities such as electrical stimulation or taping can be useful.

When nonsurgical measures fail, especially in patients with normal patellofemoral mechanics and in whom the dislocation was secondary to an acute traumatic episode, proximal or distal realignment of the extensor mechanism may be indicated, or repair of the medial patellofemoral ligament.

Adverse Outcomes of Treatment

NSAIDs can cause gastric, renal, or hepatic complications. The most common adverse outcome of treatment is residual instability or patellofemoral pain. This may be due to failure of treatment, incorrect use of isolated lateral release for instability, or articular cartilage damage that is untreated. Patellar instability may recur after lateral retinacular release, proximal realignment, or distal bony realignment. Even when successful stabilization of the patella is achieved, patellofemoral pain may persist, particularly with concomitant degenerative articular cartilage.

Referral Decisions/Red Flags

Patients with a significant effusion after a traumatic knee injury require further evaluation, as do patients with an osteochondral fracture from an acute patellar dislocation. Patients with patellofemoral malalignment or pain that fails to respond to nonsurgical measures also require further evaluation.

SECTION 6 KNEE AND LOWER LEG

Patellofemoral Pain

ICD-9 Codes

717.7
Chondromalacia of patella

719.46
Pain in joint, knee

Synonyms

Anterior knee pain

Chondromalacia

Patellofemoral (pain) syndrome

Definition

Patellofemoral syndrome refers to a constellation of problems characterized by diffuse, aching anterior knee pain that increases with activities that place additional loads across the patellofemoral joint, such as running, climbing up or down stairs, kneeling, and squatting. Forces on the articular surface of the patella can vary from three to eight times body weight in activities ranging from walking to running. The etiology of this syndrome is multifactorial and in many situations is related to overuse and overloading of the patellofemoral joint. Although patellar malalignment sometimes causes anterior knee pain, it is not a necessary component.

The term chondromalacia should not be used to describe this condition because chondromalacia indicates that pathologic changes are present in the articular surface of the patella, which may not necessarily be true. In addition, many patients who undergo arthroscopy are found to have degenerative changes on the undersurface of the patella consistent with chondromalacia, yet they have no symptoms referable to the patellofemoral joint. For this reason, the terms patellofemoral pain syndrome or anterior knee pain are preferable.

Clinical Symptoms

Patients most commonly report diffuse, aching anterior knee pain that is worse after prolonged sitting (movie theater sign), climbing stairs, jumping, or squatting. Some patients report a sense of instability or a retropatellar catching sensation. Usually no history of swelling is reported. Often the pain develops after an increase in activity level or in weight training. In most instances, patients will report no preexisting trauma, but on occasion there may be a history of a direct blow to the patella.

Tests

Physical Examination

When the patellofemoral joint is thought to contribute to the patient's pain, its evaluation should be deferred until the end of the examination; otherwise, the patient likely will resist the entire examination.

The patient should first be examined in weight-bearing stance. Watch the patient walk to see whether the patellae point toward each other (a sign of increased femoral anteversion or gluteus medius weakness). Check alignment. Look for genu valgum (knock-knees) and for foot pronation, which may result in a functional increase in genu valgum. Also check for inadequate development of the vastus medialis obliquus muscle at the distal and medial thigh. Observe the patient stepping up and down.

Tracking of the patella as the knee moves through flexion and extension should be observed. As the knee nears full extension, the patella may move laterally more than 1 cm (the J sign) or might even subluxate (a sign of instability). Soft-tissue restraints to medial and lateral patellar translation also should be evaluated. With the knee fully extended, the examiner should be able to elevate the lateral patellar facet to at least a neutral position. At 30° of flexion, the examiner should be able to translate the patella at least one quadrant medially but not more than two quadrants laterally.

The patellar apprehension sign (see page 638) may be performed to evaluate the possibility of patellar instability. Palpate the patella as the patient moves the knee through a range of motion to determine whether crepitus occurs and, if so, at what position. Hamstring muscle tightness can be evaluated by assessing resistance to passive knee extension with the hip flexed to 90° in the supine position. Quadriceps tightening can be assessed by evaluating resistance to knee flexion with the hip fully extended.

Diagnostic Tests

AP, lateral, and bilateral axial patellofemoral views are necessary. The axial patellofemoral view helps to rule out malalignment and arthritis (**Figure 1**).

Differential Diagnosis

- Meniscal tear (joint line tenderness, possible locking)
- Patellar malalignment (malalignment seen clinically and on radiographs)
- Patellar osteoarthritis (in older patients; effusion, crepitus, and evidence on axial radiograph)
- Patellar tendinitis (jumper's knee) (inferior pole tenderness, local tenderness at patellar tendon)

SECTION 6 KNEE AND LOWER LEG

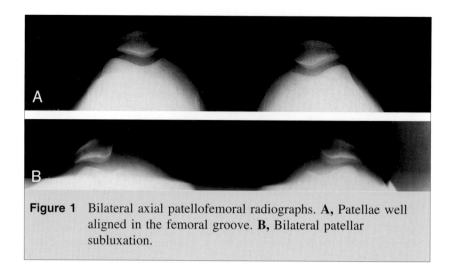

Figure 1 Bilateral axial patellofemoral radiographs. **A,** Patellae well aligned in the femoral groove. **B,** Bilateral patellar subluxation.

- Pathologic plica (medial parapatellar pain and tenderness, palpable cord in the medial parapatellar region)
- Quadriceps tendinitis (local tenderness at insertion)

Adverse Outcomes of the Disease

Pain and dysfunction are the principal problems.

Treatment

Activity should be adjusted to a pain-free level. A program of quadriceps strengthening and quadriceps and hamstring flexibility should be initiated. Quadriceps exercises need to be individually modified as necessary to avoid causing knee pain and to avoid shear forces or excessive pressure on the patella (short-arc open or closed chain, or isometric). Using a patellar pad or knee sleeve with a patellar cutout, taping the patella to decrease lateral pressure (McConnell taping), or using an infrapatellar strap may help. Some patients benefit from intermittent, short-term use of acetaminophen or NSAIDs. Weight loss is recommended for obese patients. Patients with persistent pain and/or recurrent effusions despite nonsurgical treatment may be candidates for surgery.

Rehabilitation Prescription

A home exercise program (see page 708) should include exercises to strengthen the quadriceps and gain full flexion range of motion to strengthen the hamstrings. Such exercises include straight-leg raises and prone straight-leg raises.

If pain persists after 3 to 4 weeks, formal rehabilitation may be ordered. The prescription should include an assessment of the hip and trunk muscles, patellar mobility, and quadriceps/

hamstring muscle group strength. In addition to exercises, mobilization is an important component in the treatment of patellofemoral pain.

Adverse Outcomes of Treatment

NSAIDs may cause gastric, renal, or hepatic complications. Aggressive full-arc quadriceps exercises typically aggravate the symptoms.

Referral Decisions/Red Flags

Persistent symptoms, including pain or recurrent effusions, or findings suggestive of patellar instability indicate the need for further evaluation.

SECTION 6 | KNEE AND LOWER LEG

Home Exercise Program for Patellofemoral Pain

- Perform the exercises in the order listed. Gentle quadriceps and hamstring stretches should be performed first.
- To prevent inflammation, apply a bag of crushed ice or frozen peas along the sides of the kneecap for 20 minutes or until numb after completing the exercises.
- If the pain worsens or does not improve, call your doctor.

Exercise Type	Muscle Group	Number of Repetitions/Sets	Number of Days per Week	Number of Weeks
Standing quadriceps stretch	Quadriceps	Hold for 30 to 60 seconds/2 to 3 sets	4 to 5	3 to 4
Supine hamstring stretch	Hamstrings	Hold for 30 to 60 seconds/2 to 3 sets	4 to 5	3 to 4
Hamstring curls	Hamstrings	15 repetitions/3 sets, progressing to 25 repetitions/3 sets	4 to 5	3 to 4
Straight-leg raises	Quadriceps	10 repetitions/3 sets	4 to 5	3 to 4
Straight-leg raises (prone)	Quadriceps	10 repetitions/3 sets	4 to 5	3 to 4

Standing Quadriceps Stretch

- Stand supported.
- Bend your knee up toward your buttock and grasp your ankle.
- Pull up gently and hold this position for 30 to 60 seconds.
- Repeat with the opposite leg.
- Perform 2 to 3 sets, 4 to 5 days a week, continuing for 3 to 4 weeks.

Supine Hamstring Stretch

- Lie on the floor with one leg straight and one leg bent. Clasp your hands behind the thigh of the bent leg, near the knee.
- Straighten the leg and then pull it gently toward your head, until you feel a stretch. (If you have difficulty clasping your hands behind your leg, loop a towel around your thigh. Grasp the ends of the towel and pull the leg toward you.)
- Hold this position for 30 to 60 seconds.
- Repeat with the opposite leg.
- Perform 2 to 3 sets, 4 to 5 days a week, continuing for 3 to 4 weeks.

Hamstring Curls

- Stand on a flat surface with your weight evenly distributed on both feet.
- Hold onto the back of a chair or the wall for balance.
- Bend the affected knee, raising the heel of the affected leg toward the ceiling as far as possible without pain.
- Hold this position for 5 seconds and then relax.
- Perform 3 sets of 15 repetitions, progressing to 3 sets of repetitions.
- Perform the exercise 3 to 4 days a week, continuing for 3 to 4 weeks.

Seated version:
- Sit on a chair with your feet flat on the floor.
- Slide the foot on the injured side back and hold the position for 5 seconds.

Straight-Leg Raises

- Lie on the floor, supporting your torso with your elbows as shown.
- Keep the affected leg straight and bend the other leg at the knee so that the foot is flat on the floor.
- Tighten the thigh muscle of the affected leg and slowly raise it 6 to 10 inches off the floor.
- Hold this position for 5 seconds and then relax.
- Perform 3 sets of 10 repetitions 4 to 5 days a week, continuing for 3 to 4 weeks.

Straight-Leg Raises (Prone)

- Lie on the floor on your stomach with your legs straight.
- Tighten the hamstrings of the affected leg and raise the leg toward the ceiling as far as you can.
- Hold this position for 5 seconds.
- Lower the leg and rest it for 2 seconds.
- Perform 3 sets of 10 repetitions 4 to 5 days a week, continuing for 3 to 4 weeks.

Plica Syndrome

Definition

A plica is a normal fold in the synovium of the knee. The synovium of the knee joint has five basic plicae. Three of them (suprapatellar, medial, and infrapatellar) are considered distinct structures, and two are considered minor folds. The suprapatellar plica extends from the undersurface of the quadriceps tendon to the medial or lateral capsule of the knee. The medial plica extends from the medial joint capsule to the medial anterior fat pad. The infrapatellar plica (ligamentum mucosa) extends anterior to, and may sometimes cover, the anterior cruciate ligament.

A plica that becomes inflamed and thickened from trauma or overuse may interfere with normal joint motion because the pathologic structure "bowstrings" over the femoral condyle or other structures. Plica syndromes usually result from a combination of trauma and mechanical malalignment and may occur at any age. The medial plica is the plica that most often becomes pathologic.

ICD-9 Codes
717.9 Unspecified internal derangement of knee
727.00 Synovitis and tenosynovitis, unspecified
727.83 Plica syndrome

Clinical Symptoms

The onset of pain is often insidious but may be related to a fall or injury. Patients most often describe activity-related aching in the anterior or anteromedial aspect of the knee. Some patients note a painful snapping or popping in the knee. Buckling or a sense of instability may occur, but true giving way, locking, or obvious effusion is uncommon.

Tests

Physical Examination

Inspect the knee for tenderness. With a pathologic medial plica, tenderness is localized to the medial aspect of the patella. With the knee flexed, a pathologic plica may be palpated as a thickened band. Place the knee in 90° of flexion and then extend the knee. With a pathologic plica, a pop may occur at about 60° of flexion. Other conditions, such as patellofemoral disorders, may present with similar symptoms and should be excluded.

Diagnostic Tests

AP, lateral, and axial patellofemoral views will be normal with plica syndrome but should be obtained to rule out other conditions.

Differential Diagnosis

- Meniscal tear (giving way, joint line tenderness, pain with circumduction)
- Osteochondritis dissecans (spontaneous onset, evident on radiographs)
- Patellofemoral instability (positive apprehension sign)
- Prepatellar bursitis (location)
- Quadriceps or patellar tendinitis (tenderness at tendon insertion sites)
- Septic arthritis (severe pain, fever, effusion, diagnostic joint aspiration)

Adverse Outcomes of the Disease

Continued discomfort and interference with running activities can occur, as well as erosive changes in the femoral condyle cartilage, because of the snapping of the thickened plica over the condyle.

Treatment

Initial management is aimed at decreasing the inflammation and thickening of the plica. Activity modifications and NSAIDs should be considered. An injection of local anesthetic and corticosteroid preparation into the plica can be both diagnostic and therapeutic. Based on the physical examination, an appropriate flexibility and strengthening program should be initiated. With persistent symptoms, and no other evidence of other intra-articular disorders, arthroscopic resection of the plica should be considered.

Rehabilitation Prescription

Early rehabilitation should include rest, ice, compression, and elevation (RICE) of the affected knee. The home exercise program (see page 714) should include quadriceps strengthening exercises to reduce pain and prevent joint stiffness. In addition, atrophy of the quadriceps muscle can be prevented with early isometric exercises such as straight-leg raises.

If symptoms do not respond to the home program after 3 to 4 weeks, a more complex problem involving abnormal patellofemoral mechanics is usually present, and formal rehabilitation should be ordered. The prescription should include an evaluation of foot mechanics, patellofemoral mobility, and strength of the hip and trunk muscles. After determining the extent of the muscle imbalances and mechanics, the rehabilitation specialist can develop a treatment plan.

Adverse Outcomes of Treatment

NSAIDs may cause gastric, renal, or hepatic complications. Repeated intra-articular corticosteroid injections may lead to accelerated destruction of articular cartilage and/or iatrogenic sepsis. Surgical resection may be ineffective or complicated by infection and stiffness.

Referral Decisions/Red Flags

Continued discomfort and symptoms of instability indicate the need for further evaluation.

Home Exercise Program for Plica Syndrome

- Perform the exercises in the order listed.
- Gentle quadriceps and hamstring stretching should be performed first.
- To prevent inflammation, apply a bag of crushed ice or frozen peas to the injured side of the knee for 20 minutes or until numb after completing the exercises. You should experience improved range of motion and less pain in your knee.
- If the pain does not change or becomes worse, call your doctor.

Exercise Type	Muscle Group	Number of Repetitions/Sets	Number of Days per Week	Number of Weeks
Standing quadriceps stretch	Quadriceps	10 to 20 repetitions/2 to 3 sets	4 to 5 days	3 to 4 weeks
Supine hamstring stretch	Hamstrings	Hold for 30 to 60 seconds/2 to 3 sets	4 to 5 days	3 to 4 weeks
Straight-leg raises	Quadriceps	Work up to 10 repetitions/ 3 sets	Daily	3 to 4

Standing Quadriceps Stretch

- Stand supported.
- Bend your knee up toward your buttock and grasp your ankle.
- Pull up gently and hold this position for 30 to 60 seconds.
- Repeat with the opposite leg.
- Perform 2 to 3 sets, 4 to 5 days a week, continuing for 3 to 4 weeks.

Supine Hamstring Stretch

- Lie on the floor with one leg straight and one leg bent. Clasp your hands behind the thigh of the bent leg, near the knee.
- Straighten the leg and then pull it gently toward your head, until you feel a stretch. (If you have difficulty clasping your hands behind your leg, loop a towel around your thigh. Grasp the ends of the towel and pull the leg toward you.)
- Hold this position for 30 to 60 seconds.
- Repeat with the opposite leg.
- Perform 2 to 3 sets, 4 to 5 days a week, continuing for 3 to 4 weeks.

Straight-Leg Raises

- Lie on the floor, supporting your torso with your elbows as shown.
- Keep the affected leg straight and bend the other leg at the knee so that the foot is flat on the floor.
- Tighten the thigh muscle of the affected leg and slowly raise it 6 to 10 inches off the floor.
- Hold this position for 5 seconds and then relax.
- Work up to 3 sets of 10 repetitions daily, continuing for 3 to 4 weeks.

SECTION 6   KNEE AND LOWER LEG

Popliteal Cyst

Synonyms

Baker cyst

Synovial cyst

Definition

A popliteal cyst, commonly known as a Baker cyst, is the most common benign synovial cyst in the knee. It develops in the popliteal bursa located at the posteromedial aspect of the knee joint. This normally thin bursa communicates with the knee joint and becomes more prominent (cystic) when synovitis or trauma creates excessive joint fluid that then tracks into the popliteal bursa. Popliteal cysts are associated with degenerative meniscal tears and systemic inflammatory conditions such as rheumatoid arthritis.

Clinical Symptoms

Patients present with swelling or fullness in the popliteal fossa with no history of trauma. Patients may experience mild accompanying pain or tenderness. Cysts may wax and wane in size depending on activity. Larger cysts may dissect down the posterior calf and/or rupture, but this is rare. When they rupture, these cysts may cause severe calf pain and swelling and may be mistaken for a deep vein thrombosis. Ruptures of popliteal cysts usually occur in older patients with degenerative arthritis or rheumatoid arthritis.

Tests

Physical Examination

Inspect the popliteal fossa and compare it with that of the opposite leg. Palpate the area to determine the size and consistency of the cyst and amount of tenderness. Cyst locations vary, but most are found somewhere between the medial head of the gastrocnemius muscle and the semimembranosus muscle. Examine the knee for signs of meniscal or other pathology. Effusion and accompanying mechanical signs indicate an intra-articular irritant causing the generation of excessive joint fluid. Examine the leg to determine whether the cyst has extravasated, causing swelling and tenderness in the calf. Popliteal cysts are sometimes identified as an incidental finding on a symptomatic knee examination.

Diagnostic Tests

Radiographs of the knee are usually negative but may show the outline of the cyst or show calcification present in the cyst or within the knee. MRI usually is not necessary but can demonstrate the location and character of the cystic fluid, as well as determine the presence of intra-articular pathology (**Figure 1**).

Cyst aspiration should be approached with caution because of the proximity of neurovascular structures in the popliteal fossa. Furthermore, the cyst fluid may be gelatinous and not easily retrievable with a standard-bore needle.

Figure 1 MRI shows a popliteal cyst. Areas of high signal intensity (arrows) on T2-weighted image indicate fluid, which is indicative of a cyst.

Differential Diagnosis

- Deep vein thrombosis (evident on ultrasonogram or venogram)
- Exertional compartment syndrome (evident on physical examination)
- Inflammatory arthritis (positive serologic studies)
- Medial gastrocnemius strain (evident on physical examination)
- Soft-tissue tumor (evident on MRI)
- Superficial phlebitis (superficial tenderness, negative ultrasonogram or venogram)

Adverse Outcomes of the Disease

Most popliteal cysts are asymptomatic other than causing an occasional sensation of fullness behind the knee. Rarely, a cyst rupture will cause pain in the posterior calf that, with the swelling, may mimic a deep vein thrombosis. .

Treatment

The benign nature of this condition should be emphasized. Aspiration has been suggested, but this may provide only transient relief because the cyst lining remains intact and the fluid often reaccumulates. In addition, the cyst contents may be gelatinous and quite difficult to aspirate. Treatment should be directed at the cause of increased synovial fluid. When intra-articular lesions resulting in increased production of synovial fluid can be successfully treated (usually by arthroscopic excision of a torn medial meniscus), the cyst usually resolves spontaneously and excision is unnecessary. Cysts associated with severe arthritis typically resolve after knee replacement. Rarely, cyst excision may be required in some patients. Ruptured popliteal cysts are treated symptomatically with minor analgesics, rest, and elevation.

Adverse Outcomes of Treatment

NSAIDs can cause gastric, renal, or hepatic complications. Open excision carries the risk of injury to neighboring nerves and blood vessels; dissection should be performed with caution. Recurrence rate when excision is combined with resolution of any internal derangement is low (around 5%).

Referral Decisions/Red Flags

Night pain, weight loss, fever and/or chills, or other constitutional symptoms indicate the possibility of a neoplastic process and therefore the need for further evaluation.

Posterior Cruciate Ligament Tear

Synonym

PCL sprain

ICD-9 Codes

717.84
Old disruption of posterior cruciate ligament

844.2
Acute posterior cruciate ligament tear

Definition

The posterior cruciate ligament (PCL) is a critical ligament in the knee and serves as the primary restraint to posterior translation of the tibia relative to the femur. Anatomically, it originates on the medial intercondylar wall of the femur and inserts on the posterior aspect of the tibia, running in an oblique direction. Injury to the PCL may be either a stretch injury or a complete rupture. PCL injuries are less common than injuries to the anterior cruciate ligament (ACL) and are often overlooked.

Clinical Symptoms

Four injury patterns suggest the possibility of a PCL injury:

- A dashboard injury (a posteriorly directed force to the anterior knee with the knee in flexion, as in a motor vehicle accident)
- A fall onto a flexed knee with the foot in plantar flexion, resulting in impact to the tibial tubercle; in comparison, the foot in dorsiflexion results in patellofemoral impact
- A pure hyperflexion injury to the knee
- A hyperextension injury to the knee. Typically, the ACL ruptures first; then, with sufficient force, injury to the PCL follows. This combination most commonly occurs in contact sports, secondary to a direct load on the anteromedial proximal tibia with the knee in extension. This mechanism of injury frequently results in a knee dislocation with or without spontaneous reduction.

An effusion commonly develops within the first 24 hours after injury, and range of motion usually is limited. Patients also may report pain and feelings of instability with weight bearing, especially with combined ligamentous injuries.

Tests

Physical Examination

Examination typically reveals a significant effusion and decreased range of motion. Tenderness to palpation may not be

Figure 1 The examiner's thumb palpates the position of the tibial plateau relative to the femoral condyles. With a normal PCL, the tibial plateau will be 1 cm anterior to the femoral condyles.

exhibited. A thorough examination for knee stability is required because PCL injuries are often a component of a combined ligamentous injury. In the acute setting, the physical examination may be difficult because of loss of motion and muscle guarding, which may mask increases in translation. Therefore, reexamining the patient once swelling has decreased is often helpful.

The most sensitive test is the posterior drawer test (see page 638). Be aware, though, that if increased posterior translation of the tibia relative to the femur is present, it can be easily misinterpreted as a positive anterior drawer sign when the tibia is pulled back to the anterior position. This misinterpretation is further complicated by the frequent coexistence of an ACL tear. Observe the resting position of the tibial plateau relative to the femoral condyles to help remove this uncertainty. With a PCL injury, the tibia will be in a posterior position relative to the femur because of gravity, and there will be no place to sit your thumbs on the anterior tibial plateaus (**Figure 1**). Comparison with the other knee is helpful. If the tibia sags behind the femur, a PCL injury likely is present.

In acute multiple ligament disruption, with or without spontaneous reduction, distal neurovascular status should be carefully assessed and recorded because limb-threatening vascular injury or severe neurologic deficits may be present.

Diagnostic Tests

AP and lateral radiographs of the knee obtained in the acute setting can identify bony pathology (including avulsions), aid in diagnosis, and help in planning surgical management. MRI can be useful in confirming PCL tears, as well as any concomitant injuries to ligaments, menisci, and articular cartilage.

Differential Diagnosis

- ACL tear (positive Lachman test, positive pivot shift test)
- Articular cartilage injury (pain on palpation, evident on radiographs or MRI)
- Combined ligament injury (laxity in multiple directions, evident on MRI)
- Medial or lateral collateral ligament tear (pain on palpation and varus/valgus laxity)
- Meniscal tear (joint line tenderness)
- Patellar or quadriceps tendon rupture (inability to achieve straight-leg raise)
- Patellofemoral dislocation (apprehension with lateral patellar displacement)
- Tibial plateau fracture (evident on radiographs)

Adverse Outcomes of the Disease

Limb-threatening vascular injury may be overlooked if a dislocated or hyperextended knee that has spontaneously reduced is not recognized and fully evaluated. Significant permanent peroneal or tibial nerve injury and severe knee instability may occur. Recurrent instability, subsequent meniscal tears, and osteoarthritis of the knee are all possible.

Treatment

Isolated PCL injuries typically are treated with a rehabilitation program that initially concentrates on resolving swelling and restoring range of motion. Once these goals have been achieved, progression to strengthening exercises may be initiated, with an emphasis on the quadriceps (short-arc terminal extension exercises from 30° to 0° of flexion). Functional bracing may be helpful when the patient returns to contact sports.

Failure of nonsurgical treatment typically manifests as recurrent instability and/or subsequent meniscal tears. These patients require PCL reconstruction to restore functional stability. After reconstructive procedures, instability is improved, but increased translation relative to the normal side may remain. Patients with combined injuries to the PCL and other ligaments, with or without knee dislocation, usually require surgical reconstruction.

Rehabilitation Prescription

A patient with a PCL injury who is not a candidate for surgery should start an intense rehabilitation program designed to improve range of motion and muscle strength of the quadriceps

SECTION 6 KNEE AND LOWER LEG

and hamstrings, including neuromuscular training and hip and trunk strengthening. Early rehabilitation should include rest, ice, compression, and elevation (RICE). After the initial healing stage of 1 to 5 days, range-of-motion exercises and quadriceps muscle strengthening should be started (see page 723). The patient should avoid activities that involve a high knee flexion angle until the hamstrings and quadriceps muscles become stronger. Wall slides are a safe exercise to promote increased mobility. Both prone and supine straight-leg raises are helpful in the prevention of quadriceps atrophy. Initially, hamstring curls should not be performed to avoid a posterior subluxation force. The rehabilitation prescription should include an evaluation of quadriceps, hip, and trunk muscle strength.

Adverse Outcomes of Treatment

Osteoarthritic changes involving the medial and patellofemoral compartments are well-documented sequelae to both nonsurgical and surgical management. Surgical reconstruction may be complicated by infection, graft failure, and recurrent instability.

Referral Decisions/Red Flags

Neurovascular compromise or deficits indicate the possibility of a knee dislocation. Any patient with a PCL injury and the possibility of damage to other ligamentous structures requires specialty evaluation.

Home Exercise Program for PCL Injury

■ Perform the exercises in the order listed.

■ To prevent inflammation, apply a bag of crushed ice or frozen peas to the back of the knee for 20 minutes or until numb after completing all the exercises.

■ If pain does not improve, if it worsens, or if the knee joint becomes inflamed, call your doctor.

Exercise Type	Muscle Group	Number of Repetitions/Sets	Number of Days per Week	Number of Weeks
Straight-leg raises	Quadriceps	10 repetitions/3 sets	6 to 7	3 to 4
Straight-leg raises (prone)	Quadriceps	10 repetitions/3 sets	6 to 7	3 to 4

Straight-Leg Raises

■ Lie on the floor, supporting your torso with your elbows as shown.

■ Keep the injured leg straight and bend the other leg at the knee so that the foot is flat on the floor.

■ Tighten the thigh muscle of the injured leg and slowly raise it 6 to 10 inches off the floor.

■ Hold this position for 5 seconds and then relax.

■ Perform 3 sets of 10 repetitions 6 to 7 days a week, continuing for 3 to 4 weeks.

Straight-Leg Raises (Prone)

■ Lie on the floor on your stomach with your legs straight.

■ Tighten the hamstrings of the injured leg and raise the leg toward the ceiling as far as you can.

■ Hold this position for 5 seconds.

■ Lower the leg and rest it for 2 seconds.

■ Perform 3 sets of 10 repetitions 6 to 7 days a week, continuing for 3 to 4 weeks.

SECTION 6 KNEE AND LOWER LEG

Shin-Splints

ICD-9 Codes

844.8
Sprains and strains of knee and leg, other specified sites of knee and leg

844.9
Sprains and strains of knee and leg, unspecified site of knee and leg

Definition

Shin-splints (medial tibial stress syndrome) are a condition characterized by the gradual onset of pain in the anteromedial aspect of the distal third of the leg. This condition commonly develops in response to increased exercise or activity level and probably represents inflammation of the tibial periosteum secondary to repetitive muscle contraction.

Clinical Symptoms

Shin-splints are generally associated with prolonged walking or running activity. Symptoms develop gradually with exercise, such as running on hard surfaces or early-season hill training, or with increased training intensity, pace, or distance. Pain is localized to the distal third of the medial tibia, the site of the origin of the posterior tibial muscle, and the patient may demonstrate pes planus associated with overpronation.

Tests

Physical Examination
Examination reveals tenderness along the posterior medial crest of the tibia in the middle or distal third of the leg. Some patients have pain with resisted plantar flexion.

Diagnostic Tests
AP and lateral radiographs should be obtained to rule out stress fractures.

Differential Diagnosis

- Exertional compartment syndrome (no symptoms at rest)
- Stress fracture (radiographic findings)

Adverse Outcomes of the Disease

No adverse outcomes of shin-splints are known, except continued pain and inability to walk or run.

Treatment

Mild shin-splints may be relieved by limiting activity to soft surfaces, decreasing training, and avoiding hills. NSAIDs, ice massage, and analgesic creams also may be helpful. Further

PAIN DIAGRAM
Foot and Ankle

Mallet toe
(Toe Deformities)

Sesamoiditis

Interdigital
(Morton) neuroma

Achilles tendon rupture

Peroneal
tenosynovitis/
Peroneal tendon
subluxation
*(Chronic Lateral
Ankle Pain)*

Tarsal tunnel
syndrome

Posterior
tibial tendon
dysfunction

Metatarsalgia and
callus formation

Posterior heel pain

Plantar fasciitis
Plantar fibroma
*(Soft-Tissue Masses
of the Foot and Ankle)*

Fracture of the ankle
(fibula)

Ankle sprain
Chronic lateral
ankle instability

Plantar fasciitis (proximal)

Ganglion cyst
*(Soft Tissue Masses
of the Foot and Ankle)*

Fracture of
the calcaneus

Fracture-
dislocation
of the midfoot

Subtalar arthritis
*(Arthritis of the
Foot and Ankle)*

Turf toe

Hallux valgus (bunion)

Stress fracture
(base of fifth
metatarsal)

Hallux
rigidus
Hallux
valgus
(bunion)

Bunionette

Ingrown toenail

Fracture of the
(second) metatarsal

Claw toe
(Toe Deformities)

Hammer toe
(Toe Deformities)

Corn

Ingrown
toenail

Fractures of
the phalanges

Foot and Ankle

Section Editors

Jerome M. Benavides, MD, MBA
Orthopaedic Surgeon
Foot and Ankle Center of South Texas
San Antonio, TX

Thomas O. Clanton, MD
Chief, Foot and Ankle Section
The Steadman Clinic – Vail
Vail, CO

Contributor

Michael Huxford, MEd, ATC, CSCS
Sports Medicine Coordinator
Rehabilitative Services
Institute for Sports Medicine
Children's Memorial Hospital
Chicago, IL

ANATOMY OF THE FOOT AND ANKLE

Lateral tubercle
Medial tubercle
Posterior process
Groove for tendon of flexor hallucis longus
Talus
Trochlea
Calcaneus
Body
Fibular (peroneal) trochlea
Neck
Head
Tarsal sinus
Transverse tarsal joint
Navicular
Tuberosity
Cuboid
Lateral
Intermediate
Medial
Cuneiform bones
Tuberosity of 5th metatarsal bone
Tarsometatarsal joint
Base
Metatarsal bones
5 4 3 2 1
Shaft (body)
Head
Phalanges
Proximal
Middle
Distal
Base
Shaft (body)
Head
Base
Tuberosity

Dorsal View of Right Foot

Tibia

Medial (deltoid) ligament of ankle
Posterior tibiotalar part
Tibiocalcaneal part
Tibionavicular part
Anterior tibiotalar part
Medial talocalcaneal ligament
Dorsal talonavicular ligament
Posterior process of talus
Navicular bone
Posterior talocalcaneal ligament
Dorsal cuneonavicular ligaments
Medial cuneiform bone
Calcaneal (Achilles) tendon (cut)
Dorsal intercuneiform ligament
Dorsal tarsometatarsal ligaments
Sustentaculum tali
1st metatarsal bone
Tuberosity
Tibialis anterior tendon
Short plantar ligament
Tibialis posterior tendon
Plantar calcaneo-navicular ligament
Long plantar ligament

Ankle Joint of Right Foot—Medial View

Tibia
Fibula
Posterior talofibular ligament
Calcaneofibular ligament
Anterior talofibular ligament
Components of lateral (collateral) ligament of ankle
Interosseous talocalcaneal ligament
Dorsal talonavicular ligament
Calcaneonavicular ligament
Calcaneocuboid ligament
Bifurcate ligament
Anterior and posterior tibiofibular ligaments
Dorsal cuboideonavicular ligament
Dorsal cuneonavicular ligaments
Superior fibular (peroneal) retinaculum
Dorsal intercuneiform ligaments
Calcaneal (Achilles) tendon (cut)
Dorsal tarsometatarsal ligaments
Inferior fibular (peroneal) retinaculum
Lateral talocalcaneal ligament
Dorsal metatarsal ligaments
Long plantar ligament
Dorsal cuneocuboid ligament
Fibularis (peroneus) longus tendon
Cuboid bone
Fibularis (peroneus) brevis tendon
Dorsal calcaneocuboid ligament

Ankle Joint of Right Foot—Lateral View

Bones of the Foot and Ankle

Overview of the Foot and Ankle

During standing and gait, the foot provides support, shock absorption, adaptation to uneven surfaces, balance, power, and direction. During more complex motions such as running and jumping, the functions provided by the foot and ankle increase. Therefore, it is not surprising that more than 20% of musculoskeletal problems affect the foot and ankle. Most of these disorders can be treated in the office setting.

The key to the successful diagnosis of foot and ankle pathology is to find the exact location of the problem. This requires an understanding of the anatomy of the foot and ankle. Furthermore, certain systemic illnesses such as diabetes mellitus, peripheral vascular disease, neuropathy, and inflammatory arthritis may affect the foot and therefore should be evaluated in the medical history. A history of bilateral foot pain should prompt a search for a possible systemic or spinal etiology.

Most patients with foot problems report pain. Chronic pain (more than 2 weeks' in duration) is more common than acute pain. A fracture, sprain, or infection should be suspected if the patient presents with acute pain. Always consider a stress fracture when a patient reports recent onset of pain over the metatarsals, especially in the distal aspects of the second or third metatarsals.

Foot problems can result from overuse, trauma, congenital abnormalities, systemic illness, or ill-fitting shoes. The standard radiographic views of the foot for all these problems are the AP, lateral, and 45° oblique views.

Forefoot Problems

Forefoot problems occur nine times more often in women than in men, a fact that is directly attributable to women wearing high-heeled and ill-fitting shoes. Shoe modification (lower heels, wider shoes) is always the first line of treatment. Bunions, hammer toes, claw toes, ingrown toenails, metatarsalgia, and interdigital neuromas account for most instances of forefoot pain. These problems are detailed in subsequent chapters.

Other common problems in the forefoot are hallux rigidus (arthritis of the metatarsophalangeal [MTP] joint of the great toe) and stress fractures. Limited extension (dorsiflexion) of the great toe is consistent with hallux rigidus. Pain and tenderness directly over the second or third metatarsals suggest a stress fracture. Synovitis of the lesser MTP joints is common in patients with hallux valgus (caused by pressure from the great toe against the second MTP joint) and inflammatory disorders. Synovitis of the MTP joint causes pain over the affected joint and is often confused with the pain of an interdigital neuroma (pain in the web space).

Midfoot Problems

Chronic dorsal pain at the midfoot most commonly occurs secondary to degenerative arthritis involving one or more of the midfoot joints. Patients are often able to pinpoint the exact location of the pain. A bony prominence, or osteophyte, referred to as dorsal bossing, can be palpated and corresponds to the underlying arthritic joint. Pain on the plantar aspect of the midfoot, which is unusual, occurs with plantar fasciitis or plantar fibromas.

Hindfoot Problems

Plantar heel pain secondary to plantar fasciitis is the most common problem in the hindfoot. The pain associated with this condition is often severe with the first few steps taken in the morning; patients normally are pain free during rest. Patients have focal tenderness directly over the plantar medial heel (the origin of the plantar fascia); often, on examination, considerable pressure must be applied in this area to duplicate the patient's symptoms.

Posterior heel pain may be related to irritation from shoes and associated with a prominent superior process of the calcaneus (Haglund deformity) and/or pathology in the Achilles tendon at its insertion. Often an associated superficial bursitis of the posterior heel is present. When evaluating a patient with posterior heel pain, make sure that the problem is not more proximal within the Achilles tendon; otherwise, a partial or even complete rupture of the tendon might be missed.

A commonly overlooked problem in the hindfoot is posterior tibial tendon dysfunction. This condition is characterized by pain and tenderness posterior and distal to the medial malleolus in the region of the posterior tibial tendon. Progressive dysfunction results in an acquired unilateral flatfoot that may be associated with pain on the lateral side of the ankle as the tip of the fibula abuts the collapsing foot.

Ankle Problems

More than 25,000 ankle sprains occur each day in the United States. Acute anterolateral ankle pain, swelling, and, frequently, ecchymosis are the hallmarks of this condition.

A history of the ankle "giving way" suggests a diagnosis of ankle instability. Patients with this history often report pain only when the ankle gives way and not at other times. On the other hand, patients with chronic ankle pain, which commonly occurs at the anterolateral aspect of the ankle, may have constant low-grade pain. Chronic pain and swelling on the posterolateral aspect of the ankle are consistent with injury to the peroneal tendons. An occult fracture (osteochondral lesion) of the ankle joint may present with diffuse ankle pain and an intra-articular effusion. Subtalar synovitis or arthritis also may present in a similar fashion.

Arthritis of the ankle is most often secondary to previous trauma. Rheumatoid arthritis may also affect the ankle. Tarsal tunnel syndrome may cause chronic medial ankle pain but almost always is associated with neurologic symptoms and pain that radiates into the plantar aspect of the foot.

Musculoskeletal Conditioning of the Foot and Ankle

A conditioning program consists of three basic phases: strengthening exercises, to improve muscle power; stretching exercises, to improve range of motion; and proprioception, to enhance balance and agility. In addition, the exercise session should begin with an active warm-up, and plyometric exercises may be added for power after basic strength and flexibility have been achieved. Patient handouts are provided here and on the DVD for the strengthening and stretching exercises. Advanced proprioceptive exercises and plyometric exercises should be done under the supervision of a rehabilitation specialist or other exercise professional.

The goal of a conditioning program is to enable people to live a fit and healthier lifestyle by being more active. A well-structured conditioning program also will prepare the individual for participation in sports and recreational activities. The greater the intensity of the activity that the individual wishes to engage in, the greater the intensity of the conditioning that will be required. If the individual participates in a supervised rehabilitation program that provides instruction in a conditioning routine—instead of using only an exercise handout such as provided here—the focus should be on developing and committing to a home exercise fitness program. A conditioning program for the body as a whole that includes exercises for the shoulder, hip, knee, and spine as well as the foot and ankle is described in Musculoskeletal Conditioning: Helping Patients Prevent Injury and Stay Fit, beginning on page 183.

The foot is the first part of the lower kinetic chain to hit the ground during weight-bearing activities and is therefore the first input to the neuromuscular system of the lower kinetic chain. Dynamic joint stability is critical for injury prevention and improved performance during sports activities. Whether an individual experiences a single-episode lateral ankle sprain or develops chronic ankle instability most likely depends on rehabilitation of the individual's proprioception.

Strengthening Exercises

Strengthening exercises for the foot and ankle include calf raises, ankle dorsiflexion/plantar flexion, and ankle inversion/eversion exercises.

Stretching Exercises

Perform stretching to maintain or increase flexibility. Heel cord stretches performed with the knee both straight and bent are good stretching exercises for the gastrocnemius-soleus muscle complex.

Toe Strengthening Exercises

The toe strengthening program is helpful for patients with the particular conditions listed, including bunions, hammer toes, plantar fasciitis, and toe cramps.

Proprioceptive Exercises

Optimizing the proprioceptive system is important in preventing injuries such as ankle sprains in both athletes and nonathletes. Balance, or postural control, is the result of the integration of visual, vestibular, and proprioceptive afferent inputs. The goal of proprioceptive training is to enhance the activity of the proprioceptors, thereby improving their ability to protect the ligaments of the foot and ankle. Several commercial devices, such as tiltboards and proprioceptive disks, are available for proprioceptive training. Perturbation training is another way to optimize the proprioceptive system, especially in athletes. Perturbation exercises are performed on an unstable surface with perturbing forces applied in all directions. Perturbation training and advanced balance training should be performed under the supervision of a rehabilitation specialist or other exercise professional.

Plyometrics

Explosive power is necessary for a high level of athletic performance. Plyometrics facilitate the development of power. Examples of plyometric exercises are jumping rope and jumping from side to side over a 6-inch-high barrier. More advanced exercises should be performed under the supervision of a rehabilitation specialist or other trained exercise professional.

Home Exercise Program for Foot and Ankle Conditioning

- Performing active warm-up exercises prior to athletic activities is important for optimal neuromuscular control and for maintaining normal range of motion.

- Before beginning the conditioning program, warm up the muscles of the lower extremities by riding a stationary bicycle or jogging for 10 minutes and performing leg swings as follows: While standing, swing one leg forward/backward 10 times and then side-to-side 10 times. Repeat with the opposite leg. Place one hand against a wall for balance if needed.

- Perform the exercises indefinitely or as directed by your physician. Contact your physician if the exercises cause pain.

Strengthening and Stretching Exercises for the Foot and Ankle

Exercise	Muscle Group	Number of Repetitions/Sets	Number of Days per Week
Strengthening			
Calf raises	Gastrocnemius-soleus complex	10 repetitions/3 sets	3
Ankle dorsiflexion/plantar flexion	Anterior tibialis Gastrocnemius-soleus complex	10 repetitions/3 sets	3
Ankle eversion/inversion	Posterior tibialis Peroneus longus and peroneus brevis	10 repetitions/3 sets	3
Stretching			
Heel cord stretch	Knee straight: Gastrocnemius Knee bent: Soleus	4 to 5 repetitions/ 2 to 3 sets	Daily

Toe Strengthening Program

Exercise	Recommended For	Repetitions or Duration	Number of Days Per Week
Toe squeeze	Hammer toes, toe cramps	10 repetitions	Daily
Big toe pulls	Bunions, toe cramps	10 repetitions	Daily
Toe pulls	Bunions, hammer toes, toe cramps	10 repetitions	Daily
Golf ball roll	Plantar fasciitis, arch strain, foot cramps	2 minutes	Daily
Marble pickup	Pain in ball of foot, hammer toes, toe cramps	Until all marbles have been picked up	Daily
Towel curls	Hammer toes, toe cramps, pain in ball of foot	5 repetitions	Daily

Strengthening Exercises

Calf Raises

- Stand with your weight evenly distributed over both feet. Hold onto the back of a chair or the wall for balance.
- Lift one foot so that all your weight is on the other foot.
- Then lift the heel off the floor as high as you can.
- Repeat on the other side.
- Work up to 3 sets of 10 repetitions.
- Perform the exercise 3 days per week.

Ankle Dorsiflexion/Plantar Flexion

- Find a position where your weight is off your feet, such as lying on a bed or on the floor with your legs straight out in front of you.
- For dorsiflexion, wrap an elastic band or tubing around your foot and anchor the other end to a door or bedpost or have someone hold it. Pull your toes toward you; then return slowly to the starting position. Repeat 10 to 15 times.
- For plantar flexion, wrap an elastic band or tubing around your foot and hold the other end in your hand. Gently point your toes; then return slowly to the starting position. Repeat 10 to 15 times.
- Perform 3 sets of 10 repetitions; 3 days per week.

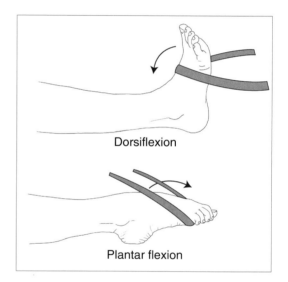

Dorsiflexion

Plantar flexion

Ankle Eversion/Inversion

- Find a position where your weight is off your feet, such as lying on a bed or on the floor with your legs straight out in front of you.
- For inversion, wrap an elastic band or tube around the inside of your foot and anchor the other end to a door or bedpost or have someone hold it. Pull your foot inward against the resistance; then return slowly to the starting position. Repeat 10 to 15 times.
- For eversion, wrap an elastic band or tube around the inside of your foot and anchor the other end to a door or bedpost or have someone hold it. Pull your foot outward against the resistance; then return slowly to the starting position. Repeat 10 to 15 times.

Strengthening Exercises

Heel Cord Stretch

- Support yourself against a wall with your feet pointed straight ahead.
  Stretch with knee straight: Keeping the heel in contact with the ground and the knee straight, place the foot as far back as possible until a stretch is felt in the calf.
  Stretch with knee flexed: Same position but bend the knee of the leg being stretched.
- Hold the stretch for 30 seconds; then relax for 30 seconds.
- Repeat on the other side.
- Perform 2 to 3 sets of 4 to 5 repetitions of each exercise daily.

Toe Strengthening Exercises

Toe Squeeze

- Place small sponges or corks between the toes.
- Squeeze and hold for 5 seconds.
- Repeat 10 times.

Big Toe Pulls

- Place a thick rubber band around both big toes and pull the big toes away from each other and toward the small toes.
- Hold for 5 seconds.
- Repeat 10 times.

SECTION 7 FOOT AND ANKLE

Toe Pulls

- Put a thick rubber band around all your toes and spread them.
- Hold this position for 5 seconds.
- Repeat 10 times.

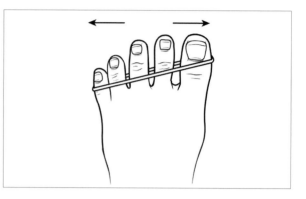

Golf Ball Roll

- Roll a golf ball under the ball of your foot for 2 minutes to massage the bottom of the foot.

Marble Pickup

- Place 20 marbles on the floor. Pick up one marble at a time and put it in a small bowl.
- Repeat until you have picked up all 20 marbles.

Towel Curls

- Place a small towel on the floor and curl it toward you, using only your toes. You can increase the resistance by putting weight on the end of the towel.
- Relax and repeat 5 times.

Physical Examination of the Foot and Ankle

INSPECTION/PALPATION

Anterior View, Standing

Observe the anterior aspect of both feet. Inspect the foot and ankle from the front. Observe the alignment of the great and lesser toes, the position of the foot in relation to the limb, and the medial curvature of the forefoot (metatarsus adductus).

Medial View

Observe the medial aspect of both feet. Inspect for a high arch (cavus foot), flatfoot posture (pes planus), or undue prominence of the medial midfoot (accessory navicular). The arches of both feet should be symmetric.

Lateral View

Observe the lateral aspect of both feet. Inspect for callosities, ankle swelling, or prominence of the posterior calcaneus.

Posterior View

Observe the posterior aspect of both feet. Assess heel alignment. Normal alignment is neutral or slight valgus (turned-out heel), with no more than one or two lateral toes visible from behind. A patient with an acquired flatfoot from posterior tibial tendon dysfunction will have increased valgus of the calcaneus and more than two visible toes ("too many toes" sign). A varus calcaneus (turned-in heel) occurs with a cavus foot.

Standing on Toes

With the patient standing on the toes, look to see that the heels move into a normal varus (inward) position. A patient with an acquired flatfoot secondary to posterior tibial tendon dysfunction will not be able to rise up on the toes of the affected foot.

Gait

Gait is best observed with the patient barefoot. Have the patient walk across the room as you observe from the side. Look for deviations from normal while the patient walks. Normal gait demonstrates equal stride length, foot position, and weight distribution. At heel strike, the heel everts and the ankle plantar flexes. The weight transfers along the lateral side of the foot. Pronation occurs in the foot with dorsiflexion of the ankle and internal rotation at the leg, knee, and hip. As the body and leg move forward, supination begins with plantar flexion of the ankle.

Analyze alignment of the foot during the different phases of gait. These phases include heel strike, midstance, toe-off, and swing phase. Look for obvious limp, lurch, dragging of the feet, intoeing, outtoeing, and drop-foot gait.

Angle of Gait

Assess the angle of gait, which is the angle of the foot in relation to the axis of the limb when the patient is walking, to identify problems of intoeing and outtoeing. When walking, the foot is normally positioned in 0° to 20° of external rotation. Because tibial torsion is typically asymmetric, one foot is normally positioned in more external rotation.

SECTION 7   FOOT AND ANKLE

SECTION 7   FOOT AND ANKLE

is extended
flexed, con
Charcot-M
involved, a
langeal joi
Inspect the
ingrown to

Kleiger Test (External Rotation Test)

With the patient seated and the knee flexed approximately 90° and the ankle relaxed, use one hand to grasp and stabilize the leg from behind, making sure not to compress the fibula and tibia together. Use your other hand to fully dorsiflex the ankle and then externally rotate the foot. If this causes pain, determine the specific location of the pain. Pain over the location of the anterior inferior tibiofibular ligament is indicative of a syndesmosis sprain. Depending on the severity, the interosseous membrane may be involved, and pain may be radiated further up between the distal fibula and tibia. This test is also sensitive for fractures of the fibula.

Spread To

Ask the pat
the toes as
Look for co
between the
actively spr
indicate los
function. Be
cious lesion
occur in the

Thompson Test

With the patient prone and relaxed, use your fingers and thumb to squeeze the medial and lateral aspect of the mid calf together. If the foot does not plantar flex, the test is positive for an Achilles tendon rupture.

Eversion Stress Test

The eversion stress test evaluates the integrity of the deltoid ligament. With the patient seated and the knee flexed approximately 90°, place the ankle in neutral. Use one hand to stabilize the lateral aspect of the leg just above the lateral malleolus (**A**). Place your other hand somewhat inferomedial on the calcaneus and evert the hindfoot. Pain over the deltoid ligament and increased eversion as compared to the uninvolved side indicates possible injury to the mid portion of the deltoid or a possible avulsion fracture of the medial malleolus. This test should be repeated while holding the ankle in full dorsiflexion (**B**) to evaluate the posterior aspect of the deltoid and then repeated again in plantarflexion to evaluate the anterior aspect of the deltoid ligament. When performing this test, always compare the affected ankle with the opposite side.

Inversion Stress Test

The inversion stress test evaluates laxity of the calcanofibular ligament. With the patient seated and the knee flexed approximately 90°, use one hand to stabilize the medial aspect of the leg just above the medial malleolus. Place your other hand somewhat inferolateral on the calcaneus (**A**) and invert the hindfoot (**B**). An end point should normally be appreciated upon reaching full inversion, and absence of one indicates moderate to severe injury to the calcanofibular ligament. Excessive or asymmetric motion will occur with chronic laxity of the calcanofibular ligament. When performing this test, always compare the affected ankle with the opposite side. If the patient has pain during this test, the results may be unreliable.

Sensitivity Test

Use a 0.10-g (5.07-mm) filament to identify protective sensation in a patient with diabetes mellitus.

Achilles Tendon Tear

Synonyms

Heel cord rupture

Tendoachilles rupture

Definition

Disruption of the Achilles tendon (heel cord) usually occurs 5 to 7 cm proximal to the insertion of the tendon on the calcaneus. This condition commonly affects middle-aged men who play quick, stop-and-go sports such as tennis and basketball. Partial tears of the tendon can also occur at the calcaneal insertion.

Clinical Symptoms

The sudden, severe calf pain typically is described as a "gunshot wound" or as a "direct hit from a racquet." Partial tears can be described as strains or a "calf pull." The severe acute pain may resolve quickly, and the injury may be misdiagnosed as an ankle sprain. When the rupture is missed, significant weakness develops, impairing ambulation.

Tests

Physical Examination

Swelling in the lower calf is common. The patient often has difficulty bearing weight and often has a palpable defect in the tendon. With the patient lying prone and the foot hanging off the edge of the table, the foot with a ruptured Achilles tendon will rest at a 90° angle to the tibia, whereas a foot with an intact Achilles tendon will rest in slight plantar flexion because of the resting tension in the tendon. Perform the Thompson test (see page 754) by placing the patient prone with the knee and ankle at 90°. The test also can be done with the patient kneeling on a chair. Squeezing the calf normally results in passive plantar flexion of the ankle; a positive test result is the absence of plantar flexion. The Thompson test is most reliable within 48 hours of the rupture.

Diagnostic Tests

None usually are needed.

Differential Diagnosis

- Achilles tendinitis or tendinosis (thick, tender Achilles tendon or crepitus may be noted on palpation)
- Deep vein thrombosis (no history of injury, negative Thompson test)
- Medial gastrocnemius tear (pain on palpation over the medial head of the gastrocnemius-soleus complex)
- Plantaris rupture (pain but little loss of function)
- Stress fracture of the tibia (constant pain over a localized area of the tibia)

Adverse Outcomes of the Disease

Weakness during the stance phase of gait and decreased athletic function are possible. Patients note that when they are walking, they feel as if they are on soft sand.

Treatment

Nonsurgical treatment consists of a program of gradual casting or bracing in plantar flexion with subsequent casting in a lesser degree of plantar flexion until the foot reaches a neutral position. Surgical repair typically requires a brief period of immobilization as well to allow the wound to heal. The surgeon may elect to use a tapered heel lift for several weeks following the immobilization. Rehabilitation may be necessary if full range of motion and balance are not attained by 6 months after surgery, but by this time almost all patients attain full range of motion, especially dorsiflexion. The decision whether to treat the patient surgically or nonsurgically is based on the degree of tendon retraction as well as the patient's activity level, age, medical condition, and surgical risk. When either treatment is delayed beyond a few days, Achilles tendon rupture becomes significantly more complicated to treat because retraction of the proximal muscle widens the gap. Whatever treatment modality is selected, a progressive strength and conditioning program is recommended during the rehabilitation phase, followed by a gradual return to sports.

Rehabilitation Prescription

An Achilles tendon rupture can be very painful and debilitating. The type of rehabilitation depends on the extent of the tendon tear. For both severe and minor tears, pain-free immobilization and rest, ice, compression, and elevation (RICE) are indicated for the first 5 or 6 days postinjury. Use of crutches is also helpful to prevent further injury. The home exercise program for minor tears (see page 760) may be started on day 7. Minor tears usually do well with gentle active mobilization. Stretching may be initiated on day 14. The stretch should be pain free. If the patient has difficulty achieving pain-free ankle range of motion, formal rehabilitation may be ordered. The prescription should include an evaluation of the mobility of the tendon, the ankle, and the subtalar and midtarsal joints. The therapist should be careful to respect the stage of soft-tissue healing.

Adverse Outcomes of Treatment

Surgical risks include infection and wound problems such as delayed healing. A second rupture may occur with either type of treatment but is more common after nonsurgical treatment.

Referral Decisions/Red Flags

A history of a sudden pop with pain and swelling in the calf indicates probable rupture of the Achilles tendon and the need for further evaluation within 24 hours.

Home Exercise Program for Achilles Tendinosis or Tendinitis

- Begin gentle ankle range of motion on day 7 after the injury.
- Add the towel stretch, heel cord stretch, and calf raises on day 14 after the injury. Before stretching, warm up the tissues by applying moist heat or riding a stationary bicycle for 10 minutes.
- To prevent inflammation, apply a bag of crushed ice or frozen peas to the heel for 20 minutes after exercising.
- You should not experience pain with the exercises. If you are unable to perform the exercises because of pain or stiffness, or if your symptoms do not improve in 3 to 4 weeks, call your doctor.

Exercise	Muscle Group	Number of Repetitions/Sets	Number of Days per Week	Number of Weeks
Ankle range of motion	Dorsiflexors Plantar flexors Invertors Evertors	2 sets	Daily	2 to 3
Towel stretch	Gastrocnemius-soleus complex	4 repetitions/2 or 3 sets	Daily	3 to 4
Heel cord stretch	Gastrocnemius-soleus complex	4 repetitions/2 or 3 sets	Daily	3 to 4
Calf raises	Gastrocnemius-soleus complex	10 repetitions/2 or 3 sets	Daily	3 to 4

Ankle Range of Motion

- Sit on a chair or the edge of a bed so your feet don't touch the floor.
- Leading with the big toe, write each letter of the alphabet in the air. Keep your knee flexed.
- Perform 2 sets daily, for 2 to 3 weeks.

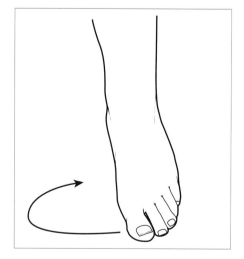

Towel Stretch

- Sit on the floor with your injured leg straight.
- Loop a towel around the ball of your foot.
- Grasp the ends of the towel and pull toward you, keeping the knee straight.
- Hold this stretch for 30 seconds and then relax for 30 seconds. Repeat 3 times.
- Perform this exercise 2 or 3 times per day, 6 or 7 days per week, for 3 to 4 weeks.

Heel Cord Stretch

- Stand facing a wall with the knee of the unaffected limb bent for support, the affected limb straight, and the toes pointed in slightly.
- Keeping the heels of both feet flat on the floor, lower your hips toward the wall.
- Hold this stretch for 30 seconds and then relax for 30 seconds. Repeat 4 times.
- Perform this exercise 2 or 3 times per day, 6 or 7 days per week, for 3 to 4 weeks.

Calf Raises

- Stand on a flat surface with your weight evenly distributed over both feet.
- Hold the back of a chair or place your hands against a wall for balance.
- Raise the heel of your uninjured leg off the floor as high as you can, using your body weight as resistance. Repeat 10 times.
- Perform 2 or 3 sets daily for 3 to 4 weeks.

Ankle Sprain

ICD-9 Codes

845.00
Sprains and strains of ankle and foot, ankle, unspecified site

845.01
Sprains and strains of ankle and foot, deltoid (ligament), ankle

845.02
Sprains and strains of ankle and foot, calcaneofibular (ligament)

845.03
Sprains and strains of ankle and foot, tibiofibular (ligament), distal

Synonyms

Inversion injury

Lateral collateral ligament tear of the ankle

Definition

More than 25,000 ankle sprains occur every day in the United States. Ankle sprains are not always simple injuries. Residual symptoms occur in up to 40% of patients.

The lateral ligaments (anterior talofibular and calcaneofibular) are the only structures injured in most ankle sprains, but other ligament tears may occur with an inversion injury (**Figure 1**). Additional injury to the anterior tibiofibular syndesmosis, the thick ligaments connecting the distal tibia and fibula, also may occur. This combined injury, referred to as a "high" ankle sprain, increases recovery time. Injury to the subtalar joint is commonly associated with a severe ankle sprain. The most common injury to the subtalar joint after an inversion injury is a tear of one of the interosseous ligaments. Associated injuries to the medial deltoid ligament also occur but are less common.

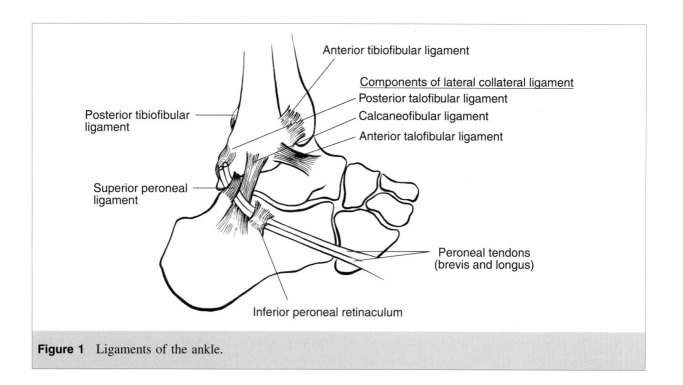

Figure 1 Ligaments of the ankle.

Clinical Symptoms

Pain over the injured ligaments, swelling, and loss of function are common. A severe sprain is more common in patients who report feeling a pop, followed by immediate swelling and the inability to walk. Determine whether the patient has a history of ankle sprains and giving way to identify whether an acute injury is superimposed on chronic ankle instability.

Tests

Physical Examination

Examination often reveals ecchymosis and swelling around the entire ankle joint, not just the lateral side. Tenderness on palpation over the anterior talofibular and calcaneofibular ligaments can help identify which ligaments are injured. Palpate the lateral and medial malleoli and the base of the fifth metatarsal; crepitus or tenderness suggests a fracture.

Injury to the tibiofibular syndesmosis is suggested by two tests: the squeeze test (**Figure 2**) and the external rotation test. The squeeze test is performed by compressing the tibia and fibula at midcalf. The external rotation test is performed by placing the ankle in dorsiflexion and then externally rotating the foot. A positive result is the presence of pain over the distal tibiofibular syndesmosis.

After an injury to the subtalar joint, tenderness over the sinus tarsi is present; ecchymosis also may be observed on the medial aspect of the heel.

Diagnostic Tests

When tenderness is present over the distal fibula, ankle joint, tibiofibular syndesmosis, or other bony structure, radiographs of the ankle and/or foot are needed to rule out a fracture or syndesmosis disruption. Radiographs also are indicated when the patient has marked swelling and cannot bear weight on the affected extremity. The Ottawa ankle rules provide a guideline on when to obtain radiographs of the ankle.

Figure 2 The squeeze test for injury to the tibiofibular syndesmosis. Pain over the distal tibiofibular syndesmosis when the examiner squeezes the tibia and fibula at midcalf is a positive result.

SECTION 7 FOOT AND ANKLE

Differential Diagnosis

- Fracture of the calcaneus, talus, lateral malleolus, or base of the fifth metatarsal (focal tenderness over the fractured anatomic structure, evident on radiographs)
- Fracture of the lateral process of the talus (focal tenderness, swelling below the fibula)
- Fracture of the proximal fibula (Maisonneuve fracture associated with tear of deltoid and disruption of syndesmotic ligament) (focal tenderness, crepitus over the proximal fibula)

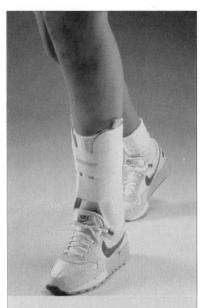

Figure 3 An air stirrup–type ankle brace.

- Osteochondral fracture of the talar dome (evident on ankle radiographs, bone scan, or MRI)
- Peroneal tendon tear or subluxation (retrofibular tenderness and swelling)

Adverse Outcomes of the Disease

An untreated severe sprain may result in chronic pain, instability, and the possibility of ankle arthritis. Chronic pain may result from subtalar stiffness. Chronic instability is most common after incomplete rehabilitation.

Treatment

The goal of treatment is to prevent chronic pain and instability. A three-phase treatment program is recommended.

Phase 1 consists of NSAIDs, rest, ice, compression, and elevation (RICE). The use of a functional ankle brace or air stirrup is indicated for protection and to promote soft-tissue healing (**Figure 3**). Encourage weight bearing as tolerated, with crutch use as needed. For severe sprains or sprains in children, the use of a cast or cast boot for 2 to 3 weeks may facilitate walking and healing.

Phase 2 begins when the patient can bear weight without increased pain or swelling, usually 2 to 4 weeks after the injury. Continue use of the air stirrup or functional ankle brace. Begin exercises to increase peroneal and dorsiflexor strength; also, the Achilles tendon should be stretched. Continue this phase until the patient has full range of motion and 80% of normal ankle strength. Plantar flexion exercises are not included in the exercise program because they place the ankle in a position of minimal stability.

Phase 3 usually begins 4 to 6 weeks after injury. This phase of functional conditioning includes proprioception, agility, and endurance training. Exercises that are helpful for proprioception include standing on the sprained ankle with the opposite foot elevated and the eyes closed. Balance boards are very useful during this phase of treatment. Running in progressively smaller figures-of-8 is excellent for agility and peroneal strength. During this time, the patient should be weaned from the air stirrup or functional ankle brace.

This three-phase treatment program may take only 2 weeks to complete for minor sprains, or up to 6 to 8 weeks for severe injuries. For athletes with moderate to severe sprains who are returning to sports, the use of a functional ankle brace or air stirrup, or taping on a long-term basis, will help prevent recurrent injury. The use of a brace is particularly indicated for athletes in sports associated with a high risk for ankle sprains such as basketball, volleyball, and soccer. Long-term exercises should include peroneal strengthening in both dorsiflexion and plantar flexion, as well as continued Achilles tendon stretching.

Rehabilitation Prescription

The most important part of early rehabilitation is to control the inflammation with RICE for the first 5 or 6 days postinjury. Use of crutches during this same period can be helpful to control further damage to the healing ligament. Early mobilization of the ankle can begin as part of a home program of active pain-free exercises beginning on day 7 (see page 766). If the patient continues to have pain and limited mobility of the ankle after 2 to 3 weeks on a home exercise program, formal rehabilitation may be ordered. The prescription should include an evaluation by the rehabilitation specialist to determine the mobility of the ankle and subtalar joints. Strengthening exercises combined with balance training may be initiated at the rehabilitation specialist's discretion.

Adverse Outcomes of Treatment

Casting and ankle immobilization for more than 3 weeks may cause stiffness and a slower return to normal activity. Incomplete rehabilitation is the most common cause of chronic instability after an ankle sprain. Subtalar stiffness may result in persistent anterolateral pain.

Referral Decisions/Red Flags

Fractures of the foot and ankle, tears or subluxation of the peroneal tendons, nerve injury, a history of repeated giving way (chronic instability), and failure to improve in 6 weeks with appropriate treatment all indicate serious injury and the need for further evaluation.

Home Exercise Program for Ankle Sprain

- To prevent inflammation, apply a bag of crushed ice or frozen peas to the ankle for 20 minutes after performing the exercises.

- You should not experience pain with the exercises.

- If you continue to experience pain or limited mobility of the ankle after performing the exercises for 2 to 3 weeks, call your doctor.

Exercise	Muscle Group	Number of Repetitions/Sets	Number of Days per Week	Number of Weeks
Ankle range of motion	Dorsiflexors Plantar flexors Invertors Evertors	2 sets	Daily	3 to 4
Ankle dorsiflexion/ plantar flexion	Anterior tibialis Gastrocnemius-soleus complex	10 to 15 repetitions/3 sets	Daily	3 to 4
Ankle eversion/ inversion	Posterior tibialis Peroneus longus and peroneus brevis	25 repetitions/3 sets, progressing to 45 repetitions/3 sets	Daily	3 to 4

Ankle Range of Motion

- Sit on a chair or the edge of a bed so your feet do not touch the floor.

- Leading with the big toe, write each letter of the alphabet in the air. Keep your knee flexed.

- Perform 2 sets daily, for 3 to 4 weeks.

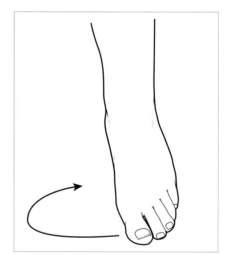

Ankle Dorsiflexion/Plantar Flexion

- Find a position where your weight is off your feet, such as lying on a bed or on the floor with your legs straight out in front of you.

- For dorsiflexion, wrap an elastic band or tubing around your foot and anchor the other end to a door or bedpost or have someone hold it. Pull your toes toward you; then return slowly to the starting position. Repeat 10 to 15 times.

- For plantar flexion, wrap an elastic band or tubing around your foot and hold the other end in your hand. Gently point your toes; then return slowly to the starting position. Repeat 10 to 15 times.

- Perform 2 to 3 sets daily, for 3 to 4 weeks.

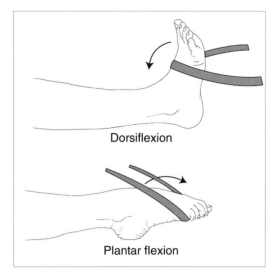

Dorsiflexion

Plantar flexion

Ankle Eversion/Inversion

- Find a position where your weight is off your feet, such as lying on a bed or on the floor with your legs straight out in front of you.

- For inversion, wrap an elastic band or tube around the inside of your foot and anchor the other end to a door or bedpost or have someone hold it. Pull your foot inward against the resistance; then return slowly to the starting position. Repeat 10 to 15 times.

- For eversion, wrap an elastic band or tube around the inside of your foot and anchor the other end to a door or bedpost or have someone hold it. Pull your foot outward against the resistance; then return slowly to the starting position. Repeat 10 to 15 times.

- Perform 2 to 3 sets daily, for 3 to 4 weeks.

SECTION 7 FOOT AND ANKLE

Arthritis of the Foot and Ankle

Synonyms

Osteoarthritis

Posttraumatic arthritis

Definition

The most common types of arthritis of the foot and ankle are osteoarthritis (degenerative arthritis) and posttraumatic arthritis. Frequent locations of arthritis in the foot and ankle are the first metatarsophalangeal (MTP) joint (MTP joint of the great toe), the midfoot (tarsometatarsal joint), the talonavicular joint, the subtalar (talocalcaneal) joint, and the ankle (talonavicular) joint (**Figure 1**).

Clinical Symptoms

Patients with arthritis of the first MTP joint report pain, loss of dorsiflexion, and swelling of the great toe joint (see page 816).

Figure 1 Common sites of foot and ankle arthritis. C = calcaneus, T = tibia, Ta = talus, M = metatarsal, MTP = metatarsophalangeal.

Midfoot osteoarthritis commonly occurs in older patients and also after a Lisfranc (tarsometatarsal) dislocation. The patient usually reports diffuse aching in the midfoot that worsens with prolonged walking or standing as well as difficulty pushing off with the foot.

Talonavicular arthritis causes focal pain over the joint (medial aspect of the hindfoot). This is a common site for rheumatoid arthritis.

Subtalar arthritis produces pain over the subtalar joint and frequently follows calcaneal fractures. Difficulty walking on uneven surfaces (such as sand or rocky terrain) results because the motion of this joint primarily involves inversion and eversion of the foot.

Most patients with ankle arthritis have a history of trauma. Pain, swelling, and stiffness in the anterior ankle are common symptoms. Patients with ankle arthritis have difficulty flexing and extending the ankle and therefore tend to walk with the leg externally rotated.

Tests

Physical Examination

With hallux rigidus, loss of motion in the first MTP joint and difficulty pushing off with the great toe are common. In patients with midfoot arthritis, palpation reveals tenderness and often a dorsal bump on the midfoot. Patients with talonavicular or subtalar arthritis may show a loss of inversion and eversion of the hindfoot compared with the opposite foot; however, ankle joint motion is relatively normal. Patients with ankle joint arthritis have swelling and loss of ankle motion, and they often walk with the leg externally rotated.

Diagnostic Tests

Weight-bearing radiographs reveal the typical signs of degenerative or posttraumatic arthritis, including osteophytes (spurs) and joint space narrowing. The first MTP joint usually shows dorsal osteophytes protruding from the metatarsal head. In midfoot arthritis, joint space narrowing is especially evident at the second tarsometatarsal joint (**Figure 2**). Talonavicular arthritis is best viewed on an AP radiograph of the foot. With subtalar arthritis, the lateral view of the foot reveals loss of the normal talocalcaneal joint space. Ankle joint arthritis usually causes loss of joint space, which can be seen on both AP (**Figure 3**) and lateral ankle views, as well as spur formation anteriorly and posteriorly.

When the extent of arthritis is uncertain, CT can be helpful, especially in the midfoot, where the bony anatomy is sometimes difficult to view on plain radiographs.

Figure 2 AP view shows primary degenerative arthritis of the midfoot. Note the joint space narrowing at the second tarsometatarsal joint (arrow). (Reproduced from Beaman DN, Saltzman CL: Arthritis of the midfoot, in Mizel MS, Miller RA, Scioli MW, eds: *Orthopaedic Knowledge Update: Foot and Ankle*, ed 2. Rosemont, IL, American Academy of Orthopaedic Surgeons, 1998, p 294.)

Figure 3 AP view of ankle showing ankle arthritis with asymmetric loss of joint space (arrows).

Differential Diagnosis

- Charcot arthropathy (history of diabetes mellitus, swelling that is disproportionate to symptoms)
- Gout (redness and swelling)
- Tendinitis (normal radiographs)

Adverse Outcomes of the Disease

Pain and difficulty with ambulation are common with untreated foot and ankle arthritis.

Treatment

Initial therapy consists of shoe modifications, orthotic inserts, and NSAIDs.

A stiff-soled shoe with a rocker bottom will help relieve symptoms in patients with hallux rigidus.

Midfoot arthritis can be treated nonsurgically with a rigid custom orthotic insert or a steel shank inserted into the sole of the shoe. Patients with refractory symptoms will benefit from a surgical midfoot fusion.

Symptoms of talonavicular and subtalar arthritis can be improved with a medial longitudinal arch support or the more rigid UCBL (University of California Biomechanics Laboratory) orthoses. Corticosteroid injections and NSAIDs may be helpful. Predictable pain relief can be obtained with subtalar arthrodesis (fusion), which retains ankle motion.

Ankle arthritis is treated initially with a custom-molded ankle-foot orthosis and NSAIDs. Injection of a corticosteroid also may be beneficial (see page 771). In mild to moderate cases, débridement of the joint may defer the need for fusion. Ankle arthrodesis will benefit patients with refractory symptoms. An ankle fused in a neutral position functions well, and the function of the surrounding joints is preserved. Ankle replacement surgery has shown great promise in patients with appropriate indications.

Adverse Outcomes of Treatment

Infection, nonunion, and persistent pain may occur after foot and ankle fusions.

Referral Decisions/Red Flags

Persistent and disabling pain requires further evaluation. Chronic symptoms can be relieved by surgical débridement or fusion.

Procedure: Ankle Joint Injection

Step 1
Wear protective gloves at all times during this procedure and use sterile technique.

Step 2
Cleanse the skin with a bactericidal skin preparation.

Step 3
Palpate the soft spot over the ankle joint just medial to the anterior tibial tendon (**Figure 1**). Using a 3-mL syringe with a 22-gauge needle, inject 2 mL of the 1% lidocaine anesthetic into the subcutaneous tissue of the soft spot.

Step 4
Advance the needle into the joint by directing it slightly laterally and superiorly. Inject the last 1 mL of the 1% lidocaine anesthetic. If the needle is in the joint, injection of the fluid meets no resistance. Leave the needle in place and exchange the syringe.

Materials
- Sterile gloves
- Bactericidal skin preparation solution
- Two 3-mL syringes
- One 22-gauge needle
- 3 mL of 1% lidocaine
- 1 mL of 40 mg/mL corticosteroid preparation without epinephrine
- Sterile adhesive dressing

Fibula
Tibia
Medial malleolus
Anterior tibial tendon
Talus

Figure 1 Proper location for ankle joint injection.

Step 5
Inject 1 mL of 40 mg/mL depocorticosteroid preparation. Injection of the fluid should meet no resistance. Withdraw the needle.

Step 6
Dress the puncture site with a sterile adhesive dressing.

Adverse Outcomes
Injury to the distal branch of the saphenous nerve is possible. Slow atrophy at the site of the injection is possible secondary to subcutaneous steroid deposition.

Aftercare/Patient Instructions
Remind the patient that one third of patients experience a flare-up of symptoms, with increased joint pain for 1 to 2 days. NSAIDs or analgesics may be given during this period. Ice may be helpful for the first 24 hours.

Bunionette

Synonym

Tailor's bunion

ICD-9 Code

727.1
Bunion

Definition

A bunionette, sometimes referred to as a tailor's bunion, is a deformity of the fifth metatarsophalangeal (MTP) joint that is analogous to a bunion (hallux valgus) deformity of the great toe. A bunionette is characterized by prominence of the lateral aspect of the fifth metatarsal head and medial deviation of the small toe. A bunionette is associated with frequent wearing of tight, narrow, pointed-toe shoes.

Clinical Symptoms

Patients report pain and problems finding comfortable shoes.

Tests

Physical Examination

Deformity is evident on physical examination. An overlying hard corn is frequently present.

Diagnostic Tests

Weight-bearing AP radiographs will show medial deviation of the fifth proximal phalanx and lateral deviation of the fifth metatarsal shaft and/or a prominence on the lateral aspect of the fifth metatarsal head (**Figure 1**). The joint usually is normal.

Differential Diagnosis

- Cavovarus foot deformity (excessive weight bearing on the lateral side of the foot and pain over the fifth metatarsal noted on physical examination)
- Inflammatory arthropathy (painful, swollen fifth MTP joint with deviation of the small toe often noted)

Adverse Outcomes of the Disease

The most common problem is persistent pain aggravated by shoe wear. Patients also may have associated hard and soft corns, with possible ulceration and infection.

Figure 1   Typical deformities associated with a bunionette. (Reproduced from Coughlin MJ: Etiology and treatment of the bunionette deformity. *Instr Course Lect* 1990;39:37-48.)

Treatment

Patients should be advised to select proper shoes with a soft upper and a roomy toe box. A shoe repair shop can stretch the shoe in the area over the bunionette. A modified metatarsal pad also can help shift pressure off the fifth metatarsal head. Pads can be applied to the lateral aspect of the toe box to float the painful fifth metatarsal head (see page 775). A medial longitudinal arch support can help a patient who has a flexible flatfoot. This orthotic device rotates the forefoot slightly, which decreases direct pressure over the bunionette prominence.

With continued symptoms, surgical excision of the bunionette or realignment osteotomy of the fifth metatarsal may be required.

Adverse Outcomes of Treatment

Pain may persist despite the application of a metatarsal pad. Surgical risks include persistent pain, infection, incomplete correction, painful surgical scar, and neuroma formation from injury to the cutaneous nerves in the surgical field.

Referral Decisions/Red Flags

Failure of nonsurgical treatment indicates the need for further evaluation.

Procedure: Application of a Metatarsal Pad

Step 1
Ask the patient to mark the painful spot on the bottom of the foot with a material that transfers easily, such as lipstick or eyeliner (**Figure 1A**). The mark should be approximately 0.5 cm².

Step 2
Instruct the patient to stand in a shoe without wearing a sock, to transfer the mark to the inside of the shoe.

Step 3
Place a metatarsal pad in the shoe about 5 mm proximal to (toward the heel), not directly under, the mark (**Figure 1B**). This ensures that the painful area is suspended by the proximally placed pad. Prefabricated, off-the-shelf felt or gel pads are easy to use, inexpensive, and effective, and they come in different sizes to accommodate different-size lesions and feet.

Materials
• Felt, silicone, or gel metatarsal pad
• Temporary marker (lipstick, eyeliner)

Figure 1 Application of a metatarsal pad. **A,** Marking the painful area. **B,** Proper placement of the metatarsal pad in the shoe.

Aftercare/Patient Instructions

If the pad is effective, continue the use of the pad and replace when worn. A custom-made orthosis also may be fabricated and can be transferred from shoe to shoe.

Chronic Lateral Ankle Pain

Definition

Chronic pain on the lateral aspect of the ankle is a common symptom that often follows an inversion injury. Several conditions may cause chronic lateral ankle pain after an inversion injury to the ankle, and they should be considered in the differential diagnosis.

Clinical Symptoms

Patients typically report pain on the lateral aspect of the ankle. Episodes of giving way and repeated sprains are typically associated with instability. Between sprains, however, the patient will have periods that are symptom free. In contrast, patients with a bone, cartilage, or tendon lesion often report constant, dull pain over the involved area.

ICD-9 Codes
715.17 Osteoarthritis, localized, primary, foot and ankle
715.27 Osteoarthritis, localized, secondary, ankle and foot
718.87 Ankle/foot instability
719.47 Pain in joint; foot and ankle
726.79 Peroneal tenosynovitis
727.06 Tenosynovitis and synovitis of foot and ankle

Tests

Physical Examination

Asking the patient to identify focal tenderness using one finger is the key element of the examination and can often identify the source of the problem. Identify any area of swelling. Range of motion should be assessed for both the ankle and subtalar joints. Assess laxity of the ankle and subtalar joints. Test sensation of the sural and superficial peroneal nerves.

Lidocaine injections can be very helpful in differentiating the source of a patient's symptoms. An intra-articular injection of 5 mL of 1% lidocaine into the ankle joint, for example, should provide transient pain relief in a patient with anterolateral impingement syndrome. Other common areas for differential injection include the subtalar joint and peroneal sheath.

Diagnostic Tests

AP, lateral, and mortise radiographs of the ankle joint are obtained for suspected ankle pathology. AP, lateral, and oblique radiographs of the foot are obtained for suspected foot pathology. If ankle or subtalar joint laxity is suspected, varus and anterior stress radiographs are helpful and should often include comparison stress views of the opposite, uninjured side. If the radiographs are normal and occult bony pathology is suspected, technetium Tc 99m bone scans, limited to AP and lateral views of both feet and ankles, will identify the lesion.

Although the bone scan is not specific, it is very sensitive and will detect most bony lesions, including occult fractures, arthritic changes, and tumors. If the bone scan is abnormal and an occult fracture is suspected, CT with thin cuts through the area in question should be diagnostic. If a soft-tissue or tendon injury is suspected (eg, tenosynovitis, a partial tear, or rupture of a tendon), MRI is appropriate. In these cases, the radiologist should be directed to the specific area of the tendon in question.

Differential Diagnosis

Anterolateral Impingement Syndrome of the Ankle

Anterolateral impingement of the talus with inversion (lateral gutter syndrome) occurs after an inversion ankle sprain. The borders of the lateral gutter of the ankle include the talus medially, the fibula laterally, and the tibia superiorly. Following a sprain, chronic scar tissue in the lateral gutter causes the anterolateral impingement. This condition is common in athletes, who often report pain and tenderness along the anterolateral aspect of the ankle. The pain is absent at rest and present with activities (especially dorsiflexion). These patients usually do not report buckling or giving way and do not show any signs of instability. Examination reveals tenderness and swelling along the anterior talofibular ligament and lateral gutter. Radiographs, MRIs, ^{99m}Tc bone scans, and CT scans appear normal, so this condition is often overlooked. An intra-articular injection of lidocaine will provide transient pain relief. Initial treatment should include an anti-inflammatory medication, rehabilitation, and possibly a steroid injection. Arthroscopic débridement of the lateral gutter provides definitive treatment.

Chronic Ankle/Subtalar Instability

Following an inversion sprain, chronic instability of the ankle and/or the subtalar joint may develop. These patients report frequent giving way and generalized weakness in the ankle and an inability to return to full sports or daily activities. The cause may be inadequate rehabilitation or inadequate healing, with subsequent attenuation of one or more ligaments. After a moderate to severe inversion injury, a patient will often lose proprioception, range of motion, and muscle strength. A mild contracture of the Achilles tendon also may develop. Six weeks of rehabilitation, directed specifically at increasing proprioception and range of motion, will often benefit these patients. The use of an ankle brace during sports activities also can be of significant benefit. If symptoms persist, further evaluation is required. The anterior drawer test (see page 752) and the varus stress test (see page 752) should be administered. Stress radiographs may be helpful. Surgical management options are reconstruction of the ligaments or checkrein tenodesis transfers.

Nerve Injury

Injury by direct blow, stretch, entrapment, or even transection of the superficial peroneal or sural nerves may be a cause of chronic lateral ankle pain. Repetitive stretching or nerve compression typically causes symptoms over the site of a fascial band or bony ridge. Patients report diffuse, dull, achy pain on the lateral aspect of the ankle, and burning, tingling, or radiating pain in the nerve distribution. Plantar flexion and inversion of the ankle and foot will often aggravate the symptoms. Focal tenderness and radiating paresthesias with percussion over the site of nerve injury (Tinel sign) is diagnostic. A more generalized neurologic examination should include an evaluation of the L4, L5, and S1 nerve roots to rule out a proximal nerve lesion. Electromyography and nerve conduction velocity studies often are not helpful in the diagnosis of superficial peroneal or sural nerve lesions. Many of these injuries resolve spontaneously, but some require surgical intervention.

Occult Bony Pathology

Routine radiographs identify most fractures in the foot and ankle, but osteochondral lesions of the talus, avulsion fractures of the calcaneus, lateral process fractures of the talus, and stress fractures of the fibula may not be obvious. A bone scan is an excellent initial study if these injuries are suspected. Once diagnosed, an occult bony lesion often can be treated with 4 to 6 weeks of immobilization. For persistent symptoms, excision of a loose bone fragment, arthroscopic débridement of an osteochondral lesion, or surgical fusion of an arthritic joint may be required.

Peroneal Tenosynovitis/Peroneal Tendon Subluxation

A common cause of chronic lateral ankle pain is tenosynovitis from a tear or subluxation of one of the peroneal tendons. The peroneus brevis is most commonly affected by a tear, usually just posterior to the tip of the fibula. Patients report chronic retromalleolar swelling, pain, and tenderness. Recurrent subluxation of the peroneal tendons over the lateral ridge of the fibula also may be associated with this condition. MRI is helpful in the evaluation of peroneal pathology. Simple tenosynovitis may be treated with cast immobilization for 4 to 6 weeks. A tear or chronic subluxation of the tendon, however, usually requires surgical treatment.

Subtalar Joint Arthritis

Early arthritis of the subtalar joint may be difficult to identify. These patients present with chronic lateral ankle pain that is aggravated by standing and walking, particularly on uneven terrain. Examination reveals limited inversion and eversion. Special radiographic views and/or diagnostic injections may be required to confirm early arthritis in this joint.

Subtalar Joint Synovitis/Subtalar Impingement Lesion

Similar to anterolateral impingement syndrome, subtalar joint synovitis/subtalar impingement lesion (STIL) is characterized by a chronic synovitis of the subtalar joint, often following an inversion injury. The interosseous ligaments of the ankle that insert on the floor of the sinus tarsi tear, creating thick scar tissue and impinging in the subtalar joint. Examination reveals focal pain over the lateral entrance to the sinus tarsi, which is the lateral entrance to the subtalar joint. Patients often have slight restriction and discomfort with passive subtalar motion. Diagnostic studies usually are normal, although MRI may detect chronic inflammation or fibrosis within the subtalar joint. The treatment is similar to that for anterolateral impingement syndrome. Surgical débridement of the subtalar joint usually produces good results.

Corns and Calluses

Synonyms

Callosity
Clavus
Heloma durum
Heloma molle

ICD-9 Code

700
Corns and calluses

Definition

A callus is a hyperkeratotic lesion of the skin that forms in response to excessive pressure over a bony prominence. When the callus forms on a toe, it is called a corn. When it forms elsewhere (as under a metatarsal head), it is called a callus (**Figure 1**). A persistent callus on the sole of the forefoot also is referred to as intractable plantar keratosis.

A callus usually occurs beneath the metatarsal heads and is associated with metatarsalgia, a general term for pain overlying one or several of the metatarsal heads. Pain may be caused by the callus itself or by some other manifestation of chronic pressure overload of the metatarsal head, such as synovitis of the joint, attritional tearing of the metatarsophalangeal (MTP) ligaments, or claw toe deformity. Pressure overload also may be secondary to a cavus foot, long toe (typically, the second), or wearing high-heeled shoes.

Corns usually are the result of toe deformities—hammer toe, bunionette, claw toe—caused by inappropriately tight footwear. Hard corns (heloma durum) occur over exposed bony prominences, whereas soft corns (heloma molle) develop between the toes in the web space as well as over bony prominences (**Figure 2**). Periungual corns are small but painful lesions that occur at the edge of a nail, often in association with a mallet toe or improper shoe fit.

Figure 1 Clinical appearance of a diffuse callus beneath the second metatarsal head.

Clinical Symptoms

Patients with corns and calluses typically report pain with walking or when wearing shoes.

Figure 2 **A,** Soft interdigital corn on the medial aspect of the small toe. **B,** Corn on the plantar aspect of the small toe.

Tests

Physical Examination

The pared surface of a callus has a uniform, waxy appearance. Warts and calluses generally can be distinguished by palpation. Warts are tender when pinched from side to side, whereas corns and calluses are tender with direct pressure. Plantar warts usually do not develop over a bony prominence. Corns occur over or between the toes.

When tenderness exists over the dorsal surface of the MTP joint, perform the MTP instability test (see page 753) to assess joint instability.

Diagnostic Tests

None

Differential Diagnosis

- Foreign body (history of penetrating wound)
- Interdigital (Morton) neuroma (location between the third and fourth metatarsal heads or second and third metatarsal heads, no callus)
- Plantar warts (occur on non–weight-bearing areas, may have a nearby satellite lesion, pared surface has multiple tiny points of hemorrhage near the base)
- Synovitis of the MTP joint (tenderness over the dorsal MTP joint, no plantar callus, painful MTP instability test)

Adverse Outcomes of the Disease

Persistent pain or ulceration of the skin may develop. Metatarsalgia, when caused by ligament tears or MTP synovitis, may result in gradual subluxation of the joint and deformity of the toe.

Treatment

Paring and pressure relief are the principal treatment (see page 784). Paring involves shaving the lesion layer by layer with a scalpel after the skin has been prepared with alcohol or iodine. The goal is to remove enough of the avascular keratin to restore a more normal contour to the skin without drawing blood. When performed gradually and with care, this can be accomplished using a #15 blade, without anesthetic. Paring also provides excellent short-term pain relief. Patients then should be instructed in self-care, using a pumice stone or callus file to regularly débride the lesion after soaking the foot or after a shower.

Treatment of metatarsalgia includes use of a metatarsal pad (see page 775), trimming the callus/corn, and correction of associated problems, such as improper shoe fit and claw toe deformities. Pressure is relieved by wearing roomier shoes, using commercially available silicone cushions, or inserting small foam donut pads or metatarsal pads to shift pressure from the lesion. For soft corns, a small amount of lamb's wool or a silicone spacer between the toes can wick away moisture and help cushion the area.

When nonsurgical measures fail, surgical treatment to remove the underlying bony prominences is indicated. With soft corns, syndactylization (creating a partial webbing of the involved toes) may be required.

Adverse Outcomes of Treatment

Infection and bleeding can occur from excessively deep paring. Paring a soft corn can be especially difficult because of its awkward location in the web space. Medicated keratolytic corn pads often cause maceration and can result in infection; therefore, these pads are probably best avoided.

Referral Decisions/Red Flags

Failure to respond to nonsurgical treatment and presence of ulceration and/or infection are indications for further evaluation of hyperkeratotic lesions. Deformity or persistent metatarsalgia also requires further evaluation.

SECTION 7 FOOT AND ANKLE

Procedure: Trimming a Corn or Callus

CPT Code

11055
Paring or cutting of benign hyperkeratotic lesion (eg, corn or callus); single lesion

Current Procedural Terminology © 2010 American Medical Association. All rights reserved.

Materials

- Sterile gloves
- Scalpel with #15 or #17 blade

Figure 1 Trimming a callus.

Step 1
Wear protective gloves at all times during the procedure, and use excellent lighting and sterile technique.

Step 2
Anesthesia is not required to trim a corn or callus; however, prior to the procedure, the patient should soak the foot in water for several minutes to soften the skin.

Step 3
Holding the blade almost parallel to the lesion, shave the excess skin (**Figure 1**). Bleeding should not occur.

   Note: Take special care with a corn on the toe because the skin is thin and may be fragile. Shell out several millimeters of the hard central core of a plantar callus with the sharp tip of the blade.

Adverse Outcomes
Paring down a corn or callus too deeply may expose subcutaneous tissue. If bleeding occurs, the corn or callus has been trimmed too deeply. A wart, on the other hand, tends to bleed because of its hypervascularity.

Aftercare/Patient Instructions
Instruct the patient to continue to pare down the lesion with a pumice stone or nail file daily after a shower or bath.

Dance Injuries to the Foot and Ankle

Definition

Dancing emphasizes flexibility, repetition, and technique, and great demands are placed on the foot and ankle. Poor technique and overuse can lead to injury.

Most dancers are girls and young women. Although many of the physical demands placed on dancers are similar to those of other athletes, several are unique. Unique to dance are the turned-out, demi-pointe, and en pointe foot positions (**Figure 1**). These positions place considerable stress on the anatomic structures of the foot and ankle and, particularly if improper technique is used or the individual has preexisting conditions, may lead to injuries and conditions commonly seen in dancers.

Management of injuries in dancers may be difficult because dancers are required to perform repetitive movements and move the joints through extreme ranges of motion as part of their training. Also, dancers often ignore injuries, especially during times of rehearsal or performance, until they become chronic.

Figure 1 Dance positions of the foot: turned-out (**A**), demi-pointe (**B**), en pointe (**C**).

ICD-9 Codes

726.71
Achilles bursitis or tendinitis

733.99
Sesamoiditis

735.0
Hallux valgus

735.2
Hallux rigidus

824.0
Fracture of ankle, medial malleolus, closed

824.1
Fracture of ankle, medial malleolus, open

824.2
Fracture of ankle, lateral malleolus, closed

824.3
Fracture of ankle, lateral malleolus, open

824.4
Fracture of ankle, bimalleolar, closed

824.50
Fracture of ankle, bimalleolar, open

825.20
Fracture of one or more tarsal and metatarsal bones, closed, unspecified bone(s) of foot [except toes], instep

825.21
Fracture of one or more tarsal and metatarsal bones, astragalus

825.22
Fracture of one or more tarsal and metatarsal bones, navicular [scaphoid], foot

825.23
Fracture of one or more tarsal and metatarsal bones, cuboid

Continued on next page

ICD-9 Codes *(continued)*

825.24
Fracture of one or more tarsal and metatarsal bones, cuneiform, foot

825.25
Fracture of one or more tarsal and metatarsal bones, closed, metatarsal bone(s)

845.00
Sprains and strains of ankle and foot, ankle, unspecified site

845.01
Sprains and strains of ankle and foot, ankle, deltoid (ligament), ankle

845.02
Sprains and strains of ankle and foot, ankle, calcaneofibular (ligament)

845.03
Sprains and strains of ankle and foot, ankle, tibiofibular (ligament), distal

845.10
Sprains and strains of ankle and foot, foot, unspecified site

845.11
Sprains and strains of ankle and foot, foot, tarsometatarsal (joint) (ligament)

845.12
Sprains and strains of ankle and foot, foot, metatarsophalangeal (joint)

Common injuries of the foot and ankle as seen in dancers are described in this chapter. For a more complete discussion of these conditions as seen in the general population, see the following chapters: Ankle Sprain, Hallux Rigidus, Hallux Valgus, Posterior Heel Pain, Sesamoiditis, and Stress Fractures of the Foot and Ankle.

Differential Diagnosis

Hallux Valgus and Hallux Rigidus

Dancing en point does not cause hallux valgus, but it may cause an existing hallux valgus to progress. Similarly, hallux rigidus may be made worse by a dancer's efforts to rise into the demi-pointe position. A dancer with hallux rigidus will "sickle," or abduct the forefoot, while attempting to assume the demi-pointe position. The proper demi-pointe position will be difficult if not impossible to achieve because it requires the great toe to be capable of at least 90° of flexion. Treatment for hallux valgus is usually limited to symptomatic care, if possible, until the end of the dancer's career, as surgery may limit the range of motion of the great toe. Treatment for hallux rigidus may be successful in many dancers. Ballet dancers are an exception because a full range of motion is necessary for the demi-pointe position, and this will most likely not be achieved with surgery.

Sesamoiditis

Sesamoiditis in dancers may result from excessive stress on the sesamoids caused by poor technique when landing from jumps, which puts excessive stress on the sesamoids. An ideal landing in ballet includes a small plié (bending of the knees) to absorb the forces of landing, whereas a poor landing is usually audible. On examination, the dancer will have pain on palpation over the involved (usually the medial) sesamoid. With dorsiflexion of the great toe, the point of maximal tenderness will move with the sesamoids and their soft-tissue attachments. Treatment includes using proper landing technique. If it fits in the shoe, a small felt pad can be added to the ballet shoe to relieve pressure on the sesamoid.

Stress Fractures

The most common site of stress fractures of the foot is at the neck of the second metatarsal, followed by the base of the second metatarsal. The second metatarsal is the longest metatarsal and is where the body weight of a dancer is centered when in the demi-pointe position. Stress fractures also may occur at the distal fibula, the sesamoids, the talus, the calcaneus, and the navicular bone. On examination, the dancer with a stress fracture will have swelling and pain to palpation over the injured bone. Occasionally, crepitus will be present as well.

Treatment of stress fractures is conservative. Because dancers, like athletes, want to heal and return to participation as quickly as possible, non–weight-bearing ambulation on crutches, followed by a gradual return to dance, may be recommended.

Osteophytes at the Anterior Ankle

Extreme plantar flexion of the ankle places stress on the anterior joint capsule. This may result in thickening of the capsule or traction osteophytes off the distal tibia. The thickened capsule or the osteophytes impinge, limit range of motion, and cause pain with dorsiflexion. On examination, a dancer with anterior impingement of the ankle will have maximal tenderness over the anterior osteophytes or the hypertrophied anterior ankle joint capsule. Pain will be exaggerated with dorsiflexion of the ankle, and occasionally dorsiflexion will be limited on the involved side.

The condition is initially treated with rest and, if that fails, surgical débridement of the thick anterior capsule and/or anterior osteophytes.

Ankle Sprain

The most common acute injury in dancers is an inversion sprain of the ankle (lateral collateral ligament injury). If the sprain occurs while the dancer is in demi-pointe, the injury may be quite severe. Care should be taken to examine and perform a stress test on each ligament. It is extremely important in a dancer to perform comparison stress tests on the opposite, uninjured side, as a dancer's range of motion may be exceptional compared with that of the general population. Most ankle sprains are treated nonsurgically, with the dancer returning to dance 2 to 4 weeks postinjury.

Retrocalcaneal Bursitis

The retrocalcaneal bursa may be compressed between the posterior aspect of the calcaneus and the Achilles tendon when the dancer rises up on the ball of the foot. Such compression results in the bursa becoming inflamed and painful. On physical examination, the patient will experience pain with side-to-side compression of the bursa, just anterior to the Achilles tendon. Most cases of retrocalcaneal bursitis resolve with rest, ice, NSAIDs, and a heel lift worn in street shoes. If the dancer ignores the pain, the problem may become chronic and require surgical excision of the bursa.

Posterior Impingement Syndrome

The posterior lateral tubercle of the talus (also known as Stieda's process) varies greatly in size and configuration. In 10% of people, the tubercle does not fuse with the body of the talus and is called the os trigonum, which projects into the posterior aspect of the ankle. Impingement of this bone on the soft tissue of the ankle, especially as the dancer assumes the en pointe and demi-pointe positions, results in posterior impingement syndrome. This syndrome is characterized by pain at the back of the ankle when rising up on the toes. Examination reveals tenderness at the posterior aspect of the ankle, deep behind the flexor tendons. Pain increases as the foot is placed into plantar flexion, compressing the soft tissues at the posterior aspect of the ankle.

Conservative treatment includes rest, NSAIDs, and, if these measures do not relieve the pain, an injection of local anesthetic into the posterior aspect of the ankle. If these measures do not provide relief, surgical excision of the posterior lateral tubercle or os trigonum is recommended.

Tendinitis of the Flexor Hallucis Longus Tendon

For dance positions requiring a turned-out foot position, turnout should take place at the hip because when the femur is externally rotated the greater trochanter of the femur clears the pelvis, allowing the leg to abduct. Some dancers, however, using poor technique, turn out only the feet. This causes the feet to roll into an everted position and puts stress on the medial side of the foot, which can lead to tendinitis of the flexor hallucis longus (FHL) tendon.

The FHL tendon passes through a fibro-osseous tunnel posterior to the talus as it travels to its insertion at the great toe. With chronic overuse, inflammation and fibrosis of the tendon may result in a nodular thickening. The inflamed, thickened tendon may catch and cause the great toe to trigger. FHL tendinitis will cause pain and occasionally clicking over the course of the tendon. The pain may increase when the FHL tendon travels through the fibro-osseous tunnel behind the talus. Pain may also increase when the dancer rises up on the toes or completes a grande plié, which puts tension on the FHL tendon.

Examination should include palpating the entire course of the FHL tendon while passively moving the great toe. Check for crepitus or a click in the fibro-osseous tunnel posterior to the talus.

Nonsurgical treatment includes ice, NSAIDs, rest, and an injection of a local anesthetic agent into the fibro-osseous tunnel. If conservative treatment fails, surgical release of the fibro-osseous tunnel and a tenosynovectomy may be recommended.

Tests

Clinical and diagnostic tests depend on the specific condition. A lateral view of the ankle in plantar flexion is recommended to examine for posterior impingement syndrome of the ankle. This view will reveal not only the position and size of the posterior lateral process of the talus (and os trigonum) but also any visible impingement. A lateral view with the ankle in full dorsiflexion is also recommended to evaluate for anterior impingement.

Adverse Outcomes of the Disease

Some conditions, such as hallux rigidus, may end a dancer's career because full range of motion of the great toe will most likely not be achieved, even with proper treatment.

Treatment

The goal of treatment is to return the dancer to a preinjury level of dance. This usually includes a sequence of rehabilitation, barre work, return to class, and then return to performance. This should be gradual and include consultation with the rehabilitation specialist, the dance instructor, and the dancer.

Referral Decisions/Red Flags

Further evaluation is indicated in any patient with an overuse injury that does not respond within 72 hours to ice, anti-inflammatory medication, and rest; an injury that is associated with a pop, click, or other audible sound; triggering of the great toe; any fracture; or any loss of range of motion.

The Diabetic Foot

ICD-9 Code

713.5
Arthropathy associated with neurologic disorders

Synonyms

Charcot arthropathy

Neuropathic foot

Definition

Diabetes is a group of metabolic disorders characterized by high blood glucose levels. The four major categories are type 1 (insulin-dependent diabetes mellitus), type 2 (non–insulin-dependent diabetes mellitus), gestational diabetes mellitus, and diabetes secondary to other conditions. Types 1 and 2 are the most common forms, with approximately 5% to 10% of all cases of diabetes in the United States identified as type 1 and 85% to 90% as type 2.

Diabetic foot problems are a major health problem in the United States and are a common cause of hospitalization and amputation. Patients present with skin ulceration, infection, and/or Charcot arthropathy. The primary etiology is peripheral nerve impairment that results in loss of protective sensation, autonomic dysfunction, and/or motor impairment. With inadequate sensory feedback, repetitive trauma is not perceived and skin breakdown results. Vascular insufficiency also may contribute to foot problems in patients with diabetes.

Patients with autonomic dysfunction have dry, scaly, and cracking skin, a condition that predisposes the skin to ulceration.

Motor neuropathy leads to weakness of the intrinsic muscles of the foot, claw toe deformities, subluxation or dislocation of the metatarsophalangeal joints, abnormal plantar positioning of the metatarsal heads, increased pressure on the sole of the foot, skin breakdown, ulcers, deep infections, and osteomyelitis. Extrinsic forces, such as tight shoes, may contribute to skin breakdown.

Charcot arthropathy results from repetitive stress in a patient in whom pain and proprioceptive sensation is not perceived normally. The result is progressive disruption of joint stability and severe bony deformities (**Figure 1**).

Figure 1 Severe deformity from Charcot breakdown of the ankle joint. (Reproduced from Harrelson JM: The diabetic foot: Charcot arthropathy. *Instr Course Lect* 1993;42;141-146.)

Clinical Symptoms

Patients may have no symptoms or they may report foot pain at night, characterized as burning and tingling, secondary to neuritis. With abnormal areas of pressure, skin breakdown follows, leading to a painless ulcer. Deep infections and osteomyelitis may subsequently develop, usually with a sudden increase in swelling, redness, and drainage, and sometimes pain.

Patients with Charcot arthropathy have noticeable swelling, warmth, and redness, even though pain is only mild or absent. Charcot arthropathy may be misdiagnosed as cellulitis, osteomyelitis, or gout.

Tests

Physical Examination

A thorough evaluation of the feet is essential when examining patients with diabetes. A significant number of amputations can be avoided by simple preventive measures and early treatment of skin lesions. Light touch should be tested. Protective foot care, including wearing well-cushioned shoes, is particularly necessary in patients below the protective sensation threshold, that is, those who cannot feel a 10-g (5.07-mm) nylon filament applied to the plantar aspect of the foot (**Figure 2**).

Diabetic ulcers are insensate and can be easily inspected and probed to determine depth and size. If bone can be probed, osteomyelitis is likely to be present.

Examination of a Charcot joint reveals a hot, red, swollen joint with intact skin. Pulses usually are strong in patients with Charcot arthropathy. A Charcot foot elevated above the heart for 1 minute will lose its redness, whereas a foot affected by cellulitis, soft-tissue abscess, and/or osteomyelitis will not.

Diagnostic Tests

Radiographs are necessary to help rule out osteomyelitis and Charcot arthropathy (**Figure 3**). Vascular studies are appropriate when pulses are absent or when the patient has a nonhealing ulcer. MRI can help confirm a deep abscess or osteomyelitis but usually is not necessary. Combined technetium-iridium bone scans have been used in difficult cases to differentiate Charcot arthropathy from osteomyelitis.

Differential Diagnosis

- Cellulitis (most likely associated with skin breakdown)
- Gout (painful lesion, increased serum uric acid)
- Osteomyelitis (usually beneath an open skin ulcer)
- Other neuropathies (Charcot-Marie-Tooth disease, alcoholic neuropathy, spinal cord neuropathy)

Figure 2 Testing for protective sensation. (Reproduced from Pinzur MS: Ankle fractures in patients with diabetes mellitus, in Nunley JA, Pfeffer GB, Sanders RW, Trepman E, eds: *Advanced Reconstruction: Foot and Ankle*, Rosemont, IL, American Academy of Orthopaedic Surgeons, 2004, p 427.)

SECTION 7 FOOT AND ANKLE

Figure 3 Lateral radiograph showing Charcot degeneration of the midfoot (arrows). (Reproduced from Harrelson JM: The diabetic foot: Charcot arthropathy. *Instr Course Lect* 1993;42;141-146.)

Adverse Outcomes of the Disease

Skin ulceration, Charcot joint, chronic osteomyelitis, and gangrene all occur in the diabetic foot. Amputation may be necessary.

Treatment

The goal of treatment is patient education and prevention (see page 794). Control of serum glucose is paramount. Once neuropathy occurs, it is irreversible. When a problem exists, aggressive treatment is needed to avoid a more serious and debilitating situation. A callus, which indicates a pressure point, is the first phase of a diabetic ulcer and signals the need for adaptive footwear (cushioned shoes and soft, molded insoles) and close follow-up.

Treatment of a diabetic ulcer requires removing the pressure causing the ulcer, allowing the ulcer to heal, and prescribing optimal footwear to prevent recurrence. Accommodative footwear, an orthotic device, and total contact casting may be used for superficial ulcerations. For deeper ulcerations, these measures are often inadequate, and surgery may be required. An associated equinus contracture should be corrected by serial casting or percutaneous heel cord lengthening.

Treatment of a deep infection must be aggressive and prompt. The infection is often polymicrobial. Skin swab cultures are inaccurate. Bone biopsy provides more definitive cultures to direct antibiotic therapy. Any abscess should be considered an emergency and drained surgically. Osteomyelitis can be treated surgically with débridement of the affected bone. Digit or ray (toe plus metatarsal) amputation is often needed to eradicate osteomyelitis of the toes or metatarsal heads.

In the initial stage of Charcot arthropathy, the foot and ankle need to be unweighted and stabilized, usually with a total contact cast. After the acute swelling and erythema have subsided, the patient can begin bearing weight with continued use of a cast or a customized clamshell-type short leg brace. The patient must be advised that the period of immobilization may be lengthy, often up to 12 months, and that a permanent brace might be required for ambulation. When Charcot arthropathy is properly recognized and treated, acceptable limb salvage can be achieved. Occasionally, surgical reconstruction by arthrodesis is needed for severe deformity that cannot be treated with bracing.

Adverse Outcomes of Treatment

The adverse outcomes of treatment are the same as those for diabetes and, in addition, include surgical complications of infection, ischemia, and death.

Referral Decisions/Red Flags

Unexplained pain in a diabetic foot, sudden onset of swelling and pain, and nonhealing ulcerations all signal the need for further evaluation.

Acknowledgment

Information regarding the sensory testing nylon filament was provided by the Filament Project, 5445 Point Clair Road, Caryville, LA 70721.

SECTION 7 FOOT AND ANKLE

Procedure: Care of Diabetic Feet

Care of the Feet

1. Never walk barefoot; always wear shoes or slippers.
2. Wash feet daily with mild soap and water.
   - Always test the water temperature with your hand or elbow before putting your feet in the water.
   - After washing, pat your feet dry; do not rub vigorously.
   - Use only one thickness of towel to dry your feet, especially between the toes.
   - Use a skin moisturizing lotion to prevent skin from getting dry and cracked; however, do not use these lotions between the toes.
3. Inspect your feet daily for puncture wounds, bruises, pressure areas and redness, and blisters.
   - Puncture wounds—Have you stepped on any nails, glass, or tacks?
   - Bruises—Feel for swelling.
   - Pressure areas and redness—Check the six major locations for pressure on the bottom of the foot:
     a. Tip of the big toe
     b. Base of the little toe
     c. Base of the middle toes
     d. Heel
     e. Outside edge of the foot
     f. Across the ball of the foot (metatarsal heads)
   - Blisters—Check the six major locations on the bottom of the foot for blisters, plus the tops of the toes and the back of the heel. *Never* pop a blister!
4. Seek treatment by a physician for any foot injuries or open wounds.
5. Do not use Lysol disinfectant, iodine, cresol, carbolic acid, kerosene, or other irritating antiseptic solutions to treat cuts or abrasions on your feet. These products will damage soft tissue.
6. Do not use sharp instruments, drugstore medications, or corn plasters on your feet. Always seek the advice of your physician for any condition that needs such care.

7. Protect your feet.
   - Wear loose bed socks while sleeping.
   - Avoid frostbite by wearing warm socks and shoes during cold weather.
   - Do not use a heating pad on your feet.
   - Do not place your feet on radiators, furnaces, furnace grills, or hot water pipes.
   - Do not hold your feet in front of the fireplace, circulators, or heaters.
   - Do not use a hair dryer on your feet.

8. Place thin pieces of cotton or lamb's wool between your toes if there is maceration of the skin between your toes or if your toes overlap.

9. Do not sit cross-legged; this position can decrease circulation to your feet.

10. Take care of your toenails in the following manner:
    - Soak or bathe feet before trimming nails.
    - Make sure that you trim your nails under good lighting.
    - Trim toenails straight across.
    - Never trim toenails into the corner.
    - If toenails are thick, see your physician for evaluation of the cause and advice on routine nail care.
    - Consult your physician when there are any signs of an ingrown toenail. Do not treat an ingrown toenail with drugstore medications; however, you can place a thin piece of cotton or waxed dental floss under the toenail. (See page 822.)

Socks and Stockings

1. Wear clean, dry socks daily. Make certain that there are no holes or wrinkles in your socks or stockings.

2. Wear thin, white cotton socks in the summer; cotton is more absorbent and porous than synthetic materials. Change them if your feet sweat excessively.

3. Wear square-toe socks; they will not squeeze your toes.

4. Wear pantyhose or stockings with a garter belt. It is important that you do not wear or use the following:
   - Elastic-top socks or stockings, or knee-high stockings
   - Circular elastic garters
   - String tied around the tops of stockings
   - Stockings that are rolled or knotted at the top

SECTION 7 FOOT AND ANKLE

Shoe Wear

1. Always wear proper shoes. Check the following components daily to ensure that your shoes fit properly and will not damage your feet:

   - Shoe width—Make sure that the shoes are wide and deep enough to give the joints of your toes breathing room. Shoes that are too narrow will cause pressure bruises and blisters on the inside and outside edges of your foot at the base of the toes.

   - Shoe length—Shoes that are too short will cause pressure and blisters on the tops of your toes.

   - Back of shoe—Looseness at the heel will cause blisters at your heels.

   - Bottom of heel—Make sure there are no nails. The presence of holes indicates that there are nails in the heels.

   - Sole—Make sure that the sole is not broken. A break in the sole will allow nails or other sharp objects to puncture the skin.

2. Be careful about the type of new shoes you purchase. Use the following guidelines:

   - Buy new shoes in the evening to allow for swelling in your feet.

   - Inspect your feet once an hour for the first few days you wear a new pair of shoes. Look for red areas, bruises, and blisters.

   - Do not wear your new shoes for more than a half day for the first few days.

   - The following features are desirable:

     a. Laces or adjustable closure

     b. Soft leather tops (to allow feet to breathe; they mold to the feet)

     c. Crepe soles (to provide a good cushion for walking)

   - Avoid the following features:

     a. Elastic across the tops of the shoes

     b. Pointed-toe styles (they constrict the toes)

     c. High heels

     d. Shoes made of plastic (they retain moisture and do not allow the feet to "breathe")

3. Put your shoes on properly.

   - Inspect the inside of each shoe before putting it on. Make sure to remove any small stones or debris. Be certain that the inside of the shoe is smooth.

   - Loosen the laces before putting on or taking off your shoes. Make sure that the tongue is flat, with no wrinkles.

   - Be certain that you do not tie your laces either too tightly or too loosely.

Fracture-Dislocations of the Midfoot

Synonym

Lisfranc fracture-dislocation

ICD-9 Codes

838.03
Closed dislocation, tarsometatarsal joint

838.13
Open dislocation, tarsometatarsal (joint)

Definition

Fracture-dislocations of the midfoot, commonly called Lisfranc fracture-dislocations, are traumatic disruptions of the tarsometatarsal joints. Injury to these joints occurs as a result of significant trauma or from an indirect mechanism, as may occur in athletics or as a result of tripping. The critical injury involves the second tarsometatarsal joint. The second metatarsal wedges into a slot in the cuneiforms and is key to stabilizing the other tarsometatarsal joints.

Clinical Symptoms

Patients often report a "sprain." Pain is localized to the dorsum of the midfoot. The swelling may be relatively mild.

Tests

Physical Examination

This injury is easily missed and is sometimes misdiagnosed as a foot or ankle sprain. Examination reveals maximum tenderness and swelling over the tarsometatarsal joint rather than the ankle ligaments. An acute injury to this joint usually presents with ecchymosis in the plantar arch.

During examination, stabilize the hindfoot (calcaneus) with one hand and rotate and/or abduct the forefoot with the other hand (**Figure 1**). This maneuver produces severe pain with a Lisfranc injury but only minimal pain with an ankle sprain.

Diagnostic Tests

AP, lateral, and oblique radiographs of the foot should be obtained. Spontaneous reduction after complete dislocation may occur. Subtle injuries may be more apparent on weight-bearing radiographs. The medial aspect of the middle cuneiform should line up with the medial aspect of the second metatarsal on an AP radiograph (**Figure 2**). The oblique view should show the medial aspect of the fourth metatarsal aligned with the medial aspect of the cuboid. Comparison views of the uninjured foot may be helpful.

Figure 1 To test for a Lisfranc fracture-dislocation, stabilize the hindfoot with one hand and rotate and/or abduct the forefoot with the other.

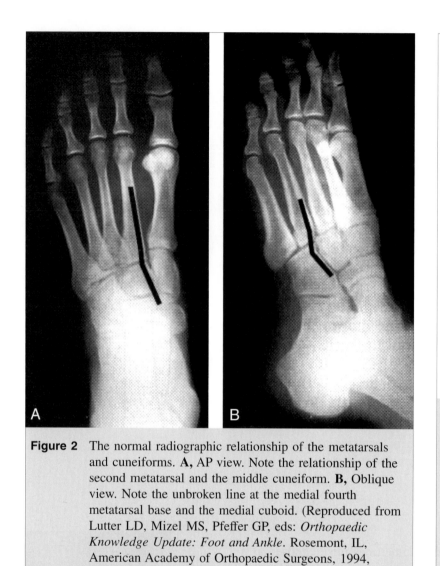

Figure 2 The normal radiographic relationship of the metatarsals and cuneiforms. **A,** AP view. Note the relationship of the second metatarsal and the middle cuneiform. **B,** Oblique view. Note the unbroken line at the medial fourth metatarsal base and the medial cuboid. (Reproduced from Lutter LD, Mizel MS, Pfeffer GP, eds: *Orthopaedic Knowledge Update: Foot and Ankle*. Rosemont, IL, American Academy of Orthopaedic Surgeons, 1994, p 261.)

Figure 3 Lisfranc fracture-dislocation, with lateral shift of the second metatarsal. (Reproduced with permission from Alexander IJ, ed: *The Foot: Examination and Diagnosis*. New York, NY, Churchill Livingstone, 1990, p 131.)

When the AP radiograph shows that the second metatarsal base has shifted laterally, even by only a few millimeters, a Lisfranc fracture-dislocation has occurred (**Figure 3**). A small avulsion fracture between the base of the first and second metatarsals indicates disruption of the ligament connecting the base of the second metatarsal and the medial cuneiform (Lisfranc ligament) and instability of the tarsometatarsal joints.

When radiographs are normal but physical examination suggests injury to the tarsometatarsal joints, stress radiographs of the midfoot under local anesthetic or sedation may be indicated. If confusion still exists, CT or MRI is helpful in confirming the diagnosis.

Differential Diagnosis

- Ankle fracture (bony tenderness over the malleolus)
- Ankle sprain (focal tenderness over the lateral ankle ligament)
- Metatarsal fracture (focal tenderness over the metatarsal)
- Midfoot arthritis (chronic pain and tenderness, no recent history of trauma)
- Navicular fracture (focal tenderness over the navicular)

Adverse Outcomes of the Disease

Adverse outcomes include midfoot instability, deformity, and arthritis. Compartment syndrome with subsequent ischemic contracture, claw toes, and sensory impairment also can occur.

Treatment

Nondisplaced injuries are treated with 6 to 8 weeks of non–weight-bearing cast immobilization, followed by use of a rigid arch support for 3 months. A fracture or fracture-dislocation with any displacement requires surgical reduction and stabilization.

Adverse Outcomes of Treatment

If the tarsometatarsal articulations are not well reduced, posttraumatic arthritis may develop.

Referral Decisions/Red Flags

Because these injuries are frequently missed, further evaluation and diagnostic testing is warranted if there is even a slight suspicion of their presence. Even a minimally displaced fracture-dislocation requires surgical reduction. Any possibility of compartment syndrome requires immediate surgical evaluation.

Fractures of the Ankle

Figure 1 Minimally displaced fracture of the lateral malleolus (white arrow). Note the small chip off the medial malleolus (black arrow).

Definition

Ankle fractures include injuries to the lateral malleolus (distal fibula), the medial malleolus, the posterior lip of the tibia (posterior malleolus), the collateral ligamentous structures, and/or the talar dome. Stable fractures involve only one side of the joint (eg, a fracture of the distal fibula without injury to the medial deltoid ligament) (**Figure 1**). Unstable ankle fractures involve both sides of the ankle joint and may be bimalleolar or trimalleolar. Bimalleolar injuries are either fractures of the lateral and medial malleolus or a fracture of the distal fibula with disruption of the deltoid ligament. Trimalleolar injuries include a fracture of the posterior malleolus (**Figure 2**). Posterior dislocation of the ankle also may be present with a trimalleolar fracture. This injury is described as a trimalleolar fracture-dislocation.

Stable injuries may be treated nonsurgically. Unstable injuries, however, are vulnerable for displacement and subsequent posttraumatic arthritis and usually require surgical management.

Clinical Symptoms

Patients usually report acute pain following trauma. The etiologies of ankle fractures are as varied as the circumstances, but usually some element of rotation or twisting has occurred.

Tests

Physical Examination

Medial, lateral, and/or posterior swelling accompanies most ankle fractures. Marked tenderness is evident at the fracture site. A palpable gap may be apparent on the medial side. External rotation or lateral displacement of the foot from the tibia may be present as well.

A fracture of the distal fibula (lateral malleolus) with tenderness over the medial deltoid ligament is presumed to be an unstable bimalleolar injury.

Palpate the proximal fibula for tenderness because tenderness in this area, coupled with swelling of the medial ankle, may indicate a Maisonneuve fracture, an unstable external rotation injury that includes fracture of the proximal fibula, a tear of the medial deltoid ligament, and a disruption of the tibiofibular syndesmotic ligaments.

Assess circulatory status and posterior tibial, superficial peroneal, and deep peroneal nerve function distal to the fracture. Lacerations over the fracture site may indicate an open fracture and should be assessed carefully.

Diagnostic Tests

AP, lateral, and mortise (AP view with the ankle internally rotated, usually 15°) views will reveal most fractures. The relationships of the tibia, fibula, and talus are clearest in the mortise view (**Figure 3**). AP and lateral views should include the proximal fibula and tibia when there is tenderness in that area.

Minimally displaced fractures may not be apparent on initial radiographs; therefore, when such a fracture is suspected, radiographs should be repeated in 10 to 14 days, when callus will usually be evident.

With a rotational injury, an osteochondral fracture of the lateral articular surface of the talus may occur. This is best seen on the mortise view. CT may be required for evaluation of complex fractures.

Differential Diagnosis

- Ankle sprain (history of inversion injury, lateral tenderness, normal radiographs)
- Charcot arthropathy (diffuse swelling, erythema, minimal tenderness)

Figure 2   Displaced trimalleolar ankle fracture. Note the fracture of the lateral malleolus (black arrow), posterior malleolus (black arrowhead), and medial malleolus (white arrow). This fracture requires immediate reduction. (Reproduced from Grantham SA: Trimalleolar ankle fractures and open ankle fractures. *Instr Course Lect* 1990;39:105-111.)

Figure 3   Mortise views of the ankle. **A,** Uninjured ankle demonstrates normal medial clear space (MCS). **B,** Ankle with lateral fibular fracture and deltoid disruption, resulting in widening of the MCS (> 5 mm). (Reproduced from Stiehl JB: Ankle fractures with diastasis. *Instr Course Lect* 1990;39:95-103.)

- Fracture of the base of the fifth metatarsal (focal tenderness)
- Maisonneuve fracture (widening of syndesmosis, tenderness over the proximal fibula)
- Osteochondral fracture of the talar dome, lateral process of the talus, or anterior process of the calcaneus (focal tenderness over the fracture site)

Adverse Outcomes of the Disease

Posttraumatic arthritis, instability, deformity, complex regional pain syndrome, nerve injury, and compartment syndrome are possible.

Treatment

Stable fractures of the distal fibula may be treated with a weight-bearing cast or brace for 4 to 6 weeks. Unstable but nondisplaced fractures require a non–weight-bearing short or long leg cast and more prolonged immobilization. Unstable, displaced fractures require either closed or open reduction. In most cases, open reduction provides better restoration of joint function. Osteochondral fragments of the talus should be removed. If the fragment is large and there is viable bone on both the fragment and the base, the fracture may be reduced and pinned. The outcome of this procedure usually is good only in young patients. Concomitant dislocation should be reduced as soon as possible to relieve pressure on the skin and neurovascular structures. Open fractures require immediate surgical débridement. Rehabilitation is indicated in elderly patients or if full range of motion and balance are not achieved by 3 months after the fracture has healed.

Adverse Outcomes of Treatment

Joint stiffness and atrophy from casting may occur.

Referral Decisions/Red Flags

Patients with unstable fractures or osteochondral fractures of the talus need further evaluation. All open fractures or open joint injuries require immediate evaluation.

Fractures of the Calcaneus and Talus

Synonyms

Aviator's fracture (talus)

Heel fracture

Definition

Fractures of the two bones of the hindfoot, the talus and calcaneus, usually occur as a result of severe trauma, such as a motor vehicle accident or a fall from a height. The two fractures seldom occur together, however. Most fractures of the talus or calcaneus involve the articular surface and are serious injuries.

Clinical Symptoms

Patients often report acute pain and inability to bear weight.

Tests

Physical Examination

Examination reveals swelling and tenderness. Assess function of the superficial peroneal, deep peroneal, sural, and medial and lateral plantar nerves distal to the fracture. With swelling, the pulses might not be palpable. Check capillary refill of the toes.

Compartment syndrome is difficult to evaluate with calcaneal and talar injuries; however, notable swelling in the area of the arch is suggestive of a plantar compartment syndrome.

Falls that fracture the calcaneus or talus may be associated with a compression fracture of the lumbar spine or other injuries to the ipsilateral lower extremity. Palpate the spine and the entire lower extremity for pain and tenderness.

Diagnostic Tests

AP and lateral radiographs of the hindfoot are indicated (**Figure 1**), along with AP and mortise views of the ankle. AP and lateral views of the spine should be obtained if spinal tenderness is present. If further evaluation is indicated (concern for associated injuries), coronal CT scans should be obtained to assess damage to the subtalar and calcaneocuboid joints, as well as tendon entrapment in the fracture fragments (**Figure 2**).

Figure 1   Lateral view of the foot demonstrates a displaced fracture of the anterior talar body (arrow). (Reproduced from Johnson TS, Steinbach LS: *Essentials of Musculoskeletal Care*. Rosemont, IL, American Academy of Orthopaedic Surgeons, 2004, p 606.)

Figure 2   Coronal CT scan of the calcaneus shows bilateral displaced, comminuted, intra-articular fractures (black arrows) and depression of the posterior facet (white arrows). (Reproduced from Johnson TS, Steinbach LS: *Essentials of Musculoskeletal Care*. Rosemont, IL, American Academy of Orthopaedic Surgeons, 2004, p 587.)

Differential Diagnosis

- Ankle fracture (ankle swelling or deformity; evident on radiographs)
- Associated lumbar spine fracture (pain and tenderness in the lower back)
- Medial or lateral ankle ligament injury (swelling and tenderness over involved ligaments)
- Talocalcaneal dislocation (deformity of the hindfoot)

Adverse Outcomes of the Disease

The adverse outcomes of either type of fracture are potentially severe and disabling, and treatment is difficult. Fractures of the talus often interrupt the blood supply to the body of the talus and may lead to osteonecrosis. Chronic pain, posttraumatic arthritis, osteonecrosis of the talus, deformity, tarsal tunnel syndrome, complex regional pain syndrome, or plantar compartment syndrome may result from either a calcaneal or a talar fracture.

Treatment

Immediate treatment consists of splinting with a well-padded posterior splint from the toe to the upper calf. The extremity should be elevated above the level of the heart, and ice should be applied for 20 minutes every 1 to 2 hours.

Many of these fractures require surgical reduction and fixation to minimize later complications. Rehabilitation to obtain range of motion of the subtalar joint is indicated after clinical healing of the fracture has occurred.

Adverse Outcomes of Treatment

Stiffness and atrophy are adverse outcomes of treatment.

Referral Decisions/Red Flags

Patients with fractures of the calcaneus or talus or a dislocation of the talocalcaneal joint need further evaluation immediately upon diagnosis.

Fracture of the Metatarsals

ICD-9 Codes

825.25
Fracture of other tarsal and metatarsal bones, closed, metatarsal bone(s)

825.35
Fracture of one or more tarsal and metatarsal bones, open, metatarsal bone(s)

Synonym

Forefoot fracture

Definition

Most fractures of the metatarsal bones heal with nonsurgical treatment; however, a zone 2 fracture of the proximal diaphysis of the fifth metatarsal (classic Jones fracture) requires more extensive immobilization, and a zone 3 fracture of this bone may result in nonunion or delayed union (**Figure 1**).

Clinical Symptoms

Swelling and pain on weight bearing are common. Stress fractures usually occur after a sudden increase in activity, such as a new training regimen (increase in intensity or distance), change in running surface, or even prolonged walking.

Tests

Physical Examination

Examination reveals swelling, ecchymosis, and tenderness over the fractured metatarsal.

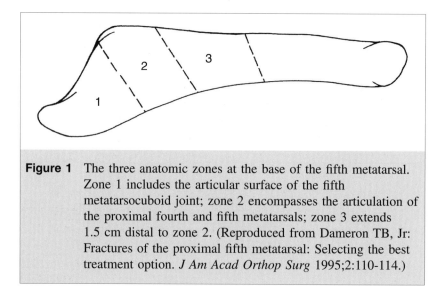

Figure 1 The three anatomic zones at the base of the fifth metatarsal. Zone 1 includes the articular surface of the fifth metatarsocuboid joint; zone 2 encompasses the articulation of the proximal fourth and fifth metatarsals; zone 3 extends 1.5 cm distal to zone 2. (Reproduced from Dameron TB, Jr: Fractures of the proximal fifth metatarsal: Selecting the best treatment option. *J Am Acad Orthop Surg* 1995;2:110-114.)

Diagnostic Tests

AP, lateral, and oblique radiographs of the foot may demonstrate the fracture. A stress fracture of a metatarsal may not show up on radiographs for 2 to 3 weeks. Follow-up radiographs are necessary if a stress fracture is suspected.

Differential Diagnosis

- Interdigital (Morton) neuroma (plantar pain and tenderness between the metatarsal heads)
- Lisfranc dislocation or sprain (location at the tarsometatarsal joint)
- Lisfranc fracture (location at the tarsometatarsal joint)
- Metatarsalgia (plantar pain and tenderness over the metatarsal head)

Adverse Outcomes of the Disease

Both malunion and nonunion are possible; however, nonunion is uncommon except in association with a fracture in zone 2 or 3 of the proximal fifth metatarsal. Malunion of a metatarsal shaft or neck fracture may result in metatarsalgia with a plantar callus. Compartment syndrome may develop after severe trauma or multiple metatarsal fractures.

Treatment

Treatment of nondisplaced metatarsal neck and shaft fractures includes the use of a short leg cast, fracture brace, or wooden-soled shoe. The device that requires the minimum amount of immobilization while providing adequate comfort should be selected. Weight bearing is permitted as tolerated. In most cases, radiographs should be repeated after 1 week to identify any displacement, and again at 6 weeks to confirm healing. Tenderness at the fracture site will diminish as the fracture heals. A fracture of the first metatarsal is often the result of a high-impact injury and may require surgery (**Figure 2**).

Multiple metatarsal fractures and fractures with more than 4 mm of displacement or an apical angulation of more than 10° (seen on the lateral view) may require either closed or open reduction to reestablish a physiologic weight-bearing position of the metatarsal head.

Fractures of the proximal fifth metatarsal may be easy or difficult to manage. Avulsion fractures of the base of the fifth metatarsal (zone 1) or proximal metaphyseal fractures (zone 2) do well with nonsurgical treatment. Immobilization with an air stirrup, wooden-soled shoe, or fracture brace is continued until symptoms subside. Acute fractures in zone 2 are more difficult

Figure 2 Radiograph shows fractures of the first metatarsal (arrow) and second metatarsal (arrowhead). (Reproduced from Shereff MJ: Fractures of the forefoot. *Instr Course Lect* 1990;39:133-140.)

to treat. Most cases will heal with cast immobilization, but treatment of these injuries should start with non–weight-bearing ambulation in a short leg cast for 6 to 8 weeks. Early internal fixation may be considered for some patients, such as athletes. Fractures in zone 3 often resemble a stress fracture with prodromal symptoms suddenly exacerbated by an inversion injury. These require surgical intervention to avoid nonunion or delayed union.

Adverse Outcomes of Treatment

Malunion with painful plantar callosities under the metatarsal heads or transfer lesions under the neighboring metatarsal heads may occur if there is displacement or shortening of the metatarsal.

Referral Decisions/Red Flags

Multiple metatarsal fractures, a metatarsal fracture with more than 4 mm of displacement or more than 10° of angulation, possible compartment syndrome, and proximal fifth metatarsal fracture in zones 2 or 3 are all indications for further evaluation. Displaced or comminuted fractures of the first metatarsal also require further evaluation. Open fractures require immediate surgical intervention.

Fractures of the Phalanges

Synonym

Broken toe

Definition

A phalangeal fracture, commonly known as a broken toe, usually involves the proximal phalanx and is caused by direct trauma. These fractures rarely result in major disability. The fifth (little) toe is the most commonly affected.

Clinical Symptoms

Patients have pain, swelling, or ecchymosis.

Tests

Physical Examination

Examination may reveal deformity of the toe, but local bony tenderness, swelling, and ecchymosis are often the only principal findings.

Diagnostic Tests

Radiographs usually confirm the diagnosis (**Figure 1**).

Differential Diagnosis

- Freiberg infraction (osteonecrosis of the metatarsal head seen on radiographs)
- Ingrown toenail/paronychia (inflammation of the fold of tissue around the toenail noted on physical examination)
- Metatarsalgia (plantar tenderness over the metatarsal head)
- Metatarsophalangeal (MTP) synovitis (tenderness over the MTP joint)

Adverse Outcomes of the Disease

Chronic swelling and deformity of the toe are possible. Permanent deformity is an uncommon possibility.

Figure 1 AP radiograph of the foot demonstrates a fracture of the proximal phalanx of the second toe.

Figure 2 Buddy taping.

Treatment

Phalangeal fractures are treated by buddy taping the fractured toe to an adjacent toe, usually the toe medial to the fractured one (**Figure 2**). A gauze pad may be placed between the toes to absorb moisture and prevent maceration of the skin from sweating. The tape and gauze should be changed as often as needed to maintain a clean, dry environment.

Closed reduction under a digital block or open reduction and pinning is rarely necessary but should be considered in several circumstances: for markedly angulated fractures, or for fractures involving the articular surface of the MTP joints of all toes or the interphalangeal joint of the great toe.

Adverse Outcomes of Treatment

The skin can become macerated from moisture under the tape.

Referral Decisions/Red Flags

Patients with an open fracture or a displaced intra-articular fracture (especially at the MTP joint) need further evaluation.

Fracture of the Sesamoid

Definition

The first metatarsophalangeal (MTP) joint has two sesamoids, one medial and one lateral (**Figure 1**). The plantar aspect of each sesamoid is surrounded by the fibers of the flexor hallucis brevis and the plantar plate, and the dorsal aspect of the sesamoid has a facet that articulates with the metatarsal head. Because of its more protected position in the lateral soft tissues, the lateral, or fibular, sesamoid is less susceptible to fracture than is the medial sesamoid. Sesamoid fractures may occur secondary to avulsion forces, such as hyperdorsiflexion of the first MTP joint; repetitive stress; or, more commonly, from direct trauma. The repetitive stress from running or dancing can result in either a stress fracture or an avulsion fracture. Accessory sesamoids also may be found under any of the lesser metatarsal heads. The most common location is under the second metatarsal head on the tibial side. Although fractures of the sesamoids of the MTP joint (**Figure 2**) are the most common, sesamoids under any metatarsal head may fracture.

A bipartite sesamoid is a normal variant (**Figure 3**). It is important to distinguish this normal condition from a fracture.

ICD-9 Codes
733.99   Other disorders of bone and cartilage
825.20   Fracture of unspecified bone(s) of foot except toes, closed
825.30   Fracture of one or more tarsal and metatarsal bones, open, unspecified bone(s) of foot [except toes], instep

Clinical Symptoms

Patients report pain under the first metatarsal head. Swelling and, rarely, ecchymosis may be present. The patient may have a

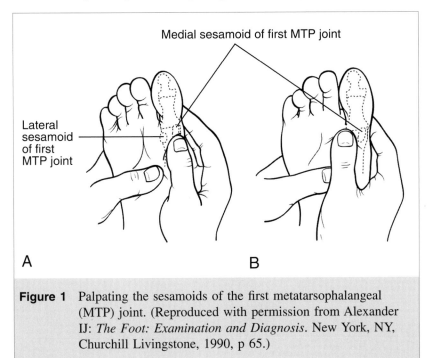

Medial sesamoid of first MTP joint

Lateral sesamoid of first MTP joint

A

B

Figure 1 Palpating the sesamoids of the first metatarsophalangeal (MTP) joint. (Reproduced with permission from Alexander IJ: *The Foot: Examination and Diagnosis*. New York, NY, Churchill Livingstone, 1990, p 65.)

Figure 2 AP view of the foot shows a fracture of the lateral sesamoid of the MTP joint.

Figure 3 AP view of a right foot shows a bipartite lateral sesamoid.

history of direct trauma, a hyperdorsiflexion injury (resulting in an avulsion fracture), or a history of repetitive stress such as running, jumping, or dancing.

Tests

Physical Examination

Patients report pain localized over the fractured sesamoid. The painful spot will move with the sesamoid as the great toe is flexed and extended. The pain may increase with dorsiflexion of the first MTP joint, as tension is applied to the flexor tendon complex. Range of motion of the first MTP joint may be restricted, especially in dorsiflexion, due to pain or guarding.

Diagnostic Tests

AP, lateral, and axial views should be obtained to establish the diagnosis. The lateral sesamoid is best visualized on an internal oblique view. A technetium Tc 99m bone scan can help differentiate an acute fracture or stress fracture from a bipartite sesamoid and is considered to be 100% sensitive. A fractured sesamoid will demonstrate increased uptake on a bone scan, whereas a bipartite sesamoid will show no increased activity. MRI can help differentiate a fracture from a bipartite sesamoid or osteonecrosis. In the presence of a fracture, MRI will show marrow edema. MRI can also help evaluate the plantar plate, the intersesamoid ligament, and the flexor tendons.

Differential Diagnosis

- Bipartite sesamoid (smooth, sclerotic edges on radiographs; negative bone scan; may be bilateral)
- Osteonecrosis (sclerotic appearance of entire sesamoid or irregularity with fragmentation seen on radiographs)
- Plantar plate disruption (proximal migration of sesamoid noted on physical examination and radiographs)

Adverse Outcomes of the Disease

The patient with an untreated sesamoid fracture will usually demonstrate pain and a limp. A nonunion may occur following an acute fracture.

Treatment

The recommended treatment for an acute sesamoid fracture is a removable short leg fracture brace or a stiff-soled shoe with a rocker bottom. Usually at 4 weeks, as the symptoms improve, the patient is allowed to wear a stiff-soled shoe with a high toe box. Once the fracture is clinically healed, a felt pad to suspend the metatarsal head is recommended for 6 months.

Adverse Outcomes of Treatment

Healing of this fracture may take 6 to 12 months, resulting in limited dorsiflexion of the first MTP joint.

Referral Decisions/Red Flags

Persistent pain is an indication for further evaluation. In more severe cases, the fractured sesamoid may have to be removed surgically.

SECTION 7 FOOT AND ANKLE

Procedure: Digital Anesthetic Block (Foot)

MATERIALS

- Sterile gloves

- Bactericidal skin preparation
  solution

- Ethyl chloride spray

- 10-mL syringe

- 18-gauge needle

- 25-gauge, 1½″ needle

- 10 mL of 1% lidocaine or 0.5%
  bupivacaine, both without
  epinephrine

- Adhesive dressing

Figure 1 Location of needle
insertion for a digital
anesthetic block.

Step 1
Wear protective gloves at all times during the procedure and use sterile technique.

Step 2
Use the 18-gauge needle to draw 10 mL of the local anesthetic into the syringe; then switch to the 25-gauge needle to preserve sterility.

Step 3
Cleanse the dorsal surface of the foot with bactericidal solution on either side of the metatarsal heads.

Step 4
Freeze the dorsal skin with ethyl chloride spray.

Step 5
Insert the 25-gauge needle into the soft-tissue space on either side of the metatarsal head until it just begins to tent the plantar skin (**Figure 1**). Remember that the sensory nerves travel along the plantar side of the metatarsal.

Step 6
Withdraw the needle approximately 1 cm or until the tip rests at the level of the plantar aspect of the metatarsal head.

Step 7
Inject 3 mL of anesthetic, then an additional 2 mL while the needle is withdrawn. Make certain that some of the anesthetic is deposited subcutaneously around the dorsal sensory nerves.

Step 8
Repeat the procedure on the other side of the metatarsal of the toe that is to be anesthetized. Within 1 to 2 minutes, the involved toe should become numb.

Step 9
Dress the puncture site with a sterile adhesive dressing.

Adverse Outcomes

Although rare, infection is possible. Necrosis of a digit is possible if epinephrine is used in the anesthetic solution.

Aftercare/Patient Instructions

Advise the patient that a collection of fluid on the plantar aspect of the foot may appear but that the fluid will dissipate within several hours after the block.

SECTION 7 FOOT AND ANKLE

Hallux Rigidus

ICD-9 Code

735.2
Hallux rigidus

Synonyms

Great toe arthritis
Hallux limitus

Definition

Hallux rigidus, or degenerative arthritis of the metatarsophalangeal (MTP) joint of the great toe, is the most common site of arthritis in the foot. The principal symptoms are pain and stiffness, especially as the toe moves into dorsiflexion. Hallux rigidus is the second most common malady of the great toe behind hallux valgus and is the most common arthritis of the foot.

Clinical Symptoms

Patients have pain in the great toe joint with activity, especially in the toe-off phase of gait as the MTP joint goes into extension. The osteophytes that develop on the dorsum of the toe may cause the overlying soft tissue to become red and irritated with shoe wear (**Figure 1**). The dorsal sensory nerves of the great toe may be irritated by the associated swelling.

Figure 1 Foot with dorsal prominence from underlying bony osteophyte (arrow). **A,** Top view. **B,** Lateral view. (Reproduced from Mann RA: Hallux rigidus. *Instr Course Lect* 1990;39:15-21.)

Figure 2 **A,** Hallux rigidus osteophytes (arrows). **B,** Loss of extension is the hallmark of this condition. (Reproduced with permission from Alexander IJ: *The Foot: Examination and Diagnosis.* New York, NY, Churchill Livingstone, 1990, p 65.)

Tests

Physical Examination

Stiffness of the great toe with loss of extension at the MTP joint is the hallmark of hallux rigidus. Osteophytes develop primarily on the dorsal portion of the first metatarsal head (**Figure 2**). The toe is usually in normal alignment.

Diagnostic Tests

AP and lateral radiographs show narrowing of the MTP joint of the great toe and osteophytes, predominantly on the dorsal and lateral aspects of the great toe (**Figure 3**).

Differential Diagnosis

- Gout (recurrent episode of erythema and swelling, positive clinical history)
- Hallux valgus (bunion and valgus angulation of the great toe)
- Turf toe (history of injury, pain on the plantar aspect of MTP joint exacerbated by extension of the toe)

Adverse Outcomes of the Disease

Pain aggravated by walking is common. Weight is transferred to the lateral side of the foot, especially during toe-off, causing increased stress and overuse on the lateral side of the foot.

Treatment

Nonsurgical treatment consists of wearing a shoe with a large, soft toe box to decrease pressure on the toe. A stiff-soled shoe modified with a steel shank or rocker bottom limits dorsiflexion of the great toe and decreases pain caused by motion in the

Figure 3 Weight-bearing AP radiograph of the feet of a patient with hallux rigidus. Note the advanced arthritic changes in the left foot (white arrow) and the small medial and lateral spurs (white arrowheads) in the right foot.

arthritic joint. Patients should be advised to avoid wearing high-heeled shoes. NSAIDs, ice, and contrast baths also can help decrease inflammation and control symptoms for a short time.

Surgical treatment consists of either excision of the dorsal osteophytes or fusion of the joint (arthrodesis). Resection of the joint may be indicated in some patients. An artificial joint implant is not recommended.

Adverse Outcomes of Treatment

NSAIDs may cause gastric, renal, or hepatic complications. No other adverse outcomes of treatment have been reported, other than the usual surgical complications.

Referral Decisions/Red Flags

Failure of nonsurgical treatment is an indication for further evaluation.

Hallux Valgus

Synonyms

Bunion

Metatarsus primus varus

ICD-9 Code

735.0
Hallux valgus (acquired)

Definition

Hallux valgus is lateral deviation of the great toe at the
metatarsophalangeal (MTP) joint that may lead to a painful
prominence of the medial aspect of the first metatarsal head,
known as a bunion (**Figure 1**). The female-to-male ratio of
symptomatic hallux valgus occurrence is approximately 10:1.

Clinical Symptoms

Pain and swelling, aggravated by shoe wear, are the principal
symptoms. A hypertrophic bursa may occur over the medial
eminence of the first metatarsal. The great toe may pronate
(rotate inward), with resultant callus on the medial aspect.
Irritation of the medial plantar sensory nerve may cause
numbness or tingling over the medial aspect of the great toe.

Tests

Physical Examination

Assess the valgus angulation at the MTP joint (normal valgus at
the MTP joint is less than 15°). Measure the range of motion at
the MTP joint. Most patients with hallux valgus have relatively
normal MTP motion (60° to 90° of extension and 30° of
flexion). Evaluate the lesser toes for associated deformities. A
second toe that overrides the laterally deviated great toe is a
common problem (**Figure 2**). Other lesser toe problems include
corns, calluses, hammer toes, and bunionette (a bunion-like
prominence on the lateral side of the fifth MTP joint).

Diagnostic Tests

The severity of a bunion deformity is graded by measuring
certain forefoot angles on weight-bearing AP radiographs of the
foot. The hallux valgus angle is measured between the first
metatarsal and the proximal phalanx. Normal is less than 15°. A
normal 1-2 intermetatarsal (IM) angle formed between the first
and second metatarsals is less than 10° (**Figure 3**). Radiographs
also are used to assess lateral subluxation of the sesamoids, the
shape of the metatarsal head, degenerative changes in the MTP
joint, valgus at the interphalangeal (IP) joint, and lesser toe

Figure 1   Anatomy of hallux
valgus. (Adapted with
permission from
Pedowitz W: Bunion
deformity, in Pfeffer
G, Frey C, eds:
*Current Practice in
Foot and Ankle
Surgery.* New York,
NY, McGraw Hill,
1993, pp 219-242.)

Figure 2   Severe hallux valgus
with dislocation of
the second toe.

Figure 3 Hallux valgus severity is assessed by measuring the hallux valgus angle and the intermetatarsal (IM) angle on a weight-bearing AP radiograph of the foot. **A**, Diagram showing the hallux valgus angle and the IM angle. **B**, AP radiograph of the feet of a patient with hallux valgus demonstrates valgus angulation of 14° in the left foot and 17° in the right foot. (Part A is adapted with permission from Pedowitz W: Bunion deformity, in Pfeffer G, Frey C, eds: *Current Practice in Foot and Ankle Surgery*. New York, NY, McGraw Hill, 1993, pp 219-242.)

abnormalities. A weight-bearing lateral radiograph of the foot is less helpful but is important for evaluating any lesser toe subluxation or arthritic changes of the great toe MTP joint.

Differential Diagnosis

- Gout (articular and periarticular inflammation and tenderness on physical examination)
- Hallux extensus (cock-up toe, or extension of the great toe) (seen on physical examination)
- Hallux interphalangeus (lateral deviation of the great toe at the IP joint) (seen on physical examination or radiographs)
- Hallux rigidus (osteoarthritis of the first MTP joint) (limited dorsiflexion of great toe)
- Hallux varus (medial deviation of the great toe at the MTP joint seen on physical examination)

Adverse Outcomes of the Disease

Chronic pain is the primary symptom.

Treatment

When bunions occur in children, they are generally observed. In adults, the initial treatment is patient education and shoe wear modifications. Nonsurgical treatment is usually successful in mild to moderate cases. Recommended shoes have adequate width at the forefoot, soft uppers, and no stitching patterns over the bunion. An orthotist or skilled shoemaker can stretch the shoe directly over the bunion. High heels increase the pressure under the ball of the foot and over the bunion deformity and therefore should be avoided. Rehabilitation, splints, and bracing are not helpful, although a medial longitudinal arch support can decrease pressure on a bunion associated with a pronated flatfoot.

No treatment is needed for asymptomatic hallux valgus, even if the deformity continues to progress. Competitive athletes should avoid surgical correction of hallux valgus deformities until after their competitive careers are over, as surgery can affect performance. For patients who have continued disability despite nonsurgical treatment, several well-established surgical procedures are available. Indications for different procedures are based on the severity of the hallux valgus, the IM angle, and joint congruity. Joint replacement is rarely indicated because of the high complication rate.

Adverse Outcomes of Treatment

Surgical treatment may result in recurrence, undercorrection, overcorrection (hallux varus), decreased function, stiffness, pain, malunion or nonunion of an osteotomy, and transfer lesions (metatarsalgia).

Referral Decisions/Red Flags

Persistent pain despite shoe modifications indicates the need for further evaluation. Patients with persistent pain may benefit from surgical correction.

Ingrown Toenail

ICD-9 Code

703.0
Diseases of nail; ingrowing nail

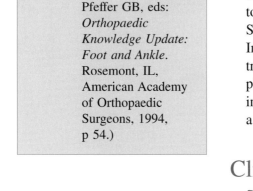

Figure 1 Ingrown toenail. (Reproduced from Lutter LD, Mizel MS, Pfeffer GB, eds: *Orthopaedic Knowledge Update: Foot and Ankle.* Rosemont, IL, American Academy of Orthopaedic Surgeons, 1994, p 54.)

Synonyms

Infected toenail

Onychocryptosis

Paronychia

Definition

With an ingrown toenail, the distal margin of the nail grows into the adjacent skin, causing irritation, inflammation, and possibly secondary bacterial or fungal infection. The condition is virtually limited to the great toe. Ingrown toenails are associated with improper trimming of the toenail, tight shoes, hereditary predisposition, subungual pathology, congenital incurved nail, thickened nail, direct trauma, or any combination of these factors (**Figure 1**).

Unlike fingernails, toenails should not be cut in a curved fashion because this allows the sharp edge of the nail to grow into the more prominent skin margins (nail fold) found at the end of toenails. Properly trimmed toenails are cut straight across to keep the lateral margin of the toenail beyond the nail fold. Some people have toenails that have a naturally incurved shape. Ingrown toenails may occur in these patients even with proper trimming techniques. Soft-tissue hypertrophy over a normal nail plate secondary to trauma or tight shoes also may cause an ingrown toenail. Skin breakthrough creates a portal of entry for a secondary bacterial or fungal infection.

Clinical Symptoms

Stage I (inflammation) is characterized by induration, swelling, and tenderness along the nail fold. In stage II (abscess), the patient has purulent or serous drainage, increased tenderness, and increased erythema. In stage III (granulation), granulation tissue grows onto the nail plate, inhibiting drainage. This stage is less painful than stage II.

Tests

Physical Examination

The diagnosis is clinical; visual inspection is the basis for staging the condition.

Diagnostic Tests

Radiographs of stage II and stage III ingrown toenails may be obtained to rule out a subungual exostosis (cartilage-capped projection from bone) and osteomyelitis.

Differential Diagnosis

- Felon (deep abscess on the plantar aspect of the toe)
- Onychomycosis (fungal infection of the nail)
- Osteomyelitis (bone infection with changes on radiograph)
- Paronychia (superficial abscess on the base of the toenail)
- Subungual exostosis (osteochondroma beneath the nail, noted radiographically)

Adverse Outcomes of the Disease

Progressive pain, paronychia, felon, nail plate deformity, and osteomyelitis are all possible. Hematogenous seeding of other organs may occur but is very uncommon.

Treatment

Stage I: Warm soaks, proper nail trimming, accommodative shoe wear, and clean socks are recommended. With a blunt instrument, insert cotton or waxed dental floss beneath the nail to lift the edge of the nail from its embedded position. Exchange packing daily until the nail has grown out sufficiently. Nonconstrictive shoes or sandals prevent extrinsic irritation of the inflamed skin.

Stage II: Initial treatment should include foot soaks along with broad-spectrum oral antibiotics (cephalosporin). Partial excision of the nail under digital block (see page 814) should be performed when the patient has severe pain, when there is a risk of secondary infection to a prosthetic joint, or when a course of oral antibiotics fails to treat associated infection. Partial nail excision is preferred (see page 825). Complete nail excision increases the risk of deformity of the nail bed, resulting in clubbing. An avulsed nail requires 3 to 4 months to regrow.

Stage III: Partial or complete nail plate excision with or without ablation of the germinal matrix of the nail is indicated.

Adverse Outcomes of Treatment

Adverse outcomes include recurrence (50% to 70% with excision alone), nail plate deformity, upturned nail or clubbed nail after complete nail plate excision, and poor cosmetic result.

Referral Decisions/Red Flags

Failure of nonsurgical treatment or the presence of stage III disease is an indication for further evaluation.

Procedure: Nail Plate Avulsion

Anatomy

A recurrent ingrown toenail or paronychial infection, which usually occurs in the great toe, makes it necessary to remove a portion of the nail plate. The lateral and/or medial margins of the nail may be involved.

Removal of the entire nail plate is described below. Because this risks nail bed deformity, however, partial removal should be performed whenever possible. Partial removal involves elevating one third of the nail on the affected (lateral or medial) side with a small scissors or hemostat, cutting the nail longitudinally with strong small scissors or an anvil nail cutter, and avulsing the freed portion of the nail adjacent to the nail fold.

Step 1

Wear protective gloves at all times during the procedure, and use sterile technique.

Step 2

Cleanse the toe with a bactericidal solution.

Step 3

Follow the steps in the procedure titled Digital Anesthetic Block (Foot) on page 814 to administer a digital block.

Step 4

Wrap a ¼″ Penrose drain or strip of rubber around the base of the toe to act as a tourniquet and control bleeding (optional).

Step 5

Using a small scissors or hemostat, elevate the nail plate from the underlying nail bed (**Figure 1**).

Step 6

Separate the proximal cuticle (nail fold) from the nail plate.

Step 7

Grasp the free portion of the nail plate with a hemostat and avulse it (**Figure 2**), then palpate the nail bed to ensure that no spikes of nail tissue remain.

Step 8

If a tourniquet was used, remove it and apply compression to stop local bleeding.

CPT Codes

11730
Avulsion of nail plate, partial or complete, simple; single

11732
Avulsion of nail plate, partial or complete, simple; each additional nail plate

(List separately in addition to code for primary procedure)

Current Procedural Terminology © 2010 American Medical Association. All rights reserved.

Materials

- Sterile gloves
- Bactericidal skin preparation solution
- ¼″ Penrose drain or a strip cut from a rubber glove (optional)
- Materials to administer a digital block (see Digital Anesthetic Block [Foot], page 814)
- Strong small scissors or anvil nail cutter
- Small hemostat
- Nonadherent sterile gauze
- Sterile dressing material

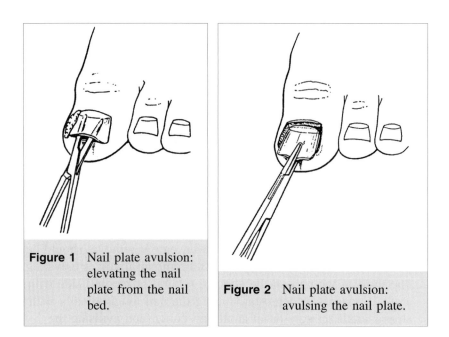

Figure 1 Nail plate avulsion: elevating the nail plate from the nail bed.

Figure 2 Nail plate avulsion: avulsing the nail plate.

Step 9

Apply nonadherent sterile gauze over the exposed nail bed and wrap the entire toe with a sterile dressing.

Adverse Outcomes

Recurrence of the ingrown toenail is common after nail plate avulsions. Permanent ablation of the nail matrix may be required.

Permanent Ablation

This procedure may be necessary and can be performed by curettage and/or phenol ablation of the nail matrix.

Interdigital (Morton) Neuroma

Synonyms

Intermetatarsal neuroma

Morton neuroma

Plantar neuroma

ICD-9 Code

355.6
Mononeuritis of lower limb; lesion of plantar nerve

Definition

A plantar interdigital neuroma, also referred to as a Morton neuroma, is not a true neuroma but rather a perineural fibrosis of the common digital nerve as it passes between the metatarsal heads. The fibrosis is secondary to repetitive irritation of the nerve. The condition most commonly occurs between the third and fourth toes (third web space) (**Figure 1**). Interdigital neuromas occur less frequently in the second web space (between the second and third toes) and rarely in either the first or fourth intermetatarsal space. The simultaneous occurrence of two neuromas is extremely uncommon. Interdigital neuroma has a female-to-male ratio of 5:1, probably related to compression of the nerve by tight shoes.

Figure 1 Interdigital neuroma between the metatarsal heads. (Adapted with permission from McElvenny RT: The etiology and surgical treatment of intractable pain about the fourth metatarsophalangeal joint (Morton toe). *J Bone Joint Surg Am* 1943;25:675-679.)

Clinical Symptoms

Plantar pain in the forefoot is the most common presenting symptom. Dysesthesias into the affected two toes or burning plantar pain that is aggravated by activity also is common. Occasionally, patients report numbness in the toes adjacent to the involved web space. Night pain is rare. Many patients state that they feel as though they are "walking on a marble" or that there is "a wrinkle in my sock." Relief often is obtained by removing the shoe and rubbing the ball of the foot. Symptoms are aggravated by wearing high-heeled or tight, restrictive shoes.

Tests

Physical Examination

Isolated pain on the plantar aspect of the web space is consistent with an interdigital neuroma. Apply direct plantar pressure to the interspace with one hand and then squeeze the metatarsals together with the other hand. If an interdigital neuroma is present, this maneuver will cause increased tenderness and pain radiating to the toes.

Inspect the plantar surface for calluses. Then palpate dorsally along the metatarsal shafts and plantarly over the metatarsal heads to evaluate for stress fractures or metatarsalgia, respectively. Evaluate sensory function of the digital nerves. Stress each tarsometatarsal joint by grasping the midfoot with one hand and moving each metatarsal dorsally and then plantarly to rule out midfoot arthritis. Similarly, grasp the metatarsal shaft and, while keeping the toe parallel to the metatarsal, try to displace the digit dorsally, then plantarly. Pain or excess motion with this maneuver indicates synovitis or inflammation of the metatarsophalangeal (MTP) joint.

Diagnostic Tests

Radiographs are normal in patients with interdigital neuroma. MRI and ultrasonography sometimes detect neuromas, but these modalities are unreliable for this purpose and their use is not commonly indicated.

Differential Diagnosis

- Hammer toe (flexion deformity of the proximal interphalangeal joint noted on physical examination)
- Metatarsalgia (plantar tenderness over the metatarsal head noted on physical examination)
- MTP synovitis (tenderness and swelling directly over the MTP joint noted on physical examination)
- Stress fracture (dorsal metatarsal tenderness noted on physical examination)

Adverse Outcomes of the Disease

Chronic, intermittent pain and the need for shoe and activity modifications are possible.

Treatment

Patients should be advised to wear a low-heeled, well-cushioned shoe with a wide toe box. A well-cushioned sandal is another option. In addition, pain relief may be obtained using metatarsal pads to spread the metatarsal heads and take pressure off the nerve (see also page 775).

Locate the neuroma on the plantar aspect of the foot in the soft tissue between the involved metatarsal heads. Ask the patient to mark the painful spot on the bottom of the foot with a material that transfers easily, such as lipstick or eyeliner. Instruct the patient to stand, without socks, in a shoe to transfer the mark to the inside of the shoe. Place the pad in the shoe just proximal to the mark, to suspend the painful area. This also ensures that the metatarsal heads are kept apart and away from the neuroma when the patient is bearing weight. Felt or gel pads are inexpensive and effective. They come in different sizes to accommodate shoes and feet of different sizes. Advise the patient that, if the pad is effective, a more permanent orthosis can be fabricated that can be transferred from shoe to shoe. Avoid using a rigid orthosis, as it may aggravate the neuroma.

A mixture of 1 to 2 mL of lidocaine without epinephrine and 1 mL (10 mg/mL) of corticosteroid injected just proximal to the metatarsal heads can be both diagnostic and therapeutic (see page 830). Multiple injections should be avoided.

If symptoms persist or recur, surgical excision of the neuroma or division of the transverse metatarsal ligament is indicated.

Adverse Outcomes of Treatment

Symptoms may persist or recur after nonsurgical treatment. Symptoms may recur or become worse after surgical excision of the neuroma if a painful stump of nerve develops.

Referral Decisions/Red Flags

Persistent pain despite shoe or insert modifications or injection of corticosteroid indicates the need for further evaluation.

Procedure: Interdigital (Morton) Neuroma Injection

CPT Code

28899
Unlisted procedure, foot or toes

Current Procedural Terminology
© 2010 American Medical
Association. All rights reserved.

Materials

- Sterile gloves
- Bactericidal skin preparation solution
- Ethyl chloride spray
- 3-mL syringe
- 18-gauge needle
- 25-gauge, 1″ to 1½″ needle
- 1 mL of 10 mg/mL corticosteroid preparation
- 2 mL of 1.0% lidocaine or 0.5% bupivacaine, both without epinephrine
- Adhesive dressing

Step 1
Wear protective gloves at all times during the procedure and use sterile technique.

Step 2
Use the 18-gauge needle to draw 1 mL of the 10 mg/mL corticosteroid preparation and 2 mL of the local anesthetic into the syringe; then switch to the 25-gauge needle to preserve sterility.

Step 3
Cleanse the dorsal skin between the metatarsal heads with bactericidal solution.

Step 4
Freeze the dorsal skin with ethyl chloride spray.

Step 5
Place the needle in line with the metatarsophalangeal joint, which is approximately 1 to 2 cm proximal to the web of the toe (**Figure 1**).

Figure 1 Proper location for injection for interdigital (Morton) neuroma.

Step 6

Insert the needle through the dorsal tissues until the tip barely tents the skin of the plantar aspect of the foot. Withdraw the needle approximately 1 cm so that the tip is where the neuroma is found, at the level of the plantar metatarsophalangeal joint.

Step 7

Inject the corticosteroid-anesthetic mixture around the neuroma, taking care not to inject into the plantar fat pad.

SECTION 7 FOOT AND ANKLE

Metatarsalgia

ICD-9 Code

726.70
Enthesopathy of ankle and tarsus, unspecified

Synonym

Forefoot pain

Definition

Metatarsalgia is a general term indicating forefoot pain localized under one or more of the lesser metatarsals. Abnormal metatarsal length with alteration of weight-bearing forces is one cause of metatarsalgia. Toe deformities such as claw or hammer toe also may lead to metatarsalgia by causing displacement of the plantar fat pad and loss of cushioning under the metatarsal heads. Callus formation occurs, and this thickened skin may be a major component of the patient's symptoms. A persistent callus on the sole of the foot is called intractable plantar keratosis.

Clinical Symptoms

Activity-related pain is localized to the plantar aspect of the forefoot directly over the metatarsal heads. The patient may complain about the diffuse callus formation.

Tests

Physical Examination

Observe the alignment of the toes. Evaluate swelling, range of motion, and stability of the metatarsophalangeal (MTP) joints. Palpate for swelling or masses along the plantar and dorsal aspects of the metatarsals as well as adjacent interspaces. Note the extent of any callus and whether it is discrete or diffuse. A discrete callus is tender with direct pressure. Evaluate digital nerve function.

Diagnostic Tests

Weight-bearing AP and lateral radiographs of the foot should be obtained to assess metatarsal and toe alignment.

Differential Diagnosis

- Claw toe–related pain (plantar displacement of the metatarsal heads and fat pad noted on physical examination)
- Interdigital neuroma (numbness in the involved web space)
- Intractable plantar keratosis (persistent callus on sole of foot)
- Metatarsal stress fracture (localized tenderness over the fracture site, radiographic findings)

- MTP synovitis (swelling of the joint, dorsal tenderness)
- Plantar wart (tender with circumferential pressure)

Adverse Outcomes of the Disease

Patients may experience progressive pain and difficulty walking.

Treatment

Accommodative shoes, a metatarsal pad (see page 775), or an orthotic device is the key to treatment. A thickened callus can be shaved (see page 784). Nonsurgical treatment usually is successful, but if these measures fail, surgery to realign the toes and/or metatarsal head may be considered. Removal of the metatarsal head should be avoided.

Adverse Outcomes of Treatment

Inadequate pain relief, delayed union, nonunion, and transfer lesions (stress with resultant pain transferred to the adjacent metatarsal) are possible complications of surgical treatment.

Referral Decisions/Red Flags

Symptoms that persist despite nonsurgical care indicate the need for further evaluation.

Nail Fungus Infection

ICD-9 Code

110.1
Dermatophytosis, of nail

Synonyms

Dermatophytic onychomycosis
Tinea ungulum

Definition

Fungal infection of the nail (onychomycosis) occurs four times more frequently in the toes than in the fingers. *Trichophyton rubrum* and *Trichophyton mentagrophytes* cause 90% of these infections. Approximately 50% of patients are older than 70 years. The problem may be primarily cosmetic, or the nail may become so hypertrophic that it interferes with shoe wear and is painful.

Clinical Symptoms

Patients report discoloration, thickening, and difficulty in trimming the nails.

Tests

Physical Examination
Thickening and chalky yellow or white discoloration of the nail is observed (**Figure 1**).

Diagnostic Tests
Diagnosis is made by microscopic examination of nail scrapings and potassium hydroxide slide preparation.

Figure 1 Toenail with fungal infection.

Differential Diagnosis

- Onychogryphosis (severe nail deformity, curling at the edge of the nail)
- Repetitive trauma (ridges and cracking of the nail with thickening)

Adverse Outcomes of the Disease

A thickened nail can make shoe wear difficult.

Treatment

Treatment options include observation with periodic trimming of the thickened nail, removal of the nail, and/or medications.

Topical medications are less effective than oral agents because topical medications cannot penetrate the thickened nail. Recently developed oral agents such as itraconazole, fluconazole, ketoconazole, and terbinafine have been shown to be effective in the treatment of onychomycosis. For example, itraconazole 200 mg per day given continuously or as a pulse dose (200 mg twice daily for 1 week per month for 3 consecutive months) has been reported to achieve a mycologic cure of 64% at 12 months, with 88% of patients showing marked improvement.

Adverse Outcomes of Treatment

Oral therapy is costly and may elevate hepatic enzyme levels. These levels should be tested periodically (especially in patients with a history of hepatic dysfunction). Rare cases of hepatobiliary dysfunction have been reported.

Orthotic Devices

Definition

Proper shoe fit, shoe modifications, inserts, pads, and orthoses can significantly relieve symptoms caused by common foot problems. An orthosis can support an area of collapse, cushion an area of pressure, accommodate fixed deformity, limit motion, equalize limb length, and reduce shear of the foot in the shoe. The appropriate use of shoe orthoses, commonly referred to as orthotics, depends on an adequate physical examination and a basic understanding of foot alignment and functions.

Foot Types and Functions

During gait, the normal foot changes from a supple, shock-absorbing structure to a rigid lever for push-off. At heel strike, the foot is supple, allowing shock absorption and accommodations to uneven ground. During midstance, the foot is converted to a rigid lever that supports full body weight while allowing continued progression of the limb (rollover).

A cavus (highly arched) foot is rigid, cannot unlock during early stance, and lacks shock absorption. A pes planus (flatfoot) foot is extremely supple and often does not supinate effectively to form a rigid lever for push-off.

Many types of simple orthotic devices can be dispensed directly from the physician's office or are available at drugstores, sporting goods stores, and shoe stores. Custom orthoses (**Figure 1**) are used for more complex problems or after off-the-shelf devices fail to correct the problem.

Types of Orthotic Devices
Pads/Inserts

1. Full-contact (full-length) insert: A prefabricated rubber or silicone insert that reduces shock by absorbing normal and shear forces.
2. Full-contact orthosis: An orthosis that is molded to the shape of the patient's foot. These are often posted with a wedge that redistributes weight to improve foot alignment and biomechanics, accommodate a deformity, and/or cushion the foot.
3. Soft orthosis: An orthosis that is used primarily for cushioning but offers little control of foot motion.
4. Semirigid orthosis: The most common type of orthosis; it provides reasonable strength and durability and is made to help control alignment of the foot during gait.

Figure 1 Custom orthoses.

Figure 2 Heel insert.

Figure 3 Custom orthoses and metatarsal pad.

Figure 4 University of California Biomechanics Laboratory orthosis.

SECTION 7 FOOT AND ANKLE

5. Rigid orthosis: An orthosis that offers maximum durability and support but requires a precise fit because it provides little flexibility.

6. Heel insert (eg, felt, foam, gel, rubber, or silicone): Prefabricated, shock-absorbing device available over the counter (**Figure 2**).

7. Heel wedge: A device that is tapered to support varus or valgus hindfoot.

8. Scaphoid pad (arch cookie): A medial longitudinal arch pad that provides support for a flatfoot.

9. Metatarsal pad: A pad that is fixed to an insert or the bottom of the shoe (**Figure 3**).

10. Toe crest: An insert that elevates a toe to relieve pressure at the tip (for mallet toe).

11. Toe separator: A pad that is placed between toes to decrease friction. It is used for calluses and corns.

12. UCBL (University of California Biomechanics Laboratory) orthosis: A type of full-contact orthosis that stabilizes the hindfoot by using medial and lateral vertical supports (**Figure 4**). Custom molded by a certified pedorthotist, this is used for subtalar arthrosis, midfoot plantar fasciitis, or a moderate pes planovalgus foot.

Shoes/Modifications

1. Extra-depth shoe: A shoe with increased depth that accommodates forefoot problems, such as a hammer toe, and allows room for inserts.

2. Shoe lift: A device that partially or fully corrects limb-length discrepancy. Typically, ¼″ of lift can be accommodated inside the shoe. Any elevation of ½″ or more must be added to the outside of the shoe.

Figure 5 Over-the-counter shoe with rocker bottom sole.

3. Metatarsal bar: An internal or external transverse bar that unloads the forefoot (for metatarsalgia).

4. Rocker bottom sole: Sole of shoe that is contoured to simulate the rollover phase of gait and therefore reduce forces on the plantar surface of the foot during walking (**Figure 5**).

5. Solid ankle–cushion heel (SACH): Soft material that replaces the posterior portion of the shoe's heel to reduce shock at heel strike.

6. Running shoes: Shoes that are designed for shock absorbency. Typically, 50% of shock absorbency is lost at 300 to 500 miles, so running shoes should be replaced at least every 6 months.

7. Shoe fit: Measure the foot by tracing the width of the forefoot while standing barefoot. The forefoot width of the shoe should be wider than this measurement. The end of the longest toe should be about ½″ from the end of the shoe.

8. Thomas heel: Medial extension of the heel to support flatfoot.

Application of Orthotic Devices and Shoe Modifications

Table 1 lists the types of orthotic therapy recommended for specific foot conditions.

Table 1 Recommended Orthotic Treatment for Specific Diagnoses

Diagnosis	Orthotic Therapy
Bunions and/or bunionettes	Wide toe box, stretch shoes, soft seamless uppers, "bunion shield" type of pad
Cavus foot (rigid)	Soft orthotic cushions to distribute pressures evenly
Flatfoot (adult)	Asymptomatic: No special orthotic or shoe treatment indicated
	Symptomatic: Semiflexible insert or longitudinal arch pad, medial heel wedge, extended medial heel counter
Flatfoot (child)	No special orthotic or shoe treatment indicated; normal in infancy, with more than 97% correcting spontaneously
Hallux rigidus	Full-length prefabricated stiff insert, Morton extension inlay, rocker bottom sole, stiff (stable) midsole
Hammer toe or claw toe	Accommodative shoe wear, toe crest
Interdigital (Morton) neuroma	Wide toe box, metatarsal pad with neuroma positioning
Metatarsalgia	Wide shoes, metatarsal pads, metatarsal bars, or rocker bottom sole; wide toe box, metatarsal pad with neuroma positioning
Neuropathic ulceration	Full-contact cushioned orthosis, extra-depth or custom shoes, rocker bottom sole to unload forefoot
Plantar fasciitis	Prefabricated heel insert (silicone, rubber, or felt)

Plantar Fasciitis

Synonyms

Heel pain syndrome

Heel spur

Plantar heel pain

ICD-9 Codes

726.73
Calcaneal spur

728.71
Plantar fascial fibromatosis

Definition

The plantar fascia arises from the medial tuberosity of the calcaneus and extends to the proximal phalanges of the toes (**Figure 1**). The plantar fascia provides support to the foot, and as the toes extend during the stance phase of gait, the plantar fascia is tightened by a windlass mechanism, resulting in elevation of the longitudinal arch, inversion of the hindfoot, and a resultant external rotation of the leg.

Plantar fasciitis is the most common cause of heel pain in adults. The etiology is probably a degenerative tear of part of the fascial origin from the calcaneus, followed by a tendinosis-type reaction. Chronic degenerative changes in the fibers of the

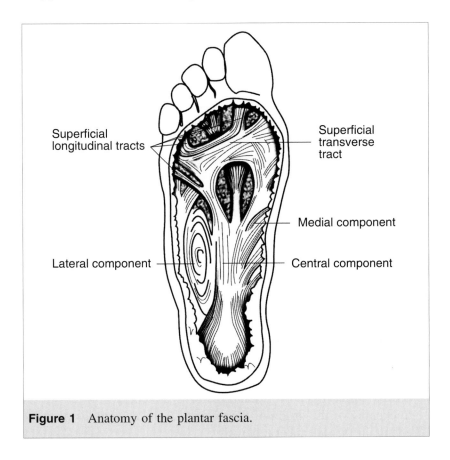

Superficial longitudinal tracts

Superficial transverse tract

Medial component

Lateral component

Central component

Figure 1 Anatomy of the plantar fascia.

plantar fascia are the predominant histologic finding. Plantar fasciitis affects women twice as often as men and is more common in overweight persons. It is not associated with a particular foot type.

Clinical Symptoms

Onset of symptoms is usually insidious and not related to a fall or twisting injury. Patients report focal pain and tenderness directly over the medial calcaneal tuberosity and 1 to 2 cm distally along the plantar fascia. Pain is usually most intense when the patient rises from a resting position, especially in the morning. This occurs because the foot is usually in plantar flexion during rest and the first few steps stretch the plantar fascia. Prolonged standing and walking also increase the pain. Sitting typically relieves symptoms.

Tests

Physical Examination

Examination reveals tenderness directly over the plantar medial calcaneal tuberosity and 1 to 2 cm distally along the plantar fascia. Often, considerable pressure must be applied to this area during the examination to reproduce weight-bearing stress and the patient's symptoms. Patients may have tightness in the Achilles tendon. Passive dorsiflexion of the toes (windlass mechanism) may cause increased pain.

Diagnostic Tests

Radiographs are not necessary as part of the initial evaluation if the patient's history and examination are consistent with a diagnosis of plantar fasciitis. Weight-bearing lateral radiographs should be obtained before an injection of corticosteroid or for patients who continue to have symptoms after 6 to 8 weeks of nonsurgical treatment. Weight-bearing lateral radiographs also may be indicated for patients with systemic symptoms or pain at rest.

A heel spur (entheseophyte) develops in the origin of the flexor brevis muscle just superior to the plantar fascia in approximately 50% of patients with plantar fasciitis (**Figure 2**). The spur is not a source of pain, however, and is present in 20% of similar-age adults who do not have plantar fasciitis.

Although not necessary for diagnosis, a bone scan may show increased uptake at the medial calcaneal tuberosity. MRI, which also is not necessary for diagnosis or treatment, will often show thickening of the origin of the plantar fascia, as well as marrow edema in the calcaneal tuberosity.

Figure 2 Radiographic appearance of a plantar heel spur (arrow).

Differential Diagnosis

- Acute traumatic rupture of the plantar fascia (ecchymosis, tenderness, swelling over the proximal plantar fascia)
- Calcaneal stress fracture (rare, tenderness with medial and lateral pressure of the calcaneus)
- Calcaneal tumor (rare, pain at rest, night pain)
- Fat pad atrophy/contusion (tenderness over an abnormally prominent calcaneal tuberosity)
- Sciatica (radicular symptoms)
- Seronegative spondyloarthropathy (typically bilateral enthesitis of the plantar fascia, other sites of enthesitis, arthralgic joints involved)
- Tarsal tunnel syndrome (paresthesias and numbness on the plantar aspect of the foot)

Adverse Outcomes of the Disease

Patients may experience chronic heel pain and a significant alteration in daily activities. Altered gait may aggravate forefoot, knee, hip, or back problems.

Figure 3 Orthotic heel pad.

Treatment

More than 95% of cases of plantar fasciitis can be managed satisfactorily with nonsurgical treatment. Patients should be informed that it commonly takes 6 to 12 months for symptoms to resolve. Avid walkers and joggers should be counseled concerning alternative exercise regimens, such as use of a stationary bike.

Initial treatment should include an over-the-counter orthotic device, such as a silicone, rubber, or felt heel pad (**Figure 3**), along with a home program of stretching exercises. Some studies suggest that a night splint should be used as part of initial treatment if the patient experiences increased pain on rising from a resting position in the morning. The night splint holds the ankle and foot in slight dorsiflexion, which maintains the Achilles tendon and plantar fascia in a stretched position during sleep.

Contrast baths, ice, NSAIDs, and/or shoes with shock-absorbing soles also can be used to decrease inflammation in the painful heel.

If symptoms persist despite nonsurgical management, injection of corticosteroid into the heel may be indicated (see page 845). A formal rehabilitation consultation may be necessary to help direct the patient's continued stretching program.

If symptoms persist, the use of a nonremovable cast or custom orthotic device should be considered. Surgical treatment typically consists of partial release of the plantar fascia.

Rehabilitation Prescription

Early rehabilitation is directed at controlling pain and increasing the range of motion of the ankle. Heel cord stretching is an important part of a home exercise program (see page 844). Use of a night splint and limited weight bearing are also important. If the symptoms do not respond to these measures, formal rehabilitation may be ordered. The prescription should include evaluation of the foot and ankle mechanics during gait. If overpronation is present, the use of foot orthoses may result in significant improvement. Continued stretching and pain-relieving modalities such as iontophoresis or laser therapy may be ordered.

Adverse Outcomes of Treatment

NSAIDs may cause gastric, renal, or hepatic complications. Fat pad necrosis or rupture of the plantar fascia may develop from improper injection of corticosteroids. Surgical treatment may not improve symptoms and also may cause complete disruption of the plantar fascia.

Referral Decisions/Red Flags

Patients whose symptoms do not respond to nonsurgical treatment require further evaluation. Surgical release should be considered only after 6 to 12 months of intense nonsurgical management. Preliminary data indicate that radial or focal shock wave treatment may be a good treatment option in some patients whose symptoms do not respond to initial nonsurgical treatment.

Home Exercise Program for Plantar Fasciitis

- Apply moist or dry heat to the painful area of the foot during the exercises.
- To prevent inflammation, apply a bag of crushed ice or frozen peas to the heel for 20 minutes after performing the exercises.
- You should not experience pain with the exercises. If you are unable to perform the exercises because of pain or stiffness or if your symptoms do not improve after performing the exercises for 3 to 4 weeks, call your doctor.

Exercise	Muscle Group	Number of Repetitions/Sets	Number of Days per Week	Number of Weeks
Heel cord stretch	Gastrocnemius-soleus complex	4 repetitions/2 or 3 sets	Daily	3 to 4
Plantar fascia massage	Plantar fascia	60 to 90 seconds/2 to 3 sets	Daily	3 to 4

Heel Cord Stretch

- Stand facing a wall with the knee of the unaffected limb bent, the affected limb straight, and the toes pointed in slightly.
- Keeping the heels of both feet flat on the floor, lower your hips toward the wall.
- Hold the stretch for 30 seconds and then relax for 30 seconds.
- Repeat 4 times.
- Perform this exercise daily, 2 or 3 times per day, for 3 to 4 weeks.

Plantar Fascia Massage

- Sit on a chair with your feet touching the floor.
- Place a tennis ball under the affected foot.
- Roll the foot back and forth and side to side over the tennis ball, applying pressure to the ball to achieve a greater massage, for 60 to 90 seconds. (This exercise might cause slight discomfort but should not be painful. If you experience pain, reduce the pressure on the tennis ball.)
- Perform the exercise 2 to 3 times per day, for 3 to 4 weeks.

Procedure: Plantar Fasciitis Injection

Step 1

Wear protective gloves at all times during the procedure and use sterile technique.

Step 2

Use the 18-gauge needle to draw 1 mL of 40 mg/mL corticosteroid preparation and 4 mL of the local anesthetic into the syringe; then switch to the 21-gauge needle to preserve sterility.

Step 3

Prepare the medial aspect of the heel.

Step 4

Spray ethyl chloride onto the heel to freeze the skin.

Step 5

Measure the soft-tissue thickness beneath the calcaneus directly on the radiograph.

Step 6

Using the measurement from the radiograph as a guide, palpate the calcaneus medially where it begins to curve upward. Insert the 21-gauge needle into this area, which is approximately 2 cm from the plantar surface of the foot (**Figure 1**).

Step 7

Advance the needle down to the calcaneus until it hits the bone. Walk the tip of the needle distally along the bone to the plantar surface of the calcaneus. The needle should be immediately superior (deep) to the plantar fascia.

Step 8

Advance the needle to its hilt and inject 3 mL of the anesthetic-corticosteroid mixture. Inject the remaining 2 mL of the preparation while withdrawing the needle 2 cm; then withdraw the needle completely. Make certain that you do not inject the anesthetic-corticosteroid preparation into the medial subcutaneous tissue or the fat pad of the heel that is superficial to the plantar fascia.

CPT Code

20550
Injection(s); single tendon sheath, or ligament, aponeurosis (eg, plantar "fascia")

Current Procedural Terminology
© 2010 American Medical Association. All rights reserved.

Materials

- Sterile gloves
- Bactericidal skin preparation solution
- Ethyl chloride spray
- Lateral radiograph of the heel
- 5-mL syringe
- 18-gauge needle
- 21-gauge, 1″ to 1½″ needle
- Mixture of 1 mL of 10 to 40 mg/mL of corticosteroid preparation and 4 mL of 1% lidocaine, without epinephrine
- Adhesive dressing

SECTION 7 FOOT AND ANKLE

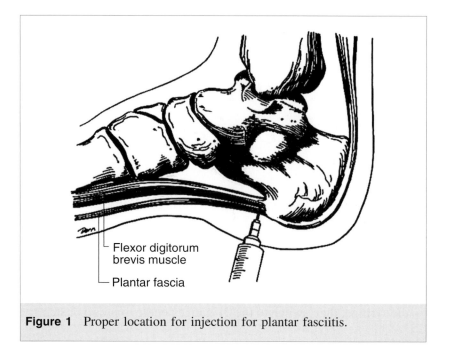

Flexor digitorum
brevis muscle

Plantar fascia

Figure 1 Proper location for injection for plantar fasciitis.

Step 9
Dress the puncture wound with a sterile adhesive bandage.

Adverse Outcomes
Injection of a corticosteroid into the superficial fat pad may cause fat necrosis, with loss of cushioning of the plantar heel. The injection may cause rupture of the plantar fascia.

Aftercare/Patient Instructions
Advise the patient that transient numbness of the heel may occur. Also explain that heel pain might return in a few hours when the anesthetic agent wears off and that the corticosteroid might take a few weeks to have an effect on the symptoms.

Plantar Warts

Synonym

Verruca vulgaris

ICD-9 Code

078.19
Viral warts, unspecified; other specified viral warts

Definition

Plantar warts are hyperkeratotic lesions on the sole of the foot caused by human papillomavirus. The peak incidence is in the second decade of life. Plantar warts are more commonly observed in athletic youngsters.

Clinical Symptoms

Patients have painful, slightly raised lesions on the sole of the foot. These lesions may occur in clusters known as "mosaic warts."

Tests

Physical Examination

Warts usually appear on non–weight-bearing areas on the sole of the foot. Normal papillary lines of the skin (fingerprint pattern) cease at the margin of the lesion (**Figure 1**). The lesions usually are very tender if pinched side to side, a finding not observed with a corn or callus. By contrast, a corn is tender with direct pressure. A plantar wart may occur anywhere on the sole, whereas a callus is associated with a bony prominence. Superficial paring of a wart with a scalpel reveals punctate hemorrhage and a fibrillated texture. A callus is avascular and on paring has a uniform texture that resembles yellow candle wax.

Figure 1 Clinical appearance of a plantar wart. (Reproduced with permission from California Pacific Medical Center, San Francisco, CA.)

Diagnostic Tests

When doubt exists, histopathologic examination of a specimen confirms the diagnosis. This type of testing is seldom necessary, however, given the characteristic gross appearance after superficial paring.

Differential Diagnosis

- Callus (hyperkeratotic lesion that forms in response to a bony prominence)
- Foreign body (history and examination)
- Plantar fibromatosis (location beneath the skin)

Adverse Outcomes of the Disease

Plantar warts are often persistent; they can spread to other areas of the foot, grow larger, and leave scars on the sole of the foot.

Treatment

Most lesions resolve spontaneously within 5 to 6 months, so aggressive treatment should be reserved for unusually large, painful, or persistent lesions. Initial treatment commonly includes superficial paring, followed by the use of a keratolytic agent, such as salicylic acid in liquid or salve form. The lesion should then be covered with occlusive tape to ensure that the medication stays within the desired area and débrides the necrotic layers of tissue upon removal of the tape. Medication should be applied twice daily for 1 month.

Warts that are resistant to initial treatment will sometimes respond to intralesional injection of approximately 1 mL of local anesthetic with epinephrine. Electrocautery, cryotherapy with liquid nitrogen, laser ablation, or curettage may be performed under local anesthetic. Care should be taken to avoid causing necrosis of the deep dermis, which may produce intractable, painful scarring on the sole of the foot. In curettage, for example, the subcutaneous fat should not be visible when the procedure is finished. Intralesional injections of bleomycin and radiation therapy also have been described for severe, recalcitrant lesions, but these options are best performed by specialists with experience in their use.

Adverse Outcomes of Treatment

Secondary infection may occur after treatment. Intractable scarring from excessively deep ablation is also a significant risk.

Referral Decisions/Red Flags

Persistent or recurring warts warrant further evaluation.

Posterior Heel Pain

Synonyms

Achilles tendinosis
Haglund syndrome
Insertional Achilles tendinitis
Pump bump

ICD-9 Code

726.71
Achilles bursitis or tendinitis

Definition

Pain in the posterior heel around the insertion of the Achilles
tendon may originate from one or more of the following
structures: the insertion of the Achilles tendon onto the
calcaneus (insertional Achilles tendinosis); the retrocalcaneal
bursa (retrocalcaneal bursitis); a prominent process of the
calcaneus impinging on the retrocalcaneal bursae and/or Achilles
tendon (Haglund syndrome); or inflammation of the bursa
between the skin and the Achilles tendon (pre-Achilles bursitis).
The exact etiology may be confusing because frequently more
than one of these areas is involved (**Figure 1**).

Clinical Symptoms

Patients with a prominent process of the calcaneus initially
develop a bursa that is irritated by shoe wear and causes a pump
bump (**Figure 2**). In older patients, insertional tendinosis with
enthesopathy, calcification, and degenerative tears of the Achilles
tendon are most often seen. A limp and pain with start-up or

Retrocalcaneal bursa

Pre-Achilles bursa

Insertion of Achilles
tendon onto calcaneus

Calcaneus

Figure 1 Sites of posterior heel pain.

Figure 2 **A,** Area of involvement. **B,** Clinical appearance. **C,** Sagittal T2-weighted MRI shows thickening of the Achilles insertion and fluid within the insertion of the tendon. **D,** Prominent Haglund deformity.

Figure 3 Pain on palpation on either side of the retrocalcaneal bursa, anterior to the Achilles tendon insertion, is indicative of retrocalcaneal bursitis.

activity are common. Shoe wear may be difficult because of the direct pressure on the posterior heel prominence.

Tests

Physical Examination

Examination reveals swelling and tenderness at the posterior heel. If a calcaneal prominence is present, it is usually larger on the lateral side of the heel. A superficial bursa (pump bump) may be present and may be inflamed by shoe wear.

If Achilles tendinosis is present, pain is present directly over the Achilles tendon and is increased by squeezing the tendon. The tendon may be thickened and have a nodule. Retrocalcaneal bursitis can cause pain anterior to the Achilles tendon that is increased by squeezing the bursa from side to side and just anterior to the Achilles tendon (**Figure 3**).

Diagnostic Tests

Lateral radiographs of the heel may show calcification of the Achilles tendon and spur formation. A prominent posterosuperior process of the calcaneus also might be apparent.

Differential Diagnosis

- Achilles tendon avulsion (palpable defect in the tendon, positive Thompson test)
- Os trigonum syndrome (posterolateral pain increased with forced dorsiflexion)
- Plantar fasciitis (pain below the calcaneus)
- Stress fracture of the calcaneus (midcalcaneal bony tenderness)

Hee

- Sta
  un
  an

- Ke
  lov

- Ho
  for

- Pei
  for

Calf

- Sta
  you

- Sta
  slo
  rea
  bac
  15

- Pei
  for

- Wl
  fee
  cor

Adverse Outcomes of the Disease

Difficulty with shoe wear and sports activities may result, as well as chronic pain and limping.

Treatment

A heel lift or open-back shoes will minimize pressure on the inflamed area. Ice massage and contrast baths will decrease inflammation. Achilles tendon stretching exercises should be started after the inflammatory phase has passed. Casting for 4 to 6 weeks may alleviate symptoms. Surgical intervention will remove the prominent bone and diseased tendon.

Rehabilitation Prescription

A home exercise program (see page 852) of heel cord stretching with the toe pointing in and the knee bent will isolate and stretch the soleus muscle; heel cord stretching with the leg straight and calf eccentrics will stretch the gastrocnemius-soleus complex. A heel lift in the shoe may be helpful in resting the tendon. If these measures are not successful, formal rehabilitation may be ordered. The prescription should include a biomechanical evaluation of the foot and ankle during ambulation. If overpronation is present, foot orthoses may be very helpful in relieving the symptoms. In addition, pain-relieving modalities such as phonophoresis, ice, or laser therapy may be ordered.

Adverse Outcomes of Treatment

Surgical removal of bone and débridement of the Achilles tendon may predispose the tendon to rupture.

Referral Decisions/Red Flags

Recalcitrant pain or failure to respond to nonsurgical management indicates the need for further evaluation.

Rheumatoid Arthritis of the Foot and Ankle

ICD-9 Code

714.0
Rheumatoid arthritis

Definition

Ninety percent of patients with rheumatoid arthritis are estimated to have symptoms that are related to the foot or ankle. The presence and severity of symptoms correlates with the longevity of the disease. Ninety percent of patients report symptoms in the forefoot and midfoot, and 67% report symptoms in the ankle and hindfoot. Chronic synovitis leads to stretching of the capsule and ligaments of the joints with subsequent malalignment of the joints, and ultimately to structural deformities such as hallux valgus, claw toes with subluxated or dislocated metatarsophalangeal (MTP) joints, and end-stage arthritis of the ankle or subtalar joint.

Clinical Symptoms

Patients present with loss of motion and pain on weight bearing. Metatarsalgia commonly occurs with subluxation/dislocation of the lesser toe MTP joints, claw toes, and distal migration of the fat pad (**Figure 1**). Severe hallux valgus often accompanies lesser toe deformities (**Figure 2**).

In the hindfoot, tenosynovitis of the posterior tibial tendon may produce medial ankle pain and swelling. Early arthritis of the talonavicular or subtalar joint also is common and typically occurs before ankle involvement.

The ankle is usually one of the last joints to be involved in rheumatoid arthritis.

Figure 1 Metatarsalgia develops as the fat pad is pulled distally and the metatarsal heads become more prominent.

Tests

Physical Examination

MTP synovitis, with focal pain and swelling over the MTP joints, may be the presenting symptom in patients with rheumatoid arthritis. Bilateral symptoms, multiple joint involvement, and the presence of nodules should lead to clinical suspicion of rheumatoid arthritis.

Diagnostic Tests

Laboratory tests reveal an elevated erythrocyte sedimentation rate and positive rheumatoid factor. Radiographs reveal soft-tissue swelling, osteopenia, subchondral erosions, and malalignment. Lateral drift occurs at the MTP joints and at the talonavicular joint (**Figure 3**).

Adverse Outcomes of the Disease

Difficulty with shoe wear and sports activities may result, as well as chronic pain and limping.

Treatment

A heel lift or open-back shoes will minimize pressure on the inflamed area. Ice massage and contrast baths will decrease inflammation. Achilles tendon stretching exercises should be started after the inflammatory phase has passed. Casting for 4 to 6 weeks may alleviate symptoms. Surgical intervention will remove the prominent bone and diseased tendon.

Rehabilitation Prescription

A home exercise program (see page 852) of heel cord stretching with the toe pointing in and the knee bent will isolate and stretch the soleus muscle; heel cord stretching with the leg straight and calf eccentrics will stretch the gastrocnemius-soleus complex. A heel lift in the shoe may be helpful in resting the tendon. If these measures are not successful, formal rehabilitation may be ordered. The prescription should include a biomechanical evaluation of the foot and ankle during ambulation. If overpronation is present, foot orthoses may be very helpful in relieving the symptoms. In addition, pain-relieving modalities such as phonophoresis, ice, or laser therapy may be ordered.

Adverse Outcomes of Treatment

Surgical removal of bone and débridement of the Achilles tendon may predispose the tendon to rupture.

Referral Decisions/Red Flags

Recalcitrant pain or failure to respond to nonsurgical management indicates the need for further evaluation.

Home Exercise Program for Posterior Heel Pain

- Apply moist or dry heat to the heel while exercising, and to prevent inflammation, apply a bag of crushed ice or frozen peas to the heel for 20 minutes after performing the exercises.
- You should not experience pain with the exercises.
- If your symptoms do not improve after performing the exercises for 3 to 4 weeks, call your doctor.

Exercise	Muscle Group	Number of Repetitions/Sets	Number of Days per Week	Number of Weeks
Heel cord stretch with knee bent	Soleus	4 repetitions/2 or 3 sets	Daily	3 to 4
Heel cord stretch	Gastrocnemius-soleus complex	4 repetitions/2 or 3 sets	Daily	3 to 4
Calf eccentrics	Gastrocnemius-soleus complex	10 to 15 repetitions/2 or 3 sets	Daily	3 to 4

Heel Cord Stretch With Knee Bent

- Stand facing a wall with the unaffected limb in front and with the knee bent for support, the affected limb in back and with the knee also bent, and the toes pointed in slightly.
- Keeping the heels of both feet flat on the floor, lower your hips toward the wall.
- Hold the stretch for 30 seconds and then relax for 30 seconds.
- Perform 2 or 3 sets of 4 repetitions daily, for 3 to 4 weeks.

Heel Cord Stretch

- Stand facing a wall with the knee of the unaffected limb bent, the affected limb straight, and the toes pointed in slightly.
- Keeping the heels of both feet flat on the floor, lower your hips toward the wall.
- Hold the stretch for 30 seconds and then relax for 30 seconds.
- Perform 2 or 3 sets of 4 repetitions daily, for 3 to 4 weeks.

Calf Eccentrics

- Stand on the bottom step of a staircase with your heels extending off the step.
- Starting up on your toes, lower your heels slowly as far as is comfortable. When you reach the lowest comfortable position, push back up to the starting position. Repeat 10 to 15 times.
- Perform the exercise 2 to 3 times daily, for 3 to 4 weeks.
- When you first perform this exercise, use both feet. As you get stronger and feel more comfortable, progress to using one foot at a time.

SECTION 7 FOOT AND ANKLE

Posterior Tibial Tendon Dysfunction

ICD-9 Codes

726.72
Posterior tibial tendinitis

734
Flat foot

Synonyms

Acquired flatfoot
Posterior tibial tendon insufficiency
Posterior tibial tendon rupture

Definition

The posterior tibial tendon is one of the main supporting structures of the medial ankle and arch. Posterior tibial tendon dysfunction is the primary cause of medial ankle pain in the middle-aged patient. Demographically, the classic presentation is an overweight woman older than 55 years. Corticosteroid injections, diabetes mellitus, hypertension, and/or previous injury to the foot are other risk factors. The posterior tibial tendon is thickened and shows degenerative changes. As a result, the posterior tibialis muscle is ineffective, and its function of supporting the medial longitudinal arch is lost. Consequently, a flatfoot develops. Initially the foot is flexible, but over time the deformity becomes fixed, and arthritic changes may occur in the hindfoot.

Clinical Symptoms

Pain and swelling on the medial aspect of the ankle are the most common symptoms. Usually patients state that they have lost the arch and that the ankle rolls in. The onset of symptoms is insidious, and there usually is no history of trauma. Although pain and tenderness initially occur along the medial aspect of the foot, lateral pain ultimately develops as the collapsed flatfoot abuts the fibula or causes impingement in the sinus tarsi.

Tests

Physical Examination

Both feet should be examined from the knee down with the patient standing. Examination shows swelling and tenderness posterior and inferior to the medial malleolus, along the course of the posterior tibial tendon. The medial arch is decreased or completely flattened. The heel shows increased valgus, and with advanced changes, the forefoot is in abduction. When viewed from behind, more than two toes will be visible on the affected foot (the "too many toes" sign) because of forefoot abduction

Figure 1 Posterior tibial tendon dysfunction. **A,** "Too many toes" sign in the left foot, caused by forefoot abduction and hindfoot valgus typical of posterior tibial tendon dysfunction. **B,** Patient is unable to rise up on the toes of the affected foot.

Figure 2 In this patient with posterior tibial tendon dysfunction of the left foot, the left heel does not rotate inward (varus) when the patient stands on her toes.

and hindfoot valgus (**Figure 1A**). Also, the patient will not be able to rise on the toes of the affected foot (**Figure 1B**).

Posterior tibial tendon strength is decreased on both manual muscle testing as well as functional maneuvers. Normally a patient with both hands placed on a wall can perform a heel rise on one leg, and during this maneuver, the posterior tibial tendon will pull the heel into inversion. Patients with dysfunction or rupture of the posterior tibial tendon cannot perform a complete heel rise on the affected leg, and when this test is performed while standing on both legs, normal inversion of the heel does not occur (**Figure 2**).

Diagnostic Tests

Weight-bearing AP and lateral radiographs of the foot reveal a flatfoot, with alignment changes at the talonavicular and other joints. MRI of the posterior tibial tendon may be useful in equivocal situations.

Differential Diagnosis

- Congenital pes planus (bilateral, present since childhood)
- Lisfranc fracture-dislocation (history of trauma, pain in the midfoot)
- Medial ankle laxity (rare, abnormal ankle radiographs)
- Medial malleolus stress fracture (focal bony tenderness)
- Tarsal coalition (fixed deformity, onset as adolescent or young adult)

Adverse Outcomes of the Disease

A progressive, painful flatfoot with gait disturbance is common. A severe flatfoot makes shoe wear or even bracing difficult.

Treatment

Tenosynovitis of the tendon without a flatfoot should be treated with a short leg cast or cast brace for 4 weeks, NSAIDs, and activity limitation. After the cast is removed, a molded ankle-foot orthosis may be used as the tendinitis resolves. A custom orthotic device with a medial longitudinal arch support and medial internal heel wedge is often recommended to help decrease the excursion of the tendon. Corticosteroid injection is not recommended as it may weaken the already pathologic tendon. When nonsurgical treatment fails, surgical débridement of the tendon may be indicated.

If a flexible flatfoot develops, use of a custom orthotic device or ankle brace should be continued. A UCBL (University of California Biomechanics Laboratory) orthotic insert or Arizona brace also can be effective. Often, surgery is required. If the deformity is flexible, a tendon transfer combined with a realignment osteotomy is usually recommended. Once a rigid flatfoot develops, however, stabilization of the hindfoot by arthrodesis is the better alternative.

Adverse Outcomes of Treatment

Tendon transfer surgery may fail, requiring an arthrodesis of the hindfoot.

Referral Decisions/Red Flags

Patients with unexplained medial ankle pain require further evaluation because a medial ankle sprain is rare and therefore other, more serious, conditions must be considered. Patients with a recent onset of flatfoot deformity also require further evaluation.

SECTION 7 FOOT AND ANKLE

Rheumatoid Arthritis of the Foot and Ankle

ICD-9 Code

714.0
Rheumatoid arthritis

Definition

Ninety percent of patients with rheumatoid arthritis are estimated to have symptoms that are related to the foot or ankle. The presence and severity of symptoms correlates with the longevity of the disease. Ninety percent of patients report symptoms in the forefoot and midfoot, and 67% report symptoms in the ankle and hindfoot. Chronic synovitis leads to stretching of the capsule and ligaments of the joints with subsequent malalignment of the joints, and ultimately to structural deformities such as hallux valgus, claw toes with subluxated or dislocated metatarsophalangeal (MTP) joints, and end-stage arthritis of the ankle or subtalar joint.

Clinical Symptoms

Patients present with loss of motion and pain on weight bearing. Metatarsalgia commonly occurs with subluxation/dislocation of the lesser toe MTP joints, claw toes, and distal migration of the fat pad (**Figure 1**). Severe hallux valgus often accompanies lesser toe deformities (**Figure 2**).

In the hindfoot, tenosynovitis of the posterior tibial tendon may produce medial ankle pain and swelling. Early arthritis of the talonavicular or subtalar joint also is common and typically occurs before ankle involvement.

The ankle is usually one of the last joints to be involved in rheumatoid arthritis.

Tests

Physical Examination

MTP synovitis, with focal pain and swelling over the MTP joints, may be the presenting symptom in patients with rheumatoid arthritis. Bilateral symptoms, multiple joint involvement, and the presence of nodules should lead to clinical suspicion of rheumatoid arthritis.

Diagnostic Tests

Laboratory tests reveal an elevated erythrocyte sedimentation rate and positive rheumatoid factor. Radiographs reveal soft-tissue swelling, osteopenia, subchondral erosions, and malalignment. Lateral drift occurs at the MTP joints and at the talonavicular joint (**Figure 3**).

Figure 1 Metatarsalgia develops as the fat pad is pulled distally and the metatarsal heads become more prominent.

Differential Diagnosis

- Posterior tibial tendon dysfunction (swelling and tenderness over the posterior tibial tendon)
- Seronegative spondyloarthropathies (enthesitis present on physical examination with pain at the insertion sites of the plantar fascia and Achilles tendon)
- Traumatic arthritis (history of preceding trauma)

Adverse Outcomes of the Disease

Pain, progressive deformity, and metatarsalgia with plantar ulcerations are common if the condition remains untreated.

Treatment

Medical management can improve symptoms and slow the progression of disease. Disease-modifying agents (eg, methotrexate and the newer pharmacotherapy agents such as disease-modifying antirheumatic drugs (DMARDs) that effect tumor necrosis factor alpha [TNF-α]) have been shown to decrease synovitis and slow progression of the disease. Corticosteroid injections may be helpful for inflamed joints and significant tenosynovitis.

An extra-depth accommodative shoe with a molded insole and rocker bottom sole often relieves metatarsalgia. A UCBL (University of California Biomechanics Laboratory) orthosis may provide significant pain relief for a patient who has a flexible hindfoot deformity. A molded ankle-foot orthosis may be used for more extensive disease involvement. (See page 836 for a discussion of various orthoses.)

The most reliable surgery for forefoot deformity involves fusion of the first MTP joint with metatarsal head resections. Implant arthroplasty of the great toe is rarely indicated.

Tenosynovectomy is only a temporizing procedure and is rarely indicated. Most patients with severe arthritis of the hindfoot joints require arthrodesis of the talocalcaneal, talonavicular, and/or calcaneocuboid joints. Patients still have dorsiflexion and plantar flexion through the ankle joint after a hindfoot arthrodesis.

Significant ankle arthritis may require arthrodesis. Patients with rheumatoid arthritis who have severe ankle destruction often have subtalar joint involvement. Injections into the joints may help determine which is more symptomatic. When both joints are involved, a hindfoot (tibiotalocalcaneal) fusion should be performed. Although new results are encouraging, total ankle replacement in patients with rheumatoid arthritis remains investigational.

Figure 2 Hallux valgus and lesser toe deformities are associated with rheumatoid arthritis.

Figure 3 AP radiograph of the foot of a patient with rheumatoid arthritis shows severe hallux valgus.

SECTION 7 FOOT AND ANKLE

Adverse Outcomes of Treatment

Incomplete correction of the deformity, inadequate pain relief, delayed union, malunion, nonunion, or adjacent joint degeneration may complicate surgical treatment.

Referral Decision/Red Flags

Persistent pain despite medical management signals the need for further evaluation.

Sesamoiditis

Synonym

Dancer's toe

ICD-9 Code

733.99
Sesamoiditis

Definition

The sesamoid bones are embedded in the flexor hallucis brevis tendon beneath the first metatarsal head (plantar surface) (**Figure 1**). Sesamoids also may be present under any of the other metatarsal heads, but this is less common. Sesamoid disorders include inflammation, fracture, and arthritis. Sesamoiditis occurs from repeated stress of the sesamoid and the subsequent inflammation.

Clinical Symptoms

Pain under the first metatarsal head is noted, with or without swelling and ecchymosis. The usual stresses involve dancing or running, but sesamoiditis also can be caused by trauma from falls or more commonly by forced dorsiflexion of the great toe with acute onset of pain.

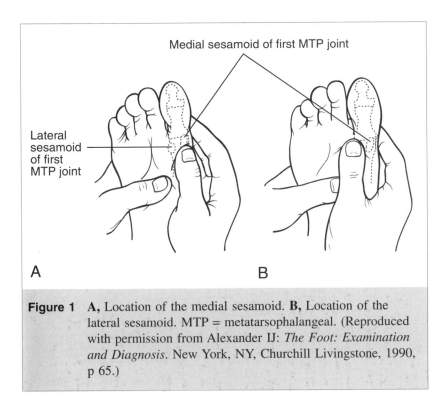

Figure 1 **A,** Location of the medial sesamoid. **B,** Location of the lateral sesamoid. MTP = metatarsophalangeal. (Reproduced with permission from Alexander IJ: *The Foot: Examination and Diagnosis.* New York, NY, Churchill Livingstone, 1990, p 65.)

Tests

Physical Examination

With both sesamoiditis and sesamoid fractures, examination reveals focal tenderness at the sesamoid bone directly beneath the metatarsal head. The tender spot will move with the sesamoid as the great toe is flexed and extended. Dorsiflexion of the toe is painful, and range of motion may be restricted.

Diagnostic Tests

AP, lateral, and axial radiographs of the sesamoid bones are indicated. An oblique view of the sesamoid also may be helpful in visualizing the entire bone and to rule out a fracture. Bipartite or multipartite sesamoid bones are common, occurring in 25% of the population. These normal variants have smooth margins and should not be confused with fractured sesamoids, which have irregular margins. Comparison views of the opposite foot or a bone scan may be helpful.

Differential Diagnosis

- Hallux rigidus (limited dorsiflexion, dorsal spur, dorsal tenderness)
- Hallux valgus (pain medially, lateral deviation of the great toe)
- Metatarsalgia (tenderness over the plantar aspect of a lesser metatarsal)
- Neuroma (pain and tenderness over the medial sensory nerve)

Adverse Outcomes of the Disease

Without treatment, the patient may have pain and a limp.

Treatment

Patients with sesamoiditis should be advised to avoid wearing high-heeled shoes. For more severe symptoms, relieving pressure on the sesamoids by taping the great toe in plantar flexion, using sesamoid pads (a felt pad used to relieve pressure on the sesamoid bone), wearing a stiff-soled or rocker bottom shoe, or wearing a removable short leg fracture brace for 4 to 6 weeks may decrease inflammation. If these measures fail, excision of the sesamoid may be required.

Adverse Outcomes of Treatment

Hallux valgus or varus rarely develops following removal of a sesamoid.

Referral Decisions/Red Flags

Persistent pain is an indication for further evaluation.

Shoe Wear

Shoes protect and cushion the feet and in many cases serve a cosmetic purpose. Improperly fitted or improperly manufactured shoes are the cause of many foot deformities. Women who consistently wear high-heeled shoes with a narrow toe box have an increased incidence of bunions, hammer toes, corns, and—ultimately—foot surgery (**Figure 1**). Foot size increases with age, but many men and women continue to buy the same size shoe throughout their adult lives without having their feet measured. Patients require instruction about the proper fitting of shoes.

Shoe Design and Lasting Techniques

The seven basic shoe styles are the pump, oxford, sandal, mule, boot, clog, and moccasin. Shoe designers create many variations of these styles, and unfortunately the design of some fashionable footwear indicates little regard for proper shoe function.

The three-dimensional form (either straight or curved) on which the base of the shoe is made is called the last. The shape of the toe box and instep and the curve of the shoe are determined by the last. The straighter the last, the straighter the shoe and the more medial support the shoe can provide.

Common methods of lasting include slip lasting, board (or flat) lasting, and combination lasting. A slip-lasted shoe is constructed by sewing together the upper, like a moccasin, and then gluing it onto the sole. This method makes a lightweight, flexible shoe with no torsional rigidity.

Figure 1   The foot takes the shape of the shoe. Common deformities include hallux valgus, hammer toes, corns, and calluses.

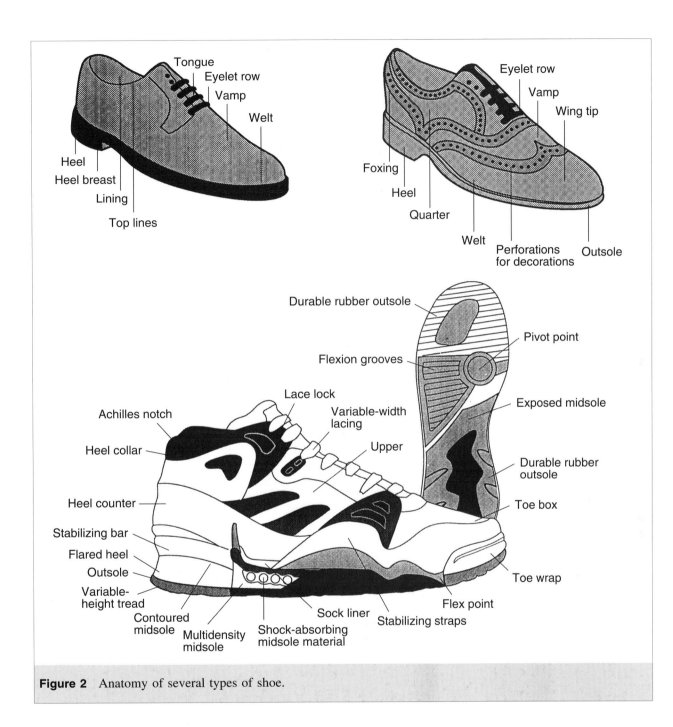

Figure 2 Anatomy of several types of shoe.

With board-lasting or flat-lasting techniques, the upper is fastened to the insole with tacks or staples. This construction makes a stable but less flexible shoe.

Combination lasting uses more than one technique for the same shoe. Shoes made in this way are typically board-lasted in the rear for stability and slip-lasted in the forefoot for flexibility.

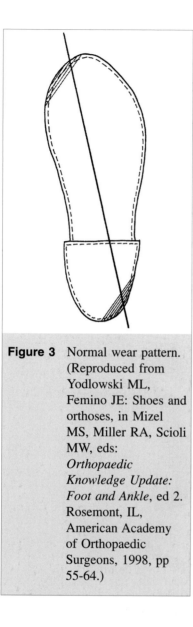

Figure 3 Normal wear pattern. (Reproduced from Yodlowski ML, Femino JE: Shoes and orthoses, in Mizel MS, Miller RA, Scioli MW, eds: *Orthopaedic Knowledge Update: Foot and Ankle*, ed 2. Rosemont, IL, American Academy of Orthopaedic Surgeons, 1998, pp 55-64.)

Shoe Anatomy

The anatomy of several types of shoe is illustrated in **Figure 2**.

Outsole

The outsole makes contact with the ground and usually is attached to the midsole. Most athletic shoes have outsoles made of hard carbon rubber or blown rubber compounds. The outsole provides pivot points and may be designed with a herringbone pattern, suction cups, radial edges, or asymmetric studs. These design patterns enhance stability and traction.

Midsole and Heel Wedge

The midsole and the heel wedge are located between the inner sole and the outsole and are attached to both. These components provide cushioning, shock absorption, lift, and control.

Heel Counter

The heel counter is a firm cup built into the rear of the shoe that holds the heel in position and helps control excessive foot motion.

Toe Box

The toe box may include a stiff material inserted between the lining and outer surface in the toe area to prevent collapse and protect the toes.

Tongue

The tongue is designed primarily to protect the dorsum of the foot from dirt, moisture, and pressure.

Sock Liners, Arch Supports, and Inserts

The sock liner covers the insole and provides comfort and appearance. This liner acts primarily as a buffer zone between the shoe and the foot. Arch supports, heel cups, and other types of padding provide additional support, cushioning, and motion control.

Welt

The welt is a strip of leather or other material that joins the upper with the outer sole.

Shoe Analysis and Fit

With any foot or ankle problem, evaluation of the patient's shoes should be an integral part of the examination. Wear patterns are generally predictable, with the normal wear pattern on the outsole slightly medial at the toe and lateral at the heel (**Figure 3**). Abnormalities in the wear pattern indicate problems with alignment and gait. A tracing of the weight-bearing foot should be compared with a tracing of the shoe (**Figure 4**).

Shoe manufacturers have added extra eyelets to many shoes so that they can be laced for a custom fit. Most people can use a conventional technique, where the laces criss-cross to the top of the shoe, aiming for a snug but comfortable fit. If foot or fit problems are present, other lacing techniques may be used (Figure 5).

Although proper fitting of shoes is not an exact science, relying on a number of easy-to-follow guidelines can help. Shoes always should be fit to the weight-bearing foot at the end of the day, when feet are at their largest. Shoes cannot be stretched to the shape of the foot. The upper should not wrinkle with flexion, and the foot should not bulge over the welt. The end of the longest toe of the larger foot should be within ⅜" to ½" of the end of the toe box. The forefoot should not be crowded, and the toes should easily extend. The shoe should provide a relatively snug grip at the counter above the heel. High heels should be avoided because this style exerts excessive pressure on the front of the foot. Above all else, shoes should be comfortable from the moment they are tried on.

Adverse Outcomes From Poor Shoe Fit

Bunions, hammer toes, neuromas, corns and calluses, and ingrown toenails are all possible.

Figure 4 A large mismatch between the contour of a patient's foot and the shoe being worn is common. Note the compression of the forefoot and the very small contact area of the high heel. Such a tracing can often disclose the cause of a patient's foot pain.

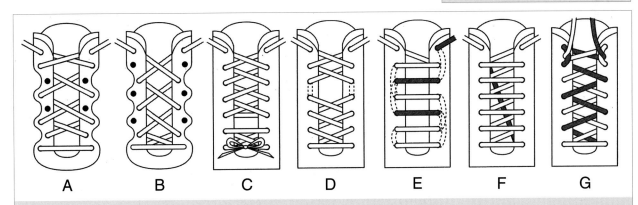

Figure 5 Lacing patterns. **A,** For narrow feet, use the eyelets set wider apart to bring up the sides of the shoe for a tighter fit. **B,** For wide feet, use the eyelets set closer to the tongue of the shoe. This has the same effect as letting out a corset. **C,** For a narrow heel and wide forefoot, use both sets of eyelets to achieve a custom fit. **D,** For dorsal pain from a bump on the top of the foot, a high arch, or pain from a dorsal nerve or tendon, leave a space in the lacing to alleviate pressure. **E,** For a high arch, avoid the normal criss-cross pattern to avoid pressure points. **F,** For hammer toes, claw toes, corns, or toenail problems, lace as shown to allow the toe box to be lifted by pulling on the lace that runs from the toe to the throat of the shoe. **G,** For heel blisters, lock the laces at the throat of the shoe to prevent excess motion of the heel in the shoe.

Soft-Tissue Masses of the Foot and Ankle

ICD-9 Codes

727.43
Ganglion and cyst of synovium, tendon, and bursa, unspecified

728.71
Plantar fascial fibromatosis

Figure 1   Ganglion cyst of the medial ankle.

Synonyms

Fibromatosis

Ledderhose disease

Mucoid cyst

Nodular fasciitis

Plantar fibroma

Definition

Ganglia and plantar fibromas are the most common soft-tissue tumors in the foot and ankle. Other lesions are not discussed in this chapter.

A ganglion is a cystic tumor that contains gelatinous fluid and arises from a joint capsule or tendon sheath (**Figure 1**). Ganglia of the foot or ankle usually are small, 2- to 3-cm masses that arise on the top or side of the foot. A common site is the lateral aspect of the foot or ankle, with the ganglion cyst arising from the subtalar or ankle joint.

A plantar fibroma is a benign thickening of the plantar fascia that may vary in size from 1 to 6 cm in diameter. Plantar fibromas may evolve to plantar fibromatosis (nodular fasciitis of the plantar fascia), a condition that is similar histologically to Dupuytren disease of the palmar fascia. Compared with Dupuytren disease, plantar fibromatosis is less likely to cause severe deformities.

Clinical Symptoms

A ganglion cyst typically is a painless, soft nodule, but it may cause problems with aching, nerve compression, or shoe wear. A plantar fibroma is a firm mass on the bottom of the foot that may be painful and is more likely to interfere with shoe wear.

Tests

Physical Examination

A ganglion cyst is a discrete mass that is usually movable with side-to-side pressure. A plantar fibroma may be focal or may have multiple, discrete masses that are hard (rubbery) and are part of the plantar fascial band.

Diagnostic Tests

Plain radiographs are typically normal. Aspiration of a ganglion with an 18-gauge needle will return a straw-colored, gelatinous material. Sophisticated diagnostic imaging generally is not necessary for either a ganglion cyst or a plantar fibroma.

Differential Diagnosis

- Giant cell tumor of the tendon sheath (solid mass, inability to aspirate soft core)
- Lipoma (subcutaneous fatty deposit, pathology diagnosis)
- Malignant sarcoma (synovial sarcoma, fibrosarcoma) (pathology diagnosis)
- Neurofibroma (often tubular along the course of the nerve, pathology diagnosis)

Adverse Outcomes of the Disease

Patients may report persistent discomfort and difficulty with shoe wear. Malignant degeneration of a plantar fibroma is possible, but the risk is small.

Treatment

Pierce the wall of the ganglion three or four times with an 18-gauge needle to release the gelatinous core and promote complete collapse of the cyst. Care should be taken to avoid any overlying sensory nerve. If the ganglion recurs and continues to be symptomatic, it should be excised. The efficacy of corticosteroid injection into a ganglion has not been proved.

A plantar fibroma is best treated with shoe modifications and an orthotic device. The orthotic device should be cushioned and designed to float the fibroma. Surgical excision is indicated in patients with significant persistent symptoms or if the fibroma has increased significantly in size.

Adverse Outcomes of Treatment

Surgical excision of a plantar fibroma should be avoided, if possible, because of the high rate of recurrence and potential for a painful plantar surgical scar.

Referral Decisions/Red Flags

If the diagnosis of the mass is not clear based on anatomy, examination, radiographs, and aspiration, further evaluation is required to rule out other etiologies. Recurrence of a ganglion following aspiration usually requires surgical excision.

Stress Fractures of the Foot and Ankle

ICD-9 Codes

824.0
Fracture of ankle, medial malleolus, closed

824.1
Fracture of ankle, medial malleolus, open

824.2
Fracture of ankle, lateral malleolus, closed

824.3
Fracture of ankle, lateral malleolus, open

824.4
Fracture of ankle, bimalleolar, closed

824.5
Fracture of ankle, bimalleolar, open

824.9
Fracture of ankle, unspecified, open

825.2
Fracture of tarsal and metatarsal bones

Synonyms

Insufficiency fracture
March fracture

Definition

A stress fracture is caused by repetitive overloading. The bone fails when the fatigue process exceeds the reparative process. Stress fractures often result from an increased level of activity or after beginning a different type of activity, such as military training or exercise walking. Conditions that weaken the bone predispose patients to stress fractures; therefore, these injuries are sometimes referred to as insufficiency fractures. Young, athletic women are at risk because of the female athlete triad of amenorrhea, osteopenia, and disordered eating. Older women are at risk because of osteoporosis.

The metatarsals (especially the second metatarsal) are the most common sites of a stress fracture, but these fractures also can be seen in other bones of the foot and ankle including the navicular, calcaneus, medial malleolus, and fibula (**Figure 1**). Theoretically, any bone exposed to repetitive stress can sustain a stress fracture.

Clinical Symptoms

Patients present with pain and swelling of insidious onset. The pain increases with weight-bearing activity and is relieved by rest. Metatarsal fractures present with a diffusely swollen dorsal forefoot, whereas fibular fractures produce a swollen lateral ankle. Some patients report hearing a crack or pop when the incomplete stress fracture became a complete break.

Tests

Physical Examination

Localized point tenderness and concomitant swelling directly over the fracture site are the most reliable physical signs. Ecchymosis occasionally is observed.

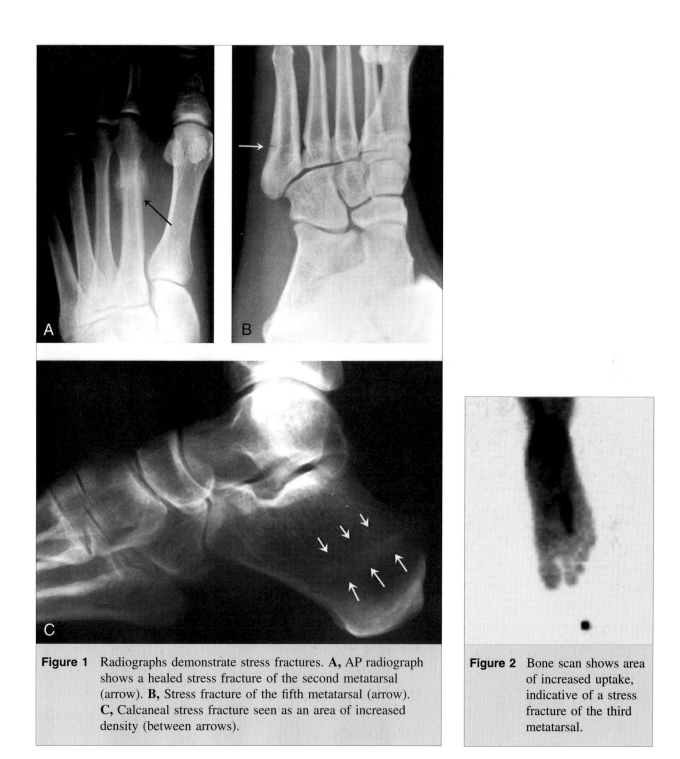

Figure 1 Radiographs demonstrate stress fractures. **A,** AP radiograph shows a healed stress fracture of the second metatarsal (arrow). **B,** Stress fracture of the fifth metatarsal (arrow). **C,** Calcaneal stress fracture seen as an area of increased density (between arrows).

Figure 2 Bone scan shows area of increased uptake, indicative of a stress fracture of the third metatarsal.

Diagnostic Tests

Early radiographs (less than 2 weeks from onset of symptoms) may be normal, but after 3 to 4 weeks, radiographs show healing callus at the fracture site. A bone scan is more sensitive than a radiograph and may be positive by 5 days postinjury (**Figure 2**). MRI can confirm the diagnosis but is not routinely used.

Differential Diagnosis

- Gout (redness, erythema)
- Interdigital (Morton) neuroma (pain and tenderness in the intermetatarsal space)
- Metabolic bone disorders (multiple stress fractures)
- Neoplasm (pain at night or at rest)
- Synovitis of the second metatarsophalangeal joint (swelling and tenderness of the joint)

Adverse Outcomes of the Disease

Chronic stress fractures may require prolonged immobilization to heal. Displacement of fractures with continued unprotected activity may lead to malunion or nonunion that requires surgical procedures. This is more likely with fifth metatarsal (Jones fracture) and navicular stress fractures. Metatarsal stress fractures may displace in the sagittal plane and lead to a painful callus.

Treatment

Treatment for most patients is based on reduced activity and protective footwear. For metatarsal stress fractures, a stiff-soled shoe, wooden-soled postoperative sandal, or removable short leg fracture brace shoe is sufficient. Most patients with calcaneal and fibular fractures benefit from 2 to 4 weeks of immobilization in a short leg walking cast. Because of the high rate of nonunion, navicular and fifth metatarsal fractures both should be casted, and the patient should use crutches and avoid bearing weight on the involved limb. Internal fixation is often a better alternative for a stress fracture of the fifth metatarsal. Patients may resume activity when they are asymptomatic and show healing radiographically. Time to healing is variable, depending on the bone involved.

Adverse Outcomes of Treatment

NSAIDs may retard osteogenesis and should be avoided during fracture healing.

Referral Decisions/Red Flags

Navicular, fifth metatarsal, and all fibular stress fractures require further evaluation early after diagnosis. Failure to heal by 4 to 6 weeks or recurrent fractures suggests the need for a metabolic workup.

Tarsal Tunnel Syndrome

Synonym

Tibial nerve entrapment

ICD-9 Code

355.5
Tarsal tunnel syndrome

Definition

Tarsal tunnel syndrome describes the symptom complex associated with compression neuropathy of the tibial nerve or its branches posterior to the medial malleolus (**Figure 1**). Although an analogy to carpal tunnel syndrome of the upper extremity has been suggested, the only real similarity is the name. In contrast with carpal tunnel syndrome, tarsal tunnel syndrome is much less common, its symptoms are more vague and intermittent, and its diagnosis is more difficult. Numerous causes of tarsal tunnel syndrome have been reported, including compression from a ganglion or bony lesion, but most cases are of unknown etiology.

Clinical Symptoms

Most patients report diffuse, poorly localized pain along the medial ankle. Paresthesias (tingling) or dysthesias (burning) along the medial ankle and into the arch are a common component of the symptom complex. The pain is often worse after walking or other exercise and also may occur at night.

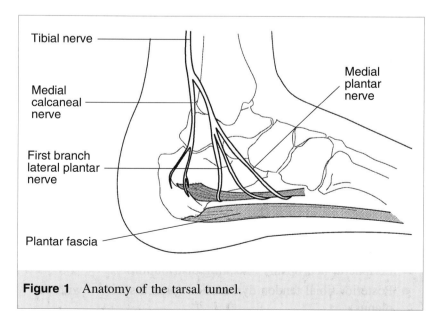

Tibial nerve

Medial plantar nerve

Medial calcaneal nerve

First branch lateral plantar nerve

Plantar fascia

Figure 1 Anatomy of the tarsal tunnel.

Toe Deformities

Synonyms

Claw toe
Hammer toe
Mallet toe

Definition

Deformities of the lesser toes are categorized as three types: hammer toes, claw toes, and mallet toes. These deformities are most commonly caused by tight, improperly fitting shoes. They also are caused by an imbalance of the intrinsic (arising from the foot) and extrinsic (arising from the leg) muscles.

A claw toe has fixed extension of the metatarsophalangeal (MTP) joint and flexion of the proximal interphalangeal (PIP) joint (**Figure 1**). A flexion contracture of the distal interphalangeal (DIP) joint may be present as well. Claw toes usually affect all of the lesser toes of the foot and often are secondary to a neurologic disorder such as Charcot-Marie-Tooth disease, or an inflammatory arthritis such as rheumatoid arthritis. Patients with diabetes mellitus who have a peripheral neuropathy commonly develop claw toes.

A hammer toe has a flexion deformity of the PIP joint with no significant deformity of the DIP or MTP joints (**Figure 2**). The flexion deformity of the PIP joint may cause some passive extension of the MTP joint when the patient is standing, but the MTP joint is in neutral alignment when the foot is examined in a non–weight-bearing position.

A mallet toe has a flexion deformity at the DIP joint with relatively normal alignment of the PIP and MTP joints (**Figure 3**). Hammer toes and mallet toes may be isolated to a single toe and are often caused by improper shoe wear. The second toe, especially if longer than the great toe, is most commonly affected.

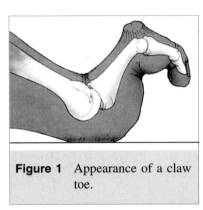

Figure 1   Appearance of a claw toe.

Figure 2   Clinical appearance of a hammer toe.

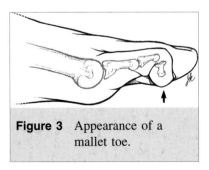

Figure 3   Appearance of a mallet toe.

Clinical Symptoms

Pain, deformity, and difficulty with shoe wear are the common symptoms of patients with lesser toe deformities. A corn may develop on the dorsum of the PIP joint or the tip of the toe. These calluses are painful and may become infected. In patients with hyperextension of the MTP joint, the metatarsal head is displaced plantarly with resultant increased pressure, callus, and pain on the plantar side of the forefoot.

Tests

Physical Examination

Examine the patient in both standing and sitting positions. Note alignment, the presence of corns, and flexibility and stability of the MTP, PIP, and DIP joints. Evaluate alignment and mobility of the ankle and hindfoot joints. Look for a cavus foot, which is associated with neurologic disorders. Evaluate sensory and motor function of the foot and lower extremities.

Diagnostic Tests

Radiographs are helpful only in planning surgery and to rule out osteomyelitis when ulceration of the toe has occurred. A neurologic workup may be indicated in patients with claw toes and a high arch.

Differential Diagnosis

- Neurologic or rheumatologic disorder (claw toes) (noted on physical examination)

Adverse Outcomes of the Disease

Without treatment, patients have difficulty with shoe wear and with persistent, painful corns and calluses. Ulceration may lead to infection and possible osteomyelitis.

Treatment

A shoe with a soft, roomy toe box to accommodate the deformity is the mainstay of treatment. A shoe repair shop can help by stretching shoes to accommodate single hammer and mallet toe deformities. Athletic shoes usually provide enough room to accommodate the deformity. Shoes with heels higher than 2¼″ should be avoided. Protective cushions sold over the counter are helpful when corns develop.

Commercially available splints to hold the toes in place may provide symptomatic relief (Figure 4). In addition, the patient can tape the toe into flexion at the MTP joint. With a narrow strip of tape, begin on the plantar aspect of the foot under the metatarsal head, looping over the dorsum of the proximal phalanx and crossing back to the starting point while holding the toe flexed at the MTP joint.

Surgical correction may be necessary for fixed deformities. The goal of surgery is not cosmetic but the proper alignment of the toes to comfortably accommodate shoe wear. Surgical correction usually achieves toes that sit flat but do not have normal range of motion. Postoperative swelling tends to last for several months.

Figure 4 Type of splint used for a claw toe.

Rehabilitation Prescription

Stretching and strengthening of the toes helps to preserve flexibility. The toe strengthening exercises on page 879 can help maintain normal range of motion in the toes and keep the intrinsic muscle of the foot strong to help prevent the condition from getting worse or recurring.

Adverse Outcomes of Treatment

Continued pain, corns, decreased range of motion, and recurrent deformity are possible.

Referral Decisions/Red Flags

Failure of nonsurgical treatment or persistent ulceration requires further evaluation. Patients with vascular insufficiency are poor candidates for surgical treatment.

Home Exercise Program for Toe Strengthening

Exercise	Condition Recommended for	Repetitions or Duration
Toe squeeze	Hammer toes Toe cramps	10 repetitions
Big toe pulls	Bunions Toe cramps	10 repetitions
Toe pulls	Bunions Hammer toes Toe cramps	10 repetitions
Golf ball roll	Plantar fasciitis Arch strain Foot cramps	2 minutes
Marble pick-up	Pain in ball of foot Hammer toes Toe cramps	Pick up all marbles once
Towel curls	Hammer toes Toe cramps Pain in ball of foot	5 repetitions

Toe Squeeze

- Place small sponges or corks between the toes.
- Squeeze and hold for 5 seconds.
- Repeat 10 times.

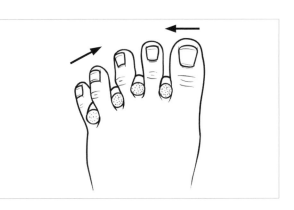

Big Toe Pulls

- Place a thick rubber band around both big toes.
- Pull the big toes away from each other and toward the small toes.
- Hold for 5 seconds.
- Repeat 10 times.

Toe Pulls

- Put a thick rubber band around all your toes and spread them.
- Hold this position for 5 seconds.
- Repeat 10 times.

Golf Ball Roll

- Roll a golf ball under the ball of your foot for 2 minutes to massage the bottom of the foot.

Marble Pick-up

- Place 20 marbles on the floor.
- Pick up one marble at a time and put it in a small bowl.
- Repeat until you have picked up all 20 marbles.

Towel Curls

- Place a small towel on the floor and curl it toward you, using only your toes. You can increase the resistance by putting weight on the end of the towel.
- Relax and repeat 5 times.

Turf Toe

Synonym

First metatarsophalangeal joint sprain

ICD-9 Code

845.12
Sprains and strains of ankle and foot; metatarsophalangeal (joint)

Definition

Turf toe is a sprain of the first metatarsophalangeal (MTP) joint that most commonly occurs with hyperextension but may occur with any forced range of motion. The term *turf toe* was coined because the incidence of these injuries increased with the use of artificial turf on athletic playing fields. Turf toe injuries are associated with significant morbidity, and in some studies these injuries accounted for more missed playing time than did ankle sprains.

Clinical Symptoms

Patients usually report swelling, tenderness, and limited motion of the first MTP joint. A grade 1 sprain is a stretch injury of the capsule, with the athlete usually able to participate in sports with mild symptoms. A grade 2 sprain is a partial tear of the plantar ligamentous complex of the MTP joint. These patients have moderate swelling, ecchymosis, and decreased range of motion. A grade 3 sprain is a complete tear of the MTP ligamentous complex. Marked swelling, bruising, and limited motion occur with grade 3 injuries. The patient can neither compete athletically nor walk normally.

Tests

Physical Examination

Assess the degree of swelling, ecchymosis, range of motion, and gait.

Diagnostic Tests

Radiographs are useful to detect associated avulsion fractures, evaluate joint congruity, and rule out preexisting arthritic changes. When the diagnosis is in question, a bone scan or MRI can help exclude other possibilities such as sesamoid or metatarsal fractures.

Differential Diagnosis

- Hallux rigidus (limited range of motion of the first MTP joint)
- Sesamoid stress fracture (focal pain over the sesamoid)

Adverse Outcomes of the Disease

Instability and arthritis (hallux rigidus) of the first MTP joint may develop. Symptomatic loose bodies and osteochondritic lesions may occur.

Treatment

Nonsurgical treatment with rest, ice, compression, and elevation (RICE) usually is sufficient. Early range of motion is started as symptoms allow. After a grade 1 or 2 sprain, a stiff-soled or rocker bottom shoe is recommended to restrict MTP joint motion and alleviate symptoms. Grade 3 injuries require protected weight bearing or immobilization for 1 to 2 weeks, with a 4- to 6-week period of rest from athletics. Taping, orthotic devices, or a stiff-soled or rocker bottom sole are then recommended. Surgical intervention is seldom necessary except in the case of displaced intra-articular or avulsion fractures.

Adverse Outcomes of Treatment

Delayed return to sports activities, hallux rigidus, and acquired hallux varus or valgus may occur.

Referral Decisions/Red Flags

Intra-articular fractures may require open reduction or excision. Urgent surgical intervention is necessary for an irreducible dislocation. Osteochondral lesions or loose bodies also require further evaluation.

PAIN DIAGRAM
Spine

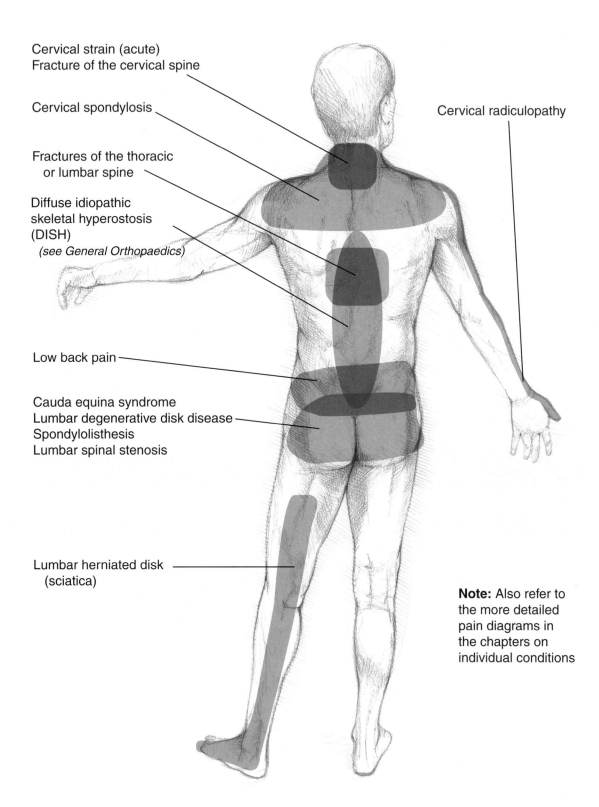

Cervical strain (acute)
Fracture of the cervical spine

Cervical spondylosis

Fractures of the thoracic
   or lumbar spine

Diffuse idiopathic
skeletal hyperostosis
(DISH)
   (see General Orthopaedics)

Low back pain

Cauda equina syndrome
Lumbar degenerative disk disease
Spondylolisthesis
Lumbar spinal stenosis

Lumbar herniated disk
   (sciatica)

Cervical radiculopathy

Note: Also refer to
the more detailed
pain diagrams in
the chapters on
individual conditions

Spine

Section Editor

Dan M. Spengler, MD
Professor and Chair
Department of Orthopaedics and Rehabilitation
Vanderbilt Orthopaedic Institute
Nashville, TN

Contributors

Sigurd H. Berven, MD

Michael Huxford, MEd, ATC, CSCS
Sports Medicine Coordinator
Rehabilitative Services
Institute for Sports Medicine
Children's Memorial Hospital
Chicago, IL

ANATOMY OF THE SPINE

12th rib

T12

Quadratus lumborum muscle

Transversus abdominis muscle (cut)

Iliohypogastric nerve

Ilioinguinal nerve

Psoas minor muscle

Psoas major muscle

Genitofemoral nerve

Lateral cutaneous nerve of thigh

Iliacus muscle

Femoral nerve

Superior pubic ramus

Greater trochanter of femur

Iliopsoas muscle passes backward to insertion on lesser trochanter

Shaft (body) of femur

L1

L2

L3

L4

L5

Origin of psoas major muscle from vertebral bodies, transverse processes, and intervertebral disks (T12-L4) and origin of psoas minor muscle from vertebral bodies (T12, L1)

Lumbar plexus

Lumbosacral trunk

Iliac crest

Anterior superior iliac spine

Iliopectineal bursa

Iliofemoral ligament of hip joint (Y ligament of Bigelow)

Pelvis: Anterior Muscles

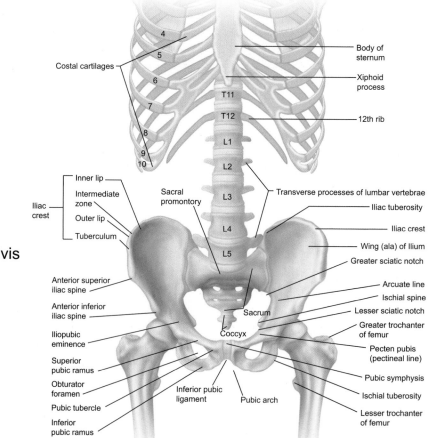

4

5

6

7

8

9

10

Costal cartilages

Body of sternum

Xiphoid process

T11

T12

12th rib

L1

L2

L3

L4

L5

Inner lip

Intermediate zone

Outer lip

Tuberculum

Iliac crest

Sacral promontory

Transverse processes of lumbar vertebrae

Iliac tuberosity

Iliac crest

Wing (ala) of Ilium

Greater sciatic notch

Arcuate line

Ischial spine

Lesser sciatic notch

Greater trochanter of femur

Pecten pubis (pectineal line)

Pubic symphysis

Ischial tuberosity

Lesser trochanter of femur

Sacrum

Coccyx

Bones of the Spine/Ribs and Pelvis

Anterior superior iliac spine

Anterior inferior iliac spine

Iliopubic eminence

Superior pubic ramus

Obturator foramen

Pubic tubercle

Inferior pubic ramus

Inferior pubic ligament

Pubic arch

Overview of the Spine

Low back pain affects 60% to 70% of adults at some time in their lives; 15% to 30% of the population is affected at any one time. Low back pain may be related to overuse/strain or age-associated degenerative changes, or it may be caused by significant pathology, such as segmental instability, neural compromise, or spinal deformity. Many pathologic disorders associated with low back pain and pain of spinal origin can have a significant and measurable impact on health-related quality of life. Low back pain and back injury are common in workers between 30 and 60 years of age and are a primary cause of absenteeism from work. In 1988, about 22.4 million people (17.6% of all US workers) missed an estimated 149 million work days as a result of low back pain. More than 30 million visits were made to physicians' offices in 2002 because of back problems.

Most individuals with low back pain experience pain for only a brief time, with near-complete resolution of symptoms within 30 days. Some patients experience persistent symptoms that progress to chronic pain, usually lasting longer than 90 days. In other patients, symptoms resolve, but the patient then experiences bouts of recurrent pain.

A complete medical history and physical examination are essential in patients with low back pain symptoms. In the absence of red flags or significant physical findings, nonsurgical treatment can begin with NSAIDs and/or rehabilitation. Initial treatment efforts should be directed toward diminishing acute symptoms; rehabilitation should be initiated as acute symptoms resolve. Rehabilitation is not immediately effective in patients with marked paraspinous dysrhythmia, limited mobility, and marked pain. Following symptom resolution, however, active rehabilitation is important to reduce recurrence.

Most patients should be able to return to work quickly, depending on presentation, but work modifications may be required. Patients unable to return to work quickly should undergo more extensive evaluation, including laboratory tests and advanced imaging studies to exclude infections, lumbar disk herniations, or other causes of pain. Other factors, such as litigation and workers' compensation claims, will significantly affect pain behavior and have impact on the motivation to return to work rapidly. These issues become clear over time. Patient education is important and requires time and patience on the part of the physician and other health care providers.

The differential diagnosis for low back pain is wide-ranging, and the patient must be evaluated to ensure that no identifiable cause for the pain is overlooked (**Table 1**). Diagnoses include

Table 1 Common Presentations of Spinal Problems

Problem	Associated Signs and Symptoms	Possible Diagnosis
Neck pain	Paravertebral discomfort relieved with rest and aggravated with activity	Acute neck strain; upper cervical disk herniation
	Limited motion or morning stiffness	Cervical spondylosis
Neck and arm pain	A younger patient with an abnormal upper extremity neurologic examination	Cervical radiculopathy due to herniated nucleus pulposus
	An older patient with limited motion and pain on extension	Cervical radiculopathy due to cervical spondylosis
	Urinary dysfunction with global sensory changes, weakness, and an abnormal gait	Cervical myelopathy secondary to cervical spondylosis or trauma; demyelinating disorder
	Shoulder pain and a positive impingement sign	Shoulder pathology; superior sulcus tumor of lung (uncommon)
	Positive Tinel sign and nondermatomal distribution of symptoms	Peripheral nerve entrapment
Back pain	Paravertebral discomfort relieved with rest and aggravated with activity	Acute low back strain
	Limited motion or stiffness	Degenerative disk disease, ankylosing spondylitis
	Unrelenting night pain and weight loss	Tumor; infection
	Fevers, chills, and sweats	Infection or intervertebral disk infection
Back and leg pain	A younger patient with an abnormal lower extremity neurologic examination	Lumbar radiculopathy due to herniated nucleus pulposus
	An older patient with poor walking tolerance and a stooped gait	Spinal stenosis
	Tenderness over the lateral hip and discomfort at night	Trochanteric bursitis

Table 2 Conditions Commonly Associated With Back Pain

Condition	Age (Years)	Position Associated With Pain	Anatomic Area Affected	Flexion/ Extension
Intervertebral disk herniation	20-50	Sitting	Leg	Flexion
Discogenic pain	20-50	Sitting	Back	Flexion
Spinal stenosis	>50	Standing	Both	Extension
Neoplasia	>50	Constant	Back	Flexion
Infection	>0	Constant	Back	Flexion

SECTION 8 SPINE

inflammation, infection, degenerative disorders, neoplasms (primary and metastatic), trauma, metabolic disorders, developmental defects, neurologic disorders, referred pain, psychologic problems, and rare conditions. Cauda equina syndrome is one of the more ominous conditions that should be considered—early recognition and treatment are critical to provide the best chance for recovery. **Table 2** lists and compares several conditions commonly associated with back pain.

Types of Pain

Night pain that interrupts or prevents sleep, along with fever and weight loss, may be an ominous symptom that indicates a more serious problem such as malignancy or infection. Night pain also may be experienced by patients with significant lumbar spinal stenosis. Acute posttraumatic pain may indicate a fracture. Patients with advanced osteoporosis may experience acute pain and may sustain a vertebral compression fracture with no history of trauma. Low back pain is uncommon in children and warrants a thorough evaluation. A pain diagram is a useful tool for communication between the patient and physician in detailing the location and quality of pain that a patient may experience (**Figure 1**).

Location of Pain

Neck Pain

Pain from strain, overuse, or an acute cervical sprain (flexion-extension or whiplash injury) is common and usually self-limiting. Pain located in the neck, trapezial, and interscapular areas commonly occurs in association with degeneration or herniation of an intervertebral disk. If the herniation occurs above the C5-6 level, the patient may not experience radiculopathy but will report only neck, trapezial, and/or interscapular pain. When injury results from a motor vehicle accident, one way to approximate the degree of injury is to ask questions regarding the severity of the crash. These patients

Table 2 *Continued*

Walking Tolerance	Night Pain/ Fevers	Valsalva Maneuver/Sneeze
No limit	No	Pain
No limit	No	Pain
Limited	No	No pain
Limited	Yes	Pain
Limited	Yes	Pain

Figure 1 Neurologic evaluation of the upper extremity (C5, C6, C7, C8). (Reproduced with permission from Klein JD, Garfin SR: History and physical examination, in Weinstein JN, Rydevik BL, Somtag VKH, eds: *Essentials of the Spine*. New York, NY, Raven Press, 1995, pp 71-95.)

require evaluation of the cervical spine with radiographs as well as a cervical MRI; a cervical myelogram/CT scan may be indicated. Other causes of neck pain that should be considered include brachial plexopathy, such as burners or stingers. With brachial plexopathy, MRI is usually normal; electromyographic tests are often positive.

Neck and Radicular Arm Pain

When accompanied by pain that radiates into the arm, neck pain may be the result of an entrapment of a cervical nerve root by a herniated disk or an osteophyte. For screening evaluation, see **Figure 1**. Many patients with a herniated cervical disk are more comfortable when they place the hand of the symptomatic arm on their head because this position reduces the tension on the nerve. In contrast, patients with intrinsic shoulder problems feel more comfortable with their arms at their sides. With peripheral nerve entrapment syndromes, such as carpal tunnel syndrome, patients may report arm pain and a lesser degree of neck pain. Other less common disorders also may cause neck and arm pain. For example, a superior sulcus tumor of the lung (Pancoast tumor) may cause neck, shoulder, and arm pain, typically in the distribution of the ulnar nerve. Clues to this less common condition include intrinsic hand weakness, Horner syndrome, and a long history of cigarette smoking.

Low Back Pain

In discussing low back pain in this section, a specific diagnosis is one that can be clearly diagnosed as a discrete entity through patient history, physical examination, imaging studies, or pathologic changes identified during surgical intervention. Conditions that meet these criteria include lumbar strain (syndrome), herniated lumbar disk, lumbar spinal stenosis, degenerative spondylolisthesis, and others.

Low back pain typically occurs in the midline (axial) at about the L4 or L5 level and may radiate to the buttocks. Back disorders that affect patients between the ages of 20 and 40 years are often related to strains (affecting muscles) of the soft-tissue structures of the back, including the ligamentous support portion of the intervertebral disk. Young adults with spondylolysis and spondylolisthesis often report episodic axial back pain that may require further evaluation and treatment. Nonsurgical treatment should be tried initially; many of these patients ultimately require surgical treatment. Job modifications also may be advised, although many patients experience resolution of their symptoms and are able to continue rigorous physical work. With seronegative spondyloarthropathies (such as ankylosing spondylitis), patients often have back pain with morning stiffness that lasts longer than 30 minutes.

SECTION 8 SPINE

With aging and degeneration of the intervertebral disk, associated arthritis may develop in the facet joints and contribute to back pain in patients older than 40 years. Most patients with physiologic aging of the spine do not develop significant symptoms that have an adverse impact on their quality of life. Back pain, with or without radiculopathy, may be associated with spinal stenosis. These symptoms are aggravated by spinal extension, as occurs during standing or walking upright or sleeping supine. Diffuse idiopathic skeletal hyperostosis (DISH), which primarily affects men, often becomes symptomatic after age 50 years (see page 87).

Extraspinal causes of back pain include pancreatitis, inflammatory bowel disease, kidney stones, pelvic infections, retroperitoneal lesions, aortic aneurysms, and tumors or cysts of the reproductive tract.

Back and Radicular Leg Pain

Unilateral leg pain is common with herniation of an intervertebral disk, usually at the L4-5 or L5-S1 vertebral levels. Herniations at the L3-4 level generally cause pain that radiates into the thigh and/or groin area. The pain is typically worse with sitting and is associated with sciatic tension signs (straight-leg raising test, supine and seated) as well as altered sensation, motor strength, and reflexes in the lower extremity (**Figure 2**). Patients with an L3-4 disk herniation may exhibit a positive reverse straight-leg raising test (positive femoral nerve stretch sign) and a diminished quadriceps reflex. Trochanteric bursitis mimics sciatica, and these two diagnoses may coexist.

Bilateral leg pain may indicate spinal stenosis, a large central disk rupture, cauda equina syndrome, or spondylolisthesis, especially after the age of 40 years. In patients older than 40 years who present with back and leg pain, degenerative spondylolisthesis is much more common than isthmic spondylolisthesis. Patients with degenerative spondylolisthesis do not have spondylolysis. Exercise-induced leg pain (unilateral or bilateral) may indicate lumbar spinal stenosis. Spinal stenosis occurs most commonly at the L3-4 and L4-5 interspaces.

Extraspinal causes of nerve root entrapment or irritation include hip disease, pyriformis syndrome, ovarian cysts, and retroperitoneal lesions. Discerning a diagnosis between a hip disorder and a spinal etiology may be difficult because both disorders occur in an aging population and both disorders frequently occur in the same patient. Thus, a physical examination and appropriate radiographs are important. Not infrequently, both conditions require surgical management after nonsurgical management fails.

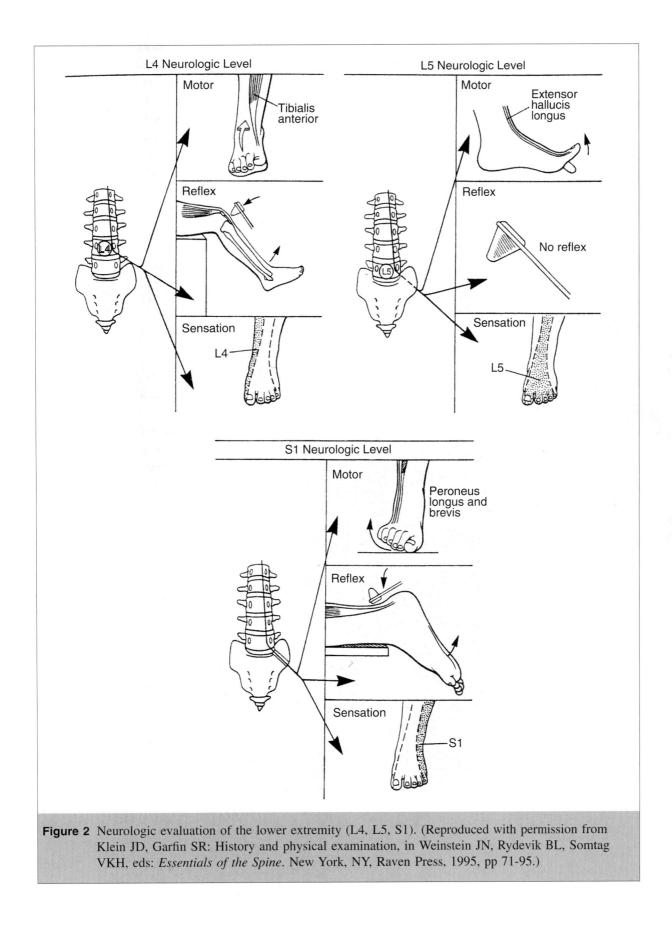

Figure 2 Neurologic evaluation of the lower extremity (L4, L5, S1). (Reproduced with permission from Klein JD, Garfin SR: History and physical examination, in Weinstein JN, Rydevik BL, Somtag VKH, eds: *Essentials of the Spine*. New York, NY, Raven Press, 1995, pp 71-95.)

SECTION 8 SPINE

Deformity

Spinal deformity may affect the sagittal, coronal, and axial planes. Sagittal plane deformity or kyphotic deformities of the spine are best seen on physical examination from the side with the patient bending forward. Sagittal plane malalignment of the spine may involve any region of the spine but is most common in the thoracic and thoracolumbar spine and is common with aging. Scoliosis is defined by coronal plane deformity, but there is a concordant rotational deformity that is apparent on examination. Shoulder asymmetry, pelvic tilt, and asymmetric abdominal or flank creases are signs of deformity in the coronal plane. Trunk rotation or rib prominence on forward bending (Adam forward bend test) is a critical measure of axial plane deformity and may be apparent earlier than coronal deformity in patients with scoliosis. In younger patients, scoliosis is usually idiopathic, but in older patients it also may occur as a result of degenerative changes. Patients with a new onset of scoliosis or rapid progression of deformity should be evaluated for syndromes or diseases that may be a cause of spinal deformity such as neurofibromatosis, spinal cord lesions, or a tethered spinal cord. Spondylolisthesis (isthmic) usually occurs at the lumbosacral joint and is accompanied by tight hamstring muscles (inability to toe-touch). Onset of a spinal deformity in adulthood, or de novo degenerative scoliosis, is common and may be associated with aging, segmental instability, and osteoporosis. A rapid progression of deformity in the adult may be an indication of neoplasm or infection. These conditions may be accompanied by compromise of the spinal nerve roots and/or the spinal cord.

Trauma

All patients who sustain spinal trauma must be thoroughly evaluated, including appropriate radiographs. Some spinal injuries may be subtle, especially in the cervical spine. Flexion-distraction injuries of the thoracolumbar spine also may be missed on radiographs because ligamentous injuries may occur without any bony injury. These injuries may be unstable, and early recognition is essential. The potential consequences of misdiagnosed spinal injuries can be devastating and include progressive deformities with or without neurologic deficits. Injuries to the spine are often associated with other life-threatening visceral, head, or skeletal injuries. For many reasons, some spinal injuries may be missed initially in the multiply injured patient, even after an appropriate evaluation. Special imaging of the spine should be deferred to the specialist to avoid duplication of these expensive tests.

Incidence by Sex

Women have an increased incidence of the following spinal conditions: scoliosis in adolescence, metastatic breast cancer, trochanteric bursitis in later adulthood, and osteoporosis with vertebral body fractures that may lead to an increased kyphosis following menopause.

Men have an increased incidence of the following spinal conditions: kyphosis in adolescence, ankylosing spondylitis in adulthood, and multiple myeloma and DISH in later adulthood. The most common metastatic spinal lesions in men include prostate and lung cancers.

Musculoskeletal Conditioning of the Lumbar Spine

The goal of a conditioning program is to enable people to live a more fit and healthy lifestyle by being more active. A well-structured conditioning program also will prepare the individual for participation in sports and recreational activities. The greater the intensity of the activity in which the individual wishes to engage, the greater the intensity of the conditioning that will be required. If the individual participates in a supervised rehabilitation program that provides instruction in a conditioning routine—instead of using only an exercise handout such as provided here—the focus should be on developing and committing to a home exercise fitness program. A conditioning program for the body as a whole that includes exercises for the shoulder, hip, knee, and foot as well as the lumbar spine is described in the chapter Musculoskeletal Conditioning: Helping Patients Prevent Injury and Stay Fit, on page 183.

Conditioning of the lumbar spine to prevent low back pain should include strengthening and stretching exercises, to improve range of motion. The focus of conditioning should be on a daily home exercise program. Because little or no muscle damage occurs with isometric exercises (unlike the concentric and eccentric exercises involved with strength training), recovery from isometric training occurs within several hours, and so isometric exercises may and should be done every day.

Strengthening Exercises

The four muscle groups that protect the spine from daily overuse and trauma include the abdominals, the quadratus lumborum (two groups, one on each side of the spine), and the back extensors. The back extensors are important because poor endurance of these muscle groups has been found in patients with low back pain. Isometric exercises for these muscle groups, such as the bird dog exercise, have an important stabilizing effect on the spine.

SECTION 8 SPINE

The quadratus lumborum is an important lateral stabilizer of the trunk. A strengthening exercise for this muscle is the side bridge, which should be repeated on both sides for maximum and symmetric lateral stability.

The abdominals are important to stabilization of the lumbar and thoracic spine. The four major muscle groups that make up the abdominals are the transverse abdominus, the internal and external obliques, and the rectus abdominus. The transverse abdominus muscle is a stabilizer of the lumbar spine through its attachment to the thoracolumbar fascia. Traditional sit-ups have been found to greatly increase the load on the lumbar disks and therefore should be avoided by patients with low back pain. A safe exercise is abdominal bracing, which activates all the abdominal muscles, including the transverse abdominus, and does not stress the lumbar spine. This exercise does not activate the transverse abdominus if a pelvic tilt is performed.

Stretching Exercises

Stretching exercises for the trunk and pelvis are helpful for improving range of motion. The cat back stretch and the kneeling back extension exercises are excellent stretching exercises for the spine in general. Flexibility of the hamstring muscles is also important for improving the mobility of the lumbar spine and reducing stress on the lumbar spine. The seat side straddle, modified seat side straddle, sitting rotation stretch, and leg crossover are all excellent stretching exercises for the lumbothoracic spine.

Home Exercise Program for Lumbar Spine Conditioning

- Perform the exercises in the order listed.
- If any of the exercises cause pain, call your doctor.

Strengthening and Stretching Exercises for the Lumbar Spine

Exercise Type	Muscle Group/ Area Targeted	Number of Repetitions	Number of Days per Week
Strengthening Exercises			
Side bridges	Quadratus lumborum	5 repetitions	Daily
Abdominal bracing	Abdominals	5 repetitions	Daily
Bird dog	Back extensors	5 repetitions	Daily
Stretching Exercises			
Cat back stretch	Middle and low back	10 repetitions	Daily
Kneeling back extension	Low back	10 repetitions	Daily
Seat side straddle	Adductor muscles Medial hamstrings Semitendinosus Semimembranosus	10 repetitions	Daily
Modified seat side straddle	Adductor muscles Hamstrings	10 repetitions	Daily
Sitting rotation stretch	Piriformis External rotators Internal rotators	10 repetitions	Daily
Leg crossover	Hamstrings	10 repetitions	Daily

Strengthening Exercises

Abdominal Bracing

- Lie on your back on the floor with your arms at your sides, your knees bent, and your feet flat on the floor.
- Contract your abdominal muscles so that your stomach is pulled away from your waistband.
- Hold this position for 15 seconds.
- Perform 5 repetitions daily.

SECTION 8 SPINE

Side Bridges

- Lie on your side on the floor (for beginners, the knees may be bent 90°).
- With your elbow bent at 90°, lift your body off the floor as shown, keeping your body straight.
- Hold this position for 15 seconds and then repeat on the other side. The goal is to hold this position for 150 seconds total on each side.
- Perform 5 repetitions daily.

Bird Dog

- Kneel on the floor on your hands and knees.
- Lift your right arm straight out from the shoulder, level with your body, at the same time you lift your left leg straight out from the hip.
- Start by holding this position for 15 seconds. The goal is to hold this position for 150 seconds (30 years or older) or 170 seconds (younger than 30 years) total.
- Repeat with the opposite arm and leg.
- Perform 5 repetitions daily.

Stretching Exercises

Cat Back Stretch

- Kneel on your hands and knees in a relaxed position.
- Raise your back up like a cat and hold for 30 seconds.
- Relax for 30 seconds.
- Repeat 10 times daily.

SECTION 8 SPINE

Kneeling Back Extension

- Crouch on your hands and knees.
- First rock forward onto your extended arms, allowing your back to sag. Hold for 5 seconds.
- Then rock back and sit on your bent knees with your arms extended and your head tucked in. Hold for 5 seconds.
- Repeat 10 times daily.

Seat Side Straddle

- Sit on the floor with your legs spread apart.
- Place both hands on the same ankle and bring your chin as close to your knee as possible.
- Hold the maximum stretch for 30 seconds and then relax for 30 seconds.
- Repeat on the other side.
- Repeat the sequence 10 times daily.

Modified Seat Side Straddle

- Sit on the floor with one leg extended to the side and the other leg bent as shown.
- Place both hands on the ankle of the extended leg and bring your chin as close to your knee as possible.
- Hold the maximum stretch for 30 seconds and then relax for 30 seconds.
- Reverse leg positions and repeat on the other side.
- Repeat the sequence 10 times daily.

SECTION 8 SPINE

Sitting Rotation Stretch

- Sit on the floor with both legs straight out in front of you.
- Cross one leg over the other, place the elbow of the opposite arm on the outside of the thigh, and support yourself with your other arm behind you.
- Rotate your head and body in the direction of the supporting arm.
- Hold the maximum stretch for 30 seconds and then relax for 30 seconds.
- Reverse positions and repeat the stretch on the other side.
- Repeat the sequence 10 times daily.

Leg Crossover

- Lie on the floor with your legs spread and your arms at your sides.
- Keeping the leg straight, bring your right toe to your left hand.
- Try to keep the other leg flat on the floor, but you may bend it slightly if needed for comfort.
- Hold the maximum stretch for 30 seconds and then relax for 30 seconds.
- Repeat with the left leg and the right hand.
- Repeat the sequence 10 times daily.

SECTION 8 SPINE

Physical Examination of the Spine

This examination is for patients who present with low back pain with or without radiculopathy.

Standing Examination

Posterior View

Inspect the spine for normal, straight alignment. Moderate to severe scoliosis will be obvious. Also inspect for muscle atrophy. A lumbar list might be present in association with a herniated disk or other condition in which the patient will lean to one side to alleviate nerve root compression. In men younger than 40 years, measure chest expansion. Expansion of less than 1 inch suggests ankylosing spondylitis.

Lateral View

With the patient standing, inspect for deviations in normal cervical lordosis, thoracic kyphosis, and lumbar lordosis. Loss of cervical lordosis or lumbar lordosis may occur with painful conditions such as acute sprains, fractures, or infectious or neoplastic processes.

Pelvic Tilt

Observe the patient standing with the feet together and the knees straight. Inspect or palpate the top of the iliac crests. A pelvis that is not level may indicate a limb-length inequality, or it may be secondary to a spinal deformity.

Gait (Barefoot)

Evaluate the patient's gait with the patient barefoot. Have the patient walk across the room as you observe. Watch for a Trendelenburg lurch. If myelopathy is suspected, have the patient perform a heel-to-toe walk, and look for the inability or difficulty to maintain the weight on the heels or toes.

Trendelenburg Test

The Trendelenberg test is used to evaluate hip abductor strength, primarily the gluteus medius. Stand behind the patient to observe the level of the pelvis as you instruct the patient to stand on one leg. With normal hip abductor strength, the pelvis will remain level. If hip abductor strength is inadequate on the stance limb side, the pelvis will drop below level on the opposite side; this is a positive Trendelenburg test. Repeat the test on the other side.

Spinous Process Palpation

Palpate the spinous processes to define the alignment of the spine. With the patient standing, palpate each vertebra in turn, starting with C7, the most prominent cervical spinous process. The cricoid cartilage is parallel to the C6 vertebral body.

The top of the thyroid cartilage is at the level of the C4 vertebral body.

Flexion, Visual Estimation

To evaluate lumbar flexion, ask the patient to stand with the hips and knees straight and the trunk in line with the lower extremities. The feet should be shoulder width apart to facilitate movement of the spine, and the arms should hang in a relaxed, extended position. While viewing from the side, with the spine at maximum flexion, measure the distance between the fingertips and the floor. If at maximum flexion the fingertips are more than 10 cm from the floor, paraspinous spasm, hamstring tightness, nerve root compression, and/or symptom amplification should be considered. Pain reported on flexion is consistent with nerve root irritation from a disk herniation.

Extension, Visual Estimation

To evaluate lumbar extension, have the patient stand with the hips and knees straight and the trunk in line with the lower extremities. The feet should be shoulder width apart to facilitate movement of the spine, and the arms should be folded comfortably across the chest. While observing from the side, have the patient bend backwards. Pain on extension suggests spinal stenosis and/or spondylolisthesis.

SECTION 8 SPINE

Lateral Bending

To evaluate lumbar lateral bending, have the patient stand with the hips and knees straight and the trunk in line with the lower extremities. The feet should be comfortably apart to facilitate movement of the spine, and the arms should hang in a relaxed, extended position. Ask the patient to bend to the right and to the left. Estimate the maximum lateral bend on each side by observing how far down the thigh the fingertips reach. Note the location of pain or muscle spasm as the patient bends laterally, and then returns to the standing position. Pain reported on lateral bending may be due to muscle spasm, typically on the contralateral side, a facet joint irritation, or possibly nerve root irritation or disk herniation.

Heel and Toe Walking

Heel walking and toe walking are used to evaluate spinal innervation. With the patient barefoot, have the patient walk first on the heels (**A**), and then on the toes (**B**), for a quick screen of the dorsiflexors (L4-L5 innervation) and plantar flexors (S1 innervation).

Seated Examination

Calf and Thigh Circumference

To evaluate for calf and thigh atrophy, a cloth tape measure is needed. With the patient seated, measure the circumference of the thigh approximately one hand breadth above the patella (**A**) and the circumference of the calf approximately one hand breadth below the patella (**B**). Atrophy may indicate chronic radiculopathy or disuse atrophy from a painful adjacent joint (knee or ankle).

Deep Tendon Reflexes

To assess deep tendon reflexes, a hammer is needed. With the patient seated, assess deep tendon reflexes at the knee. Tap the patellar tendon just below the patella (**A**). A decreased knee reflex is consistent with L3 or L4 nerve root compression. Assess deep tendon reflexes at the ankle (**B**). Tap the Achilles tendon just above the calcaneus. The ankle reflex may be diminished or absent with a decrease in function of the S1 root.

Dorsiflexion Strength Testing

To assess the strength of the dorsiflexors, grasp the posterior aspect of the leg with one hand, and use your other hand on the dorsal aspect of the foot to resist the patient's attempt to dorsiflex the ankle. Weakness may indicate L4 nerve compression.

Extensor Hallucis Longus Strength Testing

To assess the extensor hallucis longus, grasp the dorsal and plantar aspects of the midfoot medially with one hand to stabilize the foot in a neutral position, and apply resistance to the dorsal aspect of the great toe. Have the patient extend the great toe against your resistance. The extensor hallucis longus muscle is the easiest and most specific muscle to assess for L5 nerve root dysfunction.

Quadriceps Testing

Evaluate the quadriceps muscle strength by asking the seated patient to extend the knee as you apply light resistance. Weakness in the quadriceps muscle may indicate compression on the L3 or L4 nerve root or perhaps pain inhibition from a knee disorder.

Hamstrings Testing

To evaluate the hamstrings, ask the patient to pull the leg toward the table as you apply light resistance. Weakness may indicate lumbar nerve root compression or pain inhibition from a knee injury.

SECTION 8 SPINE

Iliopsoas Testing

To evaluate the iliopsoas, ask the patient to flex the hip as you apply light resistance to the anterior aspect of the distal thigh. Weakness may indicate a primary hip disorder or an upper lumbar nerve root compression.

Seated Straight-Leg Raising Test

Use the seated straight-leg test to evaluate sciatic tension. Distract the patient's attention away from the back by asking whether the patient has knee problems and then lift the foot and extend the knee. If straightening the knee to full extension on both sides does not cause the patient to lean back, no significant sciatic tension is present.

SECTION 8 SPINE

Meningeal Test (Slump Test of Maitland)

The slump test is a progressive test, which is done bilaterally, and the patient is questioned regarding symptoms at each step. Ask the seated patient to place his or her hands behind the back and then slump in a lumbar and thoracic flexed and relaxed position. Apply over pressure at shoulders, then cervical forward bending by asking the patient to actively flex the chin to chest. Apply slight over pressure to head. Then ask the patient to actively extend the knee fully. You might need to provide slight passive assistance to reach the end range. Then ask the patient to actively dorsiflex fully. Again, you may need to passively assist to maximally extend knee and dorsiflexion. As the examination has progressed to this step, impingement may be placed on the dura, spinal cord, or nerve roots, and produce radicular symptoms in the area supplied by the sciatic nerve. Upon producing the symptoms at any of the preceding steps, the examination can be checked by seeing if cervical backbending, release cervical flexion, and actively extending the head relieves the symptoms while extending the knee further.

Supine Examination

Palpation of Abdomen

Examine the patient's abdomen for tenderness, masses, or enlarged organs. Consider referring female patients to a gynecologist for a pelvic examination, especially for chronic pain.

Supine Straight-Leg Raising Test

Passively raise the leg until either the knee begins to bend or the patient reports severe pain in the buttock or back. Pain on the symptomatic side when the leg on the asymptomatic side is raised is highly suggestive of lumbar disk herniation. A markedly positive test at 20° of elevation with a negative seated straight-leg raising test is suggestive of symptom amplification rather than a true pathologic process.

Internal-External Hip Rotation in Flexion

Flex the hip and knee to 90°, with the thigh held perpendicular to the transverse line across the anterior superior iliac spines. For internal rotation, rotate the tibia away from the midline of the trunk (**A**), thus producing inward rotation of the hip. For external rotation, rotate the tibia toward the midline of the trunk (**B**), thus producing external rotation of the hip. Pain in the groin or buttocks with this maneuver suggests hip irritability.

SECTION 8   SPINE

FABER Test

The FABER (flexion-abduction-external rotation) test, sometimes called the figure-of-4 test, the Patrick test, or the Jansen test, is a stress maneuver to detect hip and sacroiliac pathology. With the patient supine, place the affected hip in flexion, abduction, and external rotation, with the patient's foot on the opposite knee. Stabilize the pelvis with your hand on the contralateral anterior superior iliac spine and press down on the thigh of the affected side. If the maneuver is painful, the hip or sacroiliac region may be affected. Increased pain with this test also may be a nonorganic finding.

Sensory Examination

Using a zero-point, 10-g filament, test for pin-prick sensation over the lateral thigh and medial femoral condyle (L3 innervation), the medial leg and medial ankle (L4 innervation), the lateral leg and dorsum of the foot (L5 innervation), and the sole of the foot and lateral ankle (S1 innervation).

Babinski Sign (Flexor Plantar Response)

To evaluate the Babinski sign, stroke lightly upward on the plantar surface of the foot and look for great toe extension (withdrawal response) and fanning of the lesser toes as a sign of long-tract spinal cord involvement.

SECTION 8 SPINE

Ankle Clonus

To evaluate ankle clonus, dorsiflex the ankle suddenly and observe for rhythmic beating, noting the duration and the number of "beats." This is another sign of long-tract spinal cord involvement.

Brudzinski-Kernig Test

Ask the supine patient to cup his or her hands behind the head and then flex the head onto the chest. Then ask the patient to flex the hip and knee of one leg. Ask the patient to extend the flexed knee until pain is felt. If the patient then flexes the knee, and if pain disappears, it is a positive test. Pain may indicate meningeal irritation, nerve root involvement, or dural irritation.

Prone Examination

Palpation of Lower Lumbar Area

To evaluate the lower lumbar area, palpate the tissues over the lower lumbar area, looking for areas of tenderness, swelling, muscle spasm, or ecchymosis.

SECTION 8 SPINE

Reverse Straight-Leg Raising Test

The reverse straight-leg raising test is a traditional way to place the L1-L4 nerve roots under tension. With the patient prone, lift the hip into extension while keeping the knee straight. Pain over the anterior thigh suggests an upper lumbar disk problem, usually above L4-5. This test would also be markedly positive in a patient with a condition that involves inflammation of the iliopsoas, such as appendicitis.

Findings Consistent With Nonorganic Pain (Waddell Signs)

The four tests shown below comprise the Waddell signs. In addition, the examiner should make a subjective evaluation of the entire history and physical examination to decide if the patient's pain behavior seems to be excessive. If the results of two or more of these tests, including the subjective evaluation, are positive, the examiner should be concerned that issues other than peripheral nociception are creating pain behavior.

Nonorganic Tenderness

With the patient standing, lightly touch the tissues over the lower lumbar spine. This procedure should not cause pain. Marked pain behavior is a positive test.

Axial Simulation

With the patient standing, apply light downward pressure on the patient's head. This maneuver should not cause pain in the lumbar spine. If the patient grimaces and moves, reporting pain, the test is positive.

Seated Straight-Leg Raising Test

Use the seated straight-leg test to evaluate sciatic tension. Distract the patient's attention away from the back by asking whether the patient has knee problems and then lift the foot and extend the knee. If straightening the knee to full extension on both sides does not cause the patient to lean back, no significant sciatic tension is present.

Sensory Examination

Using a zero-point, 10-g filament, test for pin-prick sensation over the lateral thigh and medial femoral condyle (L3 innervation), the medial leg and medial ankle (L4 innervation), the lateral leg and dorsum of the foot (L5 innervation), and the sole of the foot and lateral ankle (S1 innervation).

Cervical Spine—Range of Motion

Flexion and Extension: Zero Starting Position

To evaluate flexion and extension of the cervical spine, the patient is standing with the neck aligned with the trunk (**A**). Stabilize the trunk so that motion does not occur in the thoracic spine. Assess flexion with forward bending of the cervical spine (**B**), and extension with posterior inclination (**C**). Flexion and extension are typically estimated visually in degrees; however, limited flexion may also be measured as the distance between the chin and the sternum at maximum cervical flexion.

Lateral Bend

To evaluate the lateral bend, the nose is vertical and in line with the axis of the trunk. Stabilize the trunk so that motion occurs only at the neck. Right lateral bend is with the head inclined toward the patient's right shoulder, and left lateral bend is inclination in the opposite direction. The degree of motion is the angle between the vertical axis and the mid axis of the face.

Inspect and palpate the supraclavicular fossae for tenderness and/or masses. Superior sulcus tumors of the lung (Pancoast tumors) sometimes present as neck pain and pain in the ulnar distribution.

Rotation

To evaluate neck rotation, the nose is vertical and in line with the axis of the trunk. Rotation is estimated in degrees. To estimate upper cervical vertebral rotation, measure rotation with the neck in maximum flexion.

Spurling Test

The Spurling test is used to help diagnose cervical disk herniations or cervical spondylosis. Performing this maneuver with incorrect technique can be harmful to the patient. You should perform the Spurling test only if you are confident in your ability to perform it correctly.

Ask the seated patient to rotate and laterally flex the head to the unaffected side first, then to the affected side. Use one hand to lightly compress downward on the head to axial load the cervical spine. If this is tolerated well, the test may be repeated then in the rotated and laterally flexed position, but with extension added. This maneuver narrows the neural foramen and will increase or reproduce radicular arm pain associated with cervical disk herniations or cervical spondylosis.

SECTION 8 SPINE

Cervical Spine—Muscle Testing

C5–Deltoid Muscle (Seated)

To evaluate the strength of the deltoid muscle, with the patient seated, abduct the shoulder to 90°. Push down on the arm to resist activity of the deltoid. A ratchety, giving-way motion more than likely is a nonorganic sign. Patients with true weakness exhibit a uniform ability to sustain resistance throughout the range of motion.

C5–Biceps Brachii

With the patient seated, ask the patient to flex the elbow in a supinated position as you apply resistance. The biceps brachii also is innervated by C6, but if C5 is intact, biceps strength should be at least grade 3. Test C5 sensation by assessing light touch on the lateral aspect of the arm.

C6–Radial Wrist Extensors

Flex the patient's fingers to eliminate wrist extension activity by the finger extensor muscles, and then ask the patient to extend the wrist in a radial direction as you apply resistance. Test C6 sensation by assessing light touch on the volar aspect of the thumb.

C7–Triceps Brachii

With the patient seated and the shoulder flexed approximately 90°, ask the patient to extend the elbow as you apply light resistance.

C7–Flexor Carpi Radialis

With the patient seated, place the fingers in extension to eliminate wrist flexor activity by the finger flexor muscles, and then ask the patient to flex the wrist in a radial direction as you apply resistance. Test C7 sensation by assessing light touch on the volar aspect of the long finger.

C8–Flexor Digitorum Superficialis to Ring Finger

Stabilize the long, index, and little fingers in extension and ask the patient to flex the fingers as you apply resistance. Test C8 sensation by assessing light touch on the volar aspect of the little finger.

T1–First Dorsal Interosseous

Ask the patient to abduct the index finger as you apply resistance. Palpate the muscle belly of the first dorsal interosseous muscle to confirm activity (**A**). Test T1 sensation by assessing light touch on the medial aspect of the arm proximal to the elbow (**B**).

Hoffmann Reflex

To asses the Hoffman reflex, with the patient seated and the patient's relaxed hand cradled in yours, flick the long fingernail and look for index finger and thumb flexion as a sign of long-tract spinal cord involvement in the neck.

Cauda Equina Syndrome

Definition

The distal end of the spinal cord, the conus medullaris, terminates at the L1-2 level. Below this, the spinal canal is filled with the L2-S4 nerve roots, known as the cauda equina. Compression of roots distal to the conus causes paralysis without spasticity.

Cauda equina syndrome results from a sudden reduction in the volume of the lumbar spinal canal that causes compression of multiple nerve roots and leads to muscle paralysis. The sacral roots that control bladder and anal sphincter function (S2 to S4) are midline and are particularly vulnerable. Causes of cauda equina syndrome include central disk herniation, epidural abscess, epidural hematoma, and trauma to the spine with retropulsion of a portion of a vertebral burst fracture. Onset may be immediate (with a fracture) or may occur over a few hours or days (with other conditions). Cauda equina syndrome may require emergency surgery to relieve nerve root compression and to stop progression of neurologic deficit. Even with prompt recognition and immediate decompression, recovery of neurologic function may be incomplete and bowel and bladder function may be compromised.

Clinical Symptoms

Radicular pain and numbness involve both legs; however, symptoms are often more severe in one extremity. The presence of perineal numbness in a saddle distribution is typical for most patients with cauda equina syndrome (**Figure 1**). Lower extremity pain may diminish as the paralysis progresses. Leg weakness may present as a stumbling gait, difficulty rising from a chair, or foot drop that is often symmetric. Patients may report difficulty voiding or loss of urinary and anal sphincter control.

Patients may have a history of preexisting spinal stenosis with a sudden increase in symptoms, or the history may reveal sudden onset of pain following lifting or recent spine surgery with subsequent onset of fever, chills, and increased back and leg pain.

Tests

Physical Examination

Watch the patient walk. Inability to rise from a chair without the assistance of armrests (quadriceps and/or hip extensor weakness) and inability to walk on the heels or toes (ankle dorsiflexor and

Figure 1 Typical pain diagram for cauda equina syndrome.

SECTION 8 SPINE

plantar flexor weakness) suggest multiple nerve root dysfunction. Evaluate motor and sensory function of the lumbosacral nerve roots, including anal sphincter tone and/or perianal numbness. Patients seen in the emergency department for acute back pain may receive an injection of narcotics that may cause acute urinary retention and confuse the diagnosis of cauda equina syndrome.

Diagnostic Tests

Significant compression of the thecal sac on MRI of the lumbar spine or CT/myelogram will confirm the diagnosis of cauda equine syndrome. AP and lateral radiographs of the lumbar spine are important to identify structural problems such as a fracture and spondylolisthesis. A complete blood cell (CBC) count, C-reactive protein level, and erythrocyte sedimentation rate can assist with the diagnosis of a suspected infection.

Differential Diagnosis

- Guillain-Barré syndrome (intact sensation possible, normal MRI)
- Herniated lumbar disk (unilateral radicular symptoms and motor weakness, normal rectal tone and perineal sensation)
- Metastatic tumor (lymphoma or leukemia) (abnormal blood studies, pathologic fracture)
- Multiple sclerosis (no history of trauma, patchy numbness, diplopia, facial and/or upper extremity numbness)
- Spinal cord tumor (positive Babinski sign, patchy numbness above L2, spasticity)

Adverse Outcomes of the Disease

Permanent paralysis and loss of bladder and anal sphincter function (urinary and anal) are possible. A possible error would be to relate the bladder symptoms to age-related conditions or female cystocele or male prostatism without considering the possibility of sphincter paralysis.

Treatment

Cauda equina syndrome is a surgical emergency. Immediate decompression is almost always necessary once the anatomic lesion is defined.

SECTION 8 SPINE

Adverse Outcomes of Treatment
Wound infection and postoperative hematoma are possible.

Referral Decisions/Red Flags
Any unexplained neurologic deficit, loss of normal bowel or bladder function, increasing pain not controlled by simple analgesics, or decreasing pain in the face of increasing neurologic deficit is cause for concern.

SECTION 8 SPINE

Cervical Radiculopathy

ICD-9 Codes

722.0
Displacement of cervical intervertebral disk without myelopathy

723.4
Other disorders of cervical region, brachial neuritis or radiculitis

Figure 1 Typical pain diagram for a patient with cervical radiculo-pathy. Patients with root pressure above C5 may report scapular and inter-scapular pain with no extremity radiation.

Synonym

Herniated cervical disk

Definition

Cervical radiculopathy is referred neurogenic pain in the distribution of a cervical nerve root or roots, with or without associated numbness, weakness, or loss of reflexes. The usual cause in young adults is herniation of a cervical disk that entraps the root as it enters the foramen. In older patients, a combination of foraminal narrowing due to vertical settling of the disk space and arthritic involvement of the uncovertebral joint is the most common cause of lateral nerve root entrapment.

Clinical Symptoms

Neck pain and radicular pain with associated numbness and paresthesias in the upper extremity in the distribution of the involved root are common (**Figure 1**). Muscle spasms, or fasciculations, in the involved myotomes may occur. Other symptoms may include weakness, lack of coordination, changes in handwriting, diminished grip strength, dropping objects from the hand, and difficulty with fine manipulative tasks. Occipital headaches and pain radiating into the paraspinal and scapular regions also may occur.

Symptoms indicative of cervical myelopathy, such as trunk or leg dysfunction, gait disturbances, bowel or bladder changes, and signs of upper motor neuron involvement, occur more commonly with stenosis of the cervical spinal canal.

Patients may state that they can relieve the pain by placing their hands on top of their head, as this decreases tension on the involved nerve root.

Tests

Physical Examination

Cervical lordosis may be reduced, and the range of neck motion may be mildly restricted. Extension and axial rotation will often cause pain in the arm or shoulder. Assess motor and sensory function of the C5-T1 nerve roots as well as upper extremity reflexes and other upper motor neuron signs. Careful examination for signs of shoulder pathology, vascular disturbances, and peripheral nerve entrapment is necessary. A complete neurologic examination should be performed (**Table 1**).

Table 1 Clinical Features of Common Cervical Syndromes

Disk	Pain	Sensory Change	Motor Weakness Atrophy	Reflex Change
C4-5 (C5 root)	Base of neck, shoulder, anterolateral aspect of arm	Numbness in deltoid region	Deltoid, biceps	Biceps
C5-6 (C6 root)	Neck, shoulder, medial border of scapula, lateral aspect of arm, radial aspect of forearm	Dorsolateral aspect of thumb and index finger	Biceps, wrist extensors, pollicus longus	Biceps, brachioradialis
C6-7 (C7 root)	Neck, shoulder, medial border of scapula, lateral aspect of arm, dorsum of forearm	Index, long fingers, dorsum of hand	Triceps and/or finger extensors	Triceps

Figure 2 **A,** Axial MRI shows a cervical disk herniation (arrow) in a younger patient. **B,** Axial CT scan with intrathecal contrast shows a cervical disk herniation (arrow) in a younger patient.

Signs of upper motor neuron involvement suggest spinal cord compression.

Diagnostic Tests

Radiographs may identify regions of spondylosis or degenerative involvement of the disk and the facet joint. MRI or CT with intrathecal contrast (myelogram) confirms the diagnosis (**Figure 2**). Advanced imaging studies are necessary in patients who have not responded to nonsurgical management, in patients with profound neurologic deficits, or in patients who are considering surgical management. Electromyography and nerve conduction velocity studies help in some instances to identify the location of neurologic dysfunction. These studies are valuable to differentiate radiculopathy from peripheral neuropathy and various nerve compression syndromes, such as carpal tunnel syndrome.

SECTION 8 SPINE

Differential Diagnosis

- Adhesive capsulitis of the shoulder (restricted passive and active motion)
- Demyelinating conditions (varying symptoms, intensity, and location)
- Myocardial ischemia (abnormal electrocardiogram or stress tests)
- Peripheral nerve entrapment (positive Phalen test, positive Tinel sign at elbow or wrist)
- Rotator cuff disease (painful wince with active shoulder abduction and circumduction movements)
- Thoracic outlet syndrome (distinctly uncommon; decrease in radial pulse with shoulder abduction and external rotation may be observed)

Adverse Outcomes of the Disease

Muscle paralysis, weakness, or chronic pain syndromes may develop. Rarely, the condition may progress to a myelopathy with spinal cord involvement.

Treatment

Spontaneous resolution of all or most symptoms occurs within 2 to 8 weeks in most patients. With radicular pain, a short course of anti-inflammatory medication coupled with cervical traction in a head halter is usually beneficial. Referral to a rehabilitation specialist for cervical traction is more effective than simply providing a patient with a traction unit. Narcotic medication is best avoided and seldom warranted. Manipulation of the cervical spine should also be avoided.

Adverse Outcomes of Treatment

Quadriparesis, herniation of an intervertebral disk, stroke, or vertebral fracture may follow manipulation of the cervical spine.

Referral Decisions/Red Flags

Patients in whom nonsurgical treatment fails or who develop atrophy, motor weakness, or signs of myelopathy may require surgical evaluation. Patients with any signs that suggest a demyelinating condition, infection, or tumor require further evaluation. If radicular symptoms are accompanied by intolerable pain, early specialty evaluation should be obtained.

SECTION 8 SPINE

Cervical Spondylosis

Synonyms

Cervical arthritis

Degenerative disk disease of the cervical spine

Definition

Cervical spondylosis is degenerative disk disease in the cervical spine. This condition is produced by the ingrowth of bony spurs, buckling or protrusion of the ligamentum flavum, and/or herniation of disk material. These anatomic alterations may result in narrowing of the neural foramen and stenosis of the cervical spinal canal. Cervical spondylosis may cause neck pain, cervical radiculopathy, and/or cervical myelopathy.

Clinical Symptoms

The most common symptoms are limited mobility of the cervical spine and chronic neck pain that worsens with upright activity. Paraspinous muscle spasm may occur, as may headaches that appear to originate in the neck. Increased irritability, fatigue, sleep disturbances, and impaired work tolerance also may develop. Radicular symptoms and pain may occur in the upper extremities with lateral recess stenosis and nerve root entrapment (**Figure 1**). Radiographs are of minimal value because many radiographic changes of spondylosis occur in patients who report no significant symptoms. Therefore, careful clinical evaluations are warranted to ensure that symptoms are linked to pathologic processes and not simply to physiologic changes of aging.

Narrowing of the spinal canal and resultant myelopathy are more common in older men. Typical symptoms of early cervical myelopathy may include palmar parathesias in the upper extremities; difficulty with upper extremity dexterity, such as buttoning a shirt or blouse; and subtle gait disturbances that can usually be highlighted by asking the patient to perform a tandem walk (heel-to-toe walking). Urinary function may be abnormal as well. Loss of vibration and position sense (posterior column deficits) is more common in the feet than in the upper extremities. A concomitant radiculopathy in the upper extremity may obscure the diagnosis of cervical myelopathy. Additionally, because pain is frequently absent in patients with early cervical myelopathy, the subtle gait changes may be related to the lumbar spine, with the myelopathy being totally overlooked. The key physical findings in these patients include the presence of

ICD-9 Codes

721.0
Cervical spondylosis without myelopathy

721.1
Cervical spondylosis with myelopathy

723.0
Spinal stenosis in cervical region

SECTION 8 SPINE

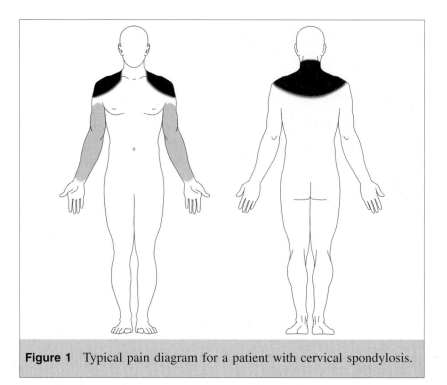

Figure 1 Typical pain diagram for a patient with cervical spondylosis.

long-tract signs (signs that indicate an upper motor neuron lesion), subtle gait disturbances, and alterations in upper extremity dexterity. These changes are not related to the common stenosis that is seen in the lumbar spine because peripheral nerves, not the spinal cord, would be involved in lumbar stenosis unless the L1-L2 area is involved.

Tests

Physical Examination

Examination may reveal tenderness along the lateral neck or along the spinous processes posteriorly. Motion may be limited or painful. Assess sensory and motor function of the upper (C5-T1) and lower (L1-S1) nerve roots. Evaluate gait and tandem walking as well as bowel and bladder function. With myelopathy, flexion may produce electric shocks that travel down the spine, arms, or legs. A Hoffmann reflex, clonus, hyperreflexia, and the Babinski sign (an extensor toe response) are possible, as are gait disturbances and global weakness.

Patients with radiculopathy may have signs that mimic a herniated cervical disk, including abnormal reflexes and motor and sensory function.

Figure 2 Lateral radiograph demonstrates advanced cervical spondylosis.

Figure 3 **A,** Axial CT myelogram of the midcervical spine demonstrates marked cervical spinal stenosis. Note the paucity of contrast material surrounding the deformed spinal cord (arrow). The anteroposterior dimension of the cervical spinal canal and the anteroposterior dimension of the cervical cord are both reduced. **B,** Lateral radiograph of a 70-year-old man with significant cervical spinal stenosis, with symptoms of cord compression and myelopathy found on examination. Note the marked narrowing of the column of contrast material (arrow).

Diagnostic Tests

AP and lateral radiographs are useful. Findings on the lateral view include bony reactive changes in the vertebral end plates, with osteophytes (bone spurs) projecting anteriorly (**Figure 2**). Osteophytes that emerge from the zygoapophyseal joints may also project into the neural foramina. In addition, osteophytes may develop on the posterior portion of the vertebral body and encroach into the spinal canal, producing stenosis of the cervical canal (**Figure 3**). Anterior subluxation of one vertebra onto the vertebra below (**Figure 4**) increases the likelihood of cervical stenosis and associated neurologic findings. Degenerative findings occur most commonly at the C5-6 and C6-7 disk spaces.

Differential Diagnosis

- Metastatic tumor (night pain that prevents sleep)
- Soft cervical disk herniation (generally seen in younger patients)
- Spinal cord tumor (extradural/metastatic, intradural/primary) (physical examination findings, confirmed by MRI and/or CT myelogram)
- Syringomyelia (loss of superficial abdominal reflexes, insensitivity to pain)
- Vertebral subluxation (in patients with advanced spondylosis or rheumatoid arthritis or following trauma)

SECTION 8 SPINE

Figure 4 Degenerative disk changes and degenerative subluxations causing canal stenosis. The arrow on the left indicates the forward slippage of C3 on C4. (Adapted with permission from Bohlmann HH: Cervical spondylosis with moderate to severe myelopathy. *Spine* 1977;2:151-162.)

Adverse Outcomes of the Disease

Chronic pain, myelopathy, or mixed myeloradiculopathy is possible. Note that these sequelae of cervical spondylosis occur more commonly when the anatomic changes are more advanced.

Treatment

Supportive treatment and reassurance may be adequate, but symptoms may last several months or become chronic. NSAIDs are often adequate. Doxepin or amitriptyline, in minimal doses, may also be useful to help with sleep. Narcotic medication should be avoided. Management should also include a cervical pillow or cervical roll and rehabilitation.

Surgical decompression and fusion may be necessary for patients with intractable pain, progressive neurologic findings, or symptoms of cervical myelopathy and spinal cord compression.

Adverse Outcomes of Treatment

NSAIDs may cause gastric, renal, or hepatic complications. Sedation from tricyclic antidepressants may occur, and adverse reactions to monoamine oxidase inhibitors are possible. Narcotic dependence is also possible, especially with the early and prolonged use of stronger narcotic medication. Monoparesis or loss of specific nerve root function may occur, and, although uncommon, quadriparesis or quadriplegia may result from progressive cervical stenosis with spinal cord compression.

Referral Decisions/Red Flags

Intractable neck pain that is not responsive to treatment, neurologic symptoms that affect either the upper or lower extremities, lack of coordination, gait disturbances, and radicular symptoms related to neck motion all indicate the need for further evaluation and referral to a specialist.

Cervical Strain

Synonym

Neck sprain

ICD-9 Code

847.0
Sprains and strains of other and unspecified parts of back, neck

Definition

Cervical strain is a common, usually self-limiting condition. By strict definition, an acute cervical strain is a muscle injury in the neck, whereas the term sprain generally refers to a ligamentous injury. These terms are often used interchangeably, however, by both the medical profession and the lay public. Moreover, because neither physical examination nor imaging can distinguish between muscle and ligament injuries in the deeply located soft-tissue structures of the neck, the term *cervical strain* includes ligamentous injuries of the facet joints and/or intervertebral disks. Regardless of which soft-tissue structures have been injured, the diagnostic and treatment protocols are similar: Evaluate the patient to identify unstable injuries and/or neurologic deficits and then provide appropriate treatment.

A whiplash mechanism (acceleration-deceleration of the neck with rapid flexion-extension) occurs commonly as a result of motor vehicle accidents. The classic mechanism is a stopped car that is struck from behind by another vehicle. These injuries may cause prolonged disability despite no apparent pathologic process. The cause may be a combination of a ligament/muscle injury and symptom amplification. On occasion, severe injuries result in definite instability patterns and/or cervical disk displacements. The concept of symptom amplification should not be advanced until after a thorough history, physical examination, and appropriate imaging studies have been performed.

Clinical Symptoms

Cervical pain may follow an incident of trauma or may be spontaneous in onset. Nonradicular, nonfocal neck pain, noted anywhere from the base of the skull to the cervicothoracic junction, is most common (**Figure 1**). Patients may also have pain in the region of the sternocleidomastoid muscles and/or the trapezius muscles. Pain is often worse with motion and may be accompanied by paraspinal spasm. Occipital headaches may occur in the early phase and may persist for months. Pain following trauma often persists longer than pain following strains or sprains of spontaneous onset. Patients may report increased irritability, fatigue, sleep disturbances, and difficulty concentrating. Work tolerance may be impaired.

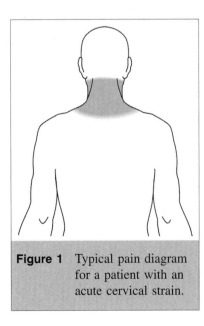

Figure 1   Typical pain diagram for a patient with an acute cervical strain.

Tests

Physical Examination

Examination may reveal areas of tenderness in the paraspinous muscles, trapezii, sternocleidomastoid muscles, spinous processes, interspinous ligaments, and/or the medial border of the scapula. Limited motion is common and may involve rotation, lateral bending, and/or flexion and extension. Pain is often noted at the extremes of motions. The neurologic examination is usually normal.

Diagnostic Tests

AP, lateral, and open-mouth (odontoid) radiographs are necessary if the patient has a history of trauma or associated neurologic deficit or if the patient is elderly. All seven cervical vertebrae must be seen. Anterior displacement of the pharyngeal air shadow indicates soft-tissue swelling that may develop following spinal fracture, injury to the intervertebral disk or anterior longitudinal ligament, or injury at the occipitocervical level. The presence of precervical swelling mandates a specialty consultation to assess the numerous possible causes. In normal adults, the width of the prevertebral soft tissue at the level of C3 should not exceed one third the width of the C3 vertebral body. The normal lordotic curve of the cervical spine may be straightened or reversed as a result of muscle spasm, but this finding is also observed in approximately 10% of normal adults. Preexisting degenerative changes may be noted; they are most commonly age related and occur most frequently at C5-6 or C6-7.

If the patient has severe pain, the screening radiographs should be examined for signs of instability that include translation of a vertebral body of more than 3.5 mm and/or more than 11° of angulation of adjacent vertebrae. Routine flexion-extension radiographs of the cervical spine should not be ordered until the patient has been evaluated by a specialist because of the risk of increased neurologic damage from the maneuvers.

Differential Diagnosis

- Cervical disk herniation (neurologic abnormality and radicular pain)
- Cervical spine tumor or infection (night pain, weight loss, history, fever, chills, sweats)
- Dislocation or subluxation of the spine (usually evident on radiographs; however, on occasion a spontaneous reduction occurs, masking the severity of the injury)
- Inflammatory conditions of the cervical spine (rheumatoid arthritis with abnormal radiographs)

- Spinal fracture (abnormal radiographs)
- Symptom amplification/secondary gain (inconsistent or exaggerated findings)

Adverse Outcomes of the Disease

Symptoms resolve completely in most patients within the first 4 to 6 weeks. With whiplash, resolution typically is delayed, but most symptoms resolve within 6 to 12 months, with few residual symptoms.

Patients with subtle disk injuries superimposed on existing degenerative conditions of the cervical spine may have intractable pain. In some instances, radiculopathy due to lateral nerve root entrapment or myelopathy due to central spinal stenosis may develop.

Treatment

Providing the patient with reassurance about the natural history of these disorders represents an important first step. Acute care (1 to 2 weeks) involves a soft cervical collar and appropriate pain medications and/or short-term NSAIDs. Muscle relaxants may help if the patient has muscle spasm. Commercially available cervical pillows help with reestablishing a normal sleep pattern.

Massage, cervical traction, and ultrasound and other modalities may help, especially in the first 4 weeks. Mild narcotic medication may be useful initially but should be restricted to the first week or two following the injury. Doxepin or amitriptyline may also be helpful for sleep. Manipulation of the cervical spine is contraindicated in patients with acute cervical injuries.

Aerobic activities, such as walking, should be initiated as soon as possible. Add isometric exercises as the patient's comfort improves, preferably in the first 2 weeks. Encourage an early return to normal activities and work.

Rehabilitation Prescription

Cervical strains secondary to limited mobility or tight muscles respond the best to stretching and strengthening exercises. A home program of exercises (see page 933) should include pain-free range-of-motion exercises such as head rolls in all directions. In addition, an upper back stretch helps to relieve tension and increase range of motion of the cervical spine. If the symptoms do not respond to the home program within 3 to 4 weeks, formal rehabilitation may be ordered. The prescription should include an evaluation to determine specific segmental limitations and muscle involvement. The rehabilitation specialist may order cervical spine traction and mobilization of the restricted segments.

SECTION 8 SPINE

Adverse Outcomes of Treatment

NSAIDs may cause gastric, renal, or hepatic complications. If the patient's condition fails to improve, depression may develop. Chronic pain syndrome and drug dependence also may develop in these patients.

Referral Decisions/Red Flags

Patients with pain refractory to treatment, nerve root deficits, or myelopathy or who present a diagnostic dilemma must be evaluated thoroughly.

SECTION 8 SPINE

Home Exercise Program for Cervical Strain

- Perform the exercises in the order listed.
- Apply heat to the painful area for 20 minutes before performing the exercises.
- If the pain worsens or does not improve, call your doctor.

Exercise Type	Area Targeted	Number of Repetitions/Sets	Number of Days per Week	Number of Weeks
Head rolls	Cervical spine	3 repetitions (all directions)/3 sets	Daily	3 to 4
Cat back stretch	Upper back	10 repetitions	Daily	3 to 4

Head Rolls

- Sit in a chair or stand with your weight evenly distributed on both feet.
- Begin by gently bowing your head toward your chest.
- Stretch your right ear toward your right shoulder (1).
- Then stretch your left ear toward your left shoulder (2).
- Next, gently roll your head in a clockwise circle three times (3).
- Switch directions and gently roll your head in a counterclockwise circle three times (4).
- Perform 3 sets daily for 3 to 4 weeks.

Cat Back Stretch

- Kneel on your hands and knees in a relaxed position.
- Raise your back up like a cat and hold for 5 seconds.
- Repeat 10 times.
- Perform the exercise daily for 3 to 4 weeks.

SECTION 8 SPINE

Fractures of the Cervical Spine

Definition

Cervical spine fractures and associated ligamentous injuries occur commonly as the result of high-energy trauma, such as a motor vehicle accident, a fall from a height, or a diving accident. These fractures must be suspected and either identified or excluded in all trauma patients who report neck pain. In addition, because in unconscious or intoxicated patients the history and physical examination are compromised, such patients must have appropriate imaging studies to evaluate the cervical spine. Most missed spinal injuries occur in patients who are obtunded from a closed head injury, unconscious, and/or intoxicated.

Clinical Symptoms

Severe neck pain, paraspinous muscle spasm, and/or point tenderness are the most common presenting symptoms. Pain that radiates into the shoulder or arm with associated numbness or tingling suggests nerve root impingement. Global sensory or motor deficits suggest spinal cord injury. In patients who have sustained multiple trauma, associated injuries may be so painful that the patient may not report every area of the body that is painful. Therefore, in these patients, the absence of neck pain on initial examination does not "clear" the patient or eliminate the possibility of a cervical spine injury.

Tests

Physical Examination

Inspect for swelling and contusions. Palpate for tenderness and paraspinal spasm. A gap or a step-off between spinous processes suggests an injury to the posterior ligamentous complex that is generally quite unstable. Evaluate motor and sensory function of the upper and lower extremities as well as the sensory status of the thoracic dermatomes. Perianal sensation, sphincter tone, and the bulbocavernosus reflex also should be assessed in any patient who is suspected of having a spinal injury.

Diagnostic Tests

Radiographs of the cervical spine should include AP and lateral views as well as an open-mouth view of the odontoid (C2). In a multiply injured patient, however, the most important view is the cross-table lateral view of the cervical spine, to include C1 through T1. In large patients, CT and/or MRI might be required to completely evaluate the cervical spine. The most commonly missed injuries are those at the upper and lower portions of the cervical spine. Lateral radiographs must include the occiput superiorly and the top of T1 inferiorly. Occasionally, a swimmer's view is required to visualize the cervicothoracic junction, although this region can usually be assessed with CT multiplanar reconstructions or with MRI.

The lateral radiograph should be evaluated for anterior soft-tissue swelling, height of the vertebral body, and alignment of the vertebral bodies, facet joints, and spinous processes. The odontoid view should be checked for odontoid fracture (often subtle), C1 lateral mass widening, and the position of the occipital condyles. The AP radiograph can show subtle malalignment of the spinous processes. This finding may indicate rotational malalignment secondary to facet fracture or dislocation.

If no fracture is seen, the radiographs should be carefully evaluated for other signs of instability, including translation of a vertebral body of more than 3.5 mm or more than 11° of angulation of adjacent vertebral bodies. Flexion-extension lateral views should be obtained only after a three-view series has been cleared and only upon recommendation by a spine consultant. Flexion-extension radiographs may not detect ligamentous instability if paraspinal spasm is present. Therefore, in the acute situation, other studies (eg, CT, MRI) may be preferable to rule out a fracture or significant ligamentous injury.

Differential Diagnosis

- Acute disk herniation (normal radiographs with or without neurologic deficit)
- Cervical sprain (normal radiographs with muscle pain/tenderness)
- High thoracic fracture (evident on swimmer's view or thoracic radiographs)

Adverse Outcomes of the Disease

Severe injury may result in complete or incomplete quadriplegia. Nerve compression with radiculopathy may also occur. Chronic neck pain and fatigue may result from deformity or associated muscle injury.

Treatment

The cervical spine must be immobilized at the time of extrication of the patient from the accident scene. In addition,

SECTION 8 SPINE

bracing of the cervical spine and the use of a spine board should be used during transport of patients who sustain high-energy trauma or who have suspected neck injuries. Immediate IV steroids (a bolus of methylprednisolone 30 mg/kg of body weight followed by a continuous drip of 5.4 mg/kg/h for 23 hours) should be initiated for patients who have sustained a spinal cord injury.

Patients whose initial radiographs and neurologic examination are normal but who have persistent pain should wear a cervical collar for 7 to 10 days. The clinical examination and radiographs should be repeated if symptoms persist. If these radiographs are normal, flexion-extension lateral radiographs and an MRI should be obtained. If these studies are normal, the patient may start a neck stretching and strengthening rehabilitation program with scapular stabilization.

Adverse Outcomes of Treatment

Neurologic deficits may develop or worsen during treatment.

Referral Decisions/Red Flags

Patients with instability or with a fracture, dislocation, subluxation, or neurologic deficit require further evaluation. A high index of suspicion for occult injury should be maintained in patients who are intoxicated, uncooperative, or unconscious.

SECTION 8 SPINE

Fractures of the Thoracic or Lumbar Spine

Definition

Fractures of the thoracic or lumbar spine generally occur as a result of high-energy trauma such as motor vehicle accidents or falls from a height. They may also occur following minimal trauma in patients who have diminished bone strength from osteoporosis, tumors, infections, or long-term steroid use.

The fracture pattern usually determines fracture stability and likelihood of neural injury. Simple compression fractures involving only the anterior half of the vertebral body are generally stable, as are some burst fractures (compression fractures extending to the posterior third of the vertebral body). Flexion-distraction injuries that disrupt the posterior ligamentous complex are highly unstable. These injuries are often associated with abdominal injuries such as bowel lacerations.

Clinical Symptoms

Moderate to severe back pain related to a traumatic event is the most common presenting symptom. The pain is exacerbated by motion. Numbness, tingling, weakness, or bowel and bladder dysfunction suggest nerve root or spinal cord injury. In addition, decreased bowel motility may occur secondary to an ileus in patients with lumbar spine fractures.

Tests

Physical Examination

Inspect the trunk, chest, and abdomen for swelling and ecchymosis. Patients with lap belt (flexion/distraction) injuries often demonstrate ecchymosis or contusions over the anterior iliac spines. Tenderness to palpation or light percussion occurs at the level of injury. Hematoma formation and a step-off (forward shift) or gap between spinous processes with swelling are the hallmarks of an unstable flexion-distraction or burst fracture. Evaluate motor and sensory function of all nerve roots distal to the injury. Diffuse numbness, weakness, loss of reflexes, ankle clonus, or a positive Babinski sign indicates spinal cord injury. Examination of perianal sensation, sphincter function, and the bulbocavernosus reflex are particularly important with an associated spinal cord injury. Evaluate the abdomen and chest for possible associated injuries.

ICD-9 Codes

805.2
Fracture of the vertebral column without mention of spinal cord injury, dorsal (thoracic), closed

805.3
Fracture of the vertebral column without mention of spinal cord injury, dorsal (thoracic), open

805.4
Fracture of the vertebral column without mention of spinal cord injury, lumbar, closed

805.5
Fracture of the vertebral column without mention of spinal cord injury, lumbar, open

SECTION 8 SPINE

Figure 1 Lateral radiograph shows a minimal compression fracture of the lumbar spine.

Figure 2 AP radiograph shows a burst fracture of the lumbar spine with widening of the interpedicular distance (double-headed arrow).

Diagnostic Tests

AP and lateral radiographs of the thoracic and lumbar spine are indicated. When a spine fracture is identified, the radiograph should be scrutinized for adjacent or nonadjacent fractures as well. CT scans with reconstructions offer the best information with respect to the need for surgical stabilization.

In the lateral view, compression and burst fractures show loss of height of the anterior wall of the vertebral body and resultant kyphotic deformity (**Figure 1**). Burst fractures involve an injury to the middle column, which can be best seen on a CT scan. Unstable flexion-distraction injuries show widening of the space between adjacent spinous processes on the AP and/or lateral view. The AP view may reveal transverse process fractures or widening of the interpedicular distance that also confirms an unstable burst fracture (**Figure 2**). Rotation of one vertebral body in relation to the one below also indicates instability. Any injury other than a simple compression fracture requires additional imaging studies.

Differential Diagnosis

- Herniated lumbar disk (no fracture, patient able to walk, single nerve root involvement)
- Thoracic or lumbar muscle strain (no neurologic findings or fractures)
- Visceral injuries (abnormal abdominal examination and radiographs, ultrasonogram, or CT scan)

Adverse Outcomes of the Disease

Loss of nerve or spinal cord function, persistent painful instability or deformity, and impaired function are serious sequelae of certain injuries to the spine.

Treatment

Preventing neurologic injury, restoring stability, and restoring normal function are the goals of treatment. Initial extrication, transportation, and evaluation in the emergency department require the use of spinal precautions, including a spine board and log rolling. If radiographs reveal no fracture or instability and no neurologic deficits are present, these precautions may be lifted after confirmation by a specialist.

Isolated transverse process fractures do not affect stability of the spine but do indicate significant injury to adjacent muscles and possible injury to the kidneys. A thoracolumbar corset may be used to decrease symptoms.

Compression fractures with wedging of less than 20° and no posterior vertebral or posterior element involvement can be managed with a thoracolumbosacral orthosis for 8 to 12 weeks, to be worn during sitting and standing activities. Pain management may require short-term oral narcotics. Walking may be encouraged, but bending, stooping, twisting, and lifting more than 20 lb should be discouraged. The patient should return to work as quickly as possible, with job modifications as needed. Exercises to strengthen trunk flexor and extensor muscles can supplement walking after the brace is removed.

Other injuries usually require more aggressive treatment. Patients with a spinal cord injury should be started on a steroid protocol as soon as possible. Patients with unstable burst fractures, flexion-distraction injuries, or fracture-dislocations are usually treated by internal fixation and spinal fusion.

Adverse Outcomes of Treatment

Progressive collapse with kyphotic deformity may occur, resulting in chronic pain and/or neurologic compromise. Chronic muscle pain may also develop if the trunk muscles are not adequately strengthened after immobilization is discontinued.

Referral Decisions/Red Flags

Any neurologic deficit is a sign of significant injury and requires further evaluation. Burst fractures, flexion-distraction injuries (or any injury to the posterior column of the spine), fractures with vertebral rotation, and fracture-dislocations all require further evaluation and treatment.

SECTION 8 SPINE

Low Back Pain: Acute

ICD-9 Codes

847.1
Sprains and strains of other and unspecified parts of back, thoracic

847.2
Sprains and strains of other and unspecified parts of back, lumbar

Synonyms

Low back strain

Lumbar sprain

Pulled low back

Definition

The term low back pain (LBP) more properly describes a symptom rather than a diagnosis. For more than 80% of patients with LBP, a more specific diagnosis is not possible.

LBP is the most frequent cause of lost work time and disability in adults younger than 45 years. Most symptoms, however, are of limited duration, with 80% of patients demonstrating significant improvement and returning to work within 1 month. The 4% of patients whose symptoms persist longer than 6 months generate 80% to 90% of the costs to society for treating LBP.

A low back strain is an injury to the paravertebral spinal muscles. The term *sprain* is used to describe ligamentous injuries that may include the facet joints or anulus fibrosus. In the latter condition, the disk does not herniate into the spinal canal, but substances may leak from the nucleus pulposus that induce inflammation and cause irritation of the lumbosacral nerve roots. Because of the deep location of the lumbar soft tissues, however, localizing an injury to a specific structure is difficult, if not impossible. Furthermore, in this area, regardless of which muscle or ligamentous structures have been injured, the treatment protocols are identical.

A history of repeated lifting and twisting or operating vibrating equipment may be associated with LBP. However, individuals who engage in little physical exertion may also report similar symptoms. Factors associated with reports of LBP include poor fitness, job dissatisfaction, smoking, and various psychosocial issues.

Figure 1 Typical pain diagram for a patient with low back pain.

Clinical Symptoms

Patients report the acute onset of LBP, often following a lifting episode. The lifting may be a trivial event, such as leaning over to pick up a piece of paper. The pain often radiates into the buttocks and posterior thighs (**Figure 1**). Patients may have difficulty standing erect and may need to change position frequently for comfort. This condition may first be experienced in the early adult years.

Tests

Physical Examination

Examination reveals diffuse tenderness in the low back or the sacroiliac region. Range of motion of the lumbar spine, particularly flexion, is typically reduced and painful. The degree of lumbar flexion and the ease with which the patient can extend the spine are good parameters by which to evaluate progress. Lower extremity reflexes and the motor and sensory function of the lumbosacral nerve roots are normal.

Diagnostic Tests

Plain radiographs usually are not helpful in diagnosing acute LBP. In adolescents and young adults, there is little or no disk space narrowing, whereas in adults older than 30 years, there is variable disk space narrowing and/or spurs. These changes are widely prevalent and are not considered pathologic but rather physiologic signs of aging.

For patients with atypical symptoms, such as pain at rest or at night or a history of significant trauma, AP and lateral radiographs should be obtained. These views help to identify pathologic processes such as infection, neoplasms (visualize up to T10), fracture, or spondylolisthesis.

Differential Diagnosis

- Ankylosing spondylitis (family history, morning stiffness, limited mobility of the lumbar spine)
- Drug-seeking behavior (symptom amplification, inconsistent and nonphysiologic examination)
- Extraspinal causes (ovarian cyst, nephrolithiasis, pancreatitis, ulcer disease, aortic aneurysm, retroperitoneal tumors)
- Fracture of the vertebral body (major trauma or minimal trauma with osteoporosis)
- Herniated disk (unilateral radicular pain symptoms that extend below the knee and are equal to or greater than the back pain)
- Infection (fever, chills, sweats, elevated erythrocyte sedimentation rate)
- Multiple myeloma (night sweats, men older than 50 years)

Adverse Outcomes of the Disease

Functional impairment is the primary disability. This can be of great significance for any patient whose normal activities are strenuous and whose general health is otherwise excellent, but young adults in particular have difficulty accepting a condition that may impair function for several weeks.

SECTION 8 SPINE

Treatment

Before any treatment is begun, a complete history is obtained and the patient is evaluated to rule out any significant neurologic findings. If signs of neurologic deficits such as dorsiflexion weakness, plantar flexion weakness, or urinary frequency are found, a referral to a specialist is indicated.

For the patient with LBP with or without sciatic symptoms and with no significant neurologic deficits, treatment has two phases: The initial phase deals with symptomatic relief; the second phase focuses on return to activity.

Phase one, or symptomatic treatment, should include avoidance of intense physical activity. Pain management can be initiated with aspirin, acetaminophen, or NSAIDs. Steroid dose packs, narcotic medication, or muscle relaxants are not recommended as primary pain management tools for most patients who present with acute LBP. It is important to inform the patient that in most cases the symptoms of acute LBP resolve quickly, with the patient able to return to work and other activities within a few days.

As the acute pain improves, phase two of treatment can begin, which focuses on helping the patient return to full activity. Initially, the patient may need lighter duty or shorter hours at work. Flexibility in allowing such arrangements benefits both the employee, in increased self-esteem, and the employer, in decreased costs. As pain diminishes and activity increases, the patient should be referred to a physical therapist for an exercise program focusing on an aerobic activity (walking, running, bicycling, swimming, using an elliptical machine) plus strengthening of trunk flexors and extensors. Once the patient is established in this program, he or she may transition to a health club or a home exercise program such as the one described below. Patients who continue to exercise and remain fit have fewer recurrences of LBP.

A patient who is unable to return to work within 4 weeks should be referred to a specialist for further evaluation and treatment.

Rehabilitation Prescription

The rehabilitation prescription should include an evaluation to determine specific segmental restrictions and muscle dysfunction. When developing a rehabilitation program, it is important to determine whether lumbar spine muscle asymmetry, especially of the multifidus, is present. Rehabilitation may include a combination of mobilization of the restricted segments and stabilization exercises emphasizing endurance. A home exercise program for LBP (see page 944) includes a combination of stretching and stabilization exercises. The kneeling back extension and knee-to-chest exercises are good general stretching exercises for the low back. Side bridges and hip bridges are excellent exercises to improve stability of the low back muscles.

Adverse Outcomes of Treatment

NSAIDs may cause gastric, renal, or hepatic complications. Although uncommon, spinal manipulation may result in a lumbar disk herniation.

Referral Decisions/Red Flags

Neurologic abnormalities, unresponsive pain syndromes, or an unusual clinical presentation indicates the need for further evaluation.

SECTION 8 SPINE

Home Exercise Program for Acute Low Back Pain

- Perform the exercises in the order listed.
- Apply heat to the low back for 20 minutes before performing the exercises.
- If the pain worsens or if it does not improve after performing the exercises for 3 to 4 weeks, call your doctor.

Exercise Type	Muscle Group/Area Targeted	Number of Repetitions/Sets	Number of Days per Week	Number of Weeks
Kneeling back extension	Low back	10 repetitions	Daily	3 to 4
Knee to chest	Low back	10 repetitions/3 sets	Daily	3 to 4
Side bridges	Quadratus lumborum	5 repetitions	Daily	3 to 4
Hip bridges	Hip extensors Low back extensors	5 repetitions	Daily	3 to 4

Kneeling Back Extension

- Crouch on your hands and knees.
- First rock forward onto your extended arms, allowing your back to sag. Hold for 5 seconds.
- Then rock back and sit on your bent knees with your arms extended and your head tucked in. Hold for 5 seconds.
- Repeat 10 times.
- Perform the exercise daily, for 3 to 4 weeks.

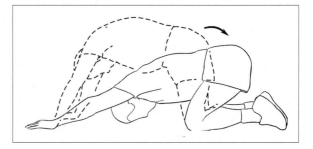

Knee to Chest

- Lie on your back on the floor.
- Grasp one knee and bring it up to your chest as far as it will go.
- Then lower your leg back to the floor.
- Repeat with the other leg.
- Then do both legs together.
- Repeat this sequence 10 times.
- Perform 3 sets daily, for 3 to 4 weeks.

Side Bridges

- Lie on your side on the floor.
- With your elbow bent at 90°, lift your body off the floor as shown, keeping your body straight.
- Hold this position for 15 seconds and then repeat on the other side.
- Perform 5 repetitions daily, for 3 to 4 weeks.

Hip Bridges

- Lie on your back on the floor with your arms at your sides, your knees bent, and your feet flat on the floor.
- Lift your pelvis so that your body is in a straight line from your shoulders to your knees.
- Hold this position for 15 seconds.
- Perform 5 repetitions daily, for 3 to 4 weeks.

SECTION 8 SPINE

Low Back Pain: Chronic

ICD-9 Codes

722.52
Degeneration of lumbar intervertebral disk, lumbar, or lumbosacral disk

724.2
Low back pain, chronic

Definition

Chronic low back pain (LBP) is used to describe LBP of more than 3 months' duration. Patients usually present between 30 and 60 years of age. Symptoms are typically recurrent and episodic, but in some patients the pain is unremitting. Once chronic LBP has been identified, an evaluation is required to exclude causes such as cancer, stenosis, deformity, osteoporosis, infection, and abdominal conditions such as aneurysm, ulcer, or retroperitoneal tumor. All patients with chronic LBP should be evaluated by a spine specialist as well as by their internist, family practitioner, or, for women, their gynecologist.

Degeneration of the intervertebral disk is a physiologic event of aging and may be modified by factors such as injury, repetitive trauma, infection, heredity, and tobacco use. As the hydrophilic properties of the nucleus pulposus degrade, the disk loses height and the segmental ligaments develop laxity. Motions such as translation and twisting may create tears within the anulus fibrosus. Chronic LBP may develop.

Clinical Symptoms

Low back pain that radiates to one or both buttocks is the hallmark symptom (**Figure 1**). The pain is often described as "mechanical" in that it is aggravated by activities such as bending, lifting, stooping, or twisting. Patients may report stiffness or have a history of intermittent sciatica (pain radiating down the back of the leg), but discomfort in the back is the predominant symptom. The pain is relieved with lying down or a night's rest. Some patients, however, have difficulty sleeping because of the symptoms.

Depression is not a primary cause of chronic LBP, but it can overlay the condition and complicate treatment. Early recognition will greatly assist with symptom resolution.

Tests

Physical Examination

Lumbar and sacroiliac tenderness is a common finding. Patients may also exhibit a side or forward list from muscle spasm. Motor and sensory function of the lower extremity nerve roots as well as the lower extremity reflexes are normal. Straight-leg raising and spinal motion may be mildly restricted. Although not characteristic, nonorganic findings such as widespread sensitivity

Figure 1 Typical pain diagram for a patient with chronic low back pain.

to light touch, nonanatomic localization of symptoms, inappropriate pain behaviors, and inconsistent actions may be seen with this condition. (See page 912.)

Diagnostic Tests

AP and lateral radiographs often show age-appropriate changes, such as anterior osteophytes and reduced height of the intervertebral disks. Often there is a "vacuum sign," with apparent air (nitrogen) in the disk space (**Figure 2**).

Differential Diagnosis (Partial List)

- Degenerative disorders (imaging abnormalities)
- Developmental defects (abnormal radiographs)
- Infection (elevated erythrocyte sedimentation rate, C-reactive protein level, temperature)
- Inflammation (other joint involvement, elevated erythrocyte sedimentation rate)
- Metabolic disease (abnormal laboratory studies)
- Neoplasms (weight loss, night pain, fatigue)
- Neurologic disorders (long tract signs)
- Psychosocial issues (depression, worker's compensation issues, positive Waddell signs)
- Referred pain (aortic aneurysm, pelvic tumor, renal disorders)
- Trauma (history of injury)

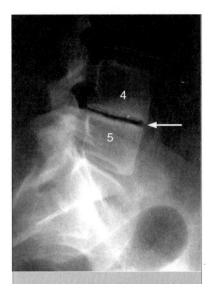

Figure 2 Lateral radiograph shows marked degenerative changes affecting the disk between L4 and L5 (arrow). Note the extreme disk space narrowing.

Adverse Outcomes of the Disease

In patients with more severe symptoms, vocational and recreational activities may be limited. Sleep disturbances, mood swings, and sexual dysfunction may occur, and concentration may be adversely affected. Deconditioning, which may be the result of reduced activity, is frequently associated with the condition and may aggravate the symptoms as well as increase any occupational dysfunction.

Treatment

Before treatment is initiated, the patient should have undergone a thorough clinical evaluation with appropriate laboratory tests and imaging studies to exclude processes other than physiologic aging. Once these conditions have been ruled out, the term *chronic benign LBP* may be used.

Narcotic abuse is a cause for concern in this population. By definition, the patient with chronic LBP has experienced pain for a lengthy period and frequently has received a variety of medications, including addictive muscle relaxants and narcotics. In addition, many of these patients are deconditioned, depressed, unemployed, angry, and demanding, so management of the condition is often challenging. Referral to a comprehensive pain management program is warranted. These programs employ a wide range of strategies, including comprehensive evaluations with thorough psychologic testing, injections, biofeedback, cognitive/behavior conditioning programs, spinal cord stimulation, psychotherapy, and detoxification programs.

In addition, a return-to-activity program is also essential to overcome the deconditioning that is typical in the patient with chronic LBP. This can be initiated on an individual or group (class) basis and is typically overseen by a rehabilitation specialist. Once a comprehensive management program has been developed, the primary care physician can follow the patient, emphasizing the need to maintain "well behavior." Pain relapses are common, and referral to the pain management center may be necessary. Because of the complexity of evaluating and managing these patients, a comprehensive team approach is highly recommended for a successful outcome.

Rehabilitation Prescription

Chronic LBP is difficult to treat using any single approach. Often the trunk muscles are weak and unable to stabilize the spine during daily activities. Therefore, a home exercise program should consist of stabilization exercises including modified side bridges, hip bridges, bird dog exercises, and abdominal bracing (see page 950). Aerobic or cardiovascular conditioning consistent with the patient's general health also is helpful. If the patient's symptoms do not improve after adhering to the home program for 3 to 4 weeks, formal rehabilitation may be ordered. The rehabilitation specialist must conduct an extensive evaluation of the mobility and strength of the lumbar spine to determine a treatment approach. Use of pain modalities is limited with chronic LBP.

Adverse Outcomes of Treatment

NSAIDs may cause gastric, renal, or hepatic complications. Avoid labeling patients as "disabled" because this may negatively affect the patient's motivation. Narcotic dependency or abuse can become a problem for these patients.

SECTION 8 SPINE

Referral Decisions/Red Flags

Further evaluation is needed for patients who have fever, chills, unexplained weight loss, a history of cancer, significant night pain, or a history of pain for more than 6 to 12 months. Other indications for additional evaluation include the presence of pathologic fractures, obvious deformity, saddle anesthesia, loss of major motor function, bowel or bladder dysfunction, abdominal pain, or visceral dysfunction.

Home Exercise Program for Chronic Low Back Pain

- Perform the exercises in the order listed.
- Apply heat to the low back for 20 minutes before performing the exercises.
- You should not experience pain with the exercises.
- If the pain worsens or if it does not improve after performing the exercises for 3 to 4 weeks, call your doctor.

Exercise Type	Muscle Group	Number of Repetitions	Number of Days per Week	Number of Weeks
Modified side bridges	Quadratus lumborum	5 repetitions	Daily	3 to 4
Hip bridges	Back and hip extensors	5 repetitions	Daily	3 to 4
Bird dog	Back extensors	5 repetitions	Daily	3 to 4
Abdominal bracing	Abdominals	5 repetitions	Daily	3 to 4

Modified Side Bridges

- Lie on your side on the floor with your knees bent.
- With your elbow bent at 90°, lift your body off the floor as shown, keeping your body straight.
- Hold this position for 15 seconds and then repeat on the other side.
- Perform 5 repetitions daily, for 3 to 4 weeks.

Hip Bridges

- Lie on your back on the floor with your arms at your sides, your knees bent, and your feet flat on the floor.
- Lift your pelvis so that your body is in a straight line from your shoulders to your knees.
- Hold this position for 15 seconds.
- Perform 5 repetitions daily, for 3 to 4 weeks.

SECTION 8 SPINE

Bird Dog

- Kneel on the floor on your hands and knees.
- Lift your right arm straight out from the shoulder, level with your body, at the same time that you lift your left leg straight out from the hip.
- Hold this position for 15 seconds.
- Repeat with the opposite arm and leg.
- Perform 5 repetitions daily, for 3 to 4 weeks.

Start

Finish

Abdominal Bracing

- Lie on your back on the floor with your arms at your sides, your knees bent, and your feet flat on the floor.
- Contract your abdominal muscles so that your stomach is pulled away from your waistband.
- Hold this position for 15 seconds.
- Perform 5 repetitions daily, for 3 to 4 weeks.

Lumbar Herniated Disk

ICD-9 Codes

722.10
Displacement of thoracic or lumbar intervertebral disk without myelopathy

724.4
Thoracic or lumbosacral neuritis or radiculitis, unspecified (Radicular syndrome of lower limb)

Synonyms

Herniated nucleus palposus (HNP)
Lumbar radiculopathy
Neurogenic leg pain
Sciatica

Definition

The intervertebral disk is composed of the nucleus pulposus, a gel-like material that cushions axial compression; the anulus fibrosus, a specialized ligamentous structure surrounding the nucleus pulposus that helps to stabilize the spine; and the superior and inferior cartilaginous end plates. Activities such as lifting and twisting increase pressure on the nucleus pulposus. Lumbar disk herniations develop over time as the weaker posterolateral portion of the anulus fibrosus develops fissures that permit the egress of other disk components that herniate into the lumbar canal adjacent to the exiting lumbar nerve root. The resultant herniated disk syndrome (commonly called sciatica) causes pain, numbness, and/or weakness in one or both lower extremities, depending on the anatomic location of the herniation. The pain results in part from direct mechanical compression of the nerve root and in part from chemical irritation of the nerve root by substances within the nucleus pulposus.

Lumbar disk herniation most commonly occurs at the L4-5 or L5-S1 levels, with subsequent irritation of the L5 or S1 nerve root. Herniations at more proximal intervertebral levels constitute only 5% of all lumbar disk herniations.

Lumbar disk herniations affect approximately 2% of the population. Even though only 10% of these patients have symptoms that persist longer than 3 months, the numbers are so great that this represents approximately 600,000 patients. Most of these patients improve with nonsurgical care, but those who remain symptomatic generally consider surgical management to improve their quality of life.

Clinical Symptoms

The onset of symptoms is often abrupt, but it also may be insidious. Unilateral radicular leg pain frequently follows the onset of acute low back pain. The theory is that the initial posterolateral disk bulge results in low back pain that then becomes sciatic pain as the herniation emerges past the anulus to the spinal canal.

The pain is often severe and is exaggerated by sitting, walking, standing, coughing, and sneezing. Typically, the pain radiates from the buttock down the posterior or posterolateral leg to the ankle or foot (**Figure 1**). Patients have a difficult time finding a position of comfort. Usually, lying on the back with a pillow under the knees or lying on the side in a fetal position provides some relief.

Upper or midlumbar radiculopathy (L1 to L4 nerve root compression) refers pain to the anterior aspect of the thigh and often does not radiate below the knee.

Tests

Physical Examination

As the patient stands, look for the presence of a trunk list to one side (**Figure 2**). The patient may also evidence limited forward flexion with dysrhythmia of the paraspinous muscles (ie, they contract asymmetrically). With the patient sitting, perform the seated straight-leg raising test (see page 907). As the knee is extended on the symptomatic side, a patient with true sciatic tension will lean back to relieve the pressure on the exiting nerve root. This sign has a high correlation with a herniated lumbar disk. Even more specific is the crossed straight-leg raising sign: when the nonsymptomatic extremity is elevated, the patient reports buttock or sciatic pain on the symptomatic side. Evaluate motor and sensory function of the lumbosacral nerve roots as well as the deep tendon reflexes.

With the patient supine, perform supine straight-leg raising on the involved and uninvolved limbs. This test places the L5 and S1 nerve roots on stretch. Ipsilateral restriction of straight-leg raising is common with a variety of lumbar spine problems, but a positive crossed straight-leg raising test (pain that occurs in the involved leg or buttock when the uninvolved leg is lifted) is highly specific for lumbar nerve root entrapment. To stretch the upper lumbar nerve roots, perform the reverse straight-leg raising test (see page 912). Classic findings (**Figure 3**) include the following:

- The L3-4 disk (L4 nerve root) may produce weakness in the anterior tibialis, numbness in the shin, pain in the thigh, and an asymmetric knee reflex. About 5% of disk ruptures occur at this level.

- The L4-5 disk (L5 nerve root) may produce weakness in the great toe extensor, numbness on the top of the foot and first web space, and pain in the posterolateral thigh and calf. There is no predictable reflex test for a herniated lumbar disk at the L4-L5 level. Thus, checking the extensor hallucis longus is especially important because this may be the only sign to confirm an L5 radiculopathy.

Figure 1 Typical pain diagram for lumbar radiculopathy.

Figure 2 Trunk shift, or "list," to the right.

SECTION 8 SPINE

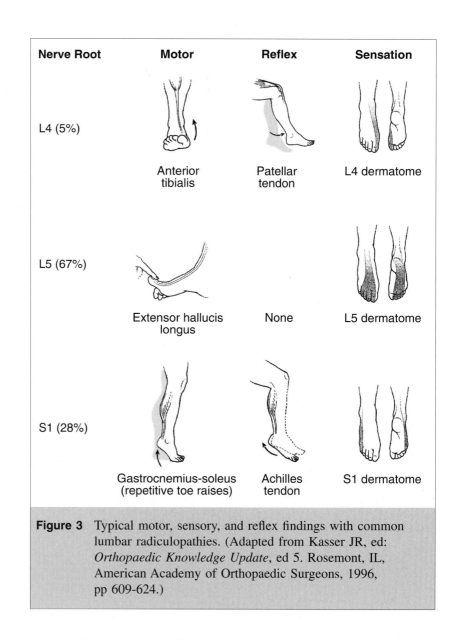

Nerve Root	Motor	Reflex	Sensation
L4 (5%)	Anterior tibialis	Patellar tendon	L4 dermatome
L5 (67%)	Extensor hallucis longus	None	L5 dermatome
S1 (28%)	Gastrocnemius-soleus (repetitive toe raises)	Achilles tendon	S1 dermatome

Figure 3 Typical motor, sensory, and reflex findings with common lumbar radiculopathies. (Adapted from Kasser JR, ed: *Orthopaedic Knowledge Update*, ed 5. Rosemont, IL, American Academy of Orthopaedic Surgeons, 1996, pp 609-624.)

- The L5-S1 disk (S1 nerve root) may produce weakness in the great toe flexor as well as in the gastrocnemius-soleus complex, with inability to sustain toe-walking, numbness in the lateral foot, pain and ache in the posterior calf, and an asymmetric ankle reflex.

Diagnostic Tests

Radiographs demonstrate age-appropriate changes with no specific findings. MRI should be ordered to confirm the diagnosis if symptoms persist longer than 4 weeks, if a significant neurologic deficit is identified, or as a part of the preoperative evaluation (**Figure 4**). MRI is otherwise not necessary unless there are progressive neurologic changes or intolerable pain.

Differential Diagnosis

- Cauda equina syndrome (perianal numbness, urinary overflow incontinence or retention, reduced anal sphincter tone, bilateral involvement)
- Demyelinating conditions (clonus)
- Extraspinal nerve entrapment (abdominal or pelvic mass)
- Hip or knee arthritis (decreased internal rotation of hip, knee deformity or effusion)
- Lateral femoral cutaneous nerve entrapment (sensory only, lateral thigh)
- Spinal stenosis (older population)
- Thoracic cord compression (clonus, spasticity, high sensory pattern, abdominal reflexes)
- Trochanteric bursitis (no tension signs, pain down lateral thigh and leg, exquisite tenderness over the trochanter)
- Vascular insufficiency (absent posterior tibial pulse, claudication, trophic changes)

Figure 4 Preoperative axial MRI shows herniated lumbar disk (arrow).

Adverse Outcomes of the Disease

Cauda equina syndrome with permanent motor loss, urinary incontinence, and sensory numbness may develop. Specific root deficit, with permanent dysesthesia, pain, or weakness, may occur.

Treatment

NSAIDs may be used in the acute phase, along with 1 to 2 days of minimal activity. Narcotic medication may be helpful in the acute phase for selected patients but typically should not be prescribed for longer than 7 days. Patients should limit sitting, prolonged standing, or walking. Patients should be reassured that most disk herniations resolve without residual problems.

Most patients who have a lumbar disk herniation will improve within 3 to 4 weeks. If they do not, an evaluation by a specialist should be obtained.

Rehabilitation as described for acute low back pain (see page 944) is also appropriate for patients with a lumbar herniated disk. Patients with true radiculopathy with a lumbar herniated disk take longer to recover, however, and usually require activity modification for at least 4 to 8 weeks. Both aerobic conditioning and trunk strengthening are essential for the best outcome. Patients whose symptoms do not improve and who experience a clear decrease in their quality of life are candidates for surgical diskectomy. Profound or progressive neurologic disorders, including cauda equina syndrome, require urgent surgery.

Epidural steroid injections (up to three in a 6-month period), which are usually administered under radiologic guidance, may

SECTION 8 SPINE

be considered. These injections should be avoided in any patient who presents with a significant neurologic deficit. Although the risk of significant complications is low, epidural steroid injections should not be recommended without consideration of these risks. Also, if the patient experiences no relief of symptoms, repeating the injections later is not warranted.

The effectiveness of manipulative therapy, traction, or acupuncture for patients with a confirmed lumbar herniated disk remains unproved in Level 1 evidence trials.

Adverse Outcomes of Treatment

NSAIDs may cause gastric, renal, or hepatic complications. Progression of neurologic deficit or persistent numbness and weakness may occur despite treatment.

Referral Decisions/Red Flags

Patients with any of the following conditions require further evaluation: cauda equina syndrome, urinary retention, perianal numbness, motor loss, severe single nerve root paralysis, progressive neurologic deficit, radicular symptoms that persist for more than 6 weeks, intractable leg pain, or recurrent episodes of sciatica that interfere with the patient's life activities.

Lumbar Spinal Stenosis

Synonym

Neurogenic claudication

ICD-9 Code

724.02
Spinal stenosis other than
cervical, lumbar region

Definition

Lumbar spinal stenosis is the narrowing of one or more levels of
the lumbar spinal canal with subsequent compression of the
nerve roots. Anatomically, lumbar stenosis affects as much as
30% of the population older than 60 years, yet only a portion of
these individuals will have symptoms. In elderly patients, spinal
stenosis is typically degenerative in origin. Younger patients
with achondroplasia or other disorders that cause a small spinal
canal may experience clinical symptoms in their 20s or 30s.

Degenerative lumbar spinal stenosis occurs most commonly at
the L3-4, L4-5, and L2-3 levels. Although central lumbar
stenosis is uncommon at L5-S1, lateral degenerative changes at
this level may cause compression of the L5 (higher) nerve root.

Clinical Symptoms

The stenosis may be quite advanced before symptoms occur.
Onset of symptoms may be insidious, or symptoms may develop
quickly without any history of injury. A common pattern of
presentation is neurogenic claudication that causes radicular
symptoms (with or without associated back pain) in one or both
legs (**Figure 1**). Neurogenic claudication differs from vascular
claudication, but these conditions may coexist in elderly patients
(**Table 1**). With neurogenic claudication, symptoms progress
from a proximal to a distal direction. Walking or prolonged
standing causes fatigue and weakness in the legs. Sitting or
lying generally relieves the pain. Vascular insufficiency may be
difficult to differentiate from lumbar spinal stenosis.

Extension of the spine narrows the lumbar spinal canal,
flexion increases the canal diameter. Therefore, patients may
obtain short-term relief by leaning forward (stooping). For
example, these patients often lean on the cart while grocery
shopping. The length of time that symptomatic relief lasts after
sitting will vary. Patients may also awaken at night with back
and/or leg pain after a few hours of sleep.

Lumbosacral pain occurs less commonly and is associated
with walking or standing. A vague aching in the legs associated
with leg weakness may also be reported.

Spondylolisthesis (degenerative or spondylolytic), vascular
insufficiency, and osteoarthritis of the hips are often associated
with spinal stenosis. Obesity may also be an associated factor.

SECTION 8 SPINE

Figure 1 Typical pain diagram for a patient with spinal stenosis. Some patients may have severe stenosis but little thigh or leg pain.

Table 1 Comparison of Vascular and Neurogenic Claudication

Evaluation	Vascular	Neurogenic
Claudication distance	Fixed	Variable
Relief of pain	Standing	Sitting-flexed
Walk uphill	Pain	No pain
Bicycle ride	Pain	No pain
Type of pain	Cramp, tightness	Numbness, ache, sharp
Pulses	Absent	Present
Bruit	Present	Absent
Skin	Loss of hair, shiny	Normal
Atrophy	Rare	Occasional
Weakness	Rare	Occasional
Back pain	Uncommon	Common
Limitations of spinal movement	Uncommon	Common

(Reproduced from Herkowitz HN: Spinal stenosis: Clinical evaluation. *Instr Course Lect* 1992;41:183-185.)

Tests

Physical Examination

True muscle weakness in the legs is uncommon. Proprioception may be impaired and result in a mildly positive Romberg test. Sensory changes are segmental if present but may involve more than one spinal level. Reflexes may be diminished. The anterior and posterior tibial pulses will be normal unless the patient has concomitant vascular disease. Some patients will have a lumbar deformity. Bowel or bladder symptoms may be reported, but anal sphincter tone is rarely decreased. Because many patients have concomitant prostate disease or stress incontinence, genitourinary evaluation is necessary to differentiate these processes.

Diagnostic Tests

AP and lateral radiographs (including up to T10 in the lateral view) may show spondylolisthesis or significant narrowing of the intervertebral disk (**Figure 2**). Osteopenia may be present.

Figure 2 Lateral radiograph of a patient with degenerative spondylolisthesis at L4 on L5 (arrow).

Differential Diagnosis

- Abdominal aortic aneurysm (palpable pulsatile mass)
- Arterial insufficiency (distance to claudication constant, recovery after rest, absent or diminished pulses)
- Diabetes mellitus (abnormal glucose metabolism, nonsegmental numbness, skin changes)
- Folic acid or vitamin B12 deficiency (confirmed by laboratory tests, anemia)
- Infection (mild temperature elevation, elevated erythrocyte sedimentation rate, elevated C-reactive protein level, intervertebral disk narrowing with reactive changes in the adjacent vertebral end plates)
- Tumor (patchy neurologic deficit, bone destruction, night pain)

Adverse Outcomes of the Disease

The rate of progression varies widely. Many patients tolerate this condition well and never develop any neurologic deficit. However, pain and limited function may become significant and lead to an adverse quality of life with secondary depression. Standing erect may become impossible, forcing the patient to adopt a stooped posture. Claudication may develop after walking only a few feet. Although cauda equina syndrome must be considered, this syndrome is rare.

SECTION 8 SPINE

Treatment

Many patients with lumbar spinal stenosis are elderly and have comorbidities that require consideration when weighing treatment options. Initial treatment generally includes NSAIDs and physical activity. Water exercise therapy is a good initial activity for the elderly, deconditioned patient with mild symptoms. Narcotic medication is rarely required. Epidural steroid injections (up to three in a 6-month period), which are usually administered under radiologic guidance, may be considered. Epidural steroid injections improve symptoms in about 50% of patients, but the improvement usually lasts only 4 to 6 months.

Patients who are becoming nonambulatory and report a decreased quality of life are candidates for surgical management. The age of the patient is less important than comorbidities in predicting surgical outcomes. Patients with degenerative spondylolisthesis and/or scoliosis in addition to lumbar spinal stenosis may require spinal fusion in addition to decompression of the stenotic segments.

Adverse Outcomes of Treatment

Neural damage during decompression is possible but unlikely with improved techniques. Prolonged use of NSAIDs may cause renal failure, hepatotoxicity, and gastrointestinal ulcer disease. The chronic use of narcotics is associated with its own set of problems when these drugs are used inappropriately.

Referral Decisions/Red Flags

Any neurologic deficit, gait disturbance, or bowel and bladder dysfunction should be evaluated further. Because these changes may not improve following surgery, the goal of treatment is to prevent progression. If nonsurgical treatment is ineffective, specialty consultation is indicated. Night pain that disturbs sleep usually indicates advanced disease for which further evaluation is indicated.

Metastatic Disease

Definition

Malignant tumors involving the spine may be either primary (rare) or metastatic (common). Metastatic disease to the vertebrae occurs at some time in the clinical course of the disease in approximately 50% of all patients who have solid tumors. The highest incidence occurs with carcinoma of the breast, lung, prostate, colon, thyroid, and kidney.

Osseous involvement of the vertebrae is much more common than involvement of the spinal cord or dura. The most likely etiology is hematogenous spread, whereby neoplastic cells in the vertebral body are deposited through the Batson plexus, a unique venous plexus of the spine characterized by collateral connections to the inferior vena cava and a general lack of valves.

Metastatic disease may become clinically evident through one of several different presentations: (1) as an incidental finding in asymptomatic patients; (2) in patients with known primary tumors who are being evaluated for possible metastatic disease by bone scan, MRI, or CT; (3) as neurologic findings in patients with or without previous history of a primary tumor; or (4) as the primary presenting symptom of cancer in patients who were not aware they had a primary tumor.

ICD-9 Codes
198.5 Secondary malignant neoplasm of other specified site, bone and bone marrow
733.13 Pathologic fracture, vertebrae

Clinical Symptoms

Pain is the most common presenting symptom. The pain may be first noted following trivial trauma, is typically constant, and worsens progressively as the days or weeks pass. This pain is usually due to minor vertebral fractures secondary to the weakness created by the metastatic process. Weight-bearing activities (standing, sitting) aggravate the pain, whereas lying down typically results in relief. Pain that prevents sleep and persists through the night is highly suspicious for a neoplasm.

With compression of the nerve roots, the pain associated with cervical or lumbar tumors also radiates to the extremities. Similar nerve root entrapment by tumors in the thoracic spine causes a band-like distribution of pain around the chest. When the compression involves a nerve root, radicular symptoms and associated sensory loss and/or motor weakness are restricted to a single extremity. If more generalized sensory and motor dysfunction occurs, and especially if the patient reports bowel or bladder dysfunction or difficulty walking, cervical or thoracic cord compression or cauda equina syndrome may be present.

The rate of disease progression and neurologic dysfunction may be slow, evolving over weeks or months, or rapid in more aggressive tumors. Progression may be more difficult to identify in patients taking high dosages of pain medication for metastatic disease elsewhere. Acute onset of quadriplegia or paraplegia may occur (infrequently) with rapid enlargement of a soft-tissue tumor mass or following a pathologic fracture that compresses the spinal cord.

Tests

Physical Examination

An area of tenderness to palpation and/or percussion along the spinous processes is common. Tumors in the posterior elements (lamina, spinous process) may be palpable. A patient with a vertebral body collapse may develop increased kyphosis at the level of fracture. Assess motor and sensory function of all nerve roots distal to the lesion. Check deep tendon and other appropriate spinal cord reflexes. If the primary tumor has not been previously diagnosed, the patient will need a complete evaluation for staging purposes with particular emphasis on the thyroid, breasts, chest, kidney, and prostate. Consultation with an oncologist is warranted.

Diagnostic Tests

Initial radiographic evaluation requires high-quality AP and lateral radiographs. Cervical spine radiographs should also include odontoid views and show all vertebrae from the occiput to T1. Lumbar spine radiographs should include the bodies of T10 to the tip of the coccyx, with a spot lateral view of the lumbosacral junction if needed for clarity. A radiopaque marker placed next to an area of percussion tenderness helps identify the area of concern. The lateral view may show collapse with loss of height of the vertebral body or areas of bony destruction with lytic or blastic lesions in the vertebral body. Often the first radiologic sign of tumor involvement is loss of integrity of a pedicle, as seen on the AP view and commonly described as the "winking owl" sign because of the asymmetry of the involved and uninvolved pedicles (**Figure 1**).

A technetium Tc 99m bone scan is the best screening study to identify widespread metastatic disease because it evaluates the spine as well as other axial (pelvis) and appendicular (extremity) bones. This study will generally be negative in patients with multiple myeloma.

Figure 1 AP radiograph of the spine demonstrates a missing pedicle (arrow), indicative of a metastatic or a primary tumor (the "winking owl" sign).

Differential Diagnosis

- Degenerative arthritis (fracture rare, bone dense)
- Infection (loss of disk space, sclerosis)
- Multiple myeloma (men older than 50 years, fracture from trivial trauma)

- Osteoporotic fracture (generalized osteopenia, pedicles intact)
- Traumatic fracture (normal bone, widening of bone in AP and lateral views)

Adverse Outcomes of the Disease

Involvement of one area of the spine with metastatic disease does not usually change the overall survival rate, but spinal deformity and/or intractable pain poses considerable problems in patient care. Spinal involvement with neurologic deficit compromises quality of life and may shorten lifespan with complications of paraplegia. Quadriplegia and paraplegia are the most serious sequelae of pathologic fractures.

Treatment

Treatment of spinal tumors is based on the type of tumor, the degree of bony involvement, the type of symptoms, and physician/patient preference. Chemotherapy, hormone therapy, or radiation is appropriate for asymptomatic tumors detected during evaluation for metastatic disease. Radiation therapy is appropriate for painful metastases without serious deformity or neural compression. Alternative methods are considered in tumors that are insensitive to radiation (renal cell carcinoma). With pain and neurologic deficit, the most effective way to improve neural function and overall function is surgical decompression and stabilization, generally with adjunctive postoperative radiation therapy. Surgical intervention results in improved neurologic function in approximately 85% of patients.

Adverse Outcomes of Treatment

Neurologic deterioration persists in some patients, despite adequate decompression, because of recurrent tumor or tumor involvement in the vascular supply to the spinal cord. Surgical wound complications are more common when the surgery follows radiation therapy or the patient is taking oral steroids.

Referral Decisions/Red Flags

Patients with known prior malignancies and spinal symptoms or patients with intractable pain require specialty evaluation, as do patients in whom trivial trauma produces a spinal fracture, even in the presence of osteoporosis.

SECTION 8 SPINE

Scoliosis in Adults

Definition

Scoliosis is a lateral curvature of the spine. In adults, the condition is classified as either a deformity that developed during childhood or a deformity that developed after skeletal maturity, usually secondary to degenerative spondylosis and/or degenerative spondylolisthesis. Changes that occur with aging, including osteoporosis, degenerative disk disease, spinal stenosis, and degenerative spondylolisthesis, may contribute to and/or confound the symptoms and progression of either condition.

Clinical Symptoms

The most common presenting symptom is pain localized to the region of the deformity. The most common overlapping syndrome is degenerative spondylosis, which may also cause lower lumbar pain. Because age-related changes in the spine are present in nearly everyone, a thorough evaluation is required to identify the most likely source of pain. Radicular pain is most commonly associated with compression of the L4 or L5 nerve root due to asymmetric hypertrophy of the facet joints, asymmetric disk degeneration, and mild rotatory subluxation. Neurologic changes are infrequent but most commonly involve the extensor hallucis longus muscle.

In some patients, the chief presenting symptom is a progressive spinal deformity. Some report that they are "getting shorter." These patients may also report that the "hump" on their back is getting bigger, or that they are leaning to the side more.

Cardiopulmonary decompensation rarely is evident in adult-onset scoliosis. Symptoms related to pulmonary compromise are associated with more severe thoracic curves, including both idiopathic and neuromuscular curves.

Tests

Physical Examination

The entire spine should be inspected and palpated with the patient standing. The relative height of the shoulders and iliac wings should be noted, as should any asymmetry at the waist. Decompensation is evaluated by measuring the distance a plumb line from C7 deviates to the right or left of the gluteal cleft. Forward bending also exaggerates the asymmetry of the posterior rib cage and thoracolumbar junction. Neurologic examination should include an evaluation of reflexes as well as motor and sensory function of the lumbosacral nerve roots. In addition, pathologic reflexes should be assessed as well as a gait analysis looking for ataxia or evidence of spinal cord compression (myelopathy).

Diagnostic Tests

Weight-bearing full-length PA and lateral radiographs should be obtained on a 36″ cassette (**Figure 1**). Electromyography is rarely indicated but occasionally may be helpful to distinguish radiculopathy from neuropathy.

Differential Diagnosis

- Congenital scoliosis (vertebral body abnormality, childhood or adolescent presentation)
- Degenerative disk disease with asymmetric disk space collapse (normal vertebral shape, sharp curve over few segments)
- Degenerative spondylolisthesis with accompanying lateral listhesis and disk degeneration (forward or backward slip of vertebral body)
- Neuromuscular scoliosis (neurologic abnormalities and weakness)
- Severe disk herniation with sciatic scoliosis and radiculopathy (unilateral neurologic signs, normal vertebral contour)
- Traumatic or pathologic vertebral fracture (wedge-shaped vertebral body, history of trauma)
- Vertebral osteomyelitis (fever, severe local pain, lysis of bone in vertebral body, narrowing of disk)

Figure 1 PA radiograph of the spine demonstrates advanced thoracolumbar kyphoscoliosis.

Adverse Outcomes of the Disease

Increased pain and deformity with diminished functional activity are possible. With increased cosmetic deformity, patients may become more introverted.

Treatment

Most cases of scoliosis in adults can be managed with NSAIDs and exercise. Exercise programs should begin with water therapy and progress to trunk strengthening as the symptoms decrease and the patient's tolerance increases. Aerobic activity is also recommended. Swimming is a particularly good exercise because it accomplishes trunk strengthening as well as aerobic conditioning.

SECTION 8 SPINE

Adverse Outcomes of Treatment

NSAIDs may cause gastric, renal, or hepatic complications. Complications of surgical management may include increased pain, increased deformity, infection, pseudarthrosis, instrumentation failure, and/or paralysis. The postoperative complication rate is much higher in adults than in adolescents. Patients must clearly understand the risks and benefits of this major surgery before undergoing the procedure. Elderly patients especially should be informed of the risks inherent in these surgeries in older patients. The physician should discuss the risks of both mortality and neurologic deficits.

Referral Decisions/Red Flags

Progressive neurologic deterioration requires emergency management. Patients who experience progressive pain and in whom the deformity progresses may be considered for major spinal fusion surgery. Patients who report that they cannot walk more than two blocks because of pain, respiratory dysfunction, or weakness require specialty evaluation. Any change in the deformity requires specialty evaluation as well.

Spinal Orthoses

Cervical

Soft Cervical Collar

This foam-covered orthosis is appropriate for short-term use in cervical sprains or intermittent use to alleviate pain in patients with cervical spondylosis. The most common error is selecting a soft cervical collar that is too wide, thus thrusting the neck into extension. A collar that positions the neck in approximately 10° of flexion maximizes the space for the nerve roots as they pass through the vertebral foramen. Patients should be on an isometric exercise program to avoid loss of intrinsic muscle support. Soft cervical collars worn at night are also helpful.

Philadelphia Collar

This molded polystyrene brace provides better control of cervical rotation and is preferred for transport and initial immobilization of patients with suspected cervical fractures. Some physicians prefer this support to the cervical collar in the treatment of acute sprains. Unless rotational control is necessary (C1-2 injury), most patients prefer the greater comfort of a soft cervical collar.

Rigid Cervical Orthoses

A hard cervical collar limits flexion and extension better than a soft cervical collar. Greater restriction of neck motion is attained by a brace that extends from the neck to the midthoracic spine. For example, the Miami J orthosis (Jerome Medical, Moorestown, NJ) is basically a Philadelphia collar that has a rigid plastic component extending to the middle of the chest. As such, it greatly restricts rotation that primarily occurs in the upper cervical spine as well as the flexion and extension and lateral bending that occur to a greater degree in the lower cervical spine.

Halo Brace

This brace provides superior immobilization of the cervical spine. The halo portion is rigidly secured to the head by four screws inserted into the outer table of the skull. Bars connect the halo to a plastic vest that surrounds the chest. Minimal cervical spinal motion occurs in a patient wearing this brace.

SECTION 8 SPINE

Thoracic

Thoracolumbosacral Corset

A standard lumbosacral corset with a proximal extension provides adequate support for patients with osteoporosis or acute thoracic sprains involving the lower thoracic spine. Some corsets are equipped with metal stays or plastic inserts that are bent to conform to the patient's spine. Women may not comply with this brace because breast irritation may occur. The orthotist may need to modify the brace to ensure patient compliance.

Three-point Spine Orthosis

The basic principle of this type of orthosis is three-point fixation, with pressure over the sternum and pubis anteriorly and over the midspine posteriorly. Most are aluminum and bendable to fit the patient. These braces limit flexion and extension of the thoracic spine but provide limited rotational control. Because of their limited contact areas and light weight, these orthoses are well tolerated by patients. This type of orthosis is useful for patients with thoracic sprains or minimal compression fractures.

Total-contact Thoracolumbosacral Orthosis

Total-contact thoracolumbosacral orthosis (TLSO) braces are either prefabricated modules that are fitted based on measurements of the torso or are made from a plaster mold of the patient's torso. The latter type provides better total contact and rotational control but is quite expensive. These braces usually are constructed of hard plastic anterior and posterior clamshells that are lined with a soft material and attach together on the sides. These braces are used primarily as definitive treatment in patients with stable fractures of the thoracolumbar spine or as a postoperative aid following spinal fusion.

Lumbar

Elastic Belts

These braces do not limit lumbar spine motion and probably do not prevent injury. With a mild lumbar strain, they do provide some abdominal support and can certainly remind the patient to be careful during various activities.

Lumbosacral Corset

The standard lumbosacral corset can be worn with or without internal stays of metal or plastic. These devices provide very little restriction of motion and are most useful as an adjunct to pain control following a lumbar sprain or acute disk herniation. The time period of bracing should be short and accompanied by an exercise program once the acute pain has subsided.

Rigid Orthoses

See the descriptions for the three-point and total-contact orthoses.

SECTION 8 SPINE

Spondylolisthesis: Degenerative

Synonym

Pseudospondylolisthesis

Definition

Degenerative spondylolisthesis is forward slippage of a lumbar vertebral body that is caused by degeneration and alterations in the facet joints in conjunction with degenerative changes in the intervertebral disk. By definition, the lamina and pars interarticularis are intact. This condition occurs most frequently between the fourth and fifth vertebral bodies. Degenerative spondylolisthesis is more common in women older than 40 years. These patients also tend to be mildly to moderately overweight.

Retrolisthesis is posterior slippage of a lumbar vertebral body on the vertebrae below. This condition also develops secondary to degenerative changes.

Clinical Symptoms

Back pain that is aggravated by bending, lifting, or twisting activities is common. Narrowing of the lateral recesses may cause a radiculopathy. Narrowing of the central canal may cause neurogenic claudication or other symptoms of spinal stenosis.

Tests

Physical Examination

Inspect and palpate the spine for any curvature, loss of lordosis, or step-off of the spinous processes. Evaluate motor and sensory function of the L1-S4 nerve roots. Diminished knee and/or ankle reflexes are often present; however, these findings are common in elderly patients. Motor examination is usually normal, but strength testing after walking may reveal weakness in toe or heel walking or in great toe dorsiflexion strength.

Diagnostic Tests

AP and lateral radiographs are important. The lateral view will show slippage of one vertebra onto another, usually with the superior vertebra displaced several millimeters relative to the one below (**Figure 1**). The involved disk space frequently shows degeneration and narrowing.

Figure 1 Lateral radiograph of a patient with degenerative spondylolisthesis at L4 on L5 (arrow).

SECTION 8 SPINE

Differential Diagnosis

- Iatrogenic instability (following diskectomy or decompression)
- Isthmic spondylolisthesis (pars defect) (findings on radiographs and single-photon emission CT [SPECT] scans)
- Pathologic fracture (from tumor)
- Posttraumatic instability (history of fracture)

Adverse Outcomes of the Disease

Disabling back pain or functional neurologic impairment associated with spinal canal stenosis or radiculopathy is possible.

Treatment

Initial management should include NSAIDs and exercise. Many patients with degenerative spondylolisthesis are overweight, and they should be advised of the benefits of weight loss. Weight loss alone is unlikely to eliminate the patient's symptoms, however, because the forces generated by the trunk and spinal muscles will not be influenced by weight reduction. Patients may find an abdominal binder to be helpful occasionally, but more rigid braces are typically poorly tolerated and are seldom worn. Patients may engage in activities as tolerated because activity will not cause injury, although it may be uncomfortable. Nonsurgical management is often successful for several years in these patients, but they usually consider surgical management eventually.

Adverse Outcomes of Treatment

NSAIDs may cause gastric, renal, or hepatic complications and may interact with other medications.

Referral Decisions/Red Flags

Patients with symptoms of spinal stenosis (neurogenic claudication) after walking two blocks or less require further evaluation. Patients with cauda equina syndrome (perianal numbness and/or bowel or bladder impairment) require immediate evaluation.

Spondylolisthesis: Isthmic

Figure 1 Typical pain diagram for a patient with isthmic spondylolisthesis. Distribution of leg symptoms will generally follow the L5 dermatome on one or both sides.

Definition

Spondylolisthesis occurs when one vertebral body slips in relation to the one below. In children this usually occurs between L5 and S1. A defect develops at the junction of the lamina with the pedicle (pars interarticularis), leaving the posterior element without a bony connection to the anterior element. Most likely this condition represents a cyclic loading event (fatigue fracture) that evolves over time in the adolescent years and fails to heal. If only the defects are present, the patient has spondylolysis. When the vertebral body slides forward, producing the "slip" or "listhesis," the condition is called spondylolisthesis and classified as isthmic. Patients who participate in activities that place stress on this area, such as gymnastics and football, have a higher incidence of this condition. For example, the incidence of spondylolysis in female gymnasts is nearly sixfold the incidence in less active age-matched females.

Clinical Symptoms

Spondylolisthesis may be asymptomatic or minimally symptomatic. However, adolescent and adult patients may also develop significant back pain that radiates posteriorly to or below the knees and worsens with standing (**Figure 1**). Frequently, patients report spasms in the hamstring muscles manifested by the inability to bend forward. In addition, markedly limited straight-leg raising is demonstrated on examination (see page 907). True nerve compression symptoms are rare, although the fibrocartilaginous tissue in the region of the pars interarticularis does compress the L5 nerve roots in patients with isthmic spondylolisthesis.

Tests
Physical Examination

Examination may reveal diminished lumbar lordosis and flattening of the buttocks. With significant spondylolisthesis, a step-off is noted, with the spinous process of the slipped vertebra that is "left behind" being more prominent than the one above.

Hamstring spasm markedly limits the patient's ability to bend forward or the height to which the examiner can raise the patient's straight leg with the patient supine (straight-leg raising test). Neurologic deficits are uncommon.

Diagnostic Tests

With forward slippage (spondylolisthesis), lateral radiographs demonstrate forward translation of L5 relative to S1 (expressed as a percentage of the AP width of the vertebral body) (**Figure 2**). A defect in the pars interarticularis (a "collar" on the "Scotty dog") is evident on the oblique views (**Figure 3**). This is the only radiographic abnormality if the condition is limited to spondylolysis.

Increasing slippage can be evaluated with radiographs taken at 6-month intervals (or sooner if symptoms increase) until skeletal maturity is achieved.

Differential Diagnosis

- Intervertebral disk injury (no step-off or slip, no defect seen on plain radiograph)
- Intervertebral diskitis (elevated erythrocyte sedimentation rate, fever)
- Osteoid osteoma (night pain, abnormal bone scan, pain relieved with aspirin)
- Spinal cord tumor (sensory findings, upper motor neuron signs)
- Tethered spinal cord (pain, hamstring tightness, upper motor neuron signs)

Adverse Outcomes of the Disease

Progressive or complete slip of the vertebral body, chronic back pain and disability, paralysis of the lower lumbar nerve roots (usually L5), or bowel and bladder involvement (cauda equina syndrome) are possible.

Treatment

Isthmic spondylolisthesis differs from degenerative spondylolisthesis in that these patients are often skeletally immature at the outset of the condition, so a single-photon emission CT (SPECT) scan should be performed in the young patient to assess metabolic activity in the area of the defect in the pars interarticularis. If the area of the defect is active and the patient is skeletally immature, some surgeons recommend surgical stabilization or fixation of the defect. Once the patient reaches skeletal maturity, fixation of the defect is not warranted.

Figure 2 Lateral radiograph of a grade 2 to 3 spondylolisthesis at the lumbosacral junction (arrow).

Figure 3 Oblique radiograph shows a normal "Scotty dog" appearance to the lamina (outlined area). In the vertebra below, the Scotty dog has a "collar" (arrow), which is the site of the pars interarticularis defect of spondylolisthesis.

SECTION 8 SPINE

Skeletally mature patients need not be restricted from any activity. Progression of this condition in an adult is rare. Most cases of progression in adults occur in patients with spondylolisthesis following decompression surgery without spinal fusion.

In adults, nonsurgical treatment with NSAIDs and exercise is recommended. Surgery is recommended only in patients with a decreased quality of life whose symptoms have not responded to a well-planned and faithfully followed nonsurgical regimen.

Adverse Outcomes of Treatment

Despite treatment, progression of the forward slip may continue.

Referral Decisions/Red Flags

Patients with significant pain and/or obvious slippage require further evaluation.

Pediatric Orthopaedics

Section Editors

David Andrew Spiegel, MD
Pediatric Orthopedic Surgeon
Children's Hospital of Philadelphia
Assistant Professor of Orthopaedic Surgery
University of Pennsylvania School of Medicine
Philadelphia, PA

John F. Sarwark, MD
Professor
Department of Orthopaedic Surgery
Northwestern University
Feinberg School of Medicine
Chicago, IL

Contributors

Michael Huxford, MEd, ATC, CSCS
Sports Medicine Coordinator
Rehabilitative Services
Institute for Sports Medicine
Children's Memorial Hospital
Chicago, IL

Lawrence Wells, MD
Attending Orthopaedic Surgeon
Department of Orthopaedic Surgery
The Children's Hospital of Philadelphia
Assistant Professor of Orthopaedic Surgery
University of Pennsylvania School of Medicine
Philadelphia, Pennsylvania

Yukiko Kimura, MD
Chief of Pediatric Rheumatology
Joseph M. Sanzari Children's Hospital
Hackensack University Medical Center
Hackensack, NJ

Overview of Pediatric Orthopaedics

The often-quoted statement "Children are not just small adults" is particularly germane to pediatric disorders of the musculoskeletal system. Fractures, soft-tissue injuries, neurologic disorders, and infections all have unique features and different considerations in children versus adults. Furthermore, the effect of growth must always be considered, as it may have a positive or negative effect depending on the underlying diagnosis.

Common Presenting Symptoms in Children

Parental concern regarding the appearance of the child's stance, posture or gait is a frequent cause for seeking medical advice. Pain from acute injuries is perhaps the most common symptom. Participation in athletics has increased both in frequency and intensity, leading to symptoms from a host of overuse injuries. When a child presents with persistent pain and local swelling and/or refuses to use a limb or bear weight on a lower extremity, a detailed physical examination is indicated to identify a specific cause and recommend effective treatment.

Age and Sex

An understanding of normal growth and development is critical to knowing whether treatment is needed. Some "deformities" in children are age-appropriate and normal for the age. Knowledge of the normal ranges for alignment and rotation of the limbs is essential to differentiate pathologic from physiologic factors. For example, genu varum (bowlegs) is normal at birth, but by the time a child reaches age 3 years, a relatively large amount of genu valgum ("knock-knee" alignment) is normal. A knowledge of the natural history of the underlying disease process helps to predict potential consequences if the condition is untreated and to define the indications for various options for treatment.

Age and sex are important factors when evaluating children. For example, a boy between the ages of 4 and 8 years who has proximal thigh pain and a limp most likely has Legg-Calvé-Perthes disease. Similar symptoms in adolescent boys might suggest a slipped capital femoral epiphysis. Female infants are more likely than male infants to have hip dysplasia, whereas clubfoot is more common in males. Adolescent girls are more likely to have scoliosis, but kyphosis of the spine is more common in adolescent boys.

Growth

Growth may benefit treatment because of its associated remodeling potential. This is particularly true in the newborn period or during infancy, when bracing a dysplastic hip for a few months will result in a normal joint that functions well for a lifetime. Certain angular deformities in pediatric fractures also may remodel completely in young children, this allows greater latitude in closed management of fractures in children when compared to adults.

On the other hand, growth may exacerbate some pediatric disorders. Fractures that damage the physis (growth plate) may cause progressive angulation and/or shortening of the limb. Progressive angulation of a weight-bearing bone (as seen in infantile tibia vara and rickets) may result from asymmetric compression on one side of the physis, which inhibits growth on the compressed side.

Neuromuscular Disorders

Many pediatric neuromuscular disorders such as cerebral palsy, myelomeningocele, and muscular dystrophy cause muscle weakness and/or imbalance (greater weakness on one side of the joint), which may result in limb deformities and impaired function. Normal longitudinal growth of the skeleton may be affected by muscle contractures, resulting in rotational and/or angular deformities. For example, in a child with cerebral palsy, the hip adductor and flexor muscles are often more spastic and therefore stronger than the opposing hip abductors and extensors. With growth, this muscle imbalance may cause progressive contracture of the adductors and flexors, as well as dysplasia of the acetabulum, valgus alignment of the proximal femur, and subluxation or dislocation of the hip.

Variables in Soft-Tissue Injuries

As children grow, their coordination and strength are developing. As a result, competitive sports require adaptation of the game to the age and size of the child. While overuse injuries in the adult primarily manifest themselves as either microscopic tears or complete rupture at the musculotendinous junction (or within the substance of the tendon), the bone-tendon junction is the weak link in children and adolescents, different types of overuse syndromes are seen in these age groups. For example, Osgood-Schlatter disease results from microscopic avulsion fractures at the insertion of the patellar tendon during adolescence when the child is relatively big and active and when the relatively weak secondary ossification center of the proximal tibia is developing.

SECTION 9 PEDIATRIC ORTHOPAEDICS

Variables in Infection and Arthritis

The higher incidence of acute hematogenous osteomyelitis (AHO) in children is related to the unique anatomy of the child's metaphyseal bone circulation. A child's spine is also more susceptible to diskitis for similar reasons. Hematogenous septic arthritis also is more common in children. Chronic inflammatory diseases such as juvenile idiopathic arthritis also are different in children.

SECTION 9 PEDIATRIC ORTHOPAEDICS

Pediatric Physical Examination

Inspection/Palpation

Anterior View

With the patient standing, inspect frontal, side, and rotational alignment of the lower extremities for genu valgum (knock-knee), genu varum (bowleg), internal femoral torsion (where the patellae point toward one another), external femoral torsion (where the patellae face away from each other and not straight ahead), and limb-length inequality (where the pelvis is not level). Also, look for increased angulation at the elbow or extreme shoulder height asymmetry. Look for asymmetry in the angle formed by the humerus and forearm (elbow carrying angle). It is normal for the elbow to be in slight valgus alignment. Unilateral deformity may indicate an acute injury or deformity from a congenital or traumatic growth disturbance.

Palpation

A young child may not be able to verbalize the site of his or her pain. Initiate palpation by touching an area that is probably not involved, slowly moving to the suspected area of involvement. Even though the child may be apprehensive and crying, a change in discomfort can be identified as the tender area is palpated.

Range of Motion

Hip Internal Rotation

Measure hip internal rotation with the hip in extension for accurate measurement of femoral torsion. With the patient prone and knees flexed to 90°, rotate the lower extremities outward. This maneuver positions the hip into internal rotation. With restricted unilateral motion, one hip will allow a greater arc of motion than the other. With increased femoral anteversion, internal rotation will exceed external rotation by 30° or more.

Hip External Rotation

Assess hip external rotation with the child prone and the knees together. Rotate the lower extremities inward while stabilizing the pelvis. This maneuver positions the hip in external rotation. Compare the two sides. Rotation of the hips is typically symmetric.

Hip Abduction—Older Children

Assess hip abduction in older children with the hip in extension and the pelvis level. With the patient supine, place one hand on the contralateral anterior superior iliac spine. This hand will sense when the pelvis starts to tilt upward (limit of hip abduction). Abduct the hip until the pelvis starts to tilt and estimate the degree of movement.

Special Tests

Limb-Length Discrepancy

Using a tape measure, measure each lower extremity from the anterior superior iliac spine to the inferior prominence of the medial malleolus. Compare the measurements of the two sides. Alternatively, with the patient in stance, different-sized wooden blocks can be placed under the short lower extremity. The thickness of the blocks under the lower extremity when the iliac crests are level indicates the amount of limb-length discrepancy.

SECTION 9   PEDIATRIC ORTHOPAEDICS

Scoliosis—Forward Bend Test

In a patient with scoliosis, the vertebral column rotates, making the chest wall posteriorly on the convex side more prominent. The resulting posterior prominence is accentuated with the forward bend test. Ask the patient to bend forward with the knees straight and with both arms and the head and neck hanging free. Examine the back from behind during the forward bend test. A prominence indicates scoliosis, a structural and rotational deformity of the spine. Measure the quantity of trunk asymmetry with an inclinometer.

Kyphosis

When assessing patients for kyphosis, inspect the thoracic spine from the side, in stance. Look for excessive rounding of the thoracic spine. Ask the patient to bend forward with the arms and the head and neck hanging free. If the patient is not able to touch the toes, consider the possibility of tight hamstrings associated with Scheuermann disease or spondylolisthesis in the lower lumbar spine.

SECTION 9 PEDIATRIC ORTHOPAEDICS

Wilson Test

The Wilson test is used to assess the presence of symptomatic osteochondritis dissecans. With the patient supine, flex the hip and knee 90° and internally rotate the tibia. Then, slowly extend the knee. The Wilson test is positive when the patient reports pain as the knee reaches full extention or near–full extension, and the pain is relieved with the external rotation of the tibia, while maintaining the same flexion angle. This maneuver causes the tibial spine to impact and then rotate away from the osteochondritis dissecans lesion located on the medial femoral condyle.

Musculoskeletal Screening Examination

The musculoskeletal screening examination is used to clear young athletes (and others) for the musculoskeletal component of sports participation. It also can be used as part of a periodic musculoskeletal physical examination of a patient with no presenting symptoms.

The preparticipation physical examination (PPE) helps detect diseases, susceptibilities, or injuries that may preclude sports participation. It is important to remember, however, that the history and questionnaire have been shown to be the most sensitive in detecting medical issues or injuries. The examiner should question the patient about prior injuries and perform a more detailed examination of affected systems. The purpose of the musculoskeletal screening examination is to look for asymmetry, strength deficits, changes in muscle mass, or limitation of joint motion.

Make sure the patient is dressed appropriately to permit adequate examination of the spine and extremities. Ideally, males should be in shorts and should remove their shirt if they are comfortable doing so. Female patients can wear a tank top or a sports bra with shorts.

PEDIATRIC ORTHOPAEDICS

SECTION 9

Gait

Observe the patient's gait. Assess for symmetry, antalgic gait, limb-length discrepancies, and abnormal mechanics. Assess for trunk shift by checking to see if the torso sways to one side. Ask the patient to walk on the toes, then the heels.

Spine

With the patient standing, inspect the spine. Observe the patient's posture to assess for normal thoracic kyphosis and lumbar lordosis. Check symmetry and height of the shoulders and hips. Perform the forward bend test and record the angle of trunk rotation (ATR).

Cervical Spine

Inspect the cervical spine. Check for asymmetry. Assess the patient's range of motion in each direction. Ask the patient to flex and extend the neck. Ask the patient to rotate the head laterally. Finally, have the patient bend the neck laterally.

Thoracic and Lumbar Spine

Inspect the thoracic and lumbar spine. Observe for asymmetry. Ask the patient to avoid movement at the hips to ensure the assessment properly evaluates the spine. Assess range of motion by having the patient bend forward, bend backward, perform side bending, and rotation.

Upper Extremity

Begin with the patient standing and shoulders visible. Inspect for asymmetry and muscle atrophy.

SECTION 9 PEDIATRIC ORTHOPAEDICS

Shoulder Range of Motion

Evaluate shoulder flexion by asking the patient to lock the elbows and extend the arms fully overhead. Evaluate shoulder abduction by having the patient lock the elbows and then (like making a snow angel) bring the thumbs together overhead. Evaluate external and internal rotation by asking the patient to place the hands behind the head, palms facing in, and then to place the hands behind the back, with palms facing outward. Shoulder motion may more accurately be assessed with the patient supine, shoulder abducted to 90°, and elbow flexed 90° so the examiner can rotate the arm. Generally, external rotation is greater on the dominant side, particularly in a throwing athlete. Total arc of motion should be symmetric.

Elbows

Inspect the elbows. Ask the patient to raise the arms parallel to the floor. Inspect the elbows from the anterior and lateral aspects of the patient. Assess for cubitus varus and cubitus valgus. Have the patient extend and flex the elbows. Ask the patient to flex the elbows to 90° with the elbows at the side. Evaluate elbow pronation and supination.

SECTION 9   PEDIATRIC ORTHOPAEDICS

Wrists

Inspect the wrists. Look for asymmetry. Ask the patient to place the palms together, then the backs of the hands together, to check wrist extension and flexion. Ask the patient to bend the wrist inward and outward to assess for ulnar and radial deviation.

Hands

Inspect the hands. Look for asymmetry. Ask the patient to make a fist with the forearms supinated. Inspect the resting arc of the fingers. Have the patient open the hands and spread the fingers.

Hips

Inspect the hips. Ask the patient to put feet together, with hips abducted (the butterfly stretch position). Ask the patient to squat down, with knees out to the side, then stand.

Knees

With the patient supine on the examination table, inspect for asymmetry. Assess knee flexion by having the patient fully flex the knees with the feet on the table.

Ankles

Inspect the ankles. With the patient seated on the examination table with the legs flexed 90°, observe the position and alignment of the heels. Have the patient dorsiflex the ankles fully by pointing the feet upward, then plantar flex the ankles by pointing the feet downward. Then have the patient evert and invert the feet.

Feet

Inspect the feet for symmetry and normal alignment. Inspect the midfoot and forefoot. Inspect the number and appearance of the toes. Look for symmetry and normal alignment.

Anterior Knee Pain

Definition

Pain about the anterior aspect of the knee is a common problem in active adolescents and preadolescents and is primarily the result of repetitive stress. The most common cause is patellar maltracking. Anterior knee pain caused by altered patellofemoral forces secondary to growth and changing patellar tracking in the trochlear groove of the femur with growth and development is common and has different names, including patellofemoral syndrome (PFS), miserable malalignment syndrome (**Figure 1**), and anterior knee syndrome.

Less common causes of anterior knee pain are pathologic plica and a symptomatic bipartite patella. A plica is a normal fold of the synovium that may become thickened and/or fibrotic secondary to a direct blow or repetitive stress. A bipartite patella is a failure of an ossification center of the patella to fuse, most commonly the superolateral corner (**Figure 2**). A bipartite patella is typically seen as an incidental finding on radiographs; however, it may become symptomatic as a result of a direct blow or following repetitive stress from flexion-extension exercises.

Clinical Symptoms

Patients with anterior knee pain typically report a history of vague peripatellar pain, frequently activity related. With PFS, the pain frequently increases with flexion-extension activities such as running, kicking, and jumping, as well as with squatting, walking downhill, descending stairs, or prolonged sitting. Giving way (falling) with these activities is occasionally reported. Infrequently, a patient will report that the knee locks, defined as a temporary inability to bend or extend the knee following an activity that places a high stress load on the patellofemoral joint (eg, squatting or kneeling). Swelling is rarely reported.

A bipartite patella may be asymptomatic until the patient falls on the knee, presumably altering the fibrous union between the unfused ossicle and the remainder of the patella. In the acute setting, tenderness and swelling are localized to the superolateral corner of the patella. In chronic cases, patients report pain after running and jumping activities.

Tests

Physical Examination

If asked to place one finger on the spot that hurts the most, adolescents with PFS often report that they cannot identify an exact spot but will state that their knee "hurts around the

ICD-9 Codes	
717.9	Pathologic plica
719.46	Patellofemoral pain
736.6	Bipartite patella

Figure 1 Clinical photograph of a patient with miserable malalignment syndrome. Note medial position of the patella, due to femoral anteversion, with outward position of foot, due to external tibial torsion.

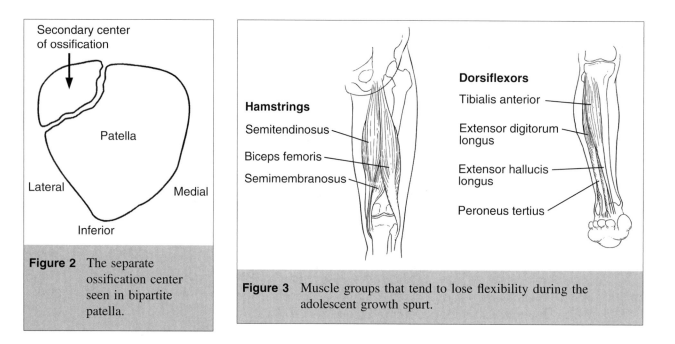

Figure 2 The separate ossification center seen in bipartite patella.

Figure 3 Muscle groups that tend to lose flexibility during the adolescent growth spurt.

kneecap" and make a sweeping gesture over the front of the knee. In contrast, a patient with symptomatic plica or bipartite patella typically localizes the symptoms. Whereas plica pain typically is localized to the medial border of the patella, pain associated with bipartite patella occurs over the junctional area, typically the upper outer border. Hip rotation should be assessed to exclude the possibility of slipped capital femoral epiphysis, which can present as anterior knee pain. Assess the overall alignment of the extremity. Patients with PFS often have hip varus, femoral anteversion knee valgus, and foot pronation, resulting in excessive lateral tracking of the patella in the femoral groove.

Strength of the abdominal and paravertebral muscles, as well as the muscles of the hip, should be evaluated, as should flexibility of the muscles of the lower leg. Tight, weak muscles of the core and leg can result in greater stress to the patellofemoral joint (**Figure 3**). A positive apprehension sign (see page 635) implies true patellar instability rather than PFS. Patellar compression may cause pain but often is nonspecific. A thorough knee examination is required to rule out other causes of pain.

In patients with a symptomatic patella plica, examination may reveal a clicking sensation with knee flexion and extension. The tender plica occasionally may be palpated along the medial border of the patella.

Diagnostic Tests

Screening radiographs include AP, lateral, and skyline views of the knee. The skyline view shows both the location of the patella in the femoral groove and the thickness of the cartilage.

Adolescents with PFS have a normal patellofemoral joint space. Special imaging studies such as CT or MRI may be required to further evaluate patients who have persistent pain.

Differential Diagnosis

- Articular cartilage defects (swelling, abnormal MRI)
- Infection (rare) (erythema, effusion, severe pain, elevated C-reactive protein level)
- Neoplasm (rare) (severe pain, night pain, abnormal bone scan)
- Osteochondritis dissecans (swelling, abnormal radiographs and MRI)
- Patellar subluxation or dislocation (marked positive apprehension sign, marked hypermobility of the patella)

Adverse Outcomes of the Disease

The long-term prognosis is good in patients treated nonsurgically for symptomatic bipartite patella, symptomatic plica, or PFS. The natural history of PFS, which is commonly seen in adolescents, is not well defined and continues to be studied. Most recover uneventfully. In the absence of true patellar subluxation or dislocation, progression to chondromalacia is rare.

Treatment

Symptoms associated with PFS improve with rest from aggravating activities, strengthening of the medial head of the quadriceps, and stretching of the muscles of the lower extremity. Core strengthening exercises also are beneficial. Strengthening the hip, abdominal, and trunk muscles helps better position the body, increases agility, and diminishes the abnormal forces across the patellofemoral joint. A brace to help elevate the patella in the trochlear groove (infrapatellar strap) or guide the patella more centrally in the groove (sleeve/pad with window) may be beneficial. Orthoses (shoe inserts) can be used to decrease foot pronation, which can enhance apparent knee valgus. Surgical management of PFS is recommended only rarely.

Treatment of symptomatic plica includes rest for 7 to 10 days with the knee in an extended position or, if symptoms are mild, activity modification. Occasionally, oral NSAIDs may be helpful in diminishing symptoms. Icing the area often provides relief. Arthroscopic excision of a symptomatic plica rarely is required in adolescents but may be considered if a prolonged trial (3 to 6 months) of nonsurgical measures fails.

SECTION 9 PEDIATRIC ORTHOPAEDICS

Treatment of a symptomatic bipartite patella is similar to that of symptomatic plica. Patients often recover after 5 to 7 days of rest or immobilization or after use of a brace with a lateral pad combined with a decrease in flexion-extension activities followed by quadriceps strengthening. In the unusual case of persistent pain over the fibrous junction of the ossicle with the patella, surgery to remove the unfused ossicle may be required.

Adverse Outcomes of Treatment

Persistent effusion of the knee may indicate inflammatory disease (eg, juvenile rheumatoid arthritis) or infection (eg, Lyme disease). Pain, hypersensitivity to touch, and limited knee motion suggest the presence of complex regional pain syndrome.

Referral Decisions/Red Flags

Pain at rest or that increases at night requires further evaluation to rule out neoplastic processes. A joint effusion, increased generalized joint laxity, or joint line pain should raise concern for internal derangement. Marked apprehension with lateral deviation of the patella suggests patellar instability, and specialty evaluation may be warranted.

Back Pain

Synonyms

Axial back pain

Backache

Low back pain

Lumbar strain

Lumbar syndrome

ICD-9 Codes

724.1
Pain in thoracic spine

724.2
Lumbago

724.5
Backache, unspecified

Definition

The prevalence of back pain in the pediatric population varies from 5% to 75% and increases with age; by 18 years of age, the prevalence mirrors that of adults. In the past, it was believed that an extensive evaluation was required for most pediatric patients with back pain. Although it is true that back pain in infants and young children is likely to be the result of a specific etiology and requires a more extensive evaluation in most cases, in older children and adolescents the likelihood of establishing a diagnosis is much lower, similar to that in the adult population. Two recent studies suggested that a definitive anatomic diagnosis was established in only 22% to 36% of older children and adolescents. All pediatric patients with back pain require a detailed history and physical examination, but the need for additional diagnostic tests (laboratory studies and advanced imaging) depends on the clinical findings and the age of the patient.

Clinical Symptoms

The nature of onset, as well as the location, character, and radiation of the pain, should be determined. Back pain that occurs during or following physical activity and is relieved by rest suggests a mechanical cause. Back pain accompanied by neurologic signs and symptoms (eg, radicular pain, muscle weakness, gait abnormalities, sensory changes, and bowel and bladder dysfunction) or systemic symptoms (eg, fever, malaise, and weight loss) suggests an organic cause. Night pain often signals a more serious problem such as neoplasm.

Tests

Physical Examination

A comprehensive physical examination includes the spine, the nervous system, and other sources of referred pain such as the abdomen or pelvis. In adolescent females, a gynecologic

SECTION 9 PEDIATRIC ORTHOPAEDICS

examination may be helpful if a diagnosis has not been established, as an ovarian cyst, endometriosis, or other diagnoses may present with pain referred to the back. Examine the spine with special emphasis on identifying any alterations in alignment or deformities, loss of motion, paraspinal muscle spasm, and areas of tenderness. Provocative tests also are important; for example, spinal hyperextension loads the posterior elements in compression (spondylolysis), and the spinal flexion loads the anterior column in compression (diskitis, compression fracture). The straight-leg raising test (and reverse straight-leg raising test) are provocative tests for lumbar nerve root compression or stretch. The neurologic assessment includes motor and sensory function, deep tendon reflexes, and pathologic reflexes (Babinski sign or clonus). The superficial abdominal reflex is tested by lightly stroking the skin in a diagonal direction toward the umbilicus. A normal reflex is deviation of the umbilicus toward the side of the test in all four quadrants. Asymmetric abdominal reflexes may be the only finding in a child with syringomyelia or other spinal cord pathology; however, this reflex may be absent or asymmetric in healthy children. Neurologic deficits may develop as a late manifestation of a tumor or other pathology; thus, a normal neurologic examination does not rule out serious problems in the early stages of disease.

Diagnostic Tests

The extent of the evaluation depends on the duration and degree of symptoms as well as the results of the physical examination. No laboratory or radiographic studies are necessary if the examination is normal and symptoms are mild and of limited duration.

For symptoms in the thoracic and lumbar regions, weight-bearing PA and lateral radiographs of the entire spine are the initial study of choice. Oblique views of the lumbar spine are considered when spondylolysis is in the differential diagnosis. AP, lateral, oblique, and open-mouth odontoid views of the cervical spine are indicated for patients with neck pain; these may be supplemented by lateral radiographs in flexion and extension to rule out instability.

The need for additional imaging studies (eg, bone scan, MRI, CT) depends on the suspected etiology. The need for and sequencing of these tests depends on the differential diagnosis. Laboratory studies are considered in many cases, especially when systemic signs or symptoms are present, and may include a complete blood count with differential, erythrocyte sedimentation rate, and C-reactive protein level. Other tests to consider are rheumatoid factor, Lyme titer, antinuclear antibody, and human leukocyte antigen B27 (HLA-B27).

Differential Diagnosis

The differential diagnosis of back pain in children is shown in **Table 1**. Muscle strain is the most common cause of thoracic and lumbar pain in children. Scheuermann kyphosis may present with pain in the thoracic and thoracolumbar regions, and spondylolysis and spondylolisthesis are common causes of pain in the lumbar and lumbosacral regions. Idiopathic scoliosis rarely causes pain in children, but scoliosis associated with syringomyelia, tethered spinal cord, or neoplasms may present as back pain.

Adverse Outcomes of the Disease

When back pain has an organic cause, failure to diagnose may result in progression of the condition. In certain conditions, such as instability of the upper cervical spine, tumors, or infections, failure to diagnose may result in spinal cord or peripheral nerve dysfunction.

Treatment

Treatment of back pain in children is specific to the diagnosis. Because of the extensive differential diagnosis for back pain, it is not possible to discuss all aspects of treatment here. For mild mechanical or activity-related discomfort, in the absence of worrisome signs or symptoms, observation with activity modifications and mild analgesics is appropriate initially. More extensive studies are necessary if the pain does not improve within 4 to 6 weeks, if the pain becomes worse, or if new symptoms and abnormal physical findings develop.

Adverse Outcomes of Treatment

Adverse outcomes of treatment also are specific to the diagnosis. The principal adverse outcome is lack of improvement or worsening of symptoms despite treatment.

Referral Decisions/Red Flags

The following factors suggest a treatable underlying etiology: (1) persistent or increasing pain; (2) night pain; (3) pain accompanied by systemic symptoms such as fever, malaise, or weight loss; (4) neurologic symptoms or findings; (5) bowel or bladder dysfunction; (6) onset of symptoms at a young age; and (7) a painful thoracic scoliosis. A more extensive evaluation is necessary in such cases.

SECTION 9 PEDIATRIC ORTHOPAEDICS

Table 1 Differential Diagnosis of Back Pain in Children

Etiology	Condition
Congenital	Intraspinal anomalies (tethered cord, diastematomyelia)
	Upper cervical spine instability
Developmental	Kyphosis (Scheuermann disease)
	Syringomyelia
	Spondylolisthesis
Injuries (acute or repetitive trauma)	Muscle strain
	Occult fractures
	Pathologic fractures (compression fractures)
	Spondylolysis
	Herniated disk or slipped vertebral apophysis
Infectious	Pyogenic (diskitis or vertebral osteomyelitis)
	Granulomatous (tuberculosis, brucellosis)
	Epidural abscess
	Pyelonephritis
	Pancreatitis
Systemic	Chronic infection
	Storage diseases
	Juvenile osteoporosis
Inflammatory disease	Ankylosing spondylitis
	Juvenile idiopathic arthritis
	Psoriatic arthritis
	Reiter syndrome
Neoplastic	
Benign	Osteoid osteoma
	Osteoblastoma
	Aneurysmal bone cyst
	Langerhan cell histiocytosis
	Ganglioneuroma
Malignant	Spinal cord tumor
	Leukemia
	Lymphoma
	Neuroblastoma
	Osteogenic sarcoma
	Metastatic disease
Psychogenic	

SECTION 9 PEDIATRIC ORTHOPAEDICS

Elbow Pain

Synonyms

Little League elbow

Overuse injury of the elbow

ICD-9 Code

719.42
Pain in joint, upper arm

Definition

Elbow pain in children most often is caused by acute or chronic injury to bone or soft tissues. Excessive throwing and the subsequent valgus stress cause most chronic elbow pain in children. The principal focus of this chapter is soft-tissue injuries. Fractures are discussed in other chapters.

Clinical Symptoms

Patients with acute conditions report pain, tenderness, swelling, and most often a history of falling on an outstretched arm. For those with chronic pain, activity-related aching pain at the involved area is common.

Tests

Physical Examination

For patients with acute conditions, evaluate the status of the median, ulnar, and radial nerves distal to the injury. Assess radial and ulnar pulses as well. With obvious deformity, position or splint for comfort and proceed with radiographs. When examining children with no obvious elbow deformity, attempt to find the site of maximum tenderness and perform a gentle evaluation of elbow motion.

For children with chronic pain, assess the point of maximum tenderness. Mild swelling and limited motion may be present. Palpate for a mass to exclude an atypical tumor. Palpate the ulnar nerve while moving the elbow to rule out a subluxating ulnar nerve.

Diagnostic Tests

AP and lateral radiographs of the elbow should be obtained for all acute injuries; additional views may better visualize medial and lateral epicondyle fractures or radial head and neck fractures. A fracture or dislocation may be obvious or subtle. The radial head should be directed toward the capitellum on all views. Comparison views are helpful with subtle injuries.

With chronic pain, AP and lateral radiographs may be normal or may show an avulsion fracture, fragmentation and heterotopic ossification of the medial epicondyle (Little League elbow), or fragmentation and irregularity of the capitellum.

Hemarthrosis

An elbow hemarthrosis is a diagnosis of exclusion. Examination demonstrates swelling of the joint, and radiographs typically show a posterior fat pad sign. Aspiration of the joint is diagnostic and may decrease discomfort in highly symptomatic cases.

Sprains

Elbow sprains are uncommon in children because the bone is the weak link. Short-term immobilization is appropriate.

Subluxation of the Radial Head

Also called a "pulled elbow" or "nursemaid's elbow," this is the most common elbow injury in children younger than 5 years. This injury is associated with increased ligamentous laxity. The mechanism of injury is pulling on the forearm when the elbow is extended and the forearm is pronated. The annular ligament, which wraps around the neck of the radius, slips proximally and becomes interposed between the radius and ulna.

Immediately after the injury, the child will react and cry, but the initial pain quickly subsides. Thereafter, the child is reluctant to use the arm but otherwise does not appear to be in great distress. The extremity is held by the side with the elbow slightly flexed and the forearm pronated. Tenderness over the radial head and resistance on attempted supination of the forearm are the only consistent findings. Radiographs are normal.

To reduce the subluxation, place your thumb over the radial head and fully supinate the forearm. If this maneuver fails to produce the snap of reduction, then flex the elbow. Resistance may be perceived just before reaching full flexion. As the elbow is pushed through that resistance, the annular ligament will slip back into normal position and a snap may be perceived as the radial head reduces. Pronation of the forearm with elbow extension or flexion has been proposed as an alternative reduction strategy. If the reduction is successful, the child will begin to use the extremity normally in a few minutes. The exception is the child who presents 1 to 2 days after injury. At this time, swelling of the annular ligament may both obscure the snap that signals a successful reduction and also prevent immediate resumption of normal function. If the elbow has full flexion and supination, however, the radial head has been reduced. Immobilization may be used but is probably not necessary, as parents report that slings are quickly discarded, except when discomfort persists. If reduction attempts are unsuccessful, splinting or casting is appropriate. Repeat evaluation, with radiographs, may reveal an occult fracture, or the child may have normal radiographs and return to full function once immobilization is discontinued. Failure of function to return warrants further investigation.

Infection

Infection (septic arthritis) as a cause of acute elbow pain is relatively uncommon; in one study of pediatric infections, the elbow accounted for only 12% of cases of septic arthritis. These conditions, however, should be considered when evaluating a child with elbow pain. The possibility of infection is more likely with an acute onset of pain, no history of injury, and an elevated temperature.

Chronic Pain

These injuries may affect either the medial (tension) or lateral (compression) side of the humerus. Medial injuries can be acute (avulsion fracture of the medial epicondyle) or gradual in onset (traction apophysitis of the medial epicondyle, better known as Little League elbow) (**Figure 3**). Lateral involvement is secondary to osteonecrosis of the capitellum. When children younger than 10 years are affected, the condition is called Panner disease and has a good prognosis.

Chronic injuries generally are self-limited. Resting the arm, with no throwing for 3 to 6 weeks, is indicated followed by rehabilitation to restore elbow motion and upper extremity strength. Osteonecrosis of the capitellum in adolescents, called osteochondritis dissecans, has a more guarded prognosis (**Figure 4**). This condition can result in an osteochondral loose body, which may cause a locking or catching sensation, and is more likely to cause residual symptoms. Surgical treatment should be considered. Surgical removal of loose bodies secondary to osteochondritis dissecans, along with débridement, is indicated if the loose bodies are causing pain and/or intermittent locking of the joint.

Tumors, although very uncommon about the elbow in children, are more likely with chronic pain, no history of injury, pain at rest, night pain, and pain that is getting worse.

Referral Decisions/Red Flags

Patients with pain that is constant or increasing, systemic signs or symptoms (fever, other pains), history of trauma, or chronic pain require further evaluation.

Figure 3 The throwing motion imposes valgus stress on the elbow.

Figure 4 AP radiograph demonstrates radiolucency typical of osteochondritis dissecans of the capitellum (arrow). (Reproduced with permission from Peterson RK, Savoie FH III, Field LD: Osteochondritis dissecans of the elbow. *Instr Course Lect* 1999;48: 393-398.)

SECTION 9 PEDIATRIC ORTHOPAEDICS

Foot and Ankle Pain

Definition

Foot and ankle pain in a child generally is caused by specific clinical conditions; however, trauma, infection, and tumors are other potential causes.

Clinical Symptoms

A history of a significant injury combined with localized findings may suggest some type of trauma. Children have numerous minor injuries to the lower extremities, however, and parents might attribute symptoms to a particular injury or episode when, in fact, the actual condition has nothing to do with trauma. Furthermore, injuries in younger children may occur without being observed by the parents or others, and young children are typically unable to give an exact account of how the injury occurred.

Determining whether the problem is acute or chronic provides information about its etiology. A recent onset of symptoms generally is associated with traumatic or infectious conditions.

Questions about systemic symptoms such as malaise, swelling, and fever are important with either acute-onset conditions or chronic symptoms. Fever and swelling are more likely to suggest infectious or possibly malignant conditions.

Tests

Physical Examination

Infections in the foot may have a history of direct penetrating injuries such as a nail puncture wound. If the incident occurred within the preceding 24 to 72 hours, the diagnosis is most likely a soft-tissue cellulitis or abscess.

Physical examination may localize the area of tenderness to a specific anatomic site. This step is extremely helpful in arriving at the correct diagnosis. Ask an older child to point with one finger to the spot that hurts the most, which helps localize the anatomic site and greatly narrows the differential diagnosis.

The foot should be examined for areas of swelling, erythema, or ecchymosis. Whereas ecchymosis is generally a sign of traumatic injury, erythema suggests an inflammatory or infectious process. The ankle and subtalar joints should be evaluated for range of motion and tenderness on range of motion. Decreased inversion and eversion of the subtalar joint can suggest a tarsal coalition; painful range of motion of the joint can indicate an inflammatory or infectious process. Ligamentous stability should be evaluated as well.

Diagnostic Tests

Radiographs are needed when a fracture or chronic process is suspected. Physical examination will determine whether the problem is in the foot or ankle. If the problem is localized to the foot, AP, lateral, and oblique views of the foot are taken. AP, lateral, and mortise views of the ankle are ordered if the ankle is the area of concern. If findings on radiographs could be a normal variant, comparison views of the opposite foot can be taken.

Advanced imaging studies are sometimes necessary. A bone scan can be helpful if a stress fracture or infectious process is suspected. CT is generally best for benign bony lesions; MRI provides better information for soft-tissue lesions and malignant processes.

Differential Diagnosis

Hindfoot

Calcaneal Apophysitis (Sever disease)

Calcaneal apophysitis is characterized by pain in the posterior aspect of the heel that occurs after play and sports activities and most commonly affects active, prepubertal children. Tenderness at the posterior aspect of the calcaneus is common. Radiographs typically are not needed. Short-term activity modification or restriction is indicated. Detailed information about calcaneal apophysitis is provided on page 1015.

Os Trigonum

The os trigonum is an accessory ossicle of the posterior talus that usually is a normal anatomic variant. This secondary center of ossification, however, may become symptomatic in older adolescents and adults, particularly those who participate in ballet or soccer. Patients commonly report posterior ankle pain that is activity related. Pain also develops secondary to posterior impingement of the os trigonum between the talus and tibia during plantar flexion. Relative rest and activity modification may relieve symptoms, although surgical excision may be required for refractory cases.

Osteochondral Lesion of the Talus

This lesion typically affects adolescents, particularly athletes. The pain is exacerbated by activity and is localized to the ankle region. Radiographs of the ankle usually confirm diagnosis, although MRI may be necessary in some cases. Osteochondritis dissecans of the talus may result in ankle pain with activity,

SECTION 9 PEDIATRIC ORTHOPAEDICS

Figure 1 Oblique radiograph demonstrates calcaneonavicular coalition.

Figure 2 Lateral radiograph of the foot shows a condensed, fragmented navicular (arrowhead). (Reproduced from Kasser JR, ed: *Orthopaedic Knowledge Update*, ed 5. Rosemont, IL, American Academy of Orthopaedic Surgeons, 1996, pp 503-514.)

swelling, and locking of the ankle joint. Treatment includes immobilization or sometimes surgery, depending on the size, location, and degree of displacement. Detailed information about osteochondral lesions of the talus is provided on page 1142.

Tarsal Coalition

Tarsal coalition is a common cause of rigid flatfeet in children (**Figure 1**). Symptoms typically develop during the second decade of life. The onset of pain generally is insidious but can be associated with an injury or change in activity or perceived as recurrent ankle sprains. Hindfoot motion is markedly restricted, and spasm of the peroneal muscles is elicited by quickly inverting the foot. Talocalcaneal bars are difficult to see on routine radiographs; CT is necessary to confirm the diagnosis. Treatment depends on the presentation of symptoms. Detailed information about tarsal coalition is provided on page 1188.

Midfoot

Osteonecrosis of the Navicular

This condition, also called Köhler disease, primarily affects children (usually boys) 4 to 8 years of age. The patient limps, turns out the foot while walking, and may report pain and prominence in the medial arch. Radiographs show a dense, fragmented, thin navicular (**Figure 2**). A short leg walking cast for 4 to 8 weeks relieves pain, improves walking (less pain), and may speed resolution of the osteonecrosis. The eventual outcome, however, is good whether casting or activity modifications are chosen.

Accessory Navicular

Accessory navicular is an anatomic variant in which a secondary center of ossification forms at the medial aspect of the navicular and may become symptomatic during adolescence. Patients report pain and swelling on the medial side of the foot. Activity or shoe wear may exacerbate the pain. Radiographs may be necessary, depending on the presentation and history of symptoms. Treatment generally is limited to short-term activity restrictions or shoe modifications; however, a walking cast or surgical excision may be necessary. Detailed information about accessory navicular is provided on page 1013.

Forefoot

Freiberg Infraction

Freiberg infraction is osteonecrosis that most commonly involves the head of the second metatarsal, most likely as a result of trauma, and typically affects adolescents. The pain is exacerbated by activity. Examination reveals tenderness under the involved metatarsal head, sometimes swelling on the dorsal aspect of the metatarsal head, and pain at the extremes of dorsiflexion and plantar flexion. Radiographs usually show evidence of the condition within 2 to 3 weeks of the onset of symptoms (**Figure 3**). Treatment options include activity modifications, a metatarsal pad, or short-term casting. Occasionally, surgical treatment is required to remove loose bodies or to realign the metatarsal head.

Hallux Valgus

Hallux valgus may develop during adolescence. At this age, most patients are asymptomatic, but some may report pain. Asymptomatic cases are treated with a night brace, otherwise, treatment principles are similar to those for adults. Detailed information about hallux valgus is provided on page 819.

Other Foot Problems

Enthesitis

Enthesitis (pain and inflammation at a bone-tendon insertion) is uncommon in children. Disorders such as Achilles tendinitis or plantar fasciitis may be the presenting symptoms of a seronegative spondyloarthropathy.

Infection

Infection in the foot commonly is secondary to a direct penetrating injury, such as a nail puncture wound. If symptoms develop within 24 to 72 hours after the injury, cellulitis or abscess usually is secondary to a *Staphylococcus aureus* infection. If swelling and erythema develop several days after the injury, the infection may be septic arthritis or osteomyelitis secondary to *Pseudomonas aeruginosa*; this requires surgical débridement and IV antibiotic therapy.

Sprains, Strains, and Fractures

Sprains, strains, and fractures of the foot and ankle occur but are relatively uncommon until late adolescence. Most of these injuries in children can be managed by nonsurgical modalities. In a child who has a history of an inversion injury and tenderness over the distal fibular physis, the most likely diagnosis is a nondisplaced type I fracture of the distal fibular physis. This injury is treated with a short leg cast.

Tumors

Tumors in the foot and ankle are uncommon at all ages. The most common benign bone tumor of the foot and ankle in children is a unicameral or aneurysmal bone cyst involving the calcaneus. Osteoid osteoma affecting the tarsal bones also occurs in children. Ewing sarcoma affecting the tarsal bones or diaphysis of metatarsals is the most common malignant bony lesion involving the foot. The pain, swelling, and radiographic

Figure 3 Radiograph demonstrates Freiberg infraction. Note flattening and fragmentation at the head of the second metatarsal (arrow).

SECTION 9 PEDIATRIC ORTHOPAEDICS

findings in this tumor may mimic osteomyelitis. Of the malignant soft-tissue lesions, synovial cell sarcoma is most common in the foot. Typical symptoms include onset during the second decade of life and a slowly enlarging mass.

Growing Pain

Definition

Growing pain is a condition for which there is no specific diagnosis. Typically, it is a diagnosis made after more specific pathologic conditions are excluded. Although its true etiology is unknown, growing pain or leg aches are often thought to be the result of overactivity (muscular strain or fatigue). The condition typically occurs in an otherwise healthy, active child. Growing pain is more common in boys, in children with ligamentous laxity, and in 2- to 5-year-old children. Older children, however, also may be affected. The pain or discomfort is commonly localized to the calf but may be perceived in the foot, ankle, knee, or thigh. The problem often is bilateral, but the patients may report that one leg seems to hurt more than the other or that one leg hurts some nights and the other leg hurts other nights.

ICD-9 Code
719.46
Arthralgia, lower leg
729.5
Pain in limb

Clinical Symptoms

Leg pain is described as mild to moderate, intermittent, and more noticeable in the evening or at night or following a day of increased activity or sport. Most children do not limp during the day. Parents report using warm or cold compresses, massage, or simple analgesics to relieve the symptoms. Constitutional symptoms such as fever, weight loss, loss of appetite, or malaise rarely are reported.

Tests

Physical Examination

Examination of the affected extremity should focus on identifying any masses, inflammation, lymphadenopathy, abnormal joint movement, instability, muscle group atrophy, or neurologic deficits. With growing pain, the examination is normal in all aspects, although the affected extremity can be tender to deep pressure. Flexible flatfeet may be noted, but the gait and pattern of shoe wear is normal.

Diagnostic Tests

Radiographs should be considered in children who have a higher intensity of pain or more prolonged symptoms, a history of pain at rest that is not relieved by simple analgesics, or an associated finding. Bone scan, CT, or MRI is considered if a specific lesion, such as a bone or soft-tissue tumor, stress fracture, bone or joint infection, or tarsal coalition, is suspected. Metabolic workup may be needed if the history and review of systems suggest conditions such as leukemia or endocrinopathy.

Differential Diagnosis

- Calcaneal apophysitis (heel pain with activity)
- Köhler disease (unilateral, pain with activity, foot turned out with walking)
- Metabolic/systemic disease (history and review of systems suggestive of leukemia, endocrine disorder, renal osteodystrophy, juvenile idiopathic arthritis, rheumatic disease)
- Subacute osteomyelitis (unilateral, activity-related symptoms)
- Trauma (unilateral, toddler's or stress fracture)
- Tumor (unilateral, pain more persistent and severe)

Adverse Outcomes of the Disease

Growing pain has a benign and self-limiting course, although the leg aches may occur intermittently for several months. Permanent long-term impairment has not been noted.

Treatment

An explanation of the natural history and expected outcome, reassurance, muscle stretches, and perhaps a recommendation about use of simple analgesics usually are sufficient to allay parental fears and to avoid overtreatment. Short-term use of NSAIDs and/or a short period of rest or immobilization before resuming activities, as the level of pain allows, also can be recommended. Surgical treatment is not indicated.

Adverse Outcomes of Treatment

Overuse of pain medication with subsequent psychologic aspects is possible. Unnecessary testing with its concomitant risk and costs also is possible.

Referral Decisions/Red Flags

Patients with a history of severe, persistent pain along with constitutional symptoms (eg, fever, night sweats, malaise, poor appetite, weight loss) require further evaluation. Findings on physical examination that indicate masses, significant inflammation, lymphadenopathy, circulatory compromise, neuropathy, or myopathy also are a concern. To make a diagnosis of growing pain or leg aches while overlooking the more specific underlying conditions listed in the differential diagnosis is a serious error.

Accessory Navicular

Definition

Accessory navicular is an anatomic variant in which a secondary center of ossification forms in the medial portion of the tarsal navicular bone at the attachment of the posterior tibialis tendon. During adolescence, this may become prominent and symptomatic by virtue of its size or as a result of repetitive sprains and microfractures at the attachment of the ossicle to the navicular. Symptoms are more common in girls. The disorder is common, with one study observing a 14% incidence of symptoms during adolescence.

ICD-9 Code

732.5
Juvenile osteochondrosis of
foot

Clinical Symptoms

Patients report pain and swelling on the medial side (arch) of the foot. The pain is exacerbated with activity or with pressure from overlying shoes. Severe pain is uncommon.

Tests

Physical Examination

Tenderness and mild swelling over the medial aspect of the navicular (insertion of the posterior tibialis tendon) is typical. Inversion of the foot against resistance may be painful. A flexible pes planus may be present.

Diagnostic Tests

Radiographs are not necessary with a typical examination and mild symptoms. With persistent or severe symptoms, AP, lateral, and oblique radiographs of the foot will document the disorder and exclude other possibilities. The AP and lateral views should be weight bearing to best demonstrate pes planus or other alignment problems. The AP view often provides the best profile of the accessory ossicle (**Figure 1**). Some patients have a cornuated navicular (shaped like a horn of plenty), resulting from fusion of the accessory ossicle to the navicular.

Differential Diagnosis

- Flexible pes planovalgus (developmental or acquired)
- Posterior tibial tendinitis (swelling in the region of the posterior tibial tendon)
- Tarsal coalition (restricted inversion, eversion of the heel)

Figure 1 AP radiograph of the foot demonstrates accessory navicular (arrow).

Adverse Outcomes of the Disease

Patients may experience persistent pain or a limp.

Treatment

Most patients can be treated with short-term restriction of activities and/or shoe modifications to relieve pressure over the prominent navicular (soft material medial to the bump and/or stretching of the shoe). A short period of time in a walking cast may permit healing of the repetitive microfractures and resolution of symptoms. In most cases, the bump is not large and symptoms resolve with cessation of growth. Excision of the prominent portion of the navicular is the treatment of choice for patients with persistent, disabling symptoms.

Adverse Outcomes of Treatment

Postoperative infection and a tender medial scar that is irritated by shoe wear are both possible.

Referral Decisions/Red Flags

Persistent pain signals the need for further evaluation.

Calcaneal Apophysitis

Synonym

Sever disease

ICD-9 Code

732.5
Juvenile osteochondrosis of
foot

Definition

Calcaneal apophysitis commonly affects active, prepubertal children and is characterized by pain in the posterior aspect of the heel that occurs after play and sports activities. This condition is caused by repetitive stress and microtrauma on the calcaneal apophysis. This weak link resolves when the apophysis fuses to the main body of the calcaneus, a process that occurs around 9 years of age in girls and 11 years of age in boys.

Clinical Symptoms

Patients have posterior heel pain and a limp that is activity related.

Tests

Physical Examination

Examination reveals tenderness at the posterior aspect of the calcaneus.

Diagnostic Tests

Radiographs are not diagnostic, and sclerosis at the secondary ossification center is common and normal (**Figure 1**). With bilateral involvement and a typical history, radiographs probably are not necessary. With unilateral involvement, a lateral view of the heel is necessary to rule out other problems, such as a unicameral bone cyst.

Differential Diagnosis

- Achilles tendinitis (can be associated with Reiter syndrome or other seronegative spondyloarthropathies)
- Infection (unilateral, elevated erythrocyte sedimentation rate, swelling)
- Tumor (unilateral, swelling, night pain)

Adverse Outcomes of the Disease

Pain, a limp, and activity modifications are possible, but there are no long-term sequelae.

SECTION 9 PEDIATRIC ORTHOPAEDICS

Figure 1 Radiograph of the feet reveals irregular calcaneal apophyses (arrows). This is a normal finding. No radiographic findings exist that are diagnostic for or consistent with calcaneal apophysitis (Sever disease).

Treatment

Treatment includes short-term modification or restriction of the precipitating activity. Shoe modifications that use a ¼″ heel lift or heel cushion and rehabilitation with Achilles tendon stretching can be helpful. Casting is needed only rarely but can be used for 4 to 6 weeks if the pain and limp are recalcitrant. Neither surgery nor steroid injection is indicated.

Adverse Outcomes of Treatment

There are no long-term sequelae.

Referral Decisions/Red Flags

Suspicion of tumor or osteomyelitis indicates the need for further evaluation. When treatment does not relieve discomfort, additional diagnostic studies are indicated to rule out infection or neoplastic disease.

Cavus Foot Deformity

Synonyms

High-arched foot

Pes cavus

ICD-9 Codes

736.73
Cavus deformity of foot

736.75
Cavovarus deformity of foot, acquired

754.59
Varus deformities of feet, other (talipes cavovarus)

Definition

Pes cavus is the term used to describe an abnormally high arch resulting from plantar flexion (equinus) of the forefoot or midfoot relative to the hindfoot. Cavovarus describes forefoot equinus in association with hindfoot varus (**Figure 1**), and equinocavovarus describes hindfoot equinus associated with hindfoot varus and forefoot equinus.

Some cases of bilateral cavus or cavovarus feet are familial, but most children with these deformities have an underlying neurologic abnormality or neuromuscular disorder. For example, a progressive unilateral cavus foot often is due to tethering of the spinal cord, and bilateral cavus feet are commonly seen in hereditary motor and sensory neuropathies such as Charcot-Marie-Tooth disease.

Figure 1   Clinical photographs demonstrating cavovarus foot include **A,** High arch typical of a cavovarus foot. **B,** The hindfoot is tilted into varus. **C,** Clawing of the toes is common.

SECTION 9   PEDIATRIC ORTHOPAEDICS

Clinical Symptoms

Progressive deformities may be associated with a number of symptoms, including problems with shoe wear, pain in the region of the metatarsal heads or forefoot (altered weight-bearing stresses) or in the region of the plantar fascia, and frequent ankle sprains. Calluses may develop underneath the prominent metatarsal heads or along the lateral border of the foot.

Tests

History and Physical Examination

The history focuses on any symptoms, whether the changes in foot shape or alignment have been progressive, and whether any associated symptoms exist (back or leg pain, bowel or bladder dysfunction). Family members should be questioned regarding a family history of similar foot deformities or neuromuscular diseases. A thorough neurologic assessment is always required. With regard to the musculoskeletal examination, inspect the lower extremity to evaluate the alignment of the ankle, heel, midfoot, and toes, and check the plantar aspect of the foot for calluses. Examine the spine for curvatures, paraspinal spasm, and midline defects such as dimpling or abnormal hairy patches. Examine the upper extremity for weakness and atrophy of the intrinsic muscles of the hand.

Diagnostic Tests

Weight-bearing AP and lateral radiographs of the foot are obtained to evaluate alignment. On the lateral view of a normal foot, a line typically passes through the axis of the talus and first metatarsal. With a cavus foot, the first metatarsal is plantar flexed relative to the talus, resulting in an increase in the angle between the axes of the talus and the first metatarsal (Meary angle) (**Figure 2**). Weight-bearing PA and lateral radiographs of the thoracolumbar spine should be considered; these may reveal abnormal curvatures, congenital anomalies, widening of the interpedicular distance (suggests diastematomyelia), or other abnormalities. Depending on the clinical findings, other diagnostic studies may be required, including electromyography, nerve conduction velocity studies, and an MRI of the spine.

Differential Diagnosis

- Clubfoot (incomplete correction)
- Friedreich ataxia (gait abnormalities, autosomal recessive)
- Hereditary motor and sensory neuropathies (Charcot-Marie-Tooth disease) (peripheral neuropathy with abnormal nerve conduction velocity studies, autosomal dominant most common)

Figure 2 Lateral radiographs of cavus feet. **A,** Foot with a positive (25°) Meary angle caused by cavus foot and associated forefoot equinus. In a normal foot, a line drawn through the long axis of the talus would go through the first metatarsal. **B,** Foot of a patient with a more severe deformity (Meary angle = 50°). Note the claw toes (arrow) and the hypertrophy of the cortices of the fifth metatarsal (arrowhead) resulting from excessive lateral forefoot weight bearing.

- Idiopathic (familial, a diagnosis of exclusion)
- Muscular dystrophy (previous diagnosis)
- Myelomeningocele (previous diagnosis)
- Neuromuscular conditions
- Poliomyelitis (previous diagnosis)
- Spinal cord tethering lesions (low-lying conus medullaris, spinal cord tumor, diastematomyelia, lipomyelomeningocele, other intraspinal anomalies)
- Trauma (residua of tendon laceration or fracture)

Adverse Outcomes of the Disease

Cavus deformities are often progressive and interfere with shoe wear and ambulation.

Treatment

Underlying neurologic or spinal cord pathology requires evaluation and possible surgical treatment—for example, release of a tethered spinal cord. The treatment of a cavus or cavovarus foot is based on the severity and flexibility of the deformity, as well as whether the deformity is expected to worsen (on the basis of the underlying diagnosis). Mild and flexible deformities can be accommodated by shoe modifications and arch supports, and rehabilitation can help with strengthening muscles and maintaining range of motion. An ankle-foot orthosis may be required to control the hindfoot and maintain ambulation. Surgical treatment is offered when these measures fail to accomodate the deformity and the symptoms are unacceptable to the patient. A variety of procedures, alone or in combination, may be required to restore range of motion and foot alignment, as well as muscle balance. These include soft-tissue releases (plantar fascia), tendon transfers (tibialis posterior and/or extensor hallucis longus), and osteotomies (medial cuneiform or first metatarsal, calcaneus) to realign the forefoot and often the hindfoot. A hindfoot fusion (triple arthrodesis) is reserved as a salvage procedure for rigid deformities in older patients.

Adverse Outcomes of Treatment

Most of these deformities occur in patients with progressive neuromuscular diseases, so recurrence or gradual progression of the foot deformity often is encountered even after surgical treatment. Additional treatment measures (surgery and/or bracing) may be required to maximize ambulatory potential. If a triple arthrodesis was required to achieve correction, increased stresses at the ankle and midfoot joints may result in degenerative changes in ambulatory patients.

Referral Decisions/Red Flags

All patients with cavus feet should be referred for further evaluation.

Child Abuse

Synonyms

Munchausen syndrome by proxy
Nonaccidental trauma
Shaken baby syndrome

ICD-9 Codes

995.50
Child abuse, unspecified

995.59
Other child abuse and neglect

Definition

Approximately 2.4 million reports of child abuse are filed annually in the United States, and 4,000 children die every year as a result of abuse or neglect. Most cases of abuse involve children younger than 3 years. Firstborn children, premature infants, stepchildren, and handicapped children are at a greater risk. Failure to recognize injuries of child abuse results in a child being returned to the environment, with a 25% risk of serious reinjury and a 5% risk of death.

A critical factor in identifying child abuse is to accurately determine whether the history given by the family adequately explains the child's injuries. Soft-tissue injuries such as bruises, burns, or scars are seen in most patients. It is normal for toddlers to have bruises over the chin, the brow, elbows, knees, and shins, but bruises on the back of the head, buttocks, abdomen, legs, arms, cheeks, or genitalia are suspicious for abuse. Fractures are common in child abuse cases, and these children are more likely to have additional injuries, including abdominal injury resulting from blunt trauma.

The Investigative Interview

The guiding principle for the conduct of the interview is to remain objective while calmly and methodically questioning family members. A single physical finding is seldom conclusive for a diagnosis of child abuse; additional injuries and risk factors in the home must be identified. Other guidelines for the investigative interview are listed in **Table 1**.

When obtaining the social history, inquire about unusual stresses on the family, such as recent loss of a job, separation or divorce, death in the family, housing problems, or inadequate funds for food. Alcohol abuse in the home is a risk factor for child abuse, and maternal cocaine use increases the risk of abuse fivefold.

If family members later change their account of how the injury occurred or any other aspect of the history, do not alter the original account, but date and record the revision as an addendum to the record.

SECTION 9 PEDIATRIC ORTHOPAEDICS

Table 1 Guidelines for Conducting an Investigative Interview

Interview individual family members in private.

Be attentive and nonjudgmental, and avoid leading questions during the history.

Carefully document the given history of injury verbatim, as well as its source.

Establish a scenario for the injury from each witness, noting carefully any inconsistencies.

Identify the person primarily responsible for feeding and disciplining the child.

Identify all family members and other individuals who have access to the child.

Identify individuals outside the family who have been with the child without family supervision.

Assess for risk factors: boyfriends, stepparents, babysitters, and even older siblings, as these individuals are often abusers.

Note any delay in seeking medical attention for injuries.

Tests

Physical Examination

Conduct a head-to-toe physical examination to evaluate the child for any suspicious soft-tissue injuries. A thorough examination is important because in many cases of confirmed abuse, evidence of prior abuse will be identified. Note in detail any suspicious soft-tissue injuries. Palpate the face, spine, and upper and lower extremities for tenderness suggestive of fracture. Examine the abdomen for swelling and tenderness. Inspect for physical signs of sexual assault such as bruising or chafing of the genitalia. Physical findings of sexual abuse may be subtle. A pediatric physician specializing in child abuse/sexual abuse may best be able to examine the child at this time.

Diagnostic Tests

If the child's mental status is abnormal, evaluate for subdural hematoma and retinal hemorrhage secondary to violent shaking. Check bleeding studies when there is bruising, and order a toxicology screening if there is a history of substance abuse or a mental status change in the family. CT of the abdomen is indicated if the head-to-toe examination shows abdominal tenderness or if liver function test levels are elevated.

AP and lateral radiographs of all long bones, the hands, the feet, the spine, and the chest, as well as a skull series, are standard. A single radiograph, or so-called baby gram, may not provide adequate detail and may miss subtle fractures. No fracture pattern predominates in child abuse, but certain fractures are more suspicious for child abuse than others. Fractures considered highly specific for child abuse include posterior rib fractures, scapular fractures, fractures of the posterior process of the spine, and fractures of the sternum.

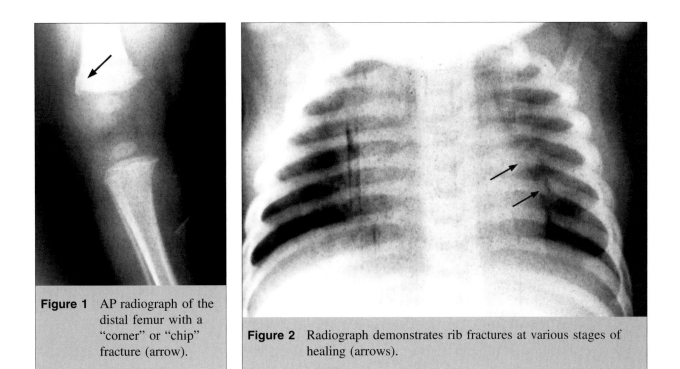

Figure 1 AP radiograph of the distal femur with a "corner" or "chip" fracture (arrow).

Figure 2 Radiograph demonstrates rib fractures at various stages of healing (arrows).

Also, one type of fracture unique to child abuse is the "corner" or "chip" fracture of the metaphysis of long bones that avulses the edge of the metaphysis from the epiphysis as a result of downward traction or pull on the extremity (**Figure 1**). Other fracture patterns are more common but also occur frequently in accidental injuries; inconsistency with the mechanism described by the caregiver should raise suspicion. Spiral fractures are caused by rotational injury, and transverse or oblique fractures are caused by a direct blow. Rib fractures also are common and, when healed, may appear only as fusiform thickening of the ribs. A bone scan may be helpful in detecting rib fractures, but it may not show skull fractures or long-bone fractures near the epiphyseal growth plates.

Fractures considered to be of moderate specificity for abuse include multiple, especially bilateral, fractures; fractures of different ages; epiphyseal separations; vertebral body fractures; fractures of the fingers; and complex skull fractures. Multiple fractures at various stages of healing without explanation strongly suggest a diagnosis of child abuse (**Figure 2**).

The age of a fracture can be estimated by radiographic appearance. From 7 to 14 days after the injury, new periosteal bone and callus formation can be seen; from 14 to 21 days after the initial injury, loss of the definition of the fracture line and maturation of the callus with trabecular formation are evident. Callus that is more dense is seen 21 to 42 days after injury. As

SECTION 9 PEDIATRIC ORTHOPAEDICS

the bone remodels to a more normal status, fractures older than 6 weeks are distinguished by subtle fusiform sclerotic thickening that is best seen when compared with a normal contralateral bone.

Fractures with low suspicion for abuse include clavicle fractures and linear skull fractures. Of note, a vague or implausible description of the mechamism of injury or the presence of other risk factors for child abuse outweighs fracture specificity in determining child abuse.

It is important to avoid misdiagnosis of child abuse. Spiral fractures of the tibia, the so-called toddler's fracture, can occur in 1- to 3-year-old children as a result of a relatively trivial fall. Spontaneous fractures can occur with diseases such as osteogenesis imperfecta. The presence of osteopenia, a family history of osteogenesis imperfecta, as well as the presence of blue sclera would suggest this disease. Pathologic fractures also are associated with osteomyelitis, benign and malignant tumors, rickets, neuromuscular disease, and other metabolic diseases.

Final Diagnosis

Once pathologic fractures are excluded, determine whether the child's fracture has been caused by accidental trauma or by inflicted trauma. A diagnosis of accidental trauma can be made when an acute injury is brought promptly to medical attention, has a plausible mechanism of injury, and lacks other risk factors for child abuse. Suspicious injuries must be reported as child abuse.

Reporting Child Abuse

In the United States, any physician who reports suspected child abuse in good faith is protected from both civil and criminal liability. Failure to report suspected child abuse exposes the physician to liability. Sexual abuse is a criminal offense and must be reported. Eliciting help from the hospital's child protection team is appropriate. In addition to making notes in the medical record, the physician may be asked to complete a notarized affidavit summarizing findings in the abuse case and stating that the child may be at risk for injury or loss of life if returned to the home environment. The child may then be placed by the courts until an investigation is completed. The physician must be prepared to explain his or her findings in custodial hearings if the family challenges the actions of child protective services.

Clubfoot

Synonyms

Congenital clubfoot

Talipes equinovarus

ICD-9 Codes

736.71
Acquired equinovarus
deformity, clubfoot, acquired

754.51
Talipes equinovarus

Definition

Clubfoot, or talipes equinovarus, is a congenital deformity of the foot/ankle characterized by four clinical components: midfoot cavus (high arch), forefoot adduction, heel varus (adduction of calcaneus), and ankle equinus (reduced dorsiflexion) or (CAVE) (**Figure 1**).

Many theories exist about the etiology of clubfoot, but none has been proven correct. Most cases are idiopathic and occur in an otherwise normal infant. An intrinsic idiopathic clubfoot is not fully correctable by passive manipulation. A positional or intrinsic clubfoot deformity may occur as a result of intrauterine molding. A positional clubfoot can be distinguished by inherent flexibility of the deformity, either spontaneous resolution or a rapid response to treatment, and the absence of calf atrophy or a difference in foot size. Clubfoot may be observed in association with a variety of neuromuscular diseases such as myelomeningocele or arthrogryposis, and also many syndromes (eg, congenital constriction band syndrome, diastrophic dysplasia). These secondary clubfeet tend to be more rigid and difficult to treat, as well as more prone to recurrence following adequate treatment.

The incidence of clubfoot worldwide is approximately 1 in 1,000 live births; it is twice as common in boys as in girls. If a family has one child with clubfoot, the risk in subsequent

Figure 1 Bilateral congenital clubfoot seen in a newborn.

SECTION 9   PEDIATRIC ORTHOPAEDICS

siblings is 3% to 4%. If one parent and one child in a family have clubfoot, the risk in subsequent children is 25%.

Clinical Symptoms

In infancy, the clubfoot is a visible deformity that is not associated with symptoms or physical limitations. Ambulatory patients with an untreated clubfoot, or with recurrent or residual deformities, often have moderate to severe gait disturbance, have difficulties wearing standard shoes, and occasionally have pain.

Tests

Physical Examination

A comprehensive physical examination is required to rule out neuromuscular disorders or syndromes (nonidiopathic clubfoot). The extremities should be examined to rule out any contractures or deformities and to assess neuromuscular function. Assessment of motor function by observation or stimulation also is important because congenital absence of the anterior compartment muscles has been associated with clubfoot in rare instances. The spine should be examined for cutaneous manifestations of an underlying intraspinal anomaly. Abnormal neurologic findings also may indicate a spinal cord disorder such as tethering due to lipomyelomeningocele, distematomyelia, or other cause. The foot examination should focus on characterizing the specific deformities (midfoot cavus, forefoot adduction, hindfoot varus, hindfoot equinus) and grading their rigidity or severity.

Diagnostic Tests

Radiographs are not usually required in infants with clubfoot. Weight-bearing AP and lateral radiographs of the foot may be required in older children with recurrent or residual deformities following treatment, or with a neglected or untreated clubfoot. An MRI of the spine may be required to rule out intraspinal pathology. Rarely, electromyography and nerve conduction studies may be needed in the diagnostic evaluation.

Differential Diagnosis

- Acquired equinovarus deformity
- Arthrogryposis (stiffness and weakness of multiple joints of the upper and/or lower extremities)
- Congenital constriction band syndrome (partial or circumferential bands of indented skin and underlying tissue, intrauterine amputations)
- Distal arthrogryposis (autosomal dominant condition, stiffness of the hands and feet)

Figure 2 Anterior (**A**) and posterior (**B**) photographs of clubfoot in an older patient.

- Metatarsus adductus (hindfoot is not in varus and equinus)
- Neuromuscular imbalance (abnormal neurologic findings)
- Secondary clubfoot
- Tethered cord (cutaneous lesions over the spine, recurrent deformity)

Adverse Outcomes of the Disease

Untreated clubfoot causes a significant disability (**Figure 2**). Not only are walking and shoe wear severely impaired, possible long-term consequences include pain and degenerative joint disease. The sociocultural implications are perhaps the greatest source of disability; in some societies patients with a clubfoot are ostracized and felt to be "cursed."

Even with adequate treatment, the affected foot will be smaller and less mobile than a normal foot. Calf atrophy is a normal finding in congenital clubfoot, and will persist despite adequate treatment of the deformity. The difference is not as obvious with bilateral involvement but is readily apparent with unilateral involvement. The foot on the affected side is typically 1 to 1½ shoe sizes smaller than the unaffected foot.

Treatment

There has been a recent paradigm shift in the treatment of clubfoot. Previously, all children were treated by serial casting, and the vast majority required a subsequent extensive surgical release to achieve correction. Long-term studies have suggested that these extensive releases are complicated by stiffness, pain, and the need for additional surgical procedures such as osteotomy or arthrodesis. The Ponseti method, which is

SECTION 9   PEDIATRIC ORTHOPAEDICS

minimally invasive, has become the treatment of choice in most centers in North America and many others throughout the world. The initial phase involves serial casting with long leg casts using a specific technique, and deformity correction that addresses the four clinical components of clubfoot represented by the CAVE mnemonic. All components except hindfoot equinus are typically corrected after four to seven casts; most patients require a percutaneous release of the tendoachilles to treat the rigid hindfoot equinus. The tendon regenerates after 3 weeks in an infant, and there is no increased risk of Achilles tendon rupture later in life. After casting is completed, patients wear a foot abduction brace for 3 months full time, and then at night for 4 to 5 years. Recurrence of deformity can occur in approximately 15% of patients, is most common within the first 2 to 3 years of life, and is very rare after 5 to 7 years of age. Most recurrences can be treated by the same method, although some patients with a dynamic equinovarus (foot inverts during swing phase of gait) from tibialis anterior overactivity will require a lateral transfer of this muscle. Approximately 95% of infants with a clubfoot can be managed with this method, avoiding the need for an extensive surgical release. Older patients with a clubfoot are commonly seen in societies with underdeveloped health infrastructure, and it appears that the Ponseti method may be of benefit in children up to 8 years of age. Older patients, and those with recurrent or persistent deformities, may require other surgical interventions such as soft-tissue release, osteotomies, or triple arthrodesis.

Adverse Outcomes of Treatment

Continuing with the serial casting in the face of rigid hindfoot equinus may result in spurious correction of the equinus through the midfoot or transverse tarsal joints, creating a "rocker bottom" foot (convex sole, flatfoot). Worsening of the deformity occurs when improper casting technique is utilized or failing to modify technique in the face of a "complex" clubfoot. Recurrent or residual deformities may require additional evaluation and treatment. Complications of the more extensive soft-tissue release and/or osteotomies or fusions include undercorrection, overcorrection, muscle weakness (especially in push off), joint stiffness and/or arthritis, and gait disturbance.

Referral Decisions/Red Flags

Patients with a clubfoot will require referral to an orthopaedic surgeon, and also may require other specialty evaluations (neurology, genetics), depending upon the history and physical findings.

Complex Regional Pain Syndrome

Synonyms

Causalgia

CRPS

Reflex sympathetic dystrophy

RSD

ICD-9 Codes

337.21
Reflex sympathetic dystrophy
of the upper limb

337.22
Reflex sympathetic dystrophy
of the lower limb

Definition

Complex regional pain syndrome (CRPS) describes a constellation of signs and symptoms of a dysfunctional, debilitating pain syndrome that is not anatomic in distribution and is disproportionate to the inciting injury. CRPS is classified as either type I (reflex sympathetic dystrophy [RSD]) or type II (causalgia). Type I CRPS is a pain syndrome that principally involves the extremities and is associated with varying degrees of autonomic dysfunction. Type I CRPS is more common in children and adolescents, particularly in children between 9 and 15 years of age. The diagnosis often is delayed because of the confusing clinical presentation of musculoskeletal, neurologic, and inflammatory symptoms.

Clinical Symptoms

An older child or adolescent with type I CRPS commonly presents after a minor injury or contusion. Signs and symptoms typically include excessive pain and hypersensitivity to light touch, cold intolerance, transient swelling, and skin discoloration in the extremity (most commonly the foot and ankle). Weight bearing, joint range of motion, and limb mobility may be severely restricted by pain, weakness, and joint stiffness.

Tests

Physical Examination

Type I CRPS is a diagnosis of exclusion. Early in the disease the physical examination can be confusing and may delay the diagnosis. The patient may be unable to bear weight on an affected lower extremity or may refuse to move an affected upper extremity. Localized soft-tissue edema and skin hyperemia are visible. Active range of motion is limited, and attempts at passive range of motion elicit severe pain. Minor sensory stimuli, such as brushing against bed sheets, cause severe burning pain in a localized but nonanatomic distribution.

Diagnostic Tests

Radiographs, three-phase bone scans, and MRIs, along with laboratory studies such as erythrocyte sedimentation rate, C-reactive protein level, and other hematologic tests are most useful to eliminate the common differential diagnoses.

In the early stages of type I CRPS, routine studies are within normal limits. Tests specific for type I CRPS such as thermography, cold testing, and sympathetic blockade (the gold standard) may help confirm the diagnosis in equivocal cases. In patients with long-standing symptoms, radiographs reveal limb osteopenia, and MRI shows edema of soft tissues and bones.

Differential Diagnosis

- Contusion (joint swelling, pain with motion)
- Inflammatory synovitis (joint swelling, pain with motion)
- Ligament sprain (history of trauma)
- Musculoskeletal infection (swelling, fever, constant pain that is increasing)
- Neoplasm (constant pain, night pain)
- Occult fracture (history of trauma)
- Spinal pathology (back pain)
- Tendinitis (history of repetitive activities, pain after activity)

Adverse Outcomes of the Disease

Long-term signs and symptoms are associated with dystrophic changes such as muscle wasting, joint contracture, thickening of the nails, and the appearance of coarse hair on the extremities. The most feared complications are chronic pain, limb dystrophy, and rare permanent limb dysfunction. Most patients, however, recover fully if diagnosed early and treated appropriately.

Treatment

Rehabilitation is the mainstay of treatment. Frequent sessions that focus on desensitization, joint mobility, and weight bearing can help to restore function within 4 to 6 weeks. Low doses of antidepressants (commonly amitriptyline) or anticonvulsants (commonly gabapentin) are effective in diminishing symptoms and facilitating rehabilitation in patients who initially are unresponsive to rehabilitation. Narcotics and other pain medications are best used under careful supervision in the earliest stages of type I CRPS and have a limited long-term role in children.

Paravertebral sympathetic chain blockade by selective injection or epidural infusion is necessary only if other treatment regimens fail. A specialized pain team approach to management enhances outcomes.

Adverse Outcomes of Treatment

Inability to resolve the pain ultimately may result in severe disability, including loss of limb function.

Referral Decisions/Red Flags

Early diagnosis and referral to a multidisciplinary pain team are most likely to result in complete resolution of the pain complex.

SECTION 9 PEDIATRIC ORTHOPAEDICS

Congenital Deficiencies of the Lower Extremity

ICD-9 Codes

755.34
Proximal femoral focal deficiency

755.36
Tibial hemimelia

755.37
Fibular hemimelia

Conditions

Longitudinal deficiency of the fibula (partial or complete)

Tibial deficiency (tibial hemimelia)

Longitudinal deficiency of the femur, partial (proximal focal femoral deficiency [PFFD])

Definition

Congenital deficiencies of the lower extremity are usually obvious at birth, and their appearance can be alarming to parents. Support and counseling provided by the physician can be critical while the parents are attempting to understand their child's condition. Treatment decisions are based on two issues: whether the foot is functional (or can be salvaged), and what the anticipated limb-length discrepancy will be at skeletal maturity. A search for anomalies in other organ systems also is required in some cases. With regard to limb-length discrepancy, the degree of growth inhibition is constant, and while the discrepancy remains proportional, the absolute difference in limb lengths increases as the child grows. Considerable variability exists in the degree of growth inhibition. Whereas some children can be treated with a simple shoe lift or an epiphysiodesis, others will require one or more limb lengthenings. Patients in whom a very large discrepancy is predicted will be best served by early amputation and prosthetic fitting. In these cases, it should be emphasized to the parents that their child can lead an active life with a prosthesis. Recent improvements in techniques for lower extremity reconstruction has made limb salvage a more viable option for a greater number of patients.

Early referral to a specialist is important, as families will need to gain an understanding of the pros and cons of all treatment options. Even though surgical treatment usually is not performed until the child is at least 9 to 12 months of age, formulating a comprehensive treatment plan takes time. Providing the parents with an opportunity to meet other affected children at a more advanced stage of growth and development is reassuring.

Figure 1 Radiographs demonstrate three types of fibular deficiency according to the Kalamchi classification. **A,** Type IA: minimal shortening of the fibula with a ball-and-socket ankle. **B,** Type IB: only partial fibula present. **C,** Type II: complete absence of the fibula.

Longitudinal Deficiency of the Fibula (Partial or Complete)

Fibular deficiency, sometimes called fibular hemimelia or congenital absence of the fibula, is a sporadic disorder of unknown etiology. Fibular deficiency is the most common long-bone deficiency (**Figure 1**). All patients require treatment for a limb-length discrepancy, but the magnitude of the projected discrepancy is quite variable.

Longitudinal deficiency of the fibula may be viewed as a "postaxial hypoplasia," as abnormalities may be noted along the lateral aspect of the limb. Coexisting problems include a common association with femoral deficiencies (congenital short femur with PFFD), patellar dysplasia, genu valgum from hypoplasia of the lateral condyle of the distal femur, absent cruciate ligaments in the knee, partial or complete absence of the fibula, anteromedial bowing of the tibia, absence of the lateral rays of the foot, tarsal coalitions, and valgus alignment of the hindfoot associated with a ball-and-socket–like ankle joint. Attention often is focused on the degree of fibular involvement, but the morphology of the fibula does not necessarily correlate with the degree of growth inhibition or the amount of foot deformity, and the associated clinical findings must be factored into the treatment plan.

SECTION 9 PEDIATRIC ORTHOPAEDICS

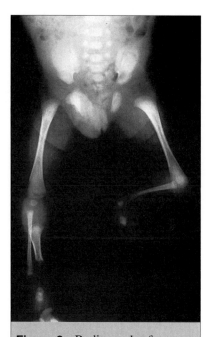

Figure 2 Radiograph of an infant with bilateral tibial deficiency. The patient's right lower limb has incomplete absence of the tibia; the left tibia is completely absent.

The goal of treatment is a normal gait with an active life. In general, a foot with more than three rays is felt to be suitable for salvage, and in some cases surgical soft-tissue release or other measures are required to achieve a plantigrade foot. The magnitude of limb-length discrepancy at skeletal maturity must be estimated. With a relatively small anticipated discrepancy and a functional foot (or one suitable for reconstruction), the treatment focuses on achieving a plantigrade foot and treating limb-length discrepancy with a shoe lift and/or an epiphysiodesis (or a single limb lengthening). When the anticipated discrepancy is extremely large and/or the foot cannot be reconstructed, consideration is given to an early Syme disarticulation (occurring at the level of the ankle) or Boyd (through the foot, but preserving part of the calcaneus) amputation and prosthetic fitting. The decision making is less straightforward for a subset of patients in whom the anticipated discrepancy would require more than a single lengthening. Multiple factors must be weighed in the decision; for example, the provision of a single straightforward procedure during infancy (amputation) versus multiple limb lengthenings and surgical procedures throughout the years of growth and development. With newer technologies, and as more experience has been gained with lengthenings for severe discrepancies, limb salvage has become an option for a greater number of patients. A situation to be avoided is having a patient undergo multiple procedures to maintain a nonfunctional foot and equalize a large limb-length discrepancy, only to realize the leg must be amputated during adolescence.

Tibial Deficiency

Tibial deficiency, also called tibial hemimelia or congenital absence of the tibia, is characterized by partial or complete absence of the tibia (**Figure 2**). This is a rare, more severe anomaly, affecting approximately 1 in 1 million live births. Most cases are sporadic, but both autosomal dominant and autosomal recessive forms have been identified in a limited number of patients. Other disorders that may be associated with tibial deficiency include congenital heart disease, cleft palate, imperforate anus, hypospadias, hernias, and gonadal malformations. Hand anomalies may be seen in up to one third of patients.

In contrast to fibular deficiencies, which have coexisting abnormalities on the lateral side of the limb (postaxial), tibial deficiencies may be viewed as a preaxial hypoplasia, with involvement on the medial side of the limb. Femoral hypoplasia may be observed, as well as patellar dysplasia and absent cruciate ligaments. The fibula is bowed, and often a dislocation at the proximal tibiofibular joint exists with proximal migration of the fibula. The foot commonly has an equinovarus deformity, with absent medial rays, and tarsal coalition. The ankle joint is absent, and the distal fibula forms a rudimentary articulation with the lateral portion of the talus and/or calcaneus.

Involvement of the medial aspect of the foot commonly manifests as talipes equinovarus (clubfoot) and absence of medial rays. Ironically, tibial deficiency also can be associated with polydactyly. Shortening of the involved limb is present and, with unilateral involvement, the anticipated discrepancy is typically large (8 to 16 cm). Knee flexion contracture exists when the tibia is totally absent or if the quadriceps is deficient, and the fibula may appear as a bony projection lateral to the lateral femoral condyle.

Treatment recommendations vary. In patients with complete absence of the tibia, the absence of both a knee and an ankle joint is associated with severe knee flexion contracture and absent quadriceps function, the anticipated limb-length discrepancy is severe, and the coexisting foot deformity often is severe. These patients are treated at an early age with through-the-knee disarticulation and prosthetic fitting. In many cases, when a proximal tibia is present, the quadriceps muscle is functional, and no knee flexion contracture exists. The proximal tibia anlagen may not be ossified at birth, and an ultrasonogram or MRI may be required to evaluate the proximal tibial anatomy. The presence of quadriceps function and the absence of a fixed knee flexion contracture suggest that a proximal tibia is present. In such cases, the main concerns include absence of a stable knee and ankle, foot deformity, and a large projected limb-length discrepancy. Most of these patients undergo an early Syme disarticulation, and later, the creation of a surgical synostosis between the proximal tibia and fibula to enhance prosthetic fit and wear. The least common form of tibial deficiency involves a distal diastasis between the tibia and fibula (the distal tibia is absent) associated with severe hindfoot equinus, and often, foot deficiencies. These cases are typically managed by early hindfoot amputation and prosthetic fitting.

Longitudinal Deficiency of the Femur

Longitudinal deficiency of the femur encompasses a spectrum of congenital abnormalities of the femur. Proximal focal femoral deficiency (PFFD) is a sporadic condition of unknown etiology characterized by dysgenesis of the proximal femur with shortening of the femoral shaft. The incidence prevalence is between 1 in 50,000 and 1 in 200,000 live births; approximately 15% of cases are bilateral. The limb assumes a characteristic position with shortening of the femoral segment, and the thigh is flexed, abducted, and externally rotated. Shortening of the femur is marked, and the limb-length discrepancy at maturity ranges from 7 to 25 cm. Associated abnormalities occur in approximately 50% of patients and include hip dysplasia, hypoplasia of the lateral femoral condyle, absent cruciate ligaments, and longitudinal deficiency of the fibula. Associated deficiencies in other organ systems, including cleft palate and congenital heart defects, are less common.

Various classifications have been proposed, but none has been universally accepted. The Aitken classification describes the spectrum of plain radiographic findings, but it does not address soft-tissue abnormalities, and it is less useful for treatment planning. The Aitken classification has four subtypes: Type A (femoral head present but delay in ossification; subtrochanteric defect, which later ossifies), type B (femoral head and acetabulum present, subtrochanteric defect with discontinuity between the femoral head and shaft), type C (absent femoral head with short tapered femoral shaft, no acetabulum), and type D (absent proximal femoral shaft, small residual distal femur, no acetabulum).

The treatment is individualized, and a host of options are available depending on the anticipated limb-length discrepancy and the status of the hip and the knee. Reconstructive surgical procedures may include femoral osteotomy and bone grafting of the pseudarthrosis, soft-tissue rebalancing, and then multiple femoral lengthenings. In cases that are not amenable to reconstruction, options include fitting with a custom prosthesis, knee fusion and Syme disarticulation (fit with a knee disarticulation prosthesis), and a Van Nes rotationplasty. In the Van Nes procedure, the knee is fused and the limb is rotated 180° so that the ankle is facing backward. The ankle joint then functions as the knee joint, and the patient can be fitted with a below-knee prosthesis. This procedure is rarely performed and is considered today to be socially unacceptable.

Referral Decisions/Red Flags

All children with absence of toes or an obviously short limb should receive early consultation with an orthopedic surgeon and appropriate additional testing for associated disorders.

Congenital Deficiencies of the Upper Extremity

Conditions

Hypoplasia/absence of the thumb
Radial deficiency
Transverse deficiency of the forearm
Ulnar deficiency

Definition

Congenital deficiencies of the upper extremity may be either longitudinal (affecting one side of the extremity) or complete transverse deficiencies. A clinical evaluation is appropriate because some patients will have abnormalities in other organ systems. Deficiency of the thumb, radial deficiency, ulnar deficiency, and transverse deficiencies of the forearm are the most common.

As a general principle, reconstructive surgery usually is not performed before the infant is 6 to 18 months of age; however, selected procedures may be required earlier than this. Early specialty evaluation is helpful to allay anxiety of the parents and grandparents. Early consultation also allows time for parents to gain an understanding and realistic expectations of the anticipated function and appearance after surgical treatment. Some of these disorders will not benefit from surgical treatment, but early discussion concerning principles of prosthetic management will be helpful.

Hypoplasia/Absence of the Thumb

The extent of the thumb deficiency is variable. A hypoplastic thumb may be small, unstable, or thin due to deficient development of the thenar musculature. Other disorders are common, including congenital heart disease (Holt-Oram syndrome), craniofacial abnormalities, and vertebral anomalies (VATER association). Fanconi anemia also can develop in later childhood.

Patients with untreated thumb deficiency adapt by using the pinch function between the index and long fingers to substitute for the deficient thumb. Patients with unilateral involvement generally have excellent overall function with minimal impairment.

Surgical management is based on the magnitude of the deficiency. Reconstruction is indicated when the hypoplastic

ICD-9 Codes	
755.21	Transverse deficiency of the forearm
755.26	Radial hemimelia
755.27	Ulnar hemimelia
755.29	Hypoplasia of the thumb

SECTION 9 PEDIATRIC ORTHOPAEDICS

thumb is of adequate size and the carpometacarpal joint is stable. Index pollicization (transfer of the index finger to the thumb position, leaving the hand with three fingers) is recommended for more severe deformities.

Radial Deficiency

Radial deficiency, sometimes called radial hemimelia or radial clubhand, is characterized by radial deviation of the hand; variable presence and stiffness of the thumb and the index and long fingers; variable shortening and bowing of the forearm segment; and variable range of motion at the elbow. Associated disorders include congenital heart disease (Holt-Oram syndrome), craniofacial abnormalities, and vertebral anomalies (VATER association). Thrombocytopenia with absent radius (TAR) syndrome also is possible. The unique aspect of TAR syndrome is the presence of an essentially normal thumb. In other syndromes, if the radius is deficient, then the thumb also is hypoplastic or absent.

Surgical management is designed to improve the alignment and appearance of the hand relative to the forearm. A centralization procedure ideally is performed between 6 and 18 months of age. Untreated patients can function surprisingly well. Surgical treatment, therefore, is contraindicated in patients with short forearms and/or limited elbow motion. These patients do better if the hand remains closer to the midline (eg, radially deviated).

Ulnar Deficiency

Ulnar deficiencies include a variety of disorders involving either a partial or complete absence of skeletal and soft-tissue elements on the ulnar (postaxial) border of the forearm and hand. Conditions range from hypoplasia of the ulna, in which the ulna is completely present but short, to total aplasia of the ulna, which may be associated with congenital fusion of the radius to the humerus (radiohumeral synostosis). Digital deficiencies are common and variable.

Unlike radial and thumb deficiencies, ulnar deficiencies are not associated with anomalies of other organ systems. Patients with ulnar deficiencies, however, are more likely to have disorders elsewhere in the skeletal system, including tibial deficiency and partial longitudinal deficiency of the femur (proximal focal femoral deficiency).

Surgical treatment is not commonly indicated for ulnar deficiency, except for associated digital deformities. Syndactyly release, web space reconstruction, and other procedures, when indicated, can improve hand function.

Transverse Deficiency of the Forearm

Transverse deficiency of the forearm, sometimes called congenital below-elbow deficiency is characterized by complete absence of the hand and wrist and a hypoplastic or partially absent forearm. Elbow function is good, even if the radial head is dislocated. This disorder is sporadic, typically unilateral, and generally is not associated with abnormalities in other organ systems, although patients may have congenital constriction band syndrome and other musculoskeletal anomalies.

Children with unilateral transverse deficiency of the forearm have minimal functional limitations. Bimanual activities are often performed using the medial aspect of the affected forearm to assist the opposite, uninvolved extremity (**Figure 1**). The principal deficit is cosmetic, which is particularly troublesome during the teenage years.

Surgical treatment is rarely necessary. Primitive digital remnants, if present, occasionally are removed to improve cosmetic acceptability.

Prosthetic management is of great interest to families of infants with this condition. The best time to introduce the prosthesis is controversial, though many centers favor an aggressive "fit when they sit" protocol. This approach is based on the developmental principle that normal bimanual activities begin when an infant is able to sit independently, at about age 6 to 8 months. Others recognize that a prosthesis often impedes an infant's ability to crawl and favor the first fitting after an infant is able to stand and walk independently.

Prosthetic options include the standard body-powered design, consisting of a shoulder harness and a hook terminal device; a myoelectric design, consisting of a mechanical hand that is opened and closed by voluntary forearm muscle activity; and a passive design, consisting of a lightweight, durable, cosmetically appealing, nonmovable hand. The optimal design is based on a number of factors and is best determined on an individual basis.

The principal benefit of prosthetic management is cosmetic, which may be more significant to the parents than the child prior to the teenage years. Function is not consistently improved by any of the prosthetic designs, leading to a high rate of prosthetic rejection.

Figure 1 Infant with unilateral transverse deficiency of the forearm using the affected limb to assist the uninvolved extremity.

SECTION 9 PEDIATRIC ORTHOPAEDICS

Congenital Deformities of the Lower Extremity

Conditions

Coxa vara
Congenital dislocation (hyperextension deformity) of the knee
Congenital dislocation of the patella
Posteromedial bowing of the tibia
Anterolateral bowing of the tibia
Calcaneovalgus foot
Congenital vertical talus
Congenital short first metatarsal
Congenital curly toe
Polydactyly

Definition

These conditions are present at birth and either may be truly congenital or may result from intrauterine molding. Some disorders, such as congenital dislocation of the patella, may not be apparent until the child is older.

Clinical Symptoms

Most of these conditions are noticed on examination of the infant, although symptoms such as pain, gait disturbance, or difficulties with shoewear may develop during infancy and early childhood.

Tests

Physical Examination

Deviations from normal should evoke suspicion, although a range of normal exists. The lower extremities of a newborn have been compressed in the uterus, and a hip flexion contracture of 40° to 60° and a knee flexion contracture of 20° to 30° are normal in newborns. Likewise, in utero, the ankles and feet are pressed into a dorsiflexed position; therefore, calcaneovalgus posture of the foot is normal.

Disproportionate shortening of the upper and lower extremities or spine suggests a generalized skeletal dysplasia. Other organ systems should be evaluated to rule out other genetic and chromosomal disorders.

Figure 1 Pelvic radiograph demonstrates congenital coxa vara in a 5-year-old child. (Reproduced from Kasser JR, ed: *Orthopaedic Knowledge Update*, ed 5. Rosemont, IL, American Academy of Orthopaedic Surgeons, 1996, p 353.)

Diagnostic Tests

AP and lateral radiographs of the affected extremity are standard.

Coxa Vara

Coxa vara is a relatively uncommon hip disorder characterized by a decrease in the neck-shaft angle of the femur (**Figure 1**). The types of coxa vara are congenital, acquired, and developmental. Congenital coxa vara is associated with a congenital short femur and proximal femoral focal deficiency. Acquired coxa vara is secondary to metabolic or traumatic conditions. Developmental coxa vara is an idiopathic condition that appears in early childhood. The diagnosis of congenital coxa vara often is made in infancy due to asymmetry in the lower extremities. Both acquired and developmental coxa vara present with gait disturbance in toddlers and young children. The bony deformity alters the mechanics of the hip and causes abductor muscle weakness, a Trendelenburg gait, and a limb-length discrepancy (unilateral disease). Untreated, the deformity and gait abnormality will progress. A realignment osteotomy can improve hip function.

SECTION 9 PEDIATRIC ORTHOPAEDICS

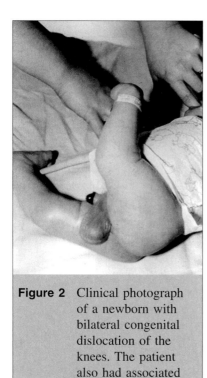

Figure 2 Clinical photograph of a newborn with bilateral congenital dislocation of the knees. The patient also had associated bilateral dislocated hips and a left clubfoot.

Congenital Dislocation of the Knee

Congenital dislocation, which is due to intrauterine positioning, presents as a hyperextension deformity of the knee at birth. The spectrum of severity ranges from a mild positional deformity that responds readily to short-term splinting, to a frank hyperextension/dislocation of the tibia on the femur that requires serial casting and occasionally an open surgical reduction (**Figure 2**). Associated abnormalities such as hip dysplasia are common, and an early ultrasound should be considered even when the hip examination is considered normal.

Congenital Dislocation of the Patella

Congenital dislocation of the patella may not be apparent for several months after birth. Persistent flexion contracture of the knee and external rotation of the leg are suggestive of the diagnosis. The patella may not be palpable in its dislocated lateral position. Ultrasound is helpful in confirming the diagnosis in a younger child whose patella has not started to ossify. Surgical treatment is necessary. It involves releasing the tight lateral structures around the knee and essentially derotating the quadriceps mechanisms; the insertion of the patellar tendon often is quite lateral, and must be surgically relocated.

Posteromedial Bowing of the Tibia

Posteromedial bowing of the tibia is an idiopathic deformity that is most obvious and rather striking at birth (**Figure 3**) and is commonly associated with a calcaneovalgus foot, which often lies along the lateral aspect of the distal tibia. The calcaneovalgus foot often resolves spontaneously, but manipulation and/or casting may be required. The posteromedial bowing of the tibia improves during growth and development, and a small subset of patients may require an osteotomy in late childhood or early adolescence if the deformity does not resolve. The major problem associated with posteromedial bowing is limb-length discrepancy, and nearly all patients will require some form of treatment. Because the mean discrepancy is approximately 4 cm at skeletal maturity, most patients will require either a shoe lift or an epiphysiodesis.

Anterolateral Bowing of the Tibia

Anterolateral bowing of the tibia is usually apparent during infancy and requires immediate specialty referral. A very limited number of cases will resolve spontaneously, but most represent a "prepseudarthrosis" of the tibia. A congenital pseudarthrosis of the tibia is extremely difficult to treat and often is associated with neurofibromatosis (genetically inherited disorders that cause tumors to grow in the nervous system), which must be ruled out (**Figure 4**). A clamshell orthosis is initially recommended in an attempt to prevent a fracture, and, although controversial, some authors recommend a prophylactic bypass graft for a prepseudarthrosis of the tibia. An established pseudarthrosis typically requires multiple surgical procedures to attempt to achieve union. A variety of surgical strategies have been successful in achieving union, including resection of the pseudarthrosis with bone grafting, intramedullary rodding, external fixation, and vascularized fibular bone grafting. Refracture is common, however, and multiple interventions are often required throughout childhood and adolescence. Even if union is achieved, patients usually require long-term bracing to prevent refracture. Some patients will elect to have an amputation after multiple attempts to achieve union, often because of dysfunction of the foot and ankle.

Calcaneovalgus Foot

Calcaneovalgus foot is a very common newborn positional abnormality or deformation characterized by marked dorsiflexion of the ankle and eversion of the foot, where the foot may be

Figure 3 Radiograph of infant with congenital posteromedial bowing of the tibia. (Reproduced from Kasser JR, ed: *Orthopaedic Knowledge Update*, ed 5. Rosemont, IL, American Academy of Orthopaedic Surgeons, 1996, p 441.)

Figure 4 AP (**A**) and lateral (**B**) radiographs show anterolateral bowing of the tibia.

SECTION 9 PEDIATRIC ORTHOPAEDICS

Figure 5 Clinical photograph of a calcaneovalgus foot in a neonate.

Figure 6 Clinical photograph of the feet of a 9-month-old infant with bilateral congenital vertical talus. (Reproduced from Kasser JR, ed: *Orthopaedic Knowledge Update*, ed 5. Rosemont, IL, American Academy of Orthopaedic Surgeons, 1996, p 507.)

pressed against the tibia (**Figure 5**). Most cases resolve spontaneously, although stretching and/or several serial casts may be required in some patients. Rarely, this deformity results from deficient activity of the plantar flexors from an underlying neurologic disorder such as a lipomyelomeningocele.

Congenital Vertical Talus

Congenital vertical talus, which appears as a flat foot with a convex sole ("rocker bottom" or "Persian slipper" foot) is diagnosed shortly after birth or in infancy; it is rare. The deformity is commonly rigid, and it does not resolve spontaneously (**Figure 6**). The condition may be idiopathic or familial, but most cases are associated with a neuromuscular disease or genetic syndrome. In addition to prompt referral to an orthopaedist, referral to a neurologist and/or geneticist should be considered. The deformity is typically rigid, and represents a dorsal dislocation of the medial column of the foot at the talonavicular joint, or of the entire midfoot on the hindfoot. A lateral radiograph of the foot obtained in maximum plantar flexion is diagnostic and will determine whether the midfoot dislocation can be reduced. Because of the rigidity of the deformity, most patients require an extensive soft-tissue release for reduction. A new technique has been reported (the "reverse Ponseti") that involves serial casting, followed by percutaneous release of the Achilles tendon. This method may reduce the need for more extensive surgical releases.

Congenital Short First Metatarsal

With congenital short first metatarsal, shortening of the great toe is obvious and often is associated with hallux varus or medial deviation of the great toe. Surgical treatment is warranted if problems with shoe wear develop. A short first metatarsal also may be seen in fibrodysplasia ossificans progressiva, a rare condition associated with progressive and diffuse ossification within various soft tissues.

Congenital Curly Toe

Congenital curly toe is an idiopathic condition characterized by flexion and medial rotation of the toe, often under the adjacent toe. Most children are asymptomatic. Strapping is ineffective. If problems develop with shoe wear, surgical treatment of the toe flexors often is successful.

Figure 7 Clinical photograph of the feet of a child with postaxial polydactyly of the right foot.

Polydactyly

Extra digits may be observed at the medial (preaxial polydactyly or duplication of the great toe) or the lateral (postaxial polydactyly) borders of the foot. In addition to cosmetic concerns, there may be difficulties with shoe wear (**Figure 7**). Extra digits should not be "tied off" in the newborn nursery. Surgical removal is best performed around 10 months of age, before the child begins to walk, and also may require soft-tissue reconstruction in some cases. An early consultation often helps the parents understand the rationale for the treatment, including the timing of surgery.

Referral Decisions/Red Flags

Calcaneovalgus foot and congenital vertical talus may look similar, but the rocker bottom and inability to plantarflex the foot, as well as lack of improvement over the first month of life, differentiates congenital vertical talus and should prompt referral to an orthopedist for treatment.

SECTION 9 PEDIATRIC ORTHOPAEDICS

Congenital Deformities of the Upper Extremity

Conditions

Congenital dislocation of the radial head
Congenital radioulnar synostosis
Polydactyly
Syndactyly ("webbing")

Definition

Congenital deformities are, by definition, present at birth. Syndactyly and polydactyly are obvious; however, congenital dislocation of the radial head and congenital radioulnar synostosis usually are not identified until the child is 3 to 10 years of age.

Syndactyly

Syndactyly is a condition characterized by the lack of normal separation between fingers or toes and occurs in about 1 in 200 live births (**Figure 1**). It can vary from simple syndactyly, in which only a skin bridge exists, to complex syndactyly, in which a bony fusion (synostosis) is located between the phalanges. The syndactyly is either complete (fingers joined to the tips) or incomplete. Other malformations occur in about 5% of patients, and a positive family history occurs in 10% to 40% of cases. Syndactyly is associated with Apert syndrome and Poland syndrome.

Because the fingers differ in length, growth may cause progressive deviation of the conjoined fingers, especially the border digits (in which case earlier surgery is considered). Use of the digits is limited, and cosmesis is an issue for patients. Therefore, children with hand syndactyly should be assessed for surgical treatment. In most cases, a skin graft will be needed. Correction of syndactyly of the toes often is not required other than for cosmetic reasons.

Polydactyly

Polydactyly is the presence of extra digits in the hand or foot, usually adjacent to the thumb or great toe (preaxial) or lateral to the little finger (postaxial) (**Figure 2**). Extra digits can vary in appearance from a vestigial digit attached by a narrow bridge of skin to a normal-appearing digit with its own metacarpal/

Figure 1 Clinical photograph of the hand of a child with complex syndactyly of the ulnar three fingers. Note how the long finger is pulled toward the shorter ring and little fingers.

metatarsal. Radiographs usually are not needed for diagnostic purposes, only for prognosis and planning surgical treatment.

Polydactyly of the hand may not cause functional difficulties, but it is a significant cosmetic deformity. Accessory digits of the foot frequently cause difficulty in shoe wear. Vestigial digits should not be ablated by application of a circumferential suture at the base of the skin bridge shortly after birth, but rather by formal excision. Removal of extra digits is typically delayed until the child is at least 6 months old. Early consultation often helps the parents understand the treatment. Surgical deletion may be performed earlier if the extra digit interferes with function or if the parents have significant concerns.

Congenital Radioulnar Synostosis

In congenital radioulnar synostosis, the proximal ends of the radius and ulna fail to separate, resulting in an inability to pronate and supinate the forearm. Children substitute shoulder motion to place the hand in a pronated or supinated position. When the condition is unilateral, fewer symptoms occur because the normal opposite extremity can be used for many activities. This abnormality often is not detected until children are old enough to start using their hands in a purposeful manner.

Limited pronation and supination of the forearm can be readily detected, even during examination of the newborn. Because many young children have lax wrist ligaments, the distal end of the radius and ulna, not the hand, should be grasped and gently pronated and supinated to assess forearm rotation.

After ossification occurs, bony union of the proximal radius and ulna can be seen on radiographs (**Figure 3**).

No treatment is needed if the forearm is in a satisfactory position. Patients with bilateral involvement are more likely to have functional limitations. Surgery to divide the synostosis and

Figure 2 Clinical photograph of the hand of a child with polydactyly expressed as a duplicated thumb.

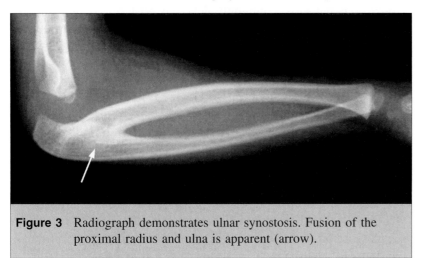

Figure 3 Radiograph demonstrates ulnar synostosis. Fusion of the proximal radius and ulna is apparent (arrow).

SECTION 9 PEDIATRIC ORTHOPAEDICS

Figure 4   Radiographs demonstrates congenital dislocation of the radial head. **A,** On the lateral view, the radial head is dislocated posteriorly and does not articulate with the humerus (arrow). **B,** On the AP view, the normal concavity of the radial head is lost and is replaced by a convexity (arrow).

restore motion has not been successful in most series. Surgical treatment usually is reserved for patients with disability secondary to a forearm positioned in either extreme pronation or supination. Osteotomy to realign the forearm can improve function. This procedure usually is not performed until the child is at least 4 years old and may be delayed until the adolescent or adult years if the degree of disability is questionable.

Congenital Dislocation of the Radial Head

Congenital dislocation of the radial head can occur in several directions but most commonly develops posteriorly; typically, it is bilateral. Elbow deformity and limited motion are the presenting symptoms, but these may not be noticed by the parents for several years. Occasionally, the child reports pain. The abnormality may also be discovered incidentally on radiographs following an injury, often being mistaken for an acute radial head dislocation.

Examination reveals that elbow motion is limited. Rotation often is more limited than flexion and extension. The dislocated radial head often presents as a palpable prominence on the lateral side of the elbow.

Radiographs of the elbow demonstrate the dislocation (**Figure 4**). The radial head is dome-shaped (convex) instead of having a normal concave appearance, differentiating it from a traumatic radial head dislocation.

The deformity and limited elbow motion associated with this condition are often well tolerated. Attempts at open reduction in young children have met with little success. Excision of the radial head, preferably after the most growth is completed, can be considered for pain relief but usually does not improve motion.

Referral Decisions/Red Flags

Limitations in pronation or supination of the forearm should prompt radiographs and referral to an orthopedic surgeon. Concavity of a dislocated radial head suggests a traumatic dislocation amenable to surgical relocation and reconstruction, whereas a convex radial head is indicative of a congenital dislocation that is unlikely to be treated surgically.

SECTION 9 PEDIATRIC ORTHOPAEDICS

Figure 3 Radiographs show developmental dysplasia of the hip (DDH), which is a spectrum of pathology. **A,** Dislocated hip. **B,** Severe subluxation with acetabular dysplasia. **C,** Dysplastic hip.

hip is dislocated, a 2- to 3-week trial in the Pavlik harness may be followed up with an ultrasound to confirm reduction because leaving an unreduced hip in the harness for longer than this may result in deformation of the posterior rim of the acetabulum and a posterior capsular contracture. The Pavlik harness is typically worn full time for 6 to 12 weeks, and then at nighttime for a variable period. If the Pavlik harness fails to reduce the dislocation, the next options for treatment are closed reduction (open reduction if a closed reduction fails) and application of a spica cast, which are performed under general anesthesia. For hips that remain unstable despite an adequate trial with the Pavlik harness, there has been recent interest in splinting with a more rigid hip abduction orthosis before considering a closed reduction. In patients older than 18 to 24 months with a developmental dislocation, a more extensive surgery is typically required to reduce the hip, including an open reduction and capsular repair, a shortening proximal femoral osteotomy, and a pelvic osteotomy. Even when the hip has been successfully reduced, patients may still require treatment for residual or progressive dysplasia of the proximal femur and/or acetabulum, most commonly realignment osteotomies on one or both sides of the joint (**Figure 3**).

Adverse Outcomes of Treatment

Failure of concentric reduction of the femoral head into the socket, persistent hip instability, and osteonecrosis of the femoral head are complications associated with treatment. Osteonecrosis can interfere with the growth of the proximal femur and the acetabulum, resulting in deformity of the proximal femur and progressive limb-length discrepancy.

Referral Decisions/Red Flags

An infant with an abnormal examination and/or significant risk factors may require specialty evaluation.

Diskitis

Definition

Diskitis and vertebral osteomyelitis are bacterial infections involving the anterior elements of the spine. Diskitis is most commonly seen in children younger than 5 years; vertebral osteomyelitis is diagnosed in older children and adolescents. This may be explained by age-dependent variations in the microcirculation within the vertebra and disk. In infants and young children, vascular channels communicate between the vertebral body and the disk space, allowing hematogenous seeding of the disk space. Once those channels have closed, the bacteria typically settle within the vertebrae. Diskitis can occur anywhere in the spine, but it most commonly affects the low thoracic and lumbar regions. The most common infecting organism is *Staphylococcus aureus*. Other organisms include *Kingella kingae*, Group A *Streptococcus*, and *Escherichia coli*.

Clinical Symptoms

A high index of suspicion is required to establish the diagnosis, as the symptoms and findings are often nonspecific. Fever and malaise are common, and patients often experience back pain. Children who are able to communicate may be able to localize the pain to the back, but they also may perceive their pain to be in the abdominal region or thigh. Toddlers frequently are first seen with a limp or refusal to walk. The differential diagnosis is extensive and includes both infectious and noninfectious processes of the spine, the abdomen/pelvis, and the lower extremities.

Tests

Physical Examination

Children rarely appear systemically ill, although a fever, usually low grade, is common. Toddlers may refuse to walk or sit unsupported. Those who will walk often lean forward and place their hands on their thighs for support (psoas sign). Percussion of the spinous processes may help localize the pain. The spine may be held in a rigid position to avoid spinal motion, and if both lower extremities are elevated simultaneously from the supine position, the back and hips are held in a rigid position. Passive spinal flexion, which compresses the anterior elements, is painful. A provocative test involves asking the patient to pick up an object from the floor; children with diskitis will avoid bending forward and will not pick up the item. The single straight-leg raising test also may be positive.

Diagnostic Tests

Laboratory studies should be obtained. The white blood cell count is within the normal range in many cases, but both the erythrocyte sedimentation rate and C-reactive protein level are usually elevated. Cultures of the blood and disk space are diagnostic in only 50% to 60% of cases. AP and lateral radiographs of the thoracolumbar spine are obtained as part of the initial assessment, recognizing that the plain radiographic findings such as irregularity of the vertebral end plates and narrowing of the disk are usually not apparent until 2 or 3 weeks after onset of symptoms. A three-phase bone scan may be helpful in establishing the diagnosis and localizing the pathology. MRI is the imaging study of choice (**Figure 1**). MRI not only confirms the diagnosis and clearly defines the extent of the process but also may help diagnose rare complications such as an epidural abscess. Because of the low diagnostic yield and the necessity for general anesthesia, a CT-guided aspiration of the disk space is usually considered only in patients who have not successfully completed empiric treatment, or when another diagnosis is likely, based on the clinical evaluation. A tuberculin skin test should be considered as well.

Figure 1 T1-weighted MRI shows signal changes characteristic of diskitis at L2-3.

Differential Diagnosis

- Epidural abscess (rare, neurologic symptoms)
- Herniated disk or slipped vertebral apophysis (teenagers, radicular symptoms)
- Pyelonephritis (flank pain, pyuria)
- Retrocecal appendicitis (systemic symptoms, pain with hip extension)
- Retroperitoneal mass (may require MRI)
- Septic arthritis of the hip (marked pain on movement of the hip)
- Spinal tuberculosis (spares the disk, involves bone, usually thoracolumbar area)
- Spine tumor (neurologic abnormalities, may require MRI to differentiate)

Adverse Outcomes of the Disease

Although persistent disk space narrowing and spontaneous fusion of the adjacent vertebrae are common, these rarely result in any symptoms or problems.

Treatment

Most patients suspected of having diskitis are treated empirically. Symptomatic treatment measures include bed rest or

SECTION 9 PEDIATRIC ORTHOPAEDICS

activity restriction, and analgesics. A spinal orthosis may provide considerable relief, and is generally worn for 4 to 6 weeks. Antibiotics effective against *S aureus* are administered for a total course of 6 weeks in most patients. Intravenous administration is typically recommended for up to 2 weeks, and the transition to oral antibiotics is based on the clinical response.

A gradual return to activities is permitted. Surgical treatment, which rarely is required, usually involves either a biopsy with or without débridement or decompression of an epidural abscess. A biopsy is considered when the clinical response to empiric therapy is inadequate (especially if a CT-guided biopsy is nondiagnostic) or when another diagnosis is suspected.

Adverse Outcomes of Treatment

Complications of intravenous antibiotics include line sepsis and an allergic reaction or intolerance to the agent selected.

Referral Decisions/Red Flags

A lack of response to empiric treatment suggests the need for additional workup and/or biopsy. Further evaluation also is indicated in the rare case in which neurologic symptoms are present, usually from an epidural abscess.

Evaluation of the Limping Child

Definition

Limping results from a host of causes. **Tables 1** through **3** present differential diagnoses based on age. There are several broad categories of gait disturbance where the child may present with a limp. An *antalgic gait* is characterized by a shortened stance phase and is caused by pain in the extremity or spine. A Trendelenburg gait, or *abductor lurch*, is characterized by shifting the trunk or shoulders toward the affected side (stance phase) to compensate for weakness of the abductor muscles; it is associated with pathology localized to the hip. An *equinus gait* is characterized by foot contact with the floor by the front of the foot; it might be due to a heel cord contracture or to compensate for a limb-length discrepancy. A *circumduction gait* is characterized by swinging the entire leg out to the side in a

ICD-9 Code

719.7
Difficulty in walking

Table 1 Causes of Limping in Infants/Toddlers

Diagnostic Category	Differential Diagnosis
Congenital	Limb-length discrepancies
Developmental	Hip dysplasia
	Developmental coxa vara
Traumatic	Toddler's fracture
	Nonaccidental injury
Infectious	Septic arthritis
	Osteomyelitis
	Pyomyositis
	Lyme disease
	Diskitis
Inflammatory	Juvenile idiopathic arthritis
	Dermatomyositis
	Reactive arthritis
Neoplastic	Leukemia
	Neuroblastoma
Neurologic	Cerebral palsy
	Muscle diseases
	Neuropathies
	Tethered cord

Table 2 Causes of Limping in Childhood

Diagnostic Category	Differential Diagnosis
Congenital	Hypermobility syndromes
	Diskoid meniscus
Developmental	Hip dysplasia
	Developmental coxa vara
	Spondylolysis or spondylolisthesis
Traumatic	Sprains or strains
	Fractures
	Overuse syndromes (Sever disease)
Infectious	Septic arthritis
	Osteomyelitis
	Pyomyositis
	Lyme disease
	Diskitis
Inflammatory	Reactive arthritis
	Juvenile idiopathic arthritis (oligoarthritis, rheumatoid factor–negative polyarthritis, systemic arthritis, psoriatic arthritis, enthesitis-related arthritis)
	Rheumatic conditions (acute rheumatic fever, lupus, dermatomyositis)
Neoplastic	Leukemia
	Neuroblastoma
Neurologic	Cerebral palsy
	Muscle diseases
	Neuropathies
	Intraspinal anomalies (spinal cord tumor, tethered cord, diastematomyelia, lipomyelomeningocele, syrinx)
Other	Transient synovitis
	Legg-Calvé-Perthes disease
	Limb-length discrepancy
	Osteochondroses (Köhler disease, Freiberg infraction)

circle during the swing phase, such as to allow clearance of a longer leg or due to spasticity. Although a large number of conditions can result in limping, a history and physical examination, supplemented by appropriate imaging studies, will facilitate diagnosis in most cases.

Unless an infection or other serious process is suspected, observation is appropriate for problems of short duration. Chronic problems, however, require further evaluation. Specific treatment strategies depend on the underlying diagnosis.

Table 3 Causes of Limping in Adolescence

Diagnostic Category	Differential Diagnosis
Congenital	Tarsal coalition
	Diskoid meniscus
Developmental	Slipped capital femoral epiphysis
	Spondylolysis or spondylolisthesis
Traumatic	Fractures, sprains/strains
	Stress fractures
	Overuse syndromes or repetitive microtrauma (Osgood-Schlatter disease, Sinding-Larsen–Johansson disease, Sever disease)
	Acetabular labral tears
	Apophyseal avulsion fractures
	Herniated disk or slipped vertebral apophysis
Infectious	Septic arthritis (gonococcus)
	Osteomyelitis
	Pyomyositis
	Lyme disease
	Vertebral osteomyelitis
Inflammatory	Reactive arthritis
	Juvenile idiopathic arthritis
	Rheumatic conditions (acute rheumatic fever, lupus, dermatomyositis)
Neoplastic	Malignant (osteogenic sarcoma)
	Benign (osteoid osteoma)
Neurologic	Cerebral palsy
	Muscle diseases
	Neuropathies
	Intraspinal anomalies (spinal cord tumor, tethered cord, diastematomyelia, lipomyelomeningocele, syrinx)
Other	Limb-length discrepancy
	Idiopathic pain syndromes (especially complex regional pain syndrome and fibromyalgia)
	Osteochondroses (Freiberg infraction, Köhler disease)

Diagnostic Evaluation

History

A history is essential, including the timing and location of any discomfort; the history of any injury (or chronic repetitive activities); the presence of systemic signs or symptoms; whether the limp is worsened by activities and relieved by rest; and the chronicity of symptoms—have they lasted for days, weeks, months, years? Ask a patient who has pain and is able to understand/cooperate to place one finger on the spot that hurts the most. Systemic signs or symptoms such as fever and malaise, weight loss, bruising, or other generalized symptoms increase the likelihood of an underlying infectious, inflammatory, or neoplastic process. Activity-related discomfort, which is relieved by rest, is characteristic for a variety of overuse syndromes of childhood and adolescence. Pain that awakens a patient from sleep (night pain) is worrisome for infection or tumor. Stiffness when the patient wakes in the morning is suggestive of an underlying inflammatory disease. A painless limp often relates to a congenital or developmental process, for example, Legg-Calvé-Perthes disease. A family history of musculoskeletal conditions (juvenile idiopathic arthritis or other inflammatory diseases, hip dysplasia) may suggest a similar disorder in the child.

Physical Examination

The assessment begins with obtaining measurements for height, weight, and vital signs. Has the child been losing weight? Is fever present? Inspect the gait by watching the patient walk (from the front, back, and side) down a long corridor, assessing the trunk/upper body, the hips, the knees, and the foot/ankle. Inspection of stance and alignment is performed. The skin is examined for signs of bruising, erythema, or other abnormalities. The spine is examined for tenderness, spasm, deformity, and cutaneous signs of dysraphism. Palpation of muscles, bones, and joints should reveal any areas of tenderness, swelling, or synovitis. A neuromuscular examination should be performed. Muscle atrophy is an important finding and limb girth is evaluated by measuring and comparing limb circumference at symmetric locations.

Diagnostic Tests

The extent to which additional studies are ordered depends on the chronicity of illness and the findings on history and physical examination. Rest, analgesics, and reevaluation may be indicated for the runner with a mild, activity-related limp of short duration, but an immediate inpatient evaluation is required for the child with night pain, fever, and multiple bruises. In most cases, the evaluation of a limping child can be conducted on an outpatient basis; a more extensive initial evaluation is justified in patients with chronic symptoms (lasting longer than 6 weeks) or when an infection or neoplastic process is in the differential diagnosis.

Radiographs are obtained when findings on the history and physical examination can be localized. Orthogonal views (radiographs taken at 90° to one another) of the area of interest must be obtained, for example, AP and lateral views; often, oblique views are also helpful. Specialized views may be required, such as a tunnel view to rule out osteochondritis dissecans in an older child with knee pain and effusions. If the clinical examination is nonfocal, a three-phase bone scan may better localize the pathology. False-negative results can occur with this test, however; for example, leukemia may have a normal or even a "cold" bone scan. When the location is known and radiographs are nondiagnostic, MRI, CT, or both may help establish the diagnosis. CT provides outstanding bony detail. MRI provides the most comprehensive evaluation, including excellent soft-tissue detail. MRI with intravenous contrast should be ordered when an infection is in the differential diagnosis.

Laboratory studies are indicated if any suggestion of infection, neoplasia, or an inflammatory disease exists. Routine studies include a complete blood cell count with a manual differential, a C-reactive protein level, and an erythrocyte sedimentation rate. Other studies to consider are a Lyme titer and antinuclear antibody (ANA), rheumatoid factor, and anti-streptolysin-O (ASO) tests.

SECTION 9 PEDIATRIC ORTHOPAEDICS

Procedure: Hip Aspiration

CPT Code

20610
Arthrocentesis, aspiration and/or injection; major joint or bursa (eg, shoulder, hip, knee joint, subacromial bursa)

Current Procedural Terminology © 2010 American Medical Association. All rights reserved.

Materials

Sterile gloves

Bactericidal skin preparation solution

10-mL syringe with a 22-gauge, 1¼″ needle Adhesive bandage

Adhesive bandage

Note: The approach for a hip aspiration in a child can be anterior, anterolateral, or medial. The medial approach is described here.

Step 1

Wear protective gloves during this procedure and use sterile technique.

Step 2

Place the patient supine with the hip flexed, maximally abducted, and externally rotated.

Step 3

Palpate the adductor longus.

Step 4

Cleanse the area with a bactericidal solution.

Step 5

Insert the syringe. The needle is placed inferior to the proximal adductor longus tendon, aiming toward the femoral head/neck junction (**Figure 1**). Placement is confirmed on AP fluoroscopic imaging. Observe fluid for gross appearance and record it.

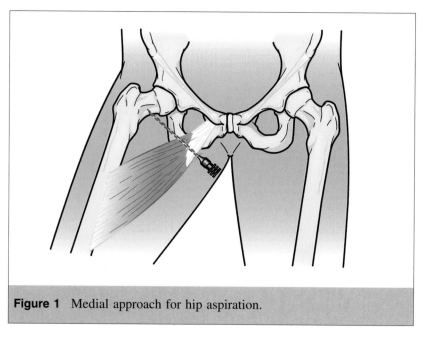

Figure 1 Medial approach for hip aspiration.

Step 6

Dress the puncture site with a sterile adhesive bandage.

Adverse Outcomes

Although rare, infection can occur.

Aftercare/Patient Instructions

Many pediatric patients undergoing this procedure are acutely, seriously ill. Many are inpatients. Aftercare includes activities as tolerated, depending on the clinical situation.

SECTION 9   PEDIATRIC ORTHOPAEDICS

Flatfoot

Synonyms

Flexible flatfoot
Peroneal spastic flatfoot
Pes planovalgus
Pes planus
Pronated foot

Definition

Flatfoot is defined as an abnormally low (or absent) longitudinal arch. In most cases, it is a normal variant. Flatfoot is common in infants and children. The longitudinal arch typically starts to develop around 4 years of age, maturing by 10 years of age. Flatfoot is present in up to 25% of the adult population, and patients often report a family history of flatfoot.

The most common diagnosis is a flexible flatfoot, which rarely is symptomatic and typically requires only reassurance. Flexible flatfoot in children is always bilateral. Patients have a visible arch when they are not standing and have normal mobility of the subtalar joint (inversion and eversion of the hindfoot). Flexible flatfoot is sometimes associated with a contracture of the Achilles tendon, and this subset of patients is most likely to be symptomatic. A rigid flatfoot is uncommon, may be unilateral or bilateral, is more often symptomatic, and usually requires a diagnostic evaluation and treatment. Flattening of the longitudinal arch occurs in non–weight-bearing positions, associated with a restriction in subtalar motion. The etiology of a rigid flatfoot may be congenital (tarsal coalition, vertical talus), neuromuscular (cerebral palsy, hypotonia), inflammatory (juvenile idiopathic arthritis), or associated with a connective tissue disease or syndrome (Ehlers-Danlos, Marfan, or Down syndrome). Idiopathic rigid flatfoot may be seen in obesity. In some of these cases the flatfoot is initially flexible but becomes more rigid over time.

Clinical Symptoms

Flexible flatfoot usually is asymptomatic, although some patients may report activity-related discomfort in the medial hindfoot region (and under the longitudinal arch) and/or the ankles and legs. These children may feel that they are unable to keep up with peers in running activities and that they become fatigued easily. Symptoms are much more common when the flatfoot is associated with a contracture of the Achilles tendon; these patients have mainly activity-related pain in the hindfoot region.

Figure 1 Medial (**A**) and posterior (**B**) views of flatfoot.

Tests

Physical Examination

The flexible flatfoot has a normal appearance when in a non–weight-bearing position. Findings in the weight-bearing position include loss of the longitudinal arch, valgus alignment of the hindfoot with prominence of the medial malleolus, and abduction of the forefoot relative to the hindfoot (**Figure 1**). With severe pes planovalgus, the medial border of the foot is convex, and the lateral border is concave. To identify the presence of an Achilles tendon contracture, ankle range of motion is assessed by dorsiflexing the foot; normal range of motion is more than 10°. During this test, the hindfoot is held in an inverted position to lock the subtalar joint and avoid "spurious" dorsiflexion through the hindfoot joints. Subtalar motion should always be assessed manually, and any restriction or asymmetry in motion between sides should be recorded. The "Jack test," or great toe extension test, re-created the arch during weight bearing in a flexible flatfoot. The flexibility of the hindfoot is assessed by asking the patient to stand on his or her tiptoes. In a flexible flatfoot, the medial longitudinal arch is restored, and the hindfoot will roll from valgus into varus in this position (**Figure 2**). The arch cannot be re-created by any means in a rigid flatfoot. A careful neurologic examination is required, as well as an assessment of connective tissue laxity.

Diagnostic Tests

Radiographs (weight-bearing AP and lateral views of the foot) are indicated only in children who are symptomatic. An oblique radiograph (and often a Harris heel view) of the foot also is obtained when the flatfoot is rigid.

SECTION 9 PEDIATRIC ORTHOPAEDICS

Figure 2 Elevation of the arches in flexible flatfeet by the Jack test (**A**) and standing on toes (**B**).

Differential Diagnosis

- Calcaneovalgus foot (infancy, abnormal molding in utero)
- Flexible flatfoot associated with a connective tissue disease or syndrome (Down syndrome, Marfan syndrome, Ehlers-Danlos syndrome, others)
- Flexible flatfoot without Achilles tendon contracture (all ages, normal hindfoot motion)
- Rigid flatfoot associated with juvenile idiopathic arthritis
- Rigid flatfoot associated with neurologic diseases (cerebral palsy, others), connective tissue disorders, or syndromes
- Rigid flatfoot caused by congenital vertical talus (infancy and early childhood, rigid, underlying neuromuscular diagnosis or associated syndrome is common)
- Rigid flatfoot caused by tarsal coalition (adolescence, activity-related hindfoot pain)

Adverse Outcomes of the Disease

Flexible flatfoot is a normal variation of the shape of the foot that rarely causes disability or requires treatment. Pain, disability, and the need for treatment are more common in children who have a contracted Achilles tendon in association with flexible flatfoot. Rigid flatfeet are commonly symptomatic because of the altered kinematics of the hindfoot joints.

Treatment

Young children typically are asymptomatic, but the parents are often concerned about the appearance of the feet. Parents should be advised that flattening of the longitudinal arch usually improves and that corrective shoes and orthoses will not have a beneficial effect on the development of the longitudinal arch or the natural history. Furthermore, it is helpful to remind parents that adults with high arches (cavus feet) are more likely to have pain, and most adults with flatfeet are asymptomatic. Children should wear shoes with a flexible sole (rigid designs should be avoided), but time without footwear should be encouraged.

Patients with symptomatic flexible flatfoot may obtain relief with a shoe insert. Generally, treatment is best begun with an over-the-counter orthosis; custom-molded devices can be used for refractory symptoms. Arch support is less important than controlling the hindfoot. For symptomatic deformities of greater severity, especially in patients with secondary flexible flatfeet, specific orthotic designs may be considered to achieve greater control of the hindfoot. A UCBL (University of California Biomechanics Laboratory) orthosis provides better control of the hindfoot. Rarely, a supramalleolar (trim lines extend above the malleoli) orthosis will be required to control the hindfoot.

Older children and adolescents with foot pain related to a contracted Achilles tendon may benefit from daily heel cord stretching exercises. Orthoses are helpful to control the hindfoot and prevent recurrence of the contracture, but the specific type or construction depends on the underlying etiology of the flatfoot and abnormal biomechanics.

Surgery is rarely indicated for flexible flatfoot. The exception is the older child with symptoms that persist despite a vigorous program of Achilles tendon stretching, orthosis use, and shoe modifications. Osteotomy to lengthen the lateral column of the foot, as opposed to arthrodesis, is a generally accepted principle for managing this condition.

Surgical treatment is often required in patients with a rigid flatfoot. The procedure depends on the underlying diagnosis and findings. Lengthening of the Achilles tendon can be considered if stretching fails to relieve symptoms associated with a flexible flatfoot with an Achilles tendon contracture. A symptomatic tarsal coalition may require excision of the connection (bone, cartilage, or fibrous tissue) between the tarsal bones in some patients, and a subset of these cases will be best managed with a hindfoot fusion, often with realignment.

Adverse Outcomes of Treatment

Numerous surgical procedures have been developed to treat flexible flatfeet in young children. Nearly all have been abandoned because of the benign natural history of the condition and because the various procedures have had inconsistent results and frequent complications.

SECTION 9 PEDIATRIC ORTHOPAEDICS

Referral Decisions/Red Flags

Children with a flexible flatfoot typically do not require referral unless they have persistent symptoms or an associated Achilles tendon contracture. Most patients with a rigid flatfoot require further evaluation, particularly if symptoms are present.

Fractures in Children

Fractures are more common in children than in adults, due in part to their play and in part to the different characteristics of their bone. The strength of bone gradually increases as a child grows, but a child's bone is not as strong as that of an adult until late adolescence. As a result, bone is the weak link in children, and ligamentous injuries are uncommon until late adolescence.

Fractures are uncommon in children younger than 3 years. Infants and young children usually are protected by their self-limiting activity, even though their bones are weaker. Nonaccidental trauma, however, is significantly higher in very young children, as described in the chapter on child abuse (page 1021). In children older than 3 years, the incidence of fractures gradually increases until it peaks during adolescence. The incidence also is higher in boys and during the summer months.

Plasticity of bone (the modulus of elasticity) is greater in children—a child's bone can bend or deform without completely breaking. As a result, torus and greenstick fractures are common fracture patterns in children, but these injuries rarely are seen in adults.

Bone healing is more rapid in children. For example, a fracture of the femur in an adult requires 16 to 20 weeks of immobilization if treated by closed means. By comparison, the same fracture requires only 2 weeks of immobilization in an infant and 4 to 6 weeks of casting in young children. Because of more rapid healing, nonunion is very uncommon in children.

Fractures involving the growth plate or physis are unique to children, accounting for 15% to 20% of all pediatric fractures. (See Fractures of the Growth Plate, page 1073).

Bone remodeling is greater in children, and some postfracture malalignments will spontaneously self-correct. The potential for remodeling is greater in younger children, in fractures close to the physis, and in fractures angulated in the plane of motion (**Figure 1**). For example, a fracture of the distal radius with 35° of volar or dorsal angulation in a 5-year-old child will completely remodel in 1 to 2 years ("a degree a month"), even if no reduction is performed. In this instance, the primary reason for reduction is to relieve pressure on adjacent soft tissues. Angular correction in other planes is less predictable, and rotational deformities typically do not correct.

Pediatric fractures present special considerations for diagnosis and management that deserve comment: A fracture might not be visible on routine radiographs when it involves only the physis and when the secondary ossification center has not ossified.

SECTION 9 PEDIATRIC ORTHOPAEDICS

Figure 1 Radiographs show remodeling of a fracture of the distal forearm in a 5-year-old child. PA (**A**) and lateral (**B**) radiographs immediately postinjury. PA (**C**) and lateral (**D**) radiographs 3 weeks postinjury. PA (**E**) and lateral (**F**) radiographs 7 months postinjury.

Young children are also less tolerant of major blood loss, and a child with a displaced femoral fracture or multiple trauma must be monitored carefully.

Most displaced fractures in children are managed with closed reduction and casting, whereas displaced fractures in adults often require internal or external fixation devices (requiring surgery). The thick periosteum in children helps in maintaining the reduction. Pediatric fractures heal more rapidly than those in adults, which reduces the duration of and complications associated with immobilization. Furthermore, unlike adults, complications of prolonged bed rest such as pneumonia and thrombophlebitis are very uncommon in children, so body casts may be used to treat complex pediatric fractures involving the spine, pelvis, and lower extremities.

Fractures of the Growth Plate

Definition

Any fracture that involves the epiphyseal growth plate (the physis) is called a physeal fracture. The Salter-Harris classification (**Figure 1**) is the system that has been most commonly used to describe these injuries, although some concern exists that a Salter-Harris type V fracture does not occur and that this system does not describe all fracture patterns.

Clinical Symptoms

Patients have acute pain and localized tenderness and swelling. They also may have deformity and restricted motion of the involved site. There is a history of trauma.

Tests

Physical Examination

Tenderness and swelling are localized and always present with maximum tenderness over the growth plate. Vascular and neurologic compromises are rare because the fracture does not involve muscle compartments.

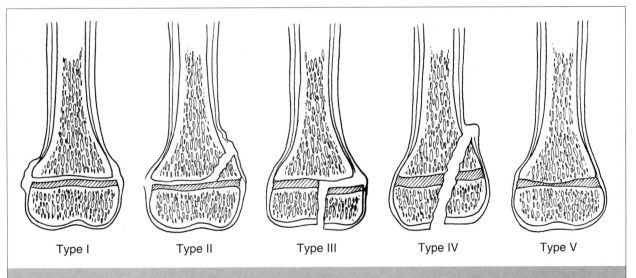

Type I   Type II   Type III   Type IV   Type V

Figure 1   Salter-Harris classification of physeal fractures. (Reproduced from Kay RM, Matthys GA: Pediatric ankle fractures: Evaluation and treatment. *J Am Acad Orthop Surg* 2001;9:268-278.)

Diagnostic Tests

AP and lateral radiographs usually identify the fracture. Oblique views will increase the ability to identify the fracture. Some nondisplaced fractures may show soft-tissue swelling only.

Differential Diagnosis

■ Contusion (swelling and ecchymosis near a joint, negative radiographs)

■ Dislocation (evident on radiographs)

■ Fracture of the metaphysis of a long bone (radiographs show no involvement of the physis)

■ Osteochondral fracture (involves articular surface but not the physis)

■ Sprain (swelling, maximum tenderness over the ligament, negative radiographs)

Adverse Outcomes of the Disease

Premature growth arrest (partial or complete) will result in diminished bone length and angulation deformity. Nonunion and overgrowth are rare.

Treatment

The goals are reduction, maintaining the reduction during the healing process, restoring normal growth, and avoiding growth arrest. These fractures heal rapidly, usually within 4 to 6 weeks.

Closed reduction and cast immobilization are indicated in Salter-Harris fracture types I, II, and III. Minimally displaced fractures require only immobilization. In boys 15 years and older and girls 13 years and older, mild displacement may be acceptable because if premature arrest occurs, these patients have little growth remaining in which significant limb-length discrepancy or deformity can develop. Conversely, in these same patients, less angular deformity can be accepted because there is less time for the fracture to remodel before the patient reaches skeletal maturity.

Salter-Harris fracture types IV and V involve the cartilage of both the growth plate and the articular surface. Therefore, anatomic reduction is required to ensure a congruous joint surface and to prevent development of a bone bridge (usually called a physeal bar) between the epiphysis and metaphysis (**Figure 2**). In most instances, open reduction and internal fixation is necessary to obtain and maintain reduction.

Open fracture requires immediate surgical attention. Physeal bars may develop after this injury and, if the patient has significant growth remaining, reconstructive surgery may be required.

Figure 2 Radiographs show a physeal bar. (Reproduced from Khoshal KI, Kiefer GN: Physeal bridge resection. *J Am Acad Orthop Surg* 2005:13;47-58.)

Adverse Outcomes of Treatment

Failure to recognize the fracture and its potential for growth arrest and failure to maintain anatomic reduction are the most common causes of a poor outcome. Physeal bars do not become evident for at least 3 months after fracture, and some not for many months. Follow-up of at least 1 year is mandatory, unless the patient reaches skeletal maturity earlier. Longer follow-up is needed for physeal fractures of the femur and tibia and for more complex injuries.

Referral Decisions/Red Flags

Displaced physeal fractures require reduction and maintenance of reduction. All patients require long-term follow-up.

SECTION 9 PEDIATRIC ORTHOPAEDICS

Fractures About the Elbow

Definition

Fractures about the elbow are common in children. Injuries involving the distal humerus account for more than 80% of these fractures (**Table 1**).

Supracondylar fractures of the distal humerus are the most common elbow fractures in children, typically affecting children between 2 and 12 years of age. This fracture does not involve the physis. Most are extension fractures, with the distal fragment angulated and/or displaced posteriorly (**Figure 1**).

The next most common injury is a fracture of the lateral condyle of the distal humerus. Fracture of the medial condyle is uncommon; however, whether on the lateral or medial side, condylar fractures are serious because the fracture typically involves the growth plate of the distal humerus and the articular surface of the elbow (**Figure 2**).

Fracture of the medial epicondyle is the third most common elbow fracture (**Figure 3**); fracture of the lateral epicondyle, however, is uncommon. The epicondyles are secondary ossification centers at sites of muscle origin. Fractures of the medial or lateral epicondyle do not involve the articular surface

Table 1 Common Sites of Elbow Fractures in Children

Distal Humerus

Supracondylar

Lateral condyle

Medial condyle

Lateral epicondyle

Medial epicondyle

Distal humeral physis

Proximal Forearm

Radial neck

Olecranon

Figure 1   Radiograph demonstrates a displaced supracondylar fracture. The humerus is outlined. (Reproduced from Sullivan JA, Anderson SJ, eds: *Care of the Young Athlete*. Rosemont, IL, American Academy of Orthopaedic Surgeons, 2000, p 317.)

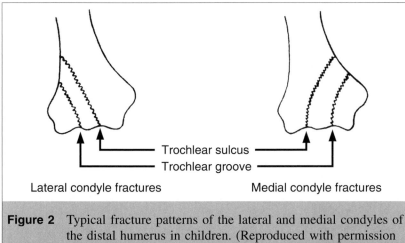

Figure 2 Typical fracture patterns of the lateral and medial condyles of the distal humerus in children. (Reproduced with permission from Milch H: Fractures and fracture-dislocations of the humeral condyles. *J Trauma* 1963;3:592-607.)

Figure 3 Radiograph demonstrates a displaced fracture of the medial epicondyle (arrow).

and do not adversely affect growth. Therefore, epicondylar fractures of the distal humerus, even when displaced, have limited consequences unless the elbow joint is concomitantly dislocated and the fragment is incarcerated in the joint. Instability under stress may result in pain, so surgical fixation is often preferred for athletes such as gymnasts and throwing athletes.

Fractures across the entire physis of the distal humerus (physeolysis) are uncommon. These injuries occur most frequently in newborns, infants, and small children as a result of child abuse.

In children, the metaphyseal portion of the radial neck is the weak link. Therefore, the valgus force that causes a fracture of the radial head in adults will result in a fracture of the radial neck in children.

Olecranon fractures are uncommon in children. These injuries usually involve the articular surface and, when displaced, require an open or closed reduction.

Clinical Symptoms

Patients have acute pain, tenderness, swelling, and most often a history of falling on an outstretched hand. The child often refuses to use the limb and holds it at the side with the elbow flexed. Swelling can be severe, but with nondisplaced or minimally displaced fractures, swelling may be mild.

SECTION 9 PEDIATRIC ORTHOPAEDICS

Figure 4 Clinical photographs demonstrate how to test for (**A**) radial, (**B**) median, and (**C**) ulnar nerve function.

Tests

Physical Examination

Evaluate the status of the median, ulnar, and radial nerves distal to the injury (**Figure 4**). Assess distal pulses and capillary filling. With obvious deformity, position or splint the limb in a position of comfort and order radiographs. In a child with no obvious deformity at the elbow, attempt to find the site of maximum tenderness and gently evaluate elbow motion.

Diagnostic Tests

AP and lateral radiographs of the elbow are necessary. The fracture may be obvious or subtle. Oblique views and comparison radiographs of the opposite elbow are helpful with subtle injuries. The radial head should be directed toward the distal humerus (capitellum) on both AP and lateral views.

An abnormal posterior fat pad sign is associated with fractures about the elbow, and the presence of this sign is particularly helpful with subtle or occult fractures. In a normal elbow, the anterior fat pad can be seen on a lateral radiograph, but the posterior fat pad is not visualized. Any process that causes an elbow effusion will elevate both anterior and posterior fat pads (**Figure 5**). The posterior fat pad is therefore often visible with elbow fractures in children (**Figure 6**), even when these injuries are not obvious on initial radiographs.

Differential Diagnosis

- Dislocation of the elbow (typically posterior, evident on radiographs)
- Hemarthrosis of the elbow (swelling, limited motion, no other positive findings)

Figure 5 Normal anterior and posterior fat pads (**A**) and anterior and posterior fat pads elevated from an effusion (**B**). (Reproduced with permission from Skaggs DL, Mirzayan R: The posterior fat pad sign in association with occult fracture of the elbow in children. *J Bone Joint Surg Am* 1999;81:1429-1433.)

Figure 6 Lateral radiograph of the elbow demonstrates a posterior fat pad sign.

- Monteggia fracture-dislocation (fracture of proximal ulna and dislocation of the radial head)
- Sprain (swelling, tenderness over the involved ligament, no evidence of fracture)
- Subluxation of the radial head (typical history and age, tenderness over radial head, negative radiographs)

Adverse Outcomes of the Disease

Supracondylar fractures have the highest incidence of neurovascular problems. Median, ulnar, and radial nerve injuries are associated with this fracture. The brachial artery may be injured, and compartment syndrome involving the volar forearm muscles may develop. Failure to recognize this problem in a

SECTION 9 PEDIATRIC ORTHOPAEDICS

timely fashion will result in necrosis of forearm muscles and subsequent contractures (Volkmann ischemic contracture). Malunion with loss of the normal carrying angle (cubitus varus) may occur.

Condylar fractures may be missed, particularly in very young children who have limited ossification of the distal humerus. In these children, only a thin wafer of metaphyseal fragment will be apparent, with the rest of the fracture involving the cartilaginous physis and trochlea and, therefore, not visible on radiographs; oblique views in internal rotation (for the lateral condyle) or external rotation (for the medial condyle) may better visualize the fracture. Fractures displaced 2 mm or more are associated with delayed union, nonunion, or malunion (rotational and/or cubitus valgus). Condylar fractures of the humerus that are initially nondisplaced may become displaced, even when immobilized, by contraction of the forearm muscles attaching at the condyle. These injuries require close follow-up and repeat radiographs.

Medial epicondyle fractures of the distal humerus do not commonly cause residual problems, even when markedly displaced, unless associated with dislocation of the elbow and a fracture fragment that is not recognized as being trapped in the joint.

Fractures across the entire distal physis of the humerus have complications that are similar but typically less severe than supracondylar fractures. In addition, the potential for child abuse should be recognized and appropriately investigated.

Fractures of the radial neck that are angulated more than 30° may be associated with loss of forearm rotation, premature closure of the growth plate, and osteonecrosis of the radial head, so reduction is preferable to preserve motion.

Fractures of the olecranon with disruption of 2 mm or more of the articular surface require reduction to prevent progressive arthritic changes.

Treatment

Nondisplaced fractures are treated with splint or cast immobilization. Condylar fractures, in particular, require repeat radiographs in 3 to 5 days. Displaced fractures require reduction and, in most cases, pinning. The exception is medial or lateral epicondyle fractures of the humerus and radial neck fractures with less than 30° of angulation.

Adverse Outcomes of Treatment

Postoperative infection can develop.

Referral Decisions/Red Flags

Any displacement or angulation, an inability to extend all fingers of the affected hand, failure of over-the-counter medications to provide pain relief, and an absent or diminished radial pulse are signs that further evaluation is necessary.

SECTION 9 PEDIATRIC ORTHOPAEDICS

Fractures of the Clavicle and Proximal Humerus

ICD-9 Codes

810.00
Clavicle fracture, closed, unspecified part

810.10
Open fracture of clavicle, unspecified part

812.00
Proximal humerus fracture, closed, unspecified part

812.2
Unspecified part of humerus

Definition

The clavicle is a common site of fracture in children. Most clavicle fractures occur in the middle third, but they can occur at either end as well. Fractures close to the sternoclavicular joint can be serious because the great vessels are located just posterior to the joint. Fractures at the distal third of the clavicle generally heal rapidly in children and typically do not require surgery.

Fractures of the proximal humerus account for about 5% of fractures in children. These fractures can occur in neonates during delivery (birth fracture) or in older children as a result of a fall. Metaphyseal fractures of the proximal humerus typically occur in children between 5 and 12 years of age; physeal fractures (those involving the growth plate) most commonly occur in children between 13 and 16 years of age. Peterson type III (Salter type II) is the most common pattern of physeal fracture.

Clinical Symptoms

Newborns with a fracture of the clavicle or proximal humerus may refuse to move the arm, a condition called pseudoparalysis. Clavicle fractures in children are characterized by acute pain, tenderness, swelling, and a palpable deformity. Fractures of the proximal humerus are less obvious because of the overlying deltoid muscle.

Tests

Physical Examination
Identify the point of maximum tenderness, and check the overlying skin for any tenting or blanching. Assess motor and sensory functions of the axillary, musculocutaneous, median, ulnar, and radial nerves. Radial and ulnar pulses should be checked as well.

Diagnostic Tests
For suspected injury to the clavicle, obtain an AP radiograph of the clavicle. AP and axillary views of the shoulder are necessary for suspected injury of the proximal humerus as well as to assess for shoulder dislocation (**Figure 1**).

Figure 1 AP radiograph demonstrates a proximal humerus fracture (arrow) in a 5-year-old boy who fell from a tree.

Differential Diagnosis

- Cleidocranial dysostosis (absence of some or all of the clavicle, frontal bossing)
- Congenital muscular torticollis (asymmetric neck motion, plagiocephaly)
- Congenital pseudarthrosis of the clavicle (atrophic ends of bone at "fracture")
- Obstetric brachial plexus palsy (inability to spontaneously move fingers/wrist/elbow)
- Pathologic fracture (injury through a bone cyst or underlying bone disorder)
- Septic arthritis/osteomyelitis of the shoulder (no visible fracture, fever, pain with range of motion)
- Shoulder dislocation (evident on radiographs)
- Soft-tissue injury to shoulder (contusion)

Adverse Outcomes of the Disease

Malunion, physeal bar and growth arrest, neurologic or vascular compromise of the involved extremity, and/or osteomyelitis in an open fracture can occur.

SECTION 9 PEDIATRIC ORTHOPAEDICS

Treatment

Newborns

Fractures in newborns and infants heal without incident and remodel well. For fractures of the clavicle, no treatment is needed. For fractures of the proximal humerus, immobilize the arm for comfort by using a swathe or pinning the sleeve to the torso of the shirt.

Young Children

Middle third clavicle fractures in young children do not require reduction, as they will remodel and straighten with time. Observation and immobilization in a sling or a figure-of-8 strap is satisfactory. Unless posterior displacement with involvement of the great vessels and/or respiratory difficulties is present, fractures of the proximal third also can be treated with a sling. Fractures of the distal third generally heal without reduction or surgery. Fractures of the proximal humerus usually are best treated with a sling. Reduction usually is not needed unless angulation of more than 40° is present.

Adolescents

Clavicle fractures in adolescents usually require only a sling or figure-of-8 strap unless the fracture is tenting or blanching the overlying skin. Shortening of more than 2 cm may indicate surgical intervention, as in adults. Fractures of the proximal humerus can be treated with a sling but may require reduction if more than 30° to 40° of angulation or less than 50% apposition of the fragments is present. Rehabilitation rarely is required unless the patient has poor range of motion or atrophy several weeks after the fracture has healed.

Adverse Outcomes of Treatment

Recurrence, malunion, growth arrest of the physis, and resulting deformity are possible.

Referral Decisions/Red Flags

Neurovascular compromise, difficulty in breathing, skin tenting or blanching over the fracture site, open fractures, displacement of more than 50%, and/or angulation of more than 40° indicate the need for further evaluation.

Fractures of the Distal Forearm

Definition

The distal third of the forearm is the most common location for fractures in children, accounting for 20% to 40% of all pediatric fractures. Types of fractures, in order of relative severity, are listed in **Table 1**. Fractures of the distal forearm are uncommon in children younger than 4 years, but torus and greenstick fractures may occur in this younger age group. In children older than 10 years, fractures involving the growth plate of the distal radial physis are more common.

A torus fracture is characterized by buckling of the cortex on only one side of the bone; it is the least complicated fracture (**Figure 1**). The most common torus fracture involves the dorsal surface of the distal radius. A metaphyseal fracture isolated to the distal radius typically is nondisplaced. In a greenstick fracture, the cortex is disrupted on the tension side but is intact or only buckled on the compression side. A Galeazzi fracture is a displaced fracture of the distal radius with a dislocation of the distal ulna or a fracture of the distal ulnar physis (**Figure 2**).

Clinical Symptoms

Patients typically report a fall on an outstretched hand. Acute pain, tenderness, and swelling are noted. With displaced fractures, the deformity is obvious. Symptoms following a torus fracture may not be immediately obvious.

ICD-9 Codes
813.42
Galeazzi fracture
Greenstick fracture of the distal radius
Metaphyseal fracture of the distal radius, complete
Physeal fracture of the distal radius
Torus fracture of the distal radius
813.44
Complete fracture of the distal radius and ulna
Greenstick fractures of the distal radius and ulna

Table 1 Types of Distal Radius Fractures in Children
Torus fracture (nondisplaced "buckle" fracture)
Metaphyseal fracture, complete
Greenstick fracture
Greenstick fractures of the distal radius and ulna
Complete fracture of the distal radius and greenstick fracture of the distal ulna
Complete fracture of the distal radius and ulna
Physeal fracture
Galeazzi fracture

Figure 1   PA (**A**) and lateral (**B**) radiographs show a torus fracture of the distal radius.

Figure 2   Lateral radiograph demonstrates a significantly displaced fracture of the distal radial physis in an 11-year-old boy who presented late. (Reproduced from Waters PM: Forearm and foot fractures, in Richards BS, ed: *Orthopaedic Knowledge Update: Pediatrics*. Rosemont, IL, American Academy of Orthopaedic Surgeons, 1996, pp 251-257.)

Tests

Physical Examination

Evaluate the status of the median, ulnar, and radial nerves distal to the fracture (see page 1076). Assess circulation at the fingertips. Examine the skin carefully, as puncture wounds are indicative of a grade I open fracture.

Diagnostic Tests

AP and lateral radiographs of the forearm should show both the wrist and elbow joints. Comparison views are rarely needed with these injuries.

Differential Diagnosis

- Child abuse (multiple injuries)
- Osteomyelitis of the distal radius or ulna (no history of injury, fever, marked tenderness)
- Pathologic fracture through a bone cyst or other tumor (evident on radiographs)
- Septic arthritis of the wrist (subacute onset, no history of injury, fever, marked swelling)
- Wrist sprain (acute symptoms, uncommon in children)

Adverse Outcomes of the Disease

Malunion or crossunion (synostosis) with loss of forearm rotation, compartment syndrome (uncommon), and osteomyelitis (in open fractures) are possible.

Figure 3 Clinical photograph of a short arm cast.

Treatment

Most of these fractures heal without incident and can be treated by closed (nonsurgical) means. Residual angulation of 10° to 15° typically will remodel completely if 1 to 2 years of growth remain. The considerable remodeling potential of distal forearm fractures is related to the large amount of growth from the distal radial and ulnar physes, which contributes approximately 80% of forearm length.

Torus fractures and nondisplaced fractures of the distal radius are stable but should be immobilized in a short arm cast or splint for comfort and to protect the bone from a second fall that could exacerbate the injury (**Figure 3**). Displaced fractures are treated initially by immobilization in a long arm cast to prevent forearm rotation. The duration of immobilization depends on the age of the child and extent of injury.

For displaced fractures of the distal forearm, the degree of angulation that is acceptable depends on the plane of angulation and the amount of growth remaining. Loss of rotational alignment is the only absolute indication for both reduction and remanipulation. Distal forearm fractures that are angulated in the volar or dorsal plane remodel well in children, even if a reduction was not performed. The principal reason for reduction is to relieve the pressure on adjacent soft tissues; therefore, closed reduction generally is indicated for angulation of 10° to 15° or more.

Unlike adults, most children with Galeazzi injuries can be treated by closed reduction.

Exploration of the fracture under general anesthesia with irrigation and débridement is critical for any open fracture, even if the wound is only a small puncture.

SECTION 9 PEDIATRIC ORTHOPAEDICS

Adverse Outcomes of Treatment

Reangulation is common in completely displaced fractures, particularly when reduction is incomplete. The decision to remanipulate the fracture depends on the age of the child (older), the degree of healing, and the plane of angulation. Significant malunion with loss of functional wrist and forearm motion can occur but is relatively uncommon. Synostosis with loss of forearm pronation and supination is rare, but it is more common with open fractures. Physeal fractures may be complicated by an arrest of growth and resulting deformity at the wrist.

Referral Decisions/Red Flags

Inability to extend all fingers, pain not relieved by over-the-counter medications, neurologic dysfunction, dislocation of the distal ulna, and/or angulation of greater than 10° to 15° requires further urgent evaluation.

Fractures of the Proximal and Middle Forearm

Definition

In children, fractures of the proximal or midportion of the forearm typically cause disruption of both the radius and the ulna (**Figure 1**). Other injury patterns include a Monteggia fracture-dislocation (radial head dislocation associated with a fracture of the ulna) (**Figure 2**), a both-bone fracture, or an isolated fracture of the ulna. An isolated ulnar fracture usually occurs secondary to a direct blow as the child places the forearm in front of the face to deflect an oncoming blow.

Clinical Symptoms

Patients have acute pain, tenderness, and swelling, usually in association with a fall on an outstretched hand.

Tests

Physical Examination

Assess median, ulnar, and radial nerve function distal to the fracture site (see page 1076). Severe or inordinate pain on passive extension of the fingers should raise concern for possible compartment syndrome.

Diagnostic Tests

Full-length AP and lateral radiographs of the forearm that include the wrist and elbow are indicated. The radial head should align with the capitellum on both views. A Monteggia injury should be excluded if a fracture of the ulna is present. In a Monteggia injury, dislocation of the radial head is usually anterior but could be posterior or lateral.

Differential Diagnosis

- Child abuse (multiple injuries)
- Osteogenesis imperfecta (previous history, thin bony cortices)
- Osteomyelitis of the proximal radius or ulna (fever, swelling)
- Pathologic fracture through a bone cyst or tumor (evident on radiographs)
- Septic arthritis of the elbow (fever, swelling, markedly restricted motion)

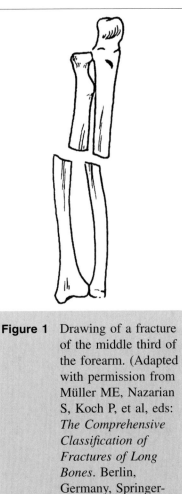

Figure 1 Drawing of a fracture of the middle third of the forearm. (Adapted with permission from Müller ME, Nazarian S, Koch P, et al, eds: *The Comprehensive Classification of Fractures of Long Bones.* Berlin, Germany, Springer-Verlag, 1990, pp 96-105.)

SECTION 9 PEDIATRIC ORTHOPAEDICS

Infant ➞ Toddler

Figure 2 Normal progression from bowlegs of infancy through slow evolution to a physiologic valgus angle of about 12° at 3 years of age. (Reproduced from Gomez JE: Growth and maturation, in Sullivan JA, Anderson SJ, eds: *Care of the Young Athlete.* Rosemont, IL, American Academy of Orthopaedic Surgeons, 1999, pp 25-32.)

(normal range, 0° to 10°) by 11 years of age. Most patients presenting for the evaluation of knock-knees will have values within the physiologic range (**Figure 3**). The goal is to identify those few patients requiring further evaluation and treatment.

Clinical Symptoms

Concern on the part of a parent or grandparent is the usual reason for the visit; children rarely have any pain or gait disturbance from variations in limb alignment. Most patients present for evaluation during the period of maximal valgus alignment, from 3 to 4 years of age. Obese children are at risk for worsening of genu valgum and should be evaluated regularly for progressive disease.

Tests

Physical Examination

The child's height and weight should be measured and plotted relative to normative data. The tibiofemoral angle may be measured with a goniometer, and the intermalleolar distance is measured as the distance between the medial malleoli with the patient standing with the medial femoral condyles touching. The lower extremity rotational alignment also should be evaluated.

Figure 3 Clinical photograph of boy referred for evaluation of "knock-knees." The patient was considered to be within normal limits. (Reproduced from Greene WB: Genu varum and genu valgum in children. *Instr Course Lect* 1994;43:151-159.)

Genu V

Synonym

Bowlegs

Definition

Genu varum (bow
the tibia medially
(**Figure 1**). Genu
spontaneously cor
limb alignment ev
age) and ultimate
The vast majority
physiologic genu
pathologic cause
adolescents. Othe
disease, posttraun
skeletal dysplasia
patients have an a
range, identifying
instituting treatme

Figure 1 AP weight
an 18-mor
Infantile ti

Diagnostic Tests

Radiographs usually are not necessary, but should be considered
when the valgus is more than 15° to 20°, or if the child is of
short stature. A weight-bearing AP radiograph on a 36 × 43–cm
cassette with the film centered at the knees and the patellae
pointing straight ahead provides screening for rickets and
skeletal dysplasia, as well as accurate measurement of the
tibiofemoral angle. Laboratory studies should be ordered when a
metabolic disease is suspected, for example with stature below
the 5th percentile or when a more generalized disorder is
suspected.

Differential Diagnosis

- Epiphyseal dysplasia (multiple epiphyseal dysplasia or
  spondyloepiphyseal dysplasia)
- Posttraumatic (history of fracture, findings of asymmetric
  growth arrest on radiographs)
- Pseudoachondroplasia (shore stature, limited range of motion,
  waddling gait)
- Rickets (nutritional, hypophosphatemic, others)

Adverse Outcomes of the Disease

Adults with excessive angulation in the frontal plane will
experience asymmetric mechanical loading of the knee and may
potentially be predisposed to early degenerative joint disease.

Treatment

Observation is the treatment of choice for an otherwise normal
3- to 4-year-old child with marked genu valgum. Shoe
modifications are ineffective, and long leg braces are not
indicated because spontaneous correction is achieved in the vast
majority of cases. In a small subset of older patients in whom
the deformity is excessive and/or symptomatic, correction may
be achieved either by growth modulation or by a realignment
osteotomy, depending on the magnitude of the deformity and the
age and skeletal maturity of the patient. Growth modulation by
hemiepiphysiodesis is an option in patients with significant
growth remaining. A reversible hemiepiphysiodesis may be
achieved by placing either a staple or a small metallic plate
across the physis on the convex side of the deformity, which
slows but does not eliminate the growth on that side. Normal
growth on the concave side will result in gradual correction of
the deformity. The device can be removed when the deformity
has been corrected and, ideally, symmetric growth is restored
and alignment is maintained. In patients who are close to the

Clinical Symptoms

Typically, medical attention is sought because parents or grandparents are concerned about how the child walks. Intoeing and outtoeing usually do not cause pain or interfere with development or stability in gait. With severe intoeing, children may stumble or trip when the foot in forward swing catches on the back of the trailing leg or the ground. With outtoeing, patients may have difficulty keeping up with their peers in running and certain sports.

Tests

Physical Examination

The examiner should recognize that a wide variation exists in what is considered normal. The physical assessment focuses on defining the magnitude and location of the intoeing or outtoeing. In addition, the family history should be reviewed. An assessment of the rotational alignment of the parents' limbs, conducted when they bring the child to the clinic, can provide helpful information to determine if any intoeing or outtoeing exists in the parents.

Measurements are compared with normative data; therefore, it is essential to know the normal range of values for these measurements for each age range. The normal rotation of an extremity about an axis is called version. A rotational value more than 2 SDs from the mean based on age-related normative data is considered torsion. The examination documents a rotational profile, which includes measuring the foot progression angle, or the angle that the foot makes relative to the line of progression as the child walks (**Figure 1**); hip rotation, or femoral rotation (**Figure 2**); thigh-foot axis, or tibial rotation (**Figure 3**); and the foot alignment. Evaluation for possible neuromuscular disorders also is important.

The foot progression angle quantifies the magnitude of intoeing or outtoeing but does not identify the location of the problem. Hip rotation is used to estimate femoral version (rotational angle of the femoral head/neck relative to the distal epicondylar axis) and is tested with the patient prone (hips extended) and the knee flexed to 90°. With one of the examiner's hands on the patients' buttocks to stabilize the pelvis, the lower leg is rotated outward to test internal (medial) rotation, and inward to test external (lateral) rotation. The degree of rotation is measured relative to the vertical axis (**Figure 4**). The average range of hip rotation for a child older than 2 years is approximately 50° of internal rotation and 40° of external rotation. An excessive amount of internal rotation (>65°) coupled with a limited degree of external rotation indicates internal femoral torsion (excessive femoral anteversion). Internal femoral torsion is classified as mild (60° to 70°),

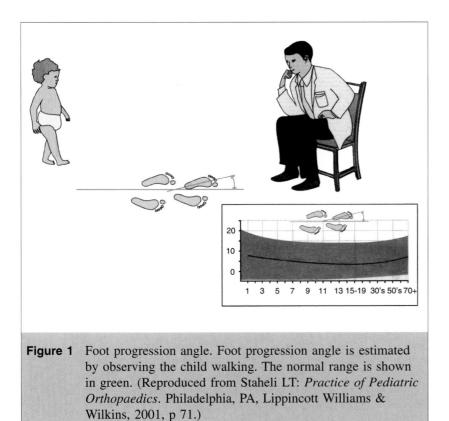

Figure 1 Foot progression angle. Foot progression angle is estimated by observing the child walking. The normal range is shown in green. (Reproduced from Staheli LT: *Practice of Pediatric Orthopaedics*. Philadelphia, PA, Lippincott Williams & Wilkins, 2001, p 71.)

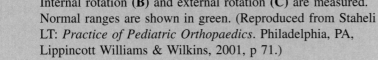

Figure 2 Hip rotation. **A,** Hip rotation is assessed with the child prone. Internal rotation (**B**) and external rotation (**C**) are measured. Normal ranges are shown in green. (Reproduced from Staheli LT: *Practice of Pediatric Orthopaedics*. Philadelphia, PA, Lippincott Williams & Wilkins, 2001, p 71.)

SECTION 9 PEDIATRIC ORTHOPAEDICS

Figure 3 Assessing rotational status of the tibia and the foot. The rotational status of the tibia and foot are best assessed by evaluating the child in the prone position. **A,** Allowing the foot to fall into a natural resting position. The thigh-foot axis (**B**) and shape of the feet (**C**) are readily determined. The range of normal is shown in green. (Reproduced from Staheli LT: *Practice of Pediatric Orthopaedics.* Philadelphia, PA, Lipponcott Williams & Wilkins, 2001, p 71.)

Figure 4 Hip rotation: Zero starting position. (Reproduced from Greene WB, Heckman JD, eds: *The Clinical Measurement of Joint Motion.* Rosemont, IL, American Academy of Orthopaedic Surgeons, 1994, pp 106-107.)

moderate (70° to 90°), or severe (more than 90°). Femoral anteversion is approximately 40° at birth and decreases to approximately 15° in adults. Infants are born with an external rotation contracture at the hip, which allows 60° to 70° of external rotation and only 20° to 30° of internal rotation. This usually improves spontaneously. Persistent or excessive external rotation represents external femoral torsion (femoral retroversion).

The lower limb axis is assessed by measuring the thigh-foot angle and the alignment of the foot. With the patient in the prone position and the knee flexed to 90° (held in neutral at the ankle and subtalar joints), the axis of the foot is measured relative to the axis of the thigh. An internal thigh-foot angle of more than 10° to 15° indicates internal tibial torsion (**Figure 5**). Foot posture is assessed for metatarsus adductus, a possible cause of intoeing, as well as hindfoot alignment. Pes planovalgus may result in outtoeing. External tibial torsion may be associated with contracture of the iliotibial band; to assess for this, the Ober test (see Physical Examination of the Knee, page 639) should be performed. For the Ober test, the patient is placed in the lateral position and the downside leg is flexed so that the thigh is touching the abdomen. The other leg is then extended, internally rotated, and adducted. The test may be

Table 1 Gross Motor Developmental Screens of Early Childhood

Age (years)	Activity
2	Stairs, one step at a time
2½	Jumps
3	Stairs, alternating feet
4	Hops on one foot
5	Skips

(Adapted from Paine RS, Oppe TE: Neurological examination of children, in *Clinics in Developmental Medicine, Nos 20/21*. London, England, William Heinemann Medical Books, 1966.)

Figure 5 Bilateral internal tibial torsion. (Adapted from Alexander IJ: *The Foot: Examination and Diagnosis*. New York, NY, Churchill Livingstone, 1990, p 115.)

positive for iliotibial band tightness if the upper leg cannot be adducted past neutral.

Patients with an underlying neuromuscular disorder may present for the evaluation of intoeing or outtoeing before the underlying disorder has been diagnosed. This is particularly common in patients with mild cerebral palsy. The patient should be assessed for appropriate motor milestones (**Table 1**) and examined for spasticity, muscle contractures, clonus, and a stiff walk or gait disturbance.

Diagnostic Tests

Radiographs are rarely needed unless the child has evidence of short stature or if the possibility of hip dysplasia exists on history or physical examination. In a subset of patients, hip dysplasia is associated with increased femoral anteversion; occasionally, it is associated with true femoral torsion.

Differential Diagnosis

- External femoral torsion (femoral retroversion)
- Internal femoral torsion (excessive femoral anteversion)
- Metatarsus adductus (forefoot adducted)
- Neuromuscular disorders (cerebral palsy or others)
- Pes planovalgus (forefoot abducted, hindfoot valgus, results in external rotation during gait)
- Skeletal dysplasias (short stature)
- Tibial torsion (increased internal or external rotation of the tibia)

Adverse Outcomes of the Disease

Children do well even if intoeing or outtoeing persists. These variations in rotational alignment have not been linked to arthritis or other problems in adulthood. Persistent intoeing may be of cosmetic concern, and toddlers and younger children may occasionally trip more frequently. Some children with internal femoral torsion also develop external tibial torsion, and this combination may result in a "miserable malalignment syndrome" with patellofemoral pain and often patellar subluxation. Patients with external torsion and/or a planovalgus foot may report being unable to keep up with other children while running and playing some sports.

Treatment

Treatment focuses on education and reassurance for the family, as most cases will improve or resolve spontaneously. Shoe modifications, braces, and exercises do not alter the normal rotational development of the femoral and tibial axes. Foot deformities may require specific treatments, such as casting for persistent or rigid metatarsus adductus; this is described more fully in the chapter on Metatarsus Adductus (page 1131) . Derotational osteotomy of the affected bone (femur or tibia) is reserved for the less than 1% of patients with severe torsional abnormalities. To allow for maximal spontaneous correction, a tibial osteotomy is usually not considered until 6 to 8 years of age, and a femoral osteotomy is delayed until at least 10 to 12 years of age. Chronic symptoms due to miserable malalignment syndrome are treated by correcting the rotational abnormalities at each level. In children with cerebral palsy and other neuromuscular disorders, abnormal femoral and tibial torsion persist in a much higher percentage of patients and are more likely to require surgical correction.

Adverse Outcomes of Treatment

Risks of surgery include failure to heal, infection, overcorrection or undercorrection of the deformity, or postoperative angular deformity. Risks of casting for metatarsus adductus are minimal.

Referral Decisions/Red Flags

Physicians who are familiar with the evaluation and examination of this problem can adequately reassure parents regarding the frequent resolution of these deformities. When metatarsus adductus persists in an infant older than 6 months, or when significant rotational problems persist beyond 4 to 6 years of age, evaluation by a specialist is sometimes necessary to allay concerns of the parents or grandparents. Asymmetric intoeing may represent spasticity on the more severe side, although tibial torsion may be asymmetric; femoral anteversion should be symmetric, so asymmetry in hip rotation may represent spasticity or underlying bony abnormalities. Asymmetric out-

SECTION 9 PEDIATRIC ORTHOPAEDICS

toeing may be due to asymmetric tibial torsion, but out-toeing is a common position of comfort in the presence of injury, infection, or other bony abnormality; a full evaluation should be conducted for pain or limitations in joint range of motion and their potential etiologies.

SECTION 9 PEDIATRIC ORTHOPAEDICS

Juvenile Idiopathic Arthritis

Synonyms

Juvenile chronic arthritis (JCA)

Juvenile rheumatoid arthritis (JRA)

Still disease

Definition

Formerly called juvenile rheumatoid arthritis (JRA) in North America and juvenile chronic arthritis (JCA) in Europe, juvenile idiopathic arthritis (JIA) is the term now used for the various forms of chronic arthritis that affect children. At least seven types of arthritis occur in children (**Table 1**), but common to all JIA types is a chronic arthritis that persists for at least 6 weeks in a joint and begins in patients younger than 16 years.

Clinical Symptoms

All JIA is characterized by the classic symptoms of inflammatory arthritis: joint pain and swelling and inactivity stiffness (stiffness, usually upon arising or after long periods of inactivity, such as after sleeping, that improves with activity). Small children may be unable to verbalize what or where the problem is, so they may just limp or be irritable when symptomatic. Each type of JIA has distinct ages of onset, associated symptoms, and sex predilection.

Systemic JIA is distinct from other types of JIA in that it is characterized by prominent systemic manifestations: daily spikes of high fever; evanescent (nonfixed) pink macular rash; and often liver, spleen, and/or lymph node enlargement, as well as serositis (usually pericarditis when it occurs). The arthritis may not be present initially in these patients, and when it is present, it can involve any number of joints. This disease affects boys and girls equally and can occur at any age. It is called Still disease in patients older than 16 years. Patients with systemic JIA are often quite ill and are anemic, with a very high white blood cell count, platelet count, erythrocyte sedimentation rate (ESR), and C-reactive protein (CRP) level. The ferritin level may be dramatically elevated.

Oligoarticular JIA (similar to what was formerly referred to as pauciarticular JRA) almost always occurs in girls and typically begins at a young age (younger than 6 years, and very often at 2 years of age), with gradual onset of discomfort and

Table 1 Types of Juvenile Idiopathic Arthritis

Type	Characteristics
Systemic	Arthritis (any number of joints) High spiking fevers Rash Other systemic manifestations (lymphadenopathy, hepatosplenomegaly, pericarditis)
Oligoarticular	Arthritis in four or fewer joints High risk of asymptomatic uveitis
RF-negative polyarticular	Usually widespread polyarthritis in five or more joints RF not present
RF-positive polyarticular	Usually widespread symmetric polyarthritis in five or more joints Highly positive for RF
Psoriatic	Arthritis in any number of joints Associated with psoriasis, psoriatic nail changes, or first-degree relative with psoriasis
Enthesitis-related	Arthritis in any number of joints Associated with enthesitis, inflammatory spine arthritis, sacroiliitis Tendency to be HLA-B27 positive
Undifferentiated	Arthritis that does not fit into other classifications

RF = rheumatoid factor, HLA-B27 = human leukocyte antigen B27.

swelling in one to four joints. The knee is the most commonly affected joint. The antinuclear antibody (ANA) test may be positive; other blood tests are almost always normal. Oligoarticular JIA patients are at very high risk of developing asymptomatic uveitis, so they must be screened every 3 months by an ophthalmologist. Some may develop more joint involvement over the first 5 years; these patients are referred to as having extended oligoarticular JIA.

Rheumatoid factor (RF)–negative polyarticular JIA most commonly occurs in patients younger than 5 years, and usually by preadolescence. It is characterized by the gradual onset of polyarthritis involving five or more small and large joints. The pattern may be symmetric or asymmetric. Girls are three times more likely to be affected than boys. The ANA test may be positive and the ESR may be elevated, but in some patients blood tests may be normal.

RF-positive polyarticular JIA occurs in older children and adolescents, almost always older than 10 years. It is much more common in females. This aggressive, symmetric polyarthritis affects small and large joints and may be associated with rheumatoid nodules. RF-positive polyarticular JIA is virtually indistinguishable from adult rheumatoid arthritis. The ANA test

SECTION 9 PEDIATRIC ORTHOPAEDICS

and the anticyclic citrullinated peptide (CCP) antibody (anti-CCP) test may be positive in these patients. The RF is positive by definition, usually in high titer. In active disease, the ESR is usually elevated.

Psoriatic JIA is arthritis associated with psoriasis and can affect any number of joints in a variable pattern (oligoarthritis, dactylitis, or polyarthritis). In children, the psoriasis may develop years after the arthritis, so a child with arthritis who has a strong family history of psoriasis or has nail changes (pitting or onycholysis) should be suspected of having this disorder. Chronic uveitis is common in this disease, so patients also need ophthalmologic screening three to four times a year.

Enthesitis-related JIA is arthritis associated with enthesitis (inflammation of tendon, fascia, or joint capsule insertions, especially around the heel). It may involve any number of joints but has a predilection for large weight-bearing joints. Boys are more often affected. Onset is usually at 6 years or older, and it occurs much more commonly in adolescents. A family history of spondyloarthropathies or inflammatory bowel disease often is present. Older children or adolescents may have inflammatory back pain and sacroiliitis, but these symptoms are often not present at onset. Most of these patients are human leukocyte antigen (HLA)-B27–positive. Acute uveitis with sudden onset of a red, painful eye may occur. In some patients, spinal involvement may evolve into ankylosing spondylitis.

Undifferentiated JIA is chronic arthritis that occurs in patients younger than 16 years and that does not fit into one of the above categories.

Tests

Physical Examination

A child with suspected arthritis or who has musculoskeletal pain or dysfunction should have all joints examined for possible arthritis because some children cannot verbalize their symptoms, and others may not report pain. Each joint should be (1) observed for obvious swelling, deformity, discoloration, surrounding muscular atrophy, and asymmetry with the opposite side; (2) palpated for warmth, tenderness, crepitus, and swelling and/or effusion; and (3) assessed for passive and active ranges of motion, including testing the ends of each arc of motion for even small amounts of loss of motion, and also assessed for pain at the ends of passive ranges of motion. The entheses around the heel and knee should be palpated for tenderness, and the spine and sacroiliac joints should be evaluated for tenderness and loss of motion. The temporomandibular joints may be affected even if they are asymptomatic, and they can become significantly deformed if untreated, so these should be examined carefully. The child's gait and strength should be evaluated. A general physical examination also should be performed, as arthritis can be a sign/symptom of many other diseases that may have other physical findings/clues.

Diagnostic Tests

A general screening panel, including a complete blood cell count with differential, ESR and/or CRP level, comprehensive metabolic panel, and urinalysis should be ordered. In addition, depending on the type of arthritis the child may have (based on the history and examination), ferritin, RF, ANA, and HLA-B27 tests may be considered; however, remember that normal blood tests do not rule out JIA, and positive tests are not diagnostic. If the child appears to have a more acute form of arthritis, blood tests that detect other infectious and noninfectious causes should be ordered. Radiographs of involved joints should generally be obtained to exclude occult fractures, malignancy, or unsuspected bony dysplasias, but these will generally be normal in children with JIA of recent onset.

Differential Diagnosis

- Acute causes of arthritis (acute rheumatic fever, Lyme disease [Lyme arthritis], reactive arthritis, viral arthritis, especially parvovirus-associated arthritis)
- Enteropathic diseases (eg, inflammatory bowel disease and celiac disease) (usually associated with abdominal pain, diarrhea, weight loss, poor growth)
- Hemophilic arthropathy (history of easy bruising or extreme bleeding)
- Leukemia and metastatic neuroblastoma (night pain, bone pain with refusal to bear weight, joint pain or effusion)
- Lupus and other rheumatic diseases (often associated with signs of other organ system involvement such as various rashes, fever, proteinuria/hematuria, weight loss, hypertension)
- Mechanical joint pain (occurs after increased activity and not after inactivity, symptoms of locking and "giving way," can be associated with hypermobility)
- Osteomyelitis (fever, severe pain with refusal to bear weight, toxic appearance and point tenderness of the involved bone)
- Septic arthritis (constant fever, usually single joint involvement, more severe pain and refusal to move joint)

SECTION 9 PEDIATRIC ORTHOPAEDICS

Adverse Outcomes of the Disease

Contrary to popular belief, spontaneous remission is uncommon, although some types of JIA have a better prognosis than others. Most patients will have chronic arthritis into adulthood and may have significant joint/bone deformities and limitations. Blindness may develop with untreated uveitis. Persistent or untreated joint inflammation may lead to progressive degenerative joint changes.

Treatment

Treatment depends on the type of JIA and the severity of the arthritis. NSAIDs are the first-line drugs. If only a few joints are involved, intra-articular steroids can be used. Unless arthritis is very mild, most patients are treated with disease-modifying anti-rheumatic drugs (DMARDs), primarily methotrexate but also anti–tumor necrosis factor (TNF) agents such as etanercept, infliximab, and adalimumab. Infliximab and adalimumab also are useful in refractory uveitis. Other biologics used for JIA include abatacept (a T-cell co-stimulation blocker), interleukin (IL)-1 blocking agents such as anakinra (especially for systemic JIA), anti–B cell antibodies such as rituximab (for RF-positive polyarticular JIA), and anti–IL-6. These treatments should be administered with the guidance of an experienced pediatric rheumatologist.

Rehabilitation is helpful in maintaining joint motion and strength when the pain has diminished. Children should be encouraged to participate in as much physical activity as tolerated. Splinting is generally not helpful unless a significant flexion contracture exists, and the splint should be used only at night. Orthoses may help maintain functional joint alignment. Regular ophthalmologic slit lamp examinations for uveitis are necessary, with the frequency of this examination dependent on the type of JIA, results of the ANA test, and the age of the child.

Adverse Outcomes of Treatment

NSAIDs can cause gastric, renal, or hepatic complications. Methotrexate requires regular safety monitoring and can cause centrally induced nausea. Increased susceptibility to infection is a concern with any biologic agent, but fungal and tuberculous infections are a particular concern with anti-TNF agents, so patients on these medications should be screened and monitored. Whether these agents can increase susceptibility to secondary malignancies is not known.

Referral Decisions/Red Flags

Atypical symptoms such as unexplained fever or severe pain and refusal to bear weight indicate the need for further evaluation. All patients suspected of having JIA should probably be referred to a pediatric rheumatologist if possible.

SECTION 9 PEDIATRIC ORTHOPAEDICS

Kyphosis

ICD-9 Codes

732.0
Scheuermann disease

737.0
Postural kyphosis

Synonyms

Juvenile kyphosis
Postural roundback
Scheuermann disease

Definition

Kyphosis is the normal spine profile of the thoracic region of the spinal column. It originates from the Greek word *kyphos,* meaning "humpbacked," and refers to a curve pointing backward (that is, the apex of the curve is posterior). The normal range of thoracic kyphosis is 20° to 50° (Cobb angle from T3 to T12), and values greater than 50° are considered hyperkyphotic. Conditions associated with hyperkyphosis in children are listed under Differential Diagnosis.

Postural kyphosis and Scheuermann disease are the most common causes of hyperkyphosis, and both present during adolescence. Postural kyphosis is a flexible deformity that is more common in girls, and patients are able to correct the kyphosis voluntarily. Scheuermann disease, in contrast, is more common in boys and is not passively correctable. Scheuermann disease is diagnosed radiographically as a hyperkyphosis associated with anterior wedging of more than 5° in at least three successive vertebrae, usually with disk space narrowing, irregularities of the vertebral end-plates, and Schmorl nodes (herniations of disk material through the vertebral end plates). Congenital kyphosis implies a structural defect in vertebral formation, and may become apparent in infants and toddlers; the other forms of kyphosis may be diagnosed throughout childhood and adolescence.

Clinical Symptoms

Most patients are seen for cosmetic concerns, poor posture, and/or activity-related discomfort in the mid to lower thoracic spine. Any discomfort is usually relieved by rest. Neurologic symptoms are very uncommon, except with congenital kyphosis.

Tests

Physical Examination

Hyperkyphosis is apparent when viewing the patient from the side, and the deformity is increased on the Adam forward bend test (**Figure 1**). Adolescents with Scheuermann disease and other

Figure 1 Adam forward bend test. **A,** Normal spine profile. **B,** Angulated spine profile seen in a patient with Scheuermann disease. (Reproduced from Staheli L, ed: *Pediatric Orthopaedic Secrets*. Hanley & Belfus, Inc, Philadelphia, PA, 1998, p 286.)

pathologic causes of kyphosis usually have a sharp angulation at the apex of the kyphosis, whereas patients with postural kyphosis have a more gentle curvature. Patients with postural kyphosis have normal flexibility (ie, the spine flattens in the supine position). The neurologic examination is usually normal in postural hyperkyphosis and Scheuermann disease but may be abnormal with other forms of kyphosis, especially when the deformity is severe. Hamstring spasm and/or contracture are common with pathologic forms of hyperkyphosis.

Diagnostic Tests

AP and lateral radiographs of the entire spine should be obtained with the patient standing. The reviewer should look for congenital abnormalities as well as irregularities of the vertebrae, disk spaces, and the end plates. The curve magnitude is measured on the lateral radiograph using the Cobb method. When the upper thoracic vertebrae cannot be well visualized, kyphosis should be measured from T5 to T12. The angle is formed by the intersection of a line drawn along the superior end plate of T5 and a line drawn on the inferior end plate of T12. Any curvature exceeding 50° is considered abnormal.

Differential Diagnosis

- Congenital
  Failure of formation (hemivertebra)
  Failure of segmentation (congenital fusion or wedge vertebra)
- Connective tissue diseases
  Marfan syndrome (ligamentous hyperlaxity)
  Osteogenesis imperfecta (frequent fractures, low bone mass)
- Dysplasias
  Achondroplasia (short stature)
  Mucopolysaccharidosis (short stature, neurologic symptoms)
  Neurofibromatosis (café-au-lait spots, subcutaneous neurofibromas, inguinal and/or axillary freckling)
- Iatrogenic (history of steroid use, radiation, or surgery)
- Infectious (fever, constant pain)
  Fungal (other fungal infections)
  Tuberculosis (Pott disease) (other mycobacterial infections)
- Inflammatory
  Juvenile idiopathic arthritis requiring prolonged steroids (multiple joint involvement, osteopenia)
- Metabolic
  Gaucher disease (stress fractures due to other etiologies)
  Osteoporosis (chronic steroid use, idiopathic osteoporosis of childhood)
  Thalassemia (other anemias)
- Neoplastic (constant pain, signs of systemic illness)
  Eosinophilic granuloma (other infections)
  Leukemia (other infections)
- Neuromuscular (cerebral palsy, spinal muscular atrophy, others)
- Postural hyperkyphosis (patient can self-correct)
- Scheuermann disease (activity-related back pain)
- Traumatic (fractures or ligamentous injuries)

Adverse Outcomes of the Disease

The natural history of flexible or postural hyperkyphosis is benign, and these curves are unlikely to progress, but other forms of kyphosis present a significant risk for progression. The consequences of a progressive kyphosis may include back pain; rarely, neurologic symptoms, usually seen with congenital kyphosis; and a decrease in pulmonary function, seen with curvatures greater than 90° to 100° (restrictive pattern).

Treatment

Postural kyphosis can be observed or treated with an exercise program. Progressive curvatures due to Scheuermann disease may be treated by a bracing program in patients who are skeletally immature (full-time wear, Milwaukee brace or equivalent), and a subset of patients with progressive and symptomatic curvatures greater than 70° are candidates for a posterior or an anterior/posterior spinal fusion with instrumentation (**Figure 2**). Congenital kyphosis is much more likely to require surgical intervention, sometimes in the first few years of life. Bracing is not effective in patients with congenital deformities, and progressive deformities often require surgical stabilization.

Adverse Outcomes of Treatment

Bracing may fail to prevent progression. Surgical treatment may be complicated by progression of deformity, nonunion of the fusion (pseudarthrosis), infection, implant-related complications such as loss of fixation or correction, medical problems such as pneumonia, and, rarely, spinal cord injury.

Referral Decisions/Red Flags

Deformities of greater magnitude, especially those associated with a structural component and/or pain, require specialty evaluation.

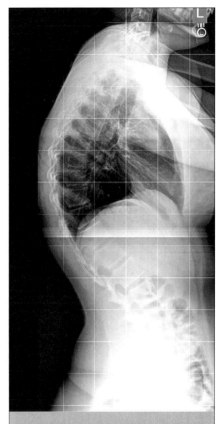

Figure 2 Radiograph of a 15-year-old girl who developed a progressive and rigid posture problem associated with back pain. The radiograph demonstrates abnormalities suggestive of thoracic Scheuermann disease. Although most patients with hyper-kyphosis can be treated nonsurgically, this patient ultimately required an instrumented posterior spinal fusion.

SECTION 9 PEDIATRIC ORTHOPAEDICS

Legg-Calvé-Perthes Disease

Synonyms

Aseptic necrosis of the femoral head

Avascular necrosis of the femoral head

(Idiopathic) osteonecrosis of the femoral head

LCPD

Definition

Legg-Calvé-Perthes disease (LCPD) is an idiopathic osteonecrosis of the femoral head in children. It is most commonly diagnosed in boys between 4 and 8 years of age. Although numerous etiologic theories have been pursued, such as heritable coagulopathy and secondhand smoke, none has been proved. Most patients (90%) with LCPD are delayed in bone age, and one third may be diagnosed with attention deficit hyperactivity disorder. A small percentage of patients has a history of transient synovitis of the hip, and 10% to 12% have bilateral disease. The physiology of the healing process in LCPD involves revascularization of the femoral head, removal of necrotic bone, and replacement with viable bone that is initially relatively weak (woven bone), followed by remodeling of woven bone to normal lamellar bone. This biologic process occurs more rapidly and with greater consistency in children, but it still takes time. The clinical symptoms often last up to 18 months, and radiographic healing and remodeling may take 4 to 5 years. The prognosis is worse in older children (because they have less potential for joint remodeling) and in patients with greater degrees of involvement of the capital femoral epiphysis. In older patients with severe involvement, deformation of the femoral head and some incongruity between the femoral head and the acetabulum may result, which may lead to premature arthritis.

Clinical Symptoms

Typically, the child has been limping for 3 to 6 weeks by the time of the initial visit. Activity worsens the limp, making symptoms more noticeable at the end of the day. If the child reports pain, it is typically an aching in the groin or proximal thigh. For knee pain, always assess the hip.

Figure 1 Radiograph of a 7-year-old boy with a 2-month history of right hip pain who was diagnosed with LCPD. The subchondral fracture (arrow) is through 75% of the femoral head. (Reproduced from Beaty JH: Legg-Calvé-Perthes disease: Diagnostic and prognostic techniques. *Instr Course Lect* 1989;38:291-296.)

Tests

Physical Examination

Range-of-motion testing will reveal restriction, especially in abduction and internal rotation, and there may be guarding at the extremes of motion. A flexion contracture also may develop. The gait examination will reveal an abductor lurch, and atrophy of the gluteal muscles also may be identified.

Diagnostic Tests

AP and frog-lateral radiographs of the pelvis should be obtained; these may be normal very early in the disease course. MRI is not needed for all cases but can be useful when the diagnosis is elusive. Findings on plain radiographs evolve over 2 to 5 years, and various stages have been described. Initial findings include a decrease in the size of the ossific nucleus and an increase in density, usually during the first 6 to 9 months. The crescent sign, which represents a subchondral fracture, is seen on frog-lateral radiographs in many patients (**Figure 1**). Next is the fragmentation stage, with collapse of the epiphysis to a variable degree. This is followed by the reossification phase, when healing takes place. The osteonecrosis often affects the physis, resulting in chronic changes in the alignment and morphology of the femoral head and neck, including shortening and widening of the femoral neck and valgus alignment of the proximal femur. Coxa magna, or enlargement of the femoral head, is a common finding as well. In patients with bilateral LCPD, the sides typically appear to be in different stages of the disease process

SECTION 9 PEDIATRIC ORTHOPAEDICS

Figure 2 Radiograph of 6-year-old boy shows bilateral LCPD. The radiographic changes are typically asymmetric, and onset of symptoms may be months apart.

(**Figure 2**). In a child with bilateral involvement, especially when radiographic changes are symmetrical, screening AP radiographs of the hand, knee, and spine are needed to rule out an epiphyseal dysplasia, and laboratory studies should be obtained to rule out hypothyroidism.

Differential Diagnosis

- Atypical septic arthritis (increasing pain and constitutional symptoms)
- Gaucher disease (osteonecrosis secondary to cerebroside and infarcts)
- Hypothyroidism (delayed development)
- Multiple epiphyseal dysplasia (bilateral, mild short stature, autosomal dominant)
- Sickle cell anemia (osteonecrosis secondary to vascular infarcts)
- Spondyloepiphyseal dysplasia (bilateral, marked short stature)
- Stickler syndrome (bilateral, short stature)
- Transient synovitis (history of recent viral illness, mild limp)
- Leukemia (constant pain, night pain)

Adverse Outcomes of the Disease

Residual deformity of the femoral head and incongruity between the femoral head and the acetabulum may result in premature degenerative changes in the hip (**Figure 3**). Limb-length discrepancy also is common.

Figure 3 AP pelvis radiographs of a patient with right-sided LCPD. **A,** Radiograph obtained on presentation shows increased density in the entire epiphysis. **B,** Radiograph obtained during the fragmentation stage shows progressive collapse of the epiphysis. **C,** Radiograph obtained at final healing several years later shows enlargement of the femoral head (coxa magna) with asphericity and shortening/widening of the femoral neck. Note that the acetabulum has remodeled as well, resulting in aspherical congruence.

Treatment

The treatment of Legg-Calvé-Perthes disease has been a subject of much controversy, and it still remains unclear what strategies

SECTION 9 PEDIATRIC ORTHOPAEDICS

will alter the natural history, especially in patients at high risk for a poor outcome (ie, older patients with significant involvement of the capital femoral epiphysis). The overall goal of any treatment is to achieve an outcome in which normal sphericity of the femoral head and congruence is maintained between the femoral head and the acetabulum. During the early phases, the patient is treated by activity restriction (with or without short periods of bedrest) and analgesics, and the symptoms and range of motion are monitored closely. Rehabilitation may help to achieve and maintain motion. Patients younger than 5 years are more likely to have an excellent outcome without the need for more intensive treatment. Patients with persistent loss of motion may benefit from an examination under anesthesia with an arthrogram to evaluate the sphericity of the femoral head. Concomitant release of the adductors is frequently performed to improve range of motion. Long leg casts with a spreader bar are then worn for 6 weeks. Patients who are considered to have a poor prognosis based on age and degree of involvement or who develop subluxation of the femoral head may be candidates for "containment" treatment. Containment is achieved when the healing femoral head is completely within the acetabulum. Containment treatment can be nonsurgical (abduction bracing) or surgical (femoral osteotomy, pelvic osteotomy, combined osteotomy). The theory is that the contained femoral head has the best chance of spherical healing. Nonsurgical containment by full-time use of a long leg abduction brace is difficult to enforce and has not been shown to alter the outcomes, and thus it is rarely recommended. At present, when containment is indicated, one of the surgical options is preferred, although insufficient evidence exists to support one particular strategy over another.

Adverse Outcomes of Treatment

In addition to surgical complications (bleeding, infection, implant-related problems), the treatment may fail to alter the natural history of the disease. Treatment also may exacerbate limb-length discrepancy and/or gait disturbance.

Referral Decisions/Red Flags

Most children younger than 6 years who have significant involvement of the femoral head or less than 40° of abduction require further evaluation. Children 6 years or older require further evaluation.

Little League Elbow

Synonyms

Medial epicondylar fracture or avulsion

Olecranon stress fracture

Osteochondritis dissecans of the elbow

Panner disease

Traction apophysitis of the elbow

Valgus-extension overload syndrome

Definition

Little League elbow is the name given to several pathologic entities that share a common etiology (overuse in the overhead throwing athlete) and a common age group (8 to 16 years). The term is too general, however; it is preferable and more accurate to use the name of specific pathologic entities when possible. These include injuries resulting from traction or tension (eg, traction apophysitis of the medial epicondyle or olecranon, medial epicondylar fragmentation or avulsion, olecranon avulsion, and ulnar collateral ligament sprains or tears) and injuries resulting from compression (eg, osteochondritis dissecans [OCD] of the capitellum, Panner disease) (**Figure 1**).

Traction apophysitis of the medial epicondyle is inflammation or injury to the unfused medial epicondyle that occurs as a result of overuse in the skeletally immature overhead throwing athlete. Fragmentation of the medial epicondyle may occur in the young athlete (8 to 12 years), whereas avulsion of the medial epicondyle typically occurs in patients closer to physeal closure (12 to 14 years). Traction apophysitis of the olecranon, likewise, is an injury to the unfused olecranon physis in the young throwing athlete. Fragmentation of the olecranon epiphysis is rare, and avulsion is less common than with the medial epicondyle. Delayed or failed closure of the olecranon physis more commonly occurs as a result of overuse and may result in chronic pain.

Injuries of the ulnar collateral ligament are now recognized with increasing frequency in the adolescent overhead throwing athlete. This injury is more completely described in the chapter on ulnar collateral ligament injuries (see page 392).

OCD occurs in adolescents (typically, older than 12 years) after the capitellum has ossified. This condition is characterized by focal osteonecrosis of the capitellum (but rarely the radial head) with varying degrees of subchondral separation and is frequently associated with overuse in the thrower (**Figure 2**).

ICD-9 Codes	
718.12	Loose body, elbow
718.92	Derangement of joint, elbow
732.3	Juvenile osteochondrosis of upper extremity (Panner disease)
732.7	Osteochondritis dissecans
812.43	Fracture of the medial epicondyle, closed
813.01	Fracture of the olecranon

SECTION 9 PEDIATRIC ORTHOPAEDICS

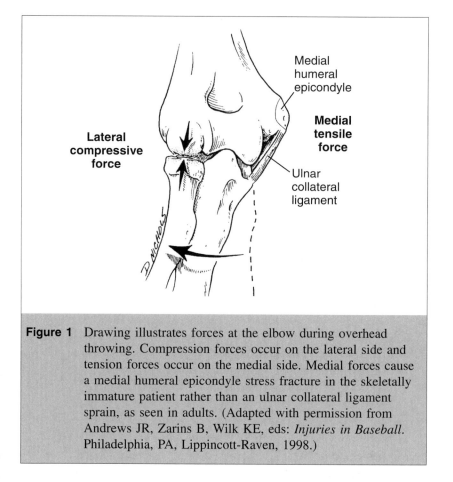

Figure 1 Drawing illustrates forces at the elbow during overhead throwing. Compression forces occur on the lateral side and tension forces occur on the medial side. Medial forces cause a medial humeral epicondyle stress fracture in the skeletally immature patient rather than an ulnar collateral ligament sprain, as seen in adults. (Adapted with permission from Andrews JR, Zarins B, Wilk KE, eds: *Injuries in Baseball.* Philadelphia, PA, Lippincott-Raven, 1998.)

Figure 2 AP radiograph of the elbow of a left-handed baseball pitcher reveals osteochondritis dissecans lesion of the capitellum (arrow) with an open medial humerus epiphysis (arrowhead). (Reproduced from Hutchinson MR, Ireland ML: Overuse and throwing injuries in the skeletally immature patient. *Instr Course Lect* 2003;52:25-36.)

Loose body formation is common, leading to mechanical signs and symptoms.

Panner disease, which often is confused with OCD, is seen in children younger than 12 years and consists of a focal avascular lesion of the capitellum that typically is self-limited and has a good prognosis.

Clinical Symptoms

These conditions occur in the young overhead throwing athlete with a history of overuse, often a history of an excessive number of pitches per game, excessive number of innings pitched per week (or year), year-round participation in the throwing sport, and the premature use of the breaking ball (curveball or slider) before adequate skeletal maturity. Pain, either chronic or acute, is the most common symptom.

Tests

Physical Examination

Tenderness to palpation is the most common physical finding and may be medial (medial epicondylar traction apophysitis, medial epicondylar fragmentation/avulsion, ulnar collateral ligament injuries), lateral (OCD, Panner disease), or posterior (olecranon traction apophysitis/avulsion). Flexion contractures are common. Instability may be seen in ulnar collateral ligament injuries or severe OCD with loss of capitellar lateral bony support.

Diagnostic Tests

Radiographs of the elbow help to establish most of these diagnoses. Obtaining a comparison view of the contralateral side is essential to better visualize subtle changes. MRI often is necessary to confirm OCD, Panner disease, and ulnar collateral ligament injuries.

Differential Diagnosis

- Cubital tunnel syndrome/ulnar neuritis (rarely seen in this age group)
- Fractures of the radial head, olecranon, or supracondylar humerus (radiographs differentiate)
- Lateral epicondylitis/tendinosis (rarely seen in this age group)
- Medial epicondylitis/tendinosis (rarely seen in this age group)

Adverse Outcomes of the Disease

Persistent pain, inability to participate in sports, chronic instability, and loss of motion are possible. Medial epicondylar avulsion may lead to late ulnar palsy. OCD may lead to loose body formation and, in more severe cases, osteoarthritis.

Treatment

Because these conditions technically are overuse injuries, the most critical component of treatment is rest. At least 3 to 6 months of rest from throwing is appropriate for these problems. In OCD, abstaining from pitching for 1 year may be necessary. Rehabilitation is helpful during this time to help maintain strength and restore motion. Immobilization should be avoided, except for possible brief periods in the acute phase, given the likelihood of significant and perhaps permanent loss of motion. Unfortunately, even with appropriate rest, the athlete may not be able to resume pitching, and a change in position or sport may be recommended. Nonsurgical care usually is appropriate, but surgical intervention is occasionally necessary.

SECTION 9 PEDIATRIC ORTHOPAEDICS

Table 1 Recommended Ages for Learning Various Pitches

Pitch	Recommended Age (Years)
Changeup	11 to 12 (or when sufficient velocity and control have been developed with the fastball)
Curveball	14.5
Slider	18

Table 2 Recommended Pitching Limits

Age Range (Years)	Maximum Number of Pitches Thrown per Game	Maximum Number of Innings Pitched per Week
8 to 10	50	6
11 to 14	75	6
15 to 18	90 to 100	10

Adverse Outcomes of Treatment

Surgery carries a small risk of infection, hardware failure, or neurovascular injury.

Referral Decisions/Red Flags

Further evaluation is needed if nonsurgical treatment fails.

Prevention

Given the increasing incidence of overuse injuries and the likelihood that results will be suboptimal despite appropriate care, prevention is emphasized. Education of athletes, parents, and coaches is critical, and governing bodies of youth baseball organizations must be willing to make rule changes for the long-term benefit of these athletes. Year-round pitching is not advised, and participation in baseball showcases should be restricted. Participation in other sports should be encouraged. General physical conditioning and proper pitching mechanics should be emphasized. Current recommendations for pitchers are given in **Tables 1** and **2**.

Metatarsus Adductus

Synonym

Metatarsus varus

ICD-9 Code

754.53
Metatarsus varus

Definition

Metatarsus adductus is a common foot deformity in infancy characterized by medial deviation (adduction) of the forefoot. It is most often due to deformation resulting from intrauterine positioning (**Figure 1**). The deformity is observed in approximately 13% of full-term infants. It resolves spontaneously in most cases. Some cases of rigid adductus of the forefoot or midfoot are caused by congenital bony abnormalities, and these deformities will persist despite nonsurgical treatment. Metatarsus adductus is commonly associated with other intrauterine positional deformations such as congenital muscular torticollis, medial tibial torsion, and, rarely, hip dysplasia.

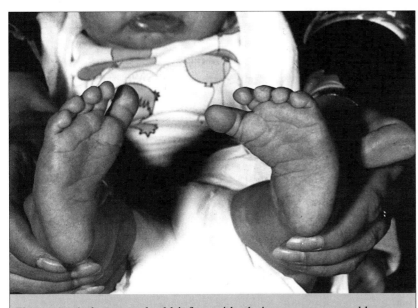

Figure 1 A three-month-old infant with obvious metatarsus adductus. The foot appears to be supinated; however, when the foot was placed in a weight-bearing position, the hindfoot alignment was normal. (Reproduced from Greene WB: Metatarsus adductus and skewfoot. *Instr Course Lect* 1994;43:161-177.)

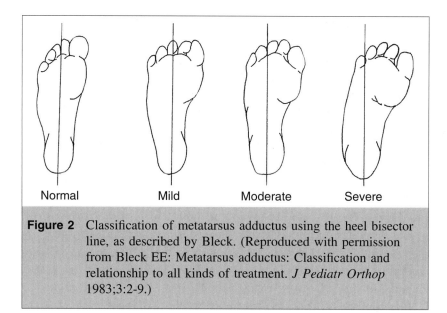

Normal	Mild	Moderate	Severe

Figure 2 Classification of metatarsus adductus using the heel bisector line, as described by Bleck. (Reproduced with permission from Bleck EE: Metatarsus adductus: Classification and relationship to all kinds of treatment. *J Pediatr Orthop* 1983;3:2-9.)

Clinical Symptoms

Most cases are asymptomatic. Parental concern is the major reason for early referral. Pain is rarely reported.

Tests

Physical Examination

The patient presents with adduction of the forefoot relative to the hindfoot, with a convexity of the lateral border of the foot. The hindfoot is in neutral or increased valgus and never demonstrates a varus posture. Normal ankle dorsiflexion also is present; these latter two findings are important because some children with severe metatarsus adductus may, at first inspection, appear to have a clubfoot deformity. Some patients also will have a mild plantar flexion deformity of the medial column of the foot, giving the appearance of an elevated longitudinal arch. A "wandering" great toe (adduction of the great toe) also may be observed in association with the condition; it typically resolves over the first several years of life.

The severity of metatarsus adductus can be assessed using the heel bisector line (**Figure 2**). Normally, a line bisecting the heel passes through the second toe or the second and third toes. Metatarsus adductus is considered mild when the heel bisector crosses the third toe, moderate when the heel bisector goes between the third and fourth toes, and severe when the heel bisector crosses between the fourth and fifth toes. The flexibility of the deformity determines the prognosis and helps identify the subset of patients who require treatment. Flexibility is assessed by first holding the hindfoot in varus to stabilize the subtalar joint, and then abducting the forefoot relative to the hindfoot. If the foot can be abducted fully, the heel bisector will fall between the great toe and the second toe, demonstrating that the deformity is fully flexible and will likely resolve spontaneously. The foot also may be moderately flexible, where the alignment improves with stress but the heel bisector cannot be brought in line with the second toe. Truly rigid deformities are rare. The deformity may have a dynamic component from overactivity of the adductor hallucis, which makes the deformity more dramatic when the patient is walking.

Diagnostic Tests

Radiographs are rarely needed, but they are indicated when the deformity cannot be passively corrected or fails to respond to nonsurgical treatment. In such cases, obliquity of the medial cuneiform may be present, resulting in adduction of the great toe. Obtaining serial photocopies of the foot is a low-cost, no-risk method of charting the progression of metatarsus adductus (**Figure 3**). A hip ultrasound may be indicated if the hip examination is abnormal or if the history and/or other physical findings (such as other intrauterine positional deformities) suggest a risk of hip dysplasia.

Figure 3 Photocopy of the feet of a 9-month-old infant with bilateral metatarsus adductus. (Reproduced from Greene WB: Metatarsus adductus and skewfoot. *Instr Course Lect* 1994;43:161-177.)

Differential Diagnosis

- Clubfoot (heel in varus; ankle in equinus)
- Hyperactive abductor hallucis (lateral border of the foot remains straight)
- Internal tibial torsion (foot rotated in; lateral border of the foot straight)
- Skeletal dysplasia (most common in diastrophic dwarfism)
- Skewfoot (Z or serpentine foot; valgus hindfoot and forefoot adduction)

Adverse Outcomes of the Disease

Cosmetic concerns and the inability to wear certain types of shoes are the most likely consequences of persistent metatarsus adductus. Abnormal shoe wear and discomfort are possible but much less likely.

Treatment

Most newborns do not require active treatment, as metatarsus adductus usually corrects spontaneously. Parents are advised to avoid positioning the infant prone with the feet turned in, a position that accentuates metatarsus adductus. If a structural component to the deformity exists (the foot does not passively overcorrect on physical examination), then serial casting should be considered. Patients with structural deformities should be referred early, as correction is easiest to achieve during the first few months of life. Casts are applied for 2-week periods, and usually three or four casts will suffice. Casting can be successful in children from 1 to 3 years of age but is more difficult at these ages and is associated with a higher rate of failure. The cast should be applied in a manner that molds the forefoot into abduction without accentuating heel valgus. Neither stretching exercises nor nighttime splints (or outflare shoes) have proven value, but they are often considered as a supplement to casting for structural deformities. Very few cases of metatarsus adductus require surgical treatment. Soft-tissue releases have not been associated with favorable outcomes; thus, an osteotomy of the midfoot or the metatarsals is required to realign the foot. Dynamic hallux varus will resolve spontaneously and requires no specific treatment.

Adverse Outcomes of Treatment

Recurrent deformity may occur despite serial casting. Complications of casting include increased heel valgus and the development of a flatfoot or skewfoot deformity. Degenerative changes at the tarsometatarsal joints have been noted after soft-tissue releases of the tarsometatarsal joints, and this procedure is no longer performed. Complications of osteotomies include undercorrection or overcorrection. Damage to the physis of the first metatarsal with subsequent shortening of that bone is a complication of a first metatarsal osteotomy.

Referral Decisions/Red Flags

Residual metatarsus adductus in an infant age 3 to 6 months or a rigid metatarsus adductus in any infant signals the need for further evaluation.

Neonatal Brachial Plexus Palsy

Synonyms

Obstetric brachial plexus palsy (OBPP)

Obstetric palsy

ICD-9 Code

767.6
Injury to brachial plexus

Definition

Neonatal brachial plexus palsy, sometimes called obstetric palsy, is a motor and sensory deficit of the upper extremity resulting from a stretch injury to the brachial plexus during labor and delivery. The incidence is between 0.4 and 4.0 per 1,000 live births. Three common patterns exist. The most common pattern is Erb palsy affecting the nerves at C5-C6, which is seen in nearly 50% of cases and results in weakness of elbow flexion and weakness of shoulder abduction, flexion, and external rotation. Patients with Erb palsy have the best prognosis for recovery. Klumpke palsy represents 30% of the cases. It is a lesion of the lower plexus (C5-C7) and affects the hand and wrist. Panplexus palsy, which represents 20% of the cases, involves the entire plexus.

The spectrum of injury ranges from a minor stretch of the nerves (temporary conduction block) to a partial or complete rupture of the nerves or avulsion of the nerve root from the spinal cord. The prognosis is based on the severity of the injury. Most cases are transient, and spontaneous recovery of antigravity strength during the first 2 months predicts a high likelihood of full recovery. Patients who do not exhibit return to biceps function after 3 months of age rarely have a full recovery. Poor prognostic factors include involvement of the entire brachial plexus, Horner syndrome, and nerve root avulsions. Subtle long-term findings such as limb shortening and reduction in limb girth also may be of concern to patients.

Clinical Symptoms

Reduced spontaneous movement, or pseudoparalysis, is commonly observed. The patient may exhibit discomfort or irritability if an associated fracture of the clavicle or humerus is present.

SECTION 9   PEDIATRIC ORTHOPAEDICS

Figure 1 Typical posture ("waiter's tip" position) of child with Erb palsy.

Tests

Physical Examination

Examination findings vary depending on the pattern of nerve injury. They include diminished spontaneous movement of the upper extremity as well as impaired reflexes (Moro reflex, symmetric and asymmetric tonic neck reflexes). Initially, the upper extremity appears to be flail. Tenderness in the supraclavicular triangle may be present during the first few weeks after birth.

The classic appearance of a neonate with Erb palsy is the "waiter's tip" position (shoulder adducted and internally rotated, elbow extended, forearm pronated, and wrist flexed) (**Figure 1**). It is important to determine whether the lesion is preganglionic (no potential for recovery) or postganglionic. Findings consistent with a preganglionic avulsion injury include involvement of the sympathetic chain (Horner syndrome), phrenic nerve paralysis, and involvement of other nerves coming off the plexus (long thoracic, dorsal scapular, suprascapular, and thoracodorsal).

Repeated examinations of muscle and sensory function are needed to correlate the physical findings with an anatomic location of injury and to assess the degree and rate of neurologic recovery. Failure to recover muscle balance results in contractures and limited motion, particularly at the shoulder and elbow.

Diagnostic Tests

Radiographs should be ordered if results of physical examination suggest a fracture of the clavicle or humerus. If the infant does not recover full function, electromyography and nerve conduction velocity studies may help guide decisions regarding surgical options. CT and MRI have been used to assess glenohumeral anatomy in patients with internal rotation contractures.

Differential Diagnosis

- Clavicle fracture (tenderness and deformity on palpation, pain on passive range of motion, possible pseudoparalysis)
- Humerus fracture (swelling, deformity, and pain with range of motion of the arm, possible pseudoparalysis)
- Proximal humeral osteomyelitis (cessation of normal motion, but infant may not appear toxic)
- Septic arthritis of the shoulder or elbow (cessation of normal motion, but infant may not appear toxic)

Adverse Outcomes of the Disease

The prognosis varies depending on the severity of the neurologic injury. Early evidence of recovery portends a good prognosis. With Erb palsy, persistent weakness and muscle imbalance may lead to progressive contractures (internal shoulder rotation), which is associated with early development of subluxation or dislocation in more than 60% of patients within the first 2 years. Radial head instability also may develop. Neurologic function may fail to improve sufficiently despite treatment. Permanent neurologic deficits may interfere with upper extremity function and may require reconstructive surgery. Bony deformities can develop and progress despite tendon transfers. Diminished overall growth potential of the extremity may occur.

Treatment

Initial treatment consists of rehabilitation to maintain joint range of motion; a supervised home exercise program may best accomplish this goal. Gentle passive range-of-motion exercise several times a day, with special attention to external rotation of the shoulder, is needed to prevent posterior subluxation of the shoulder. Motor function is evaluated at regular intervals. Early referral to a specialist is indicated if recovery is not observed within the first few weeks. The cornerstones of treatment are the detailed assessment and monitoring of neurologic function and recovery, the prevention of secondary deformities, and identifying the subset of patients that may benefit from surgical intervention to treat the neurologic impairment and/or the long-term musculoskeletal sequelae of muscle weakness/imbalance. Given the spectrum of pathology, surgical treatment needs to be individualized.

The procedures are varied and include microsurgical reconstruction (nerve grafts, nerve transfers), soft-tissue release/lengthening and/or derotational osteotomies, and tendon transfers. Although the field is advancing rapidly, many controversies remain, especially the timing and specific nature of interventions. Patients with Erb palsy who show evidence of recovery by 3 months are typically treated nonsurgically. The most recent information suggests that early microsurgical reconstruction (by 3 months) is gaining favor in patients with global lesions and Horner syndrome, based on the poor prognosis without surgical intervention. The traditional approach to reinnervation included resection of scarred areas and nerve grafting (sural nerve), but recently, nerve transfer procedures have been used with greater frequency. Nerve transfers, in which a viable nerve is anastamosed to one of the injured nerves, also may be performed in conjunction with nerve grafting procedures. Nerve transfers also have been used at a later time to improve motor strength in patients with partial recovery, whether or not early microsurgical reconstruction has been performed. Synthetic collagen nerve conduits also are under investigation as an alternative to nerve grafts.

Children with significant muscle imbalance about the shoulder, elbow, and hand should undergo appropriate muscle releases and tendon transfers to provide a balanced upper extremity. The development of an internal rotation contracture at the shoulder may rapidly lead to deformity of the glenohumeral joint, with progressive subluxation or dislocation, and early release may help to stabilize the joint and prevent deformity. In older patients with significant internal rotation contracture, a humeral derotational osteotomy will improve external rotation at the shoulder.

Referral Decisions/Red Flags

Referral is appropriate shortly after birth. Sepsis or skeletal trauma (child abuse) must be suspected if a sudden loss of function occurs in an extremity that moved well at birth.

Osgood-Schlatter Disease

Synonyms

Osteochondritis of the inferior patella
Osteochondritis of the tibial tuberosity
Tibial tubercle traction apophysitis

ICD-9 Code

732.4
Osgood-Schlatter disease

Definition

Osgood-Schlatter disease (or condition) is an overuse injury in the growing child that results from repetitive stress when a too-tight quadriceps "pulls" on the apophysis (secondary ossification center) of the tibial tubercle during a time of rapid growth (approximately age 11 to 13 years). Overuse explains the fivefold greater incidence in patients who are active in sports and the two to three times greater incidence in boys. Sinding-Larsen–Johansson disease is a similar disorder that occurs at the junction of the patellar tendon and the distal pole of the patella.

Clinical Symptoms

Patients report pain that is exacerbated by running, jumping, and kneeling activities. Pain also can occur after prolonged sitting with the knees flexed.

Tests

Physical Examination

Examination reveals tenderness and swelling at the insertion of the patellar tendon into the tibial tubercle in Osgood-Schlatter disease and at the inferior pole of the patella in Sinding-Larsen–Johansson disease. These conditions may occur in both knees simultaneously, but one side may be more symptomatic. Although knee motion usually is not restricted, kneeling is painful during the acute phase. The knee and patellofemoral joint are stable.

Diagnostic Tests

AP and lateral radiographs of the knee may be normal or show soft-tissue swelling. In Osgood-Schlatter disease, small spicules of heterotopic ossification may be seen anterior to the tibial tuberosity (**Figure 1**). In Sinding-Larsen–Johansson disease, elongation of the inferior pole of the patella may be apparent, along with fragmentation in the area, caused by repetitive stress

Figure 1 Radiograph shows symptomatic tibial tubercle ossicle (arrows) in a 13-year-old boy with Osgood-Schlatter disease. (Reproduced from Stanitski CL: Knee overuse disorders in the pediatric and adolescent athlete. *Instr Course Lect* 1993;42:483-495.)

SECTION 9 PEDIATRIC ORTHOPAEDICS

on the growth center. When a patient has bilateral symptoms, radiographs are rarely needed, but with unilateral involvement, they should be obtained to rule out tumors.

Differential Diagnosis

- Infection (rare, elevated erythrocyte sedimentation rate)
- Neoplasm (rare, unilateral)
- Patellar sleeve fracture (acute onset, inability to perform straight leg raise)
- Tibial tubercle avulsion fracture (acute pain, inability to perform straight leg raise)

Adverse Outcomes of the Disease

The long-term prognosis for patients who undergo nonsurgical treatment is good, with minimal disability in adulthood. Some residual prominence of the tibial tubercle is common, particularly in patients who have fragmentation of the epiphysis and heterotopic ossification during the active phase of the disease. These patients occasionally report discomfort when walking.

Rarely, an avulsion fracture through the tibial apophysis can occur with activity in symptomatic patients; therefore, these patients require rest from activity.

Treatment

Symptoms are often controlled adequately with intermittent use of ice after sports, coupled with occasional use of NSAIDs, use of a protective knee pad, and stretching exercises. Decreasing exercise for the muscles of the lower extremity to permit healing of the microscopic avulsion fractures is the key to treating severe symptoms.

Occasionally, immobilization is needed for severe or recalcitrant symptoms. This usually can be accomplished with a prefabricated knee immobilizer that is removed once a day for bathing and range-of-motion exercises.

Another important aspect in management is helping the parents and patient understand how long sports activities may be restricted. In patients with Osgood-Schlatter disease, activity may need to be modified for an average of 2 to 3 months or more, until symptoms subside.

Surgical treatment is not commonly needed except in the rare case of an avulsion of the ossification center or for excising a heterotopic ossification over the tibial tubercle.

SECTION 9 PEDIATRIC ORTHOPAEDICS

Adverse Outcomes of Treatment

None.

Referral Decisions/Red Flags

Unilateral pain at rest or pain not directly over the tibial tubercle should raise concerns of a neoplasm or another disorder. Acute worsening of pain, inability to perform a straight-leg raise while keeping the knee straight (patient should be able to lift his or her heel off the table without a lag, or bend, in the knee) suggests a disruption of the extensor mechanism at the patella or tibial tubercle that requires surgical fixation.

SECTION 9   PEDIATRIC ORTHOPAEDICS

Osteochondral Lesions of the Talus

Synonyms

Osteochondral fracture

Osteochondritis dissecans

Definition

Osteochondral lesions of the hyaline cartilage and underlying subchondral bone of the weight-bearing surface of the talus may occur acutely after trauma (osteochondral fracture) or may develop secondary to idiopathic subchondral avascularity (osteochondritis dissecans [OCD] of the talus), appearing similarly to OCD of the knee. These abnormalities may cause fissuring and collapse of the joint surface of the talus, delamination of joint cartilage from the underlying bone, loose fragment formation, and hyaline cartilage defects within the ankle joint.

Clinical Symptoms

Patients present with ankle pain, swelling or recurrent effusion, a sensation of catching or popping, or occasional giving way. The symptoms may occur acutely after an injury or intermittently with vigorous activities over a period of weeks to months. A history of frequent ankle swelling, often misdiagnosed as a chronic ankle sprain, is not uncommon.

Tests

Physical Examination

Examination of the ankle reveals limited, painful active and passive range of motion, a palpable effusion, and tenderness along the anterior joint line. Ligamentous stress testing and subtalar joint mobility are normal.

Diagnostic Tests

Mortise views of the ankle reveal an articular surface defect surrounded by a halo of lucent bone on the weight-bearing surface of the talus. Acute osteochondral lesions are often smaller and wafer-shaped and occur on the lateral talus; more chronic OCD lesions are deeper and cup-shaped and occur on the posteromedial talus. CT is useful for staging of medial lesions (**Figure 1**). MRI best defines the extent of the cartilage

Figure 1 AP mortise radiograph of the ankle shows nondisplaced osteochondritis of the talus (arrow).

surface disruption and its adjacent subchondral avascularity. Synovial fluid visualized between the OCD lesion and the adjacent bone of the talar body suggests an unstable lesion with little healing potential.

Differential Diagnosis

- Acute osteochondral fracture (acute onset, hemarthrosis, pain)
- Erosive osteomyelitis (rare) (subacute, joint effusion, pain with motion)
- Neoplasm (rare) (insidious onset, night pain, joint swelling)
- Osteonecrosis of the talus (joint surface collapse from previous trauma, steroid use, sickle cell disease, delayed onset, decreased ankle motion)
- Septic arthritis of the ankle with resultant chondrolysis (rare) (pain, postinfection progressive decrease in ankle motion)

Adverse Outcomes of the Disease

Long-term complications include ankle pain, stiffness, synovitis of the ankle joint, and premature osteoarthritis. When large lesions fail to heal, loose body formation and osteoarthritis of the ankle joint may develop.

Treatment

Osteochondral lesions in patients who have not reached skeletal maturity have the capacity to heal and should be evaluated for healing potential with immobilization. Osteochondral lesions in adolescents approaching skeletal maturity have a limited capacity for healing and, along with unstable lesions, usually require surgery.

Referral Decisions/Red Flags

Osteochondral lesions are best treated with early intervention and thus require early referral.

SECTION 9 PEDIATRIC ORTHOPAEDICS

and possibly a period of crutch ambulation. Immobilization is reserved for refractory symptoms or noncompliant patients.

Surgical treatment is necessary after skeletal maturity and in children in whom the lesion has progressed to the stage that the articular cartilage has partially or totally separated. If the lesion is intact (still in place), it is drilled to promote vascular ingrowth and creeping substitution. Unstable lesions require temporary internal fixation to promote healing. When the fragment is loose, treatment consists of removing the free fragment and débriding the articular surface defect.

Adverse Outcomes of Treatment

Possible complications of surgical treatment are infection or further damage to the joint caused by the hardware or failure of the hardware.

Referral Decisions/Red Flags

Children with lesions smaller than 1 cm in width usually do well with nonsurgical treatment; those with lesions larger than 2 cm usually have progressive problems. Children with lesions between 1 and 2 cm should be treated based on symptoms and radiographic findings. After the physis has closed, the prognosis for healing is significantly poorer, and these patients require further evaluation.

Osteomyelitis

Synonym

Acute hematogenous osteomyelitis

Definition

Osteomyelitis is a unique bone infection that usually develops in children as a result of hematogenous seeding (acute hematogenous osteomyelitis [AHO]); rarely, it is secondary to direct contamination, as from an open fracture or nail puncture wound. Significant disability may occur from osteomyelitis, especially if treatment is delayed and if the disease results in chronic infection.

The metaphysis of long bones is the most common location for AHO in children because small vessels are required to make a "U-turn" at the junction of the metaphysis and the physis, causing sluggish circulation in this area. The infection spreads through the medullary canal and penetrates the metaphyseal cortex, causing a subperiosteal abscess. Abscesses may result in local ischemia or bone necrosis caused by an increase in intramedullary pressure and the loss of periosteal blood supply (elevation of the periosteum), which may result in one or more necrotic fragments of bone (sequestrae). If the periosteum remains viable, new bone (involucrum) will be formed to stabilize the area, and sequestrae may be partially or completely resolved. Sequestrae that persist may result in episodes of recurrence of acute infection (chronic osteomyelitis). Local or segmental bone loss may occur if significant bone necrosis exists and/or the host response is inadequate, or following inadequate treatment of the disease.

Subacute osteomyelitis presents in a more indolent fashion. It is typically caused by organisms of lower virulence (bacteria, tuberculosis). The diagnosis often is delayed because symptoms are often vague, fever may not be present, and laboratory studies may be normal. Some lesions have an aggressive radiographic appearance that may mimic a tumor.

Chronic osteomyelitis develops when foci of necrotic and infected material remain within the bone, leading to recurrent flare-ups of infection and, often, an intermittently draining sinus.

Clinical Symptoms

Pain, swelling, tenderness, erythema, increased localized warmth, and generalized malaise are associated with acute osteomyelitis. When the lower extremity, pelvis, or spine is

ICD-9 Codes
730.00 Acute osteomyelitis, site unspecified
731.00 Chronic osteomyelitis, site unspecified

SECTION 9 PEDIATRIC ORTHOPAEDICS

involved, refusal to walk or limping is an early symptom, particularly in a young child. Pseudoparalysis (failure to use a limb despite normal neuromuscular structures) is observed when the upper extremity is affected. Subacute osteomyelitis may present with vague discomfort, but typically no fever or constitutional symptoms. Patients with chronic osteomyelitis present with periodic recurrence of sepsis and/or sinuses with chronic drainage.

Tests

Physical Examination

An elevated temperature of 100.4°F (38°C) or higher is typical for AHO, but patients with subacute or chronic osteomyelitis may have a normal temperature. Tenderness directly over the involved bone is common. Examination of the adjacent joint may be abnormal, and an effusion (reactive effusion or coexisting septic arthritis) is common. Pain with joint motion may be observed, as well as a mild restriction in range of motion, but not to the degree observed in septic arthritis.

Diagnostic Tests

Laboratory studies should include a complete blood cell count with differential, an erythrocyte sedimentation rate, and a C-reactive protein (CRP) level; the CRP level will be abnormal earliest, often within 8 hours of the onset of infection. These tests are not specific, also being elevated in a variety of other disease processes. The CRP level also is useful in monitoring the response to treatment. Neonates, children who are seen in the early stages of the disease, and those with an altered immune response may have normal laboratory studies and no fever or constitutional symptoms. A blood culture should be obtained because it will identify the infecting organism in 40% to 50% of patients. In patients clinically suspected of having AHO, consideration is given to aspiration along the metaphysis at the point of maximal tenderness. This may help to identify a subperiosteal abscess, and the metaphysis itself may be aspirated as well. In most clinical settings, this practice has been abandoned in favor of imaging modalities such as MRI. When an effusion is present and septic arthritis is in the differential diagnosis based on clinical findings (instead of a reactive effusion), aspiration of the joint should be performed. A sterile or reactive effusion accompanies many cases of AHO, but a coexisting septic arthritis also is encountered in many cases. This is most common in joints in which the metaphysis is intra-articular (proximal femur, proximal humerus, proximal radius, and distal fibula).

AP and lateral radiographs of the suspected area are necessary, but they may be normal or show only soft-tissue swelling in the early stages of AHO, as bony changes such as periosteal elevation and/or destruction of bone may take 10 to 14 days to develop. In cases of subacute osteomyelitis (**Figure 1**), the lesions are most commonly lytic and have a thin sclerotic rim and will often cross the physis (**Figure 1**). In acute hematogenous osteomyelitis, the physis is usually spared. A subset of cases of subacute osteomyelitis present a more aggressive appearance, with periosteal reaction and/or bony destruction. The changes observed in chronic osteomyelitis are well delineated on plain radiographs (**Figure 2**). Additional imaging modalities also may be useful. MRI is currently the imaging modality of choice for diagnosing AHO in the early stages (**Figure 3**); a technetium Tc-99m bone scan also may be considered. MRI demonstrates not only signal intensity change within the bone but also coexisting findings such as abscesses, effusion, and soft-tissue changes (cellulitis, myositis). MRI should be obtained with intravenous contrast when an infection or tumor is suspected.

Differential Diagnosis

- Infections

  Cellulitis (erythema and swelling of subcutaneous tissues)

  Pyomyositis (muscle pain and tenderness that gradually increases)

  Septic arthritis (joint swelling and severe restriction of motion)

- Inflammatory diseases (acute rheumatic fever, others)
- Tumors

  Benign (eosinophilic granuloma)

  Malignant (leukemia, Ewing sarcoma, osteosarcoma)

Adverse Outcomes of the Disease

A host of potential sequelae are possible, depending on the timing of diagnosis and the response to treatment. These include persistent infection (chronic osteomyelitis), focal or segmental bone loss, pathologic fracture, angular deformity, involvement of the physis leading to angular deformity and/or limb-length inequality, loss of motion at neighboring joints, and destruction of adjacent joints.

Treatment

When osteomyelitis is suspected clinically, empiric intravenous antibiotics should be started immediately after obtaining material for culture (or performing a biopsy). *Staphylococcus aureus* is the most common pathogen, and antibiotic selection should

Figure 1 Radiograph of the ankle of a patient with subacute osteomyelitis demonstrates a lytic area that extends across the physis and into the epiphysis.

Figure 2 Lateral radiograph of the leg of a patient with chronic osteomyelitis demonstrates extensive involvement of the tibial diaphysis with areas of necrotic bone (especially anterior and superior sequestrae) and areas of new bone formation (posterior involucrum).

SECTION 9 PEDIATRIC ORTHOPAEDICS

Figure 3 MRI of early-stage osteomyelitis of the distal femur demonstrates increased signal intensity within the distal femoral metaphysis with a small subperiosteal abscess posteriorly.

cover this organism in all age groups. Antibiotic selection also should cover Group B *Streptococci* and enteric rod organisms in neonates. In children ages 6 months to 4 years, *Haemophilus influenzae* also is covered if vaccination is incomplete. The typical course of antibiotics is 6 weeks but may be longer depending on clinical response and laboratory values. The indication and time to switch from intravenous to oral antibiotics is controversial at present, but an early change to oral medication (after up to 7 days of intravenous therapy) is feasible in many patients, particularly those who present early.

Surgery for acute osteomyelitis consists primarily of draining a subperiosteal or intramedullary abscess and débriding any areas of bony destruction. A biopsy is required for diagnosis in most cases of subacute osteomyelitis, which often mimics a tumor, although some evidence exists to support empiric antibiotic therapy for lesions that have a characteristic appearance and the appropriate clinical history. Chronic osteomyelitis is very difficult to treat, often requiring staged surgical procedures. Removal of all infected material provides the best chance to eradicate the disease. An extensive débridement may be required, resulting in deficiencies in the soft-tissue envelope and/or local or segmental defects within the involved bone. Additional surgical procedures are often required, including skin grafting, local rotational flaps, or free-tissue transfers to achieve soft-tissue coverage, and bone grafting or bone transport to address bony defects. Immobilization decreases pain and is considered for up to 3 to 6 weeks for comfort and to protect against a pathologic fracture. The bone is weaker not only because of the osseous destruction, but also because the woven bone that is initially formed in the healing process does not have the same strength as lamellar bone.

Adverse Outcomes of Treatment
The usual surgical risks, including infection, are possible.

Referral Decisions/Red Flags
Most patients with osteomyelitis will benefit from a team approach.

Pediatric Sports Participation

Sports participation during childhood offers a number of potential benefits that lead to lifelong habits of fitness. Children develop specific skills, learn the importance of teamwork, acquire leadership skills, and develop confidence. All of these attributes result in improved self-esteem. Physical activity also provides an appropriate outlet for releasing stress.

It is important to help children choose an activity routine that is fun, developmentally appropriate, and realistic given individual, family, and community resources. One method that is used in exercise prescriptions for adults is represented by the mnemonic FITT, which stands for frequency, intensity, time (duration), and type of activity. This can be useful for creating a physical activity prescription for children as well.

Suggestions for increasing physical activity can include walking or bicycling for transportation instead of riding in an automobile and planning physical activity rather than sedentary activities with friends. Many adolescents, especially girls, may not be active because they think organized sports are the only type of exercise that "counts." Therefore, it is important to provide education to adolescents to identify the physical activity they may already be getting (eg, walking), as well as to reinforce the benefits of other lifetime activities such as bicycling, dancing, skating, and swimming.

Potential disadvantages of organized sports include burnout, injuries, and an overemphasis on winning. Adults who lead children's sports activities should not forget that sports should be for the child and should be fun (**Table 1**).

Children are not merely small adults. They have unique needs that must be considered. For example, children are more heat-sensitive than adults and tend not to drink enough. They rarely will admit that they are tired. Therefore, practices should be scheduled during the cooler hours of the day and should include adequate breaks. Adults in charge should ensure that adequate amounts of fluids that children like to drink are readily available and are encouraged.

Readiness for Sports Participation

Overall readiness must be based on the individual child and his or her eagerness to participate, not parental desire. A variety of sport activities should be offered, and the child should be allowed to choose.

Table 1 Reasons Children Want to Play Sports

To have fun

To improve their skills

To learn new skills

To be with their friends

To make new friends

To succeed or win

To become physically fit

(Reproduced from Landry GL: Benefits of sports participation, in Sullivan JA, Anderson SJ, eds: *Care of the Young Athlete*. Rosemont, IL, American Academy of Orthopaedic Surgeons, pp 1-8.)

SECTION 9   PEDIATRIC ORTHOPAEDICS

Table 2 Developmental Skills and Sports Recommendations During Childhood

Early Childhood (2 to 5 Years)

Motor skills

    Limited fundamental skills

    Limited balance skills

Learning

    Extremely short attention span

    Poor selective attention

    Egocentric learning (trial and error)

    Visual and auditory cues are important

Vision

    Not fully mature before ages 6 to 7 (farsighted)

    Difficulty tracking and judging velocity of moving objects

Sports recommendations

    Emphasize fundamental skills with minimal variation and limited instruction

    Emphasize fun, playfulness, exploration, and experimentation rather than competition

    Activities: Running, swimming, tumbling, throwing, catching

(Adapted with permission from Nelson MA: Developmental skills and children's sports. *Phys Sportsmed* 1991;19:67-97.)

The attrition rate for youth sports participation is high: 35% annually. Many children drop out of sports because of burnout, not being able to participate, or because they are not matched to their level of skill. **Table 2** lists the developmental skills for sports and sports recommendations during childhood.

Sports programs to enhance motor development in infants and toddlers are limited, but aquatic programs for infants and toddlers are popular. A recent policy statement developed by the American Academy of Pediatrics (available at http://www.aap.org) continues to encourage swim lessons for children 4 years and older; swim instruction for younger children is no longer discouraged, as there is new evidence that drowning risk is not increased, and may be decreased, as a result of such programs. The decision to pursue swim lessons at any age should be based on the child's development, health, disabilities, and readiness to learn. Parents should be reminded that swim lessons do not eliminate all risk of drowning.

Children 3 to 5 years of age have developed the fundamental skills of crawling, walking, jumping, and running. Vision, however, is relatively imprecise. Children at this age have difficulty tracking moving objects. Therefore, the instruction to "keep your eye on the ball" is difficult to follow. Furthermore, children in this age group have shorter attention spans and are

Table 2 *(continued)*

Middle Childhood (6 to 9 Years)

Motor skills

    Continued improvement in fundamental skills

    Posture and balance become more automatic

    Improved reaction times

    Beginning transitional skills

Learning

    Short attention span

    Limited development of memory and rapid decision making

Vision

    Improved tracking

    Limited directionality

Sports recommendations

    Emphasize fundamental skills and beginning transitional skills

    Flexible rules of sports

    Allow free time in practices

    Short instruction time

    Minimal competition

    Activities: Entry-level soccer and baseball

Late Childhood (10 to 12 Years)

Motor skills

    Improved transitional skills

    Ability to master complex motor skills

    Temporary decline in balance control at puberty

Learning

    Selective attention

    Able to use memory strategies for sports such as football and basketball

Vision

    Adult patterns

Sports recommendations

    Emphasis on skill development

    Increasing emphasis on tactics and strategy

    Emphasize factors promoting continued participation

    Activities: Entry-level for complex skill sports (eg, football, basketball)

SECTION 9   PEDIATRIC ORTHOPAEDICS

egocentric in their learning. Appropriate activities for this age include running, tumbling, and throwing, but team and competitive sports are inappropriate.

At 6 to 10 years of age, children begin the transition to adult skill development. Prior to this age they could throw, but now they are ready to work on accuracy. Some children at this age are proficient; others are not. At about 7 to 8 years of age, children begin to communicate and cooperate as a group effort; however, their attention span is still limited. Team sports in this group should be modified to ensure that practices are short and fun and that skills instruction is limited to 10 to 20 minutes. Include egocentric activities to practice the material taught. Modify the rules to stress high scoring and full participation.

Adolescents develop complex sport skills that require rapid decision making. Certainly for some children, waiting until adolescence to become involved in competitive sports that require complex skills and interactions, such as football, wrestling, hockey, and basketball, prevents the burnout that occurs when these sports are pushed on the child at an earlier age. Adolescents also have fairly good attention spans, so chalk talks and the like can be used with this group.

Preparticipation Physical Evaluation

Definition

The preparticipation physical evaluation (PPE) often is the only contact an older child or adolescent has annually with a physician. Therefore, although it is not intended to substitute for a routine annual physical examination, this examination should be as comprehensive as possible.

The PPE has a number of objectives, as listed below:

Primary Objectives
- Screen for conditions that may be life-threatening or disabling
- Screen for conditions that may predispose to injury or illness

Secondary Objectives
- Determine general health
- Serve as an entry point to the health care system for adolescents
- Provide an opportunity to initiate discussion on health-related topics

Types of Evaluations

One of two types of PPE is appropriate. The first is an examination by the athlete's personal physician. This is the preferred method because it allows for continuity of care, both in regards to past medical history and coordination of necessary referrals, as well as access to other aspects of preventive care. The second is the "station" method in which athletes move through several stations for different parts of the evaluation, all of which should be coordinated and supervised by the team physician. Specialists are often available to expedite consultations, but review of the history form and the physical examination should be performed by a single physician. A standard form can be used with either of these methods. The form developed by the American Academy of Family Physicians, American Academy of Pediatrics, American College of Sports Medicine, American Medical Society for Sports Medicine, American Orthopaedic Society for Sports Medicine, and the American Osteopathic Society for Sports Medicine is reproduced on the following pages.

SECTION 9 PEDIATRIC ORTHOPAEDICS

■ PREPARTICIPATION PHYSICAL EVALUATION
HISTORY FORM

(Note: This form is to be filled out by the patient and parent prior to seeing the physician. The physician should keep this form in the chart.)

Date of Exam _____

Name _____ Date of birth _____

Sex _____ Age _____ Grade _____ School _____ Sport(s) _____

Medicines and Allergies: Please list all of the prescription and over-the-counter medicines and supplements (herbal and nutritional) that you are currently taking

_____

_____

_____

Do you have any allergies? ☐ Yes ☐ No   If yes, please identify specific allergy below.
☐ Medicines   ☐ Pollens   ☐ Food   ☐ Stinging Insects

Explain "Yes" answers below. Circle questions you don't know the answers to.

GENERAL QUESTIONS	Yes	No
1. Has a doctor ever denied or restricted your participation in sports for any reason?		
2. Do you have any ongoing medical conditions? If so, please identify below: ☐ Asthma ☐ Anemia ☐ Diabetes ☐ Infections Other: _____		
3. Have you ever spent the night in the hospital?		
4. Have you ever had surgery?		

HEART HEALTH QUESTIONS ABOUT YOU	Yes	No
5. Have you ever passed out or nearly passed out DURING or AFTER exercise?		
6. Have you ever had discomfort, pain, tightness, or pressure in your chest during exercise?		
7. Does your heart ever race or skip beats (irregular beats) during exercise?		
8. Has a doctor ever told you that you have any heart problems? If so, check all that apply: ☐ High blood pressure ☐ A heart murmur ☐ High cholesterol ☐ A heart infection ☐ Kawasaki disease Other: _____		
9. Has a doctor ever ordered a test for your heart? (For example, ECG/EKG, echocardiogram)		
10. Do you get lightheaded or feel more short of breath than expected during exercise?		
11. Have you ever had an unexplained seizure?		
12. Do you get more tired or short of breath more quickly than your friends during exercise?		

HEART HEALTH QUESTIONS ABOUT YOUR FAMILY	Yes	No
13. Has any family member or relative died of heart problems or had an unexpected or unexplained sudden death before age 50 (including drowning, unexplained car accident, or sudden infant death syndrome)?		
14. Does anyone in your family have hypertrophic cardiomyopathy, Marfan syndrome, arrhythmogenic right ventricular cardiomyopathy, long QT syndrome, short QT syndrome, Brugada syndrome, or catecholaminergic polymorphic ventricular tachycardia?		
15. Does anyone in your family have a heart problem, pacemaker, or implanted defibrillator?		
16. Has anyone in your family had unexplained fainting, unexplained seizures, or near drowning?		

BONE AND JOINT QUESTIONS	Yes	No
17. Have you ever had an injury to a bone, muscle, ligament, or tendon that caused you to miss a practice or a game?		
18. Have you ever had any broken or fractured bones or dislocated joints?		
19. Have you ever had an injury that required x-rays, MRI, CT scan, injections, therapy, a brace, a cast, or crutches?		
20. Have you ever had a stress fracture?		
21. Have you ever been told that you have or have you had an x-ray for neck instability or atlantoaxial instability? (Down syndrome or dwarfism)		
22. Do you regularly use a brace, orthotics, or other assistive device?		
23. Do you have a bone, muscle, or joint injury that bothers you?		
24. Do any of your joints become painful, swollen, feel warm, or look red?		
25. Do you have any history of juvenile arthritis or connective tissue disease?		

MEDICAL QUESTIONS	Yes	No
26. Do you cough, wheeze, or have difficulty breathing during or after exercise?		
27. Have you ever used an inhaler or taken asthma medicine?		
28. Is there anyone in your family who has asthma?		
29. Were you born without or are you missing a kidney, an eye, a testicle (males), your spleen, or any other organ?		
30. Do you have groin pain or a painful bulge or hernia in the groin area?		
31. Have you had infectious mononucleosis (mono) within the last month?		
32. Do you have any rashes, pressure sores, or other skin problems?		
33. Have you had a herpes or MRSA skin infection?		
34. Have you ever had a head injury or concussion?		
35. Have you ever had a hit or blow to the head that caused confusion, prolonged headache, or memory problems?		
36. Do you have a history of seizure disorder?		
37. Do you have headaches with exercise?		
38. Have you ever had numbness, tingling, or weakness in your arms or legs after being hit or falling?		
39. Have you ever been unable to move your arms or legs after being hit or falling?		
40. Have you ever become ill while exercising in the heat?		
41. Do you get frequent muscle cramps when exercising?		
42. Do you or someone in your family have sickle cell trait or disease?		
43. Have you had any problems with your eyes or vision?		
44. Have you had any eye injuries?		
45. Do you wear glasses or contact lenses?		
46. Do you wear protective eyewear, such as goggles or a face shield?		
47. Do you worry about your weight?		
48. Are you trying to or has anyone recommended that you gain or lose weight?		
49. Are you on a special diet or do you avoid certain types of foods?		
50. Have you ever had an eating disorder?		
51. Do you have any concerns that you would like to discuss with a doctor?		
FEMALES ONLY		
52. Have you ever had a menstrual period?		
53. How old were you when you had your first menstrual period?		
54. How many periods have you had in the last 12 months?		

Explain "yes" answers here

_____

_____

_____

_____

_____

_____

_____

I hereby state that, to the best of my knowledge, my answers to the above questions are complete and correct.

Signature of athlete _____ Signature of parent/guardian _____ Date _____

HE0503

9-2681/0410

■ PREPARTICIPATION PHYSICAL EVALUATION
THE ATHLETE WITH SPECIAL NEEDS: SUPPLEMENTAL HISTORY FORM

Date of Exam _____

Name _____ Date of birth _____

Sex _____ Age _____ Grade _____ School _____ Sport(s) _____

	Yes	No
1. Type of disability		
2. Date of disability		
3. Classification (if available)		
4. Cause of disability (birth, disease, accident/trauma, other)		
5. List the sports you are interested in playing		
6. Do you regularly use a brace, assistive device, or prosthetic?		
7. Do you use any special brace or assistive device for sports?		
8. Do you have any rashes, pressure sores, or any other skin problems?		
9. Do you have a hearing loss? Do you use a hearing aid?		
10. Do you have a visual impairment?		
11. Do you use any special devices for bowel or bladder function?		
12. Do you have burning or discomfort when urinating?		
13. Have you had autonomic dysreflexia?		
14. Have you ever been diagnosed with a heat-related (hyperthermia) or cold-related (hypothermia) illness?		
15. Do you have muscle spasticity?		
16. Do you have frequent seizures that cannot be controlled by medication?		

Explain "yes" answers here

_____
_____
_____
_____
_____

Please indicate if you have ever had any of the following.

	Yes	No
Atlantoaxial instability		
X-ray evaluation for atlantoaxial instability		
Dislocated joints (more than one)		
Easy bleeding		
Enlarged spleen		
Hepatitis		
Osteopenia or osteoporosis		
Difficulty controlling bowel		
Difficulty controlling bladder		
Numbness or tingling in arms or hands		
Numbness or tingling in legs or feet		
Weakness in arms or hands		
Weakness in legs or feet		
Recent change in coordination		
Recent change in ability to walk		
Spina bifida		
Latex allergy		

Explain "yes" answers here

_____
_____
_____
_____
_____

I hereby state that, to the best of my knowledge, my answers to the above questions are complete and correct.

Signature of athlete _____ Signature of parent/guardian _____ Date _____

SECTION 9 PEDIATRIC ORTHOPAEDICS

■ PREPARTICIPATION PHYSICAL EVALUATION
PHYSICAL EXAMINATION FORM

Name _____ Date of birth _____

PHYSICIAN REMINDERS

1. Consider additional questions on more sensitive issues
   - Do you feel stressed out or under a lot of pressure?
   - Do you ever feel sad, hopeless, depressed, or anxious?
   - Do you feel safe at your home or residence?
   - Have you ever tried cigarettes, chewing tobacco, snuff, or dip?
   - During the past 30 days, did you use chewing tobacco, snuff, or dip?
   - Do you drink alcohol or use any other drugs?
   - Have you ever taken anabolic steroids or used any other performance supplement?
   - Have you ever taken any supplements to help you gain or lose weight or improve your performance?
   - Do you wear a seat belt, use a helmet, and use condoms?
2. Consider reviewing questions on cardiovascular symptoms (questions 5–14).

EXAMINATION					
Height		Weight		☐ Male ☐ Female	
BP / (/)	Pulse	Vision R 20/	L 20/	Corrected ☐ Y ☐ N	

MEDICAL	NORMAL	ABNORMAL FINDINGS
Appearance • Marfan stigmata (kyphoscoliosis, high-arched palate, pectus excavatum, arachnodactyly, arm span > height, hyperlaxity, myopia, MVP, aortic insufficiency)		
Eyes/ears/nose/throat • Pupils equal • Hearing		
Lymph nodes		
Heart[a] • Murmurs (auscultation standing, supine, +/- Valsalva) • Location of point of maximal impulse (PMI)		
Pulses • Simultaneous femoral and radial pulses		
Lungs		
Abdomen		
Genitourinary (males only)[b]		
Skin • HSV, lesions suggestive of MRSA, tinea corporis		
Neurologic[c]		
MUSCULOSKELETAL		
Neck		
Back		
Shoulder/arm		
Elbow/forearm		
Wrist/hand/fingers		
Hip/thigh		
Knee		
Leg/ankle		
Foot/toes		
Functional • Duck-walk, single leg hop		

[a]Consider ECG, echocardiogram, and referral to cardiology for abnormal cardiac history or exam.
[b]Consider GU exam if in private setting. Having third party present is recommended.
[c]Consider cognitive evaluation or baseline neuropsychiatric testing if a history of significant concussion.

☐ Cleared for all sports without restriction

☐ Cleared for all sports without restriction with recommendations for further evaluation or treatment for _____

☐ Not cleared

    ☐ Pending further evaluation

    ☐ For any sports

    ☐ For certain sports _____

    Reason _____

Recommendations _____

I have examined the above-named student and completed the preparticipation physical evaluation. The athlete does not present apparent clinical contraindications to practice and participate in the sport(s) as outlined above. A copy of the physical exam is on record in my office and can be made available to the school at the request of the parents. If conditions arise after the athlete has been cleared for participation, the physician may rescind the clearance until the problem is resolved and the potential consequences are completely explained to the athlete (and parents/guardians).

Name of physician (print/type) _____ Date _____

Address _____ Phone _____

Signature of physician _____, MD or DO

■ PREPARTICIPATION PHYSICAL EVALUATION
CLEARANCE FORM

Name _____ Sex ☐ M ☐ F Age _____ Date of birth _____

☐ Cleared for all sports without restriction

☐ Cleared for all sports without restriction with recommendations for further evaluation or treatment for _____

_____

☐ Not cleared

    ☐ Pending further evaluation

    ☐ For any sports

    ☐ For certain sports _____

    Reason _____

Recommendations _____

_____

_____

_____

_____

_____

I have examined the above-named student and completed the preparticipation physical evaluation. The athlete does not present apparent clinical contraindications to practice and participate in the sport(s) as outlined above. A copy of the physical exam is on record in my office and can be made available to the school at the request of the parents. If conditions arise after the athlete has been cleared for participation, the physician may rescind the clearance until the problem is resolved and the potential consequences are completely explained to the athlete (and parents/guardians).

Name of physician (print/type) _____ Date _____

Address _____ Phone _____

Signature of physician _____, MD or DO

EMERGENCY INFORMATION

Allergies _____

_____

_____

_____

Other information _____

_____

_____

_____

_____

_____

_____

_____

_____

SECTION 9 PEDIATRIC ORTHOPAEDICS

Components of the PPE

Timing and Interval

Optimal timing for the PPE is 6 weeks prior to the beginning of the athletic season. This allows adequate time for further consultation, diagnostic testing, or rehabilitation of identified problems. Comprehensive evaluations should be performed at every new level of school (elementary school, middle school, high school, college) and every 2 years. On the intervening years, a comprehensive history should be obtained along with a focused evaluation of any identified issues.

History

The medical history is the most important piece in identifying relevant conditions. Often the history given by adolescents is inaccurate or incomplete; therefore, parental input is desirable. Questions should emphasize symptoms related to the cardiovascular system such as dizziness or syncope with exercise, chest pain, shortness of breath, palpitations, and fatigability. Because many important cardiovascular conditions have a hereditary component, obtaining a family history also is critical. The family history should include details about any sudden death of a close relative younger than 50 years, Marfan syndrome, long QT syndrome, or other significant cardiovascular conditions.

Additional aspects of the history should address musculoskeletal issues (prior injury, orthosis/brace use, cervical instability), asthma symptoms, infectious concerns (mononucleosis, methicillin-resistant *Staphylococcus aureus* [MRSA], herpes), neurologic disorders (seizures; headaches; radiculopathy, especially in the upper extremity), solitary organs (for example, only one kidney), visual concerns, high-risk behaviors, and heat-related concerns (sickle cell disease or trait, muscle cramping, heat intolerance). In addition, in female patients, a menstrual history should be taken.

Physical Examination

The examination component begins with a thorough general examination of all systems. The cardiovascular and musculoskeletal examinations are presented here in more detail.

Cardiovascular Examination

The cardiovascular examination includes evaluation of peripheral pulses, murmurs, and blood pressure. **Table 1** summarizes important aspects of the screening cardiovascular examination. Note that all diastolic murmurs and grade 3.6 systolic murmurs warrant further evaluation. Hypertrophic cardiomyopathy (HCM) may produce a systolic murmur that cannot be distinguished from an innocent murmur. The murmur of HCM increases in intensity with standing (decreased ventricular filling, increased

SECTION 9 PEDIATRIC ORTHOPAEDICS

Table 1 Cardiovascular Screening in Athletes

Condition	Cardiovascular Examination	Abnormailty
Hypertension	Blood pressure	Varies with age–general guideline is > 135/85 mm Hg in adolescents
Coarctation of aorta	Femoral pulses	Decreased intensity of pulse
Hypertrophic cardiomyopathy	Auscultation with provocative maneuvers (standing, supine, Valsalva)	Systolic ejection murmer that intensifies with standing or Valsalva maneuver
Marfan syndrome	Auscultation	Aortic (decrescendo diastolic murmer) or mitral (holosystolic murmer) insufficiency

(Adapted with persmission from Maron BJ, Thompson PO, Puffer JC, et al: Cardiovascular screening of competitive athletes: A statement for health professionals from the Sudden Death Committee [clinical cardiology] and Congenital Cardiac Defects Committee [cardiovascular disease in the young], American Heart Association. *Circulation* 1996;94:850-856.)

obstruction) and decreases with squatting or lying supine (increased ventricular filling, decreased obstruction), whereas that of aortic stenosis may decrease with standing but worsens with squatting.

Blood pressures obtained during the PPE often are elevated; sometimes this is due to the use of a blood pressure cuff that is too small, particularly in large adolescents. Sometimes a patient's blood pressure will be recorded as elevated because reference was not made to a table of age-based norms. At times, however, the athlete's blood pressure is truly elevated. Hypertension rarely is severe enough to disqualify an athlete from participation, but it needs to be identified and followed by the athlete's regular physician.

Musculoskeletal Examination

The musculoskeletal examination is important because it typically accounts for 50% of the abnormal physical findings identified on the PPE. A general musculoskeletal examination may be acceptable for patients without symptoms, but in patients with prior injuries or symptoms, the examination should focus on those areas. Most musculoskeletal injuries are detected on the basis of the history alone. A brief musculoskeletal screening examination that can detect problems in asymptomatic individuals is described on page 983.

Some authorities recommend a sport-specific approach to the physical examination. This method emphasizes areas that are most commonly injured or diseased in each specific sport. For example, a swimmer's examination would focus on the shoulders and ears (otitis externa); a wrestler's examination would emphasize the skin, body fat composition, and the shoulders.

SECTION 9 PEDIATRIC ORTHOPAEDICS

Diagnostic Tests

Recommendations regarding diagnostic screening tests for athletes are not provided because of the complexity of the issue. Additional tests such as electrocardiography, echocardiography, or musculoskeletal imaging should be ordered based on the history and physical examination.

Athletes With Special Needs

The PPE for athletes with physical or cognitive disabilities is the same except that there may be additional aspects to address specific to the particular athlete's disability in regard to history, physical examination, or possibly mandatory imaging.

Referral Decisions/Red Flags

Any history of the following physical findings indicates the need for further evaluation and possible specialty consultation.

- Best-corrected vision of less than 20/40 in either eye
- Early fatigue, dizziness, syncope, chest pain, shortness of breath, or palpitations with exercise or unexplained seizures
- Family history of sudden death or significant cardiovascular condition
- Murmur over left ventricular outflow tract
- Physical signs of Marfan syndrome
- Previous heat illness
- Significant head or spinal injury or persistent post-concussive symptoms
- Significant musculoskeletal problem or injury

Once the PPE has been completed, a recommendation can be made for (1) unrestricted clearance, (2) clearance with recommendations for further evaluation or treatment, (3) "not cleared" but to be reconsidered after further evaluation or treatment, or (4) "not cleared" for some or all sports. Often these decisions will be made together with the athlete, parents, and consultants. Guidelines for cardiovascular system conditions can be found in "Eligibility Recommendations for Competitive Athletes With Cardiovascular Abnormalities," published in the *Journal of the American College of Cardiology*. Blood pressure standards for children based on age, sex, and height are available from the National Institutes of Health at http://www.nhlbi.nih.gov/guidelines/hypertension/child_tbl.htm. Guidelines for most other conditions are presented in the *Preparticipation Physical Evaluation* monograph developed by the American Academy of Family Physicians, the American Academy of Pediatrics, the American College of Sports Medicine, the American Medical Society for Sports Medicine, the American Orthopaedic Society for Sports Medicine, and the American Osteopathic Academy of Sports Medicine, and published by the American Academy of Pediatrics. To obtain a copy of this monograph, contact AAP Publications at 1-888-227-1770 or go to www.aap.org/bookstore. The official *Preparticipation Physical Evaluation* forms can be accessed at http://www.aap.org/sections/sportsmedicine/PDFS/PPE-4-forms.pdf.

Scoliosis

Definition

Scoliosis is a lateral curvature of the spine greater than 10° measured using the Cobb method; the curves can occur in the thoracic or the lumbar spine (occasionally in both). Scoliosis may be accompanied by abnormalities in sagittal alignment such as excessive kyphosis or lordosis. Idiopathic scoliosis is the most common diagnosis, with a prevalence of 2% to 3%. Other diagnoses associated with scoliosis are listed in **Table 1**. This chapter focuses on idiopathic scoliosis.

The etiology of idiopathic scoliosis is most likely multifactorial. Idiopathic scoliosis may be classified according to

Table 1 Etiologic Classification of Structural Scoliosis

Type	Possible Cause
Idiopathic	Genetic and environmental factors
Congenital	Failure of formation—hemivertebra or block vertebra
	Failure of segmentation—bony bar joining one side of two or more adjacent vertebrae
	Mixed anomalies
Neuromuscular	Cerebral palsy
	Muscular dystrophy
	Myelomeningocele
	Spinal muscular atrophy
	Friedreich ataxia (spinocerebellar degeneration)
	Polio
	Myopathies
Vertebral disease	Tumor
	Infection
	Metabolic bone disease
Spinal cord disease or anomaly	Tumor
	Syringomyelia
	Spinal cord injury
Disease-associated	Neurofibromatosis
	Marfan syndrome
	Connective tissue disorders
Compensatory	Limb-length discrepancy

age at onset as follows: infantile (birth to 3 years), juvenile (3 to 11 years), and adolescent (older than 11 years). For adolescent idiopathic scoliosis, the male-to-female ratio is nearly equal for curves of less than 20°, but girls are much more likely than boys to have a curve greater than 30°. The natural history depends upon the magnitude of the curvature and the degree of skeletal maturity. Thoracic curves greater than 80° to 90° may impair pulmonary function (restrictive pattern). Curves diagnosed during the infantile and juvenile years are much more likely to be progressive and to require surgical treatment.

Neuromuscular scoliosis is associated with a host of diseases causing flaccid weakness or spasticity. The predominant impact of these deformities is a loss of sitting balance, but respiratory function also may be impaired. Patients with neuromuscular scoliosis typically have long thoracolumbar or lumbar curves.

Congenital scoliosis results from abnormalities in the shape and/or growth potential of vertebrae and can be due to a failure of formation (part of the vertebra is absent) or a failure of segmentation (two or more vertebrae partially or completely fused together); mixed anomalies are common. The risk of progression depends on the unique characteristics of each anomaly.

Clinical Symptoms

Idiopathic scoliosis is most commonly identified during a school screening program or routine examination, but it also may be noticed by family members. Pain is not common, and neurologic symptoms are very rare. Neuromuscular curves present as a loss of sitting balance. Congenital curves may present similar to idiopathic scoliosis.

Tests

Physical Examination

Idiopathic scoliosis is a diagnosis of exclusion, and a thorough history and physical examination is required to rule out other processes that may be associated with the deformity. In addition to the spinal examination, assess the trunk and lower extremities for findings of potential etiologies: skin lesions, such as café-au-lait spots, axillary freckling or lesions over the spine that may suggest neurofibromatosis or spinal disorders, respectively; cavus feet, suggestive of neuromuscular disease or spinal cord anomaly; limb-length discrepancy; abnormal joint laxity associated with Marfan syndrome or connective tissue disorders; and neuromuscular abnormalities.

The patient's spine is inspected in an upright position. The Adam forward bend test is the most sensitive clinical method of screening for scoliosis. The patient is asked to bend forward with the feet together, knees straight, and the arms hanging free.

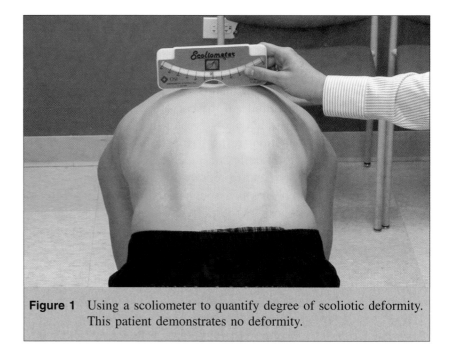

Figure 1 Using a scoliometer to quantify degree of scoliotic deformity. This patient demonstrates no deformity.

The examiner looks at the back from behind and documents any rotational asymmetry. Spinal flexion accentuates rotation of the spine, causing elevation of the posterior hemithorax and/or prominence of the lumbar paravertebral muscle mass on the convexity of the curves. The deformity can be quantified in degrees using an inclinometer such as the scoliometer (**Figure 1**); values greater than 5° to 7° have been used in the past as a benchmark for referral. School screening programs, which are widespread in the United States, have been associated with a referral rate of 3% to 30%. The efficacy of school screening remains controversial. The flexibility of the deformity also is assessed clinically.

Diagnostic Tests

PA and lateral full-length radiographs should be obtained with the patient standing and the knees straight. The x-ray tube should be positioned 6′ from the cassette, using a 14″ × 36″ grid. Positioning the patients with their backs to the x-ray source and using modern image-enhancing equipment minimizes exposure of the thyroid, breasts, and reproductive organs. The Cobb angle is the standard method of quantifying the degree of curvature and is determined by measuring the angle between lines drawn perpendicular to the end plates of the highest and lowest vertebrae in the curve (**Figure 2**). By convention, radiographs of the spine are viewed, measured, and described as if the patient were being examined from behind. The indications for MRI of the spine in patients with presumed idiopathic scoliosis include (1) age (infantile or juvenile); (2) abnormal findings on the history or physical examination (chronic pain,

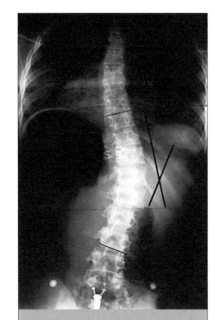

Figure 2 PA long-cassette radiograph of the entire spine demonstrates a scoliotic deformity and the Cobb method of measuring its magnitude.

neurologic symptoms or findings); and (3) selected plain radiographic findings (left-sided thoracic curve, excessive thoracic kyphosis, widening of the spinal canal, erosive vertebral changes or rib abnormalities). For patients with congenital spinal abnormalities that cause scoliosis or kyphosis, additional imaging studies include a renal ultrasound (40% have renal abnormalities), an MRI of the spine (20% have intraspinal anomalies), and an echocardiogram (15% have congenital heart abnormalities).

Differential Diagnosis

See **Table 1** for a list of differential diagnoses of potential etiologies for structural scoliosis. Leg length discrepancy may cause an apparent scoliosis (due to spinal compensation for the tilt of the pelvis) or contribute to compensation or exacerbation of a structural curve; correcting the leg length discrepancy by having the patient stand on a block resolves any compensatory curve and reveals the true degree of any underlying structural curve.

Adverse Outcomes of the Disease

Progressive idiopathic curves are associated with cosmetic concerns. The small subset of patients with progressive thoracic curves greater than 80° to 90° may develop dyspnea from restrictive pulmonary disease. A reduced life expectancy from cardiopulmonary failure (cor pulmonale) is associated with severe curves, which most commonly occur in infantile/juvenile and congenital scoliosis. An increased risk of mild to moderate back pain in untreated idiopathic curves also exists, but overall the vast majority of patients do well throughout their lives. Disabling pain is more likely to develop in patients who have decompensated lumbar or thoracolumbar curves.

Treatment

Treatment recommendations are based on the natural history of the curve, which varies based upon the underlying diagnosis, growth remaining, and other variables. Options include observation, bracing, and surgery. Observation is always appropriate for small and/or nonprogressive curves that are asymptomatic.

For progressive idiopathic scoliosis, physical therapy and electrical stimulation have not been shown to alter the natural history. Brace treatment is offered to selected patients with the goal of arresting progression of the deformity, typically skeletally immature patients with progressive curves in the range of 25° to 45°. An underarm orthosis is appropriate for most

SECTION 9 PEDIATRIC ORTHOPAEDICS

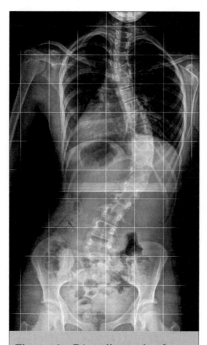

Figure 3 PA radiograph of skeletally mature adolescent girl. She had a progressive right thoracolumbar curve despite bracing and was ultimately treated with corrective surgery.

curves; the recommended time in brace varies from 18 to 23 h/day. Surgical treatment, which involves spinal fusion with instrumentation, usually is offered for skeletally immature patients with curves greater than 45° and for skeletally mature patients with curves greater than 50° to 60° (**Figure 3**). The spinal implants hold the spine in the maximally corrected position while the fusion mass develops, and usually no cast or brace is needed postoperatively. The goal is to achieve a well-balanced and stable spine while minimizing the number of vertebral segments fused (and therefore maximizing the number of mobile segments). Occasionally, an anterior spinal release (diskectomy) is required to achieve added mobility in large, rigid curves.

In neuromuscular scoliosis, deformities that do not interfere with sitting balance or function are observed. Progressive and symptomatic curves are often treated with a soft spinal orthosis. The softer materials used in this design are more comfortable, enhance the patient's sitting balance and upper extremity use, and are easy to care for. Bracing does not alter the natural history of neuromuscular scoliosis, but it may slow the progression and delay the need for more definitive treatment. Surgical stabilization by an instrumented spinal fusion is required for progressive and symptomatic curves; the decision whether to operate is made on a case-by-case basis. The risk of complications is higher in patients with neuromuscular scoliosis.

For congenital scoliosis, bracing is ineffective. Given that surgical correction carries a higher risk of complications, preemptive spinal fusion is considered for curves with a poor natural history (high likelihood of significant progression) before a significant deformity has developed. Other surgical procedures such as anterior and posterior spinal fusion or excision of a hemivertebra may be considered in selected patients. Finally, progressive spinal deformities in young children are a particular challenge, as definitive treatment (fusion) must be delayed until the pulmonary system has matured and, ideally, maximal trunk height has been achieved. Options to delay the need for fusion in this age group include bracing, serial casting followed by bracing, and surgical strategies such as "growing rods." The growing rod program, which is essentially internal bracing, involves implantation of one or two rods to anchor points at the ends of the curve. The rods are lengthened periodically to maintain correction and delay the need for definitive fusion. Progressive curves in toddlers and young children, especially when associated with rib fusions or other anomalies of the chest wall, may result in a thoracic insufficiency syndrome, in which the chest wall is unable to support normal respiration. The vertical, expandable prosthetic titanium rib (VEPTR) has been developed (and is FDA approved in the United States under the

Humanitarian Device Exemption) to treat thoracic insufficiency syndrome. The device is attached between two ribs or between the upper thoracic ribs and the lumbar spine or pelvis and is sequentially distracted to maintain expansion of the hemithorax.

Adverse Outcomes of Treatment

Surgical procedures may be complicated by infection, neurologic injury, failure of the fusion to consolidate, and/or implant-related problems such as loss of fixation.

Referral Decisions/Red Flags

Patients with idiopathic scoliosis typically are referred for specialty evaluation. Patients with pain, neurologic symptoms or findings, unilateral foot deformity, or abnormal curve patterns require further evaluation to rule out intraspinal anomalies or other diagnoses.

SECTION 9 PEDIATRIC ORTHOPAEDICS

Septic Arthritis

Synonyms

Infected joint

Pyarthrosis

Definition

Septic arthritis in children most often results from hematogenous seeding of the synovium from pneumonia, impetigo, or other skin infections. It also may be due to direct extension from an adjacent metaphyseal osteomyelitis or, rarely, from penetrating wounds. Patients often have a history of viral illness in the days to weeks preceding the joint symptoms. Septic arthritis typically affects the large joints of the lower extremities (knee and hip), but it may occur in a variety of locations, including the sacroiliac joint. Early diagnosis and treatment are essential, as damage to hyaline cartilage from the liberation of proteolytic enzymes by polymorphonuclear lymphocytes and synovial cells may be detected within 48 to 72 hours of inoculation.

Clinical Symptoms

Patients typically have an acute onset of guarding of the involved joint. The pain often is poorly localized initially. Children with lower extremity involvement often limp or refuse to walk; elbow or shoulder involvement may result in pseudoparalysis of the upper extremity. A history of mild trauma also is common. Systemic symptoms include malaise, fever, and loss of appetite.

Tests

Physical Examination

The patient typically appears ill at presentation. For comfort, the joint is held in a position that accommodates distention. When the hip is involved, patients prefer to hold the joint in a position of flexion, abduction, and external rotation. The elbow and knee are held in mild flexion. The child is apprehensive and resists attempts to examine the affected extremity. Joint movement is painful, typically throughout the range of motion. In contrast, patients with transient synovitis of the hip or Legg-Calvé-Perthes disease may only experience discomfort. Tenderness to palpation is common, as is joint swelling. An effusion may be identified on clinical examination in subcutaneous joints such as the knee, elbow, or ankle, but it may be impossible to appreciate clinically at the hip, shoulder, or sacroiliac joints.

Table 1 Typical Laboratory Results Associated with Septic Arthritis

Condition	ESR	WBC Count	Synovial WBC Count	Blood Culture	Joint Culture
Septic joint	>30 mm/h in most patients; unpredictable in neonates	>15,000/mm³ (variable), often not elevated early	> 50,000/mm³	Positive 40%-50%	Positive 50%-60%
Transient synovitis	< 50 mm/h	Normal	Normal	Negative	Negative
Juvenile idiopathic arthritis	Variable	Normal	Variable	Negative	Negative

ESR = erythrocyte sedimentation rate, WBC = white blood cell.

Diagnostic Tests

Any suspicion of joint infection requires immediate aspiration and analysis of the joint fluid. The results are corroborated with the findings on physical examination and results of other laboratory tests (**Table 1**). Inflammatory markers are usually elevated. The white blood cell count is elevated in 40% to 60% of cases, especially in older children. The erythrocyte sedimentation rate (ESR) is commonly elevated, although there may be a delay of 24 to 48 hours following the onset of symptoms. The ESR lacks specificity and will be elevated in a variety of inflammatory or infectious disease processes. The C-reactive protein (CRP) level, which becomes elevated in 6 to 8 hours, is perhaps the most helpful marker. Blood cultures are positive in 40% to 50% of cases, and cultures of joint fluid are diagnostic in 50% to 60% of patients. Plain radiographs are rarely helpful in confirming the diagnosis early in the disease process, but they are useful in excluding other disorders. Initial radiographs are often normal but may reveal joint space widening. Ultrasonography will confirm the presence of a joint effusion, and aspiration may be performed at the same time. The absence of joint effusion on ultrasound does not rule out a septic process.

Differential Diagnosis

- Hemophilia (history of bleeding)
- Infection
    Osteomyelitis (less pain with joint motion)
    Pyomyositis (muscle tenderness)
    Lyme disease (milder pain)

SECTION 9 PEDIATRIC ORTHOPAEDICS

- Inflammatory diseases

    Juvenile idiopathic arthritis (pain is less severe, subacute presentation)

    Reactive arthritis (pain is less severe, subacute presentation)

    Rheumatic fever (pain is less severe, subacute presentation)

- Legg-Calvé-Perthes disease (intermittent limp, milder pain)
- Neoplasia

    Acute leukemia (constant pain, night pain)

    Pigmented villonodular synovitis (PVNS) (painful joint swelling)

- Transient synovitis (milder pain, mild limp)
- Traumatic hemarthrosis (history of trauma)

Adverse Outcomes of the Disease

If untreated, septic arthritis causes damage to articular cartilage, which may result in progressive joint degeneration (arthritis). Capsular scarring and loss of motion also are observed. A delay in treating septic arthritis of the hip joint in a young child also may result in subluxation, dislocation, or osteonecrosis of the femoral head.

Treatment

An early diagnosis is essential. Prompt joint drainage, followed by intravenous antibiotic administration, is the treatment of choice. Empiric antibiotic therapy is directed against the most likely infecting organism (**Table 2**) and is then modified based on the culture results (**Table 3**). When the diagnosis of septic arthritis (especially of the hip) is suspected on history and physical examination, immediate aspiration should be performed, often under ultrasonographic guidance. (See Procedure: Hip Aspiration, page 1064.) When the diagnosis is highly likely based on the clinical information, then it may be advisable to take the patient to the operating room for aspiration, followed by joint drainage and irrigation even if the aspirate is equivocal. The duration and route of administration of antibiotics depends on a variety of factors, including the severity of the infection, the virulence of the organism, and the initial response to either empiric or organism-specific antibiotics. Typically, patients are treated with intravenous antibiotics for several days to 2 weeks, followed by a course of oral antibiotics.

Table 2 Causative Organisms and Preferred Antibiotics for Pending Culture Results

Age	Organism	Empiric Antibiotic
Neonates	*Staphylococcus aureus* Group B *Streptococci* Gram-negative organisms *Streptococcus pneumoniae*	Antistaphylococcal antibiotic plus cefotaxime[a]
1 month to 3 years	*S aureus* *S pneumoniae* *Streptococcus pyogenes* *Kingella kingae*[b] *Haemophilus influenzae* type B (not immunized)	Antistaphylococcal antibiotic[a] ± cefotaxime/ceftriaxone[c]
> 3 years	*S aureus* *S pneumoniae* *S pyogenes* *H influenzae* type B (not immunized)	Antistaphylococcal antibiotic[a] ± cefotaxime/ceftriaxone[c]
Adolescence	*S aureus* *Neisseria gonorrhoeae* *S pneumoniae* *S pyogenes*	Antistaphylococcal antibiotic[a] ± cefotaxime/ceftriaxone[c]

[a] Antistaphylococcal penicillins (oxacillin/nafcillin) are highly effective against *S aureus*, but vancomycin should be considered empirically if local rates of methicillin-resistant *S aureus* are high.

[b] *K kingae* has been increasingly reported in association with septic arthritis in this age group but still is relatively rare.

[c] If the history suggests *H influenzae* (patient not immunized) or *N gonorrhoeae* (sexually active patient), cefotaxime or ceftriaxone should be added empirically.

Table 3 Preferred Antibiotics for Septic Arthritis Based on Causative Organism

Organism	Initial Intravenous Antibiotic
Methicillin-sensitive *Staphylococcus aureus*	Oxacillin/nafcillin
Methicillin-resistant *S aureus*	Vancomycin
Streptococcus pyogenes or Group B *Streptococcus*	Penicillin
Streptococcus pneumoniae	Ampicillin or cefotaxime/ceftriaxone
Kingella kingae	Penicillin
Neisseria gonorrhoeae	Cefotaxime/ceftriaxone
Haemophilus influenzae	Cefotaxime/ceftriaxone

Referral Decisions/Red Flags

A high index of clinical suspicion is required to establish an early diagnosis. Patients suspected of having septic arthritis require emergent evaluation, and usually hospitalization. A multidisciplinary approach is helpful.

SECTION 9 PEDIATRIC ORTHOPAEDICS

Seronegative Spondyloarthropathies

ICD-9 Codes

696.0
Psoriatic arthritis

711.1
Reiter syndrome

713.1
Arthritis of inflammatory bowel disease

720.0
Ankylosing spondylitis

Synonyms

Ankylosing spondylitis
Psoriatic arthritis
Reiter syndrome

Definition

The seronegative spondyloarthropathies have the following characteristics in common: (1) inflammation of tendon, fascia, or joint capsule insertions (enthesitis); (2) pauciarticular arthritis, usually involving the lower extremity; (3) extra-articular inflammation involving the eye, skin, mucous membranes, heart, and bowel; and (4) association with the human leukocyte antigen B27 (HLA-B27).

Clinical Symptoms

Ankylosing Spondylitis

Ankylosing spondylitis is more likely to affect the joints of the lower extremities in children than in adults. Asymmetric pauciarticular arthritis involving the lower extremity in children 9 years or older, particularly boys, suggests the possibility of ankylosing spondylitis. The family history often is positive.

Reiter Syndrome

Reiter syndrome is characterized by the triad of conjunctivitis, enthesitis, and urethritis, although all three components of the disorder are not necessarily present in every patient, nor are they always present at the same time. In young children, it can be triggered by infectious diarrhea caused by *Yersinia*, *Campylobacter*, *Salmonella*, or *Shigella*. In adolescents, nongonococcal urethritis secondary to *Chlamydia* or trachoma may cause Reiter syndrome. The Achilles tendinitis or plantar fasciitis associated with Reiter syndrome can be extremely painful.

Psoriatic Arthritis

Psoriatic arthritis is considered uncommon in children, but in approximately one third of patients with this disease, especially girls, the onset is before the age of 15 years. Arthritis frequently antedates skin problems when this disorder occurs in childhood. A family history of psoriasis is a helpful clue when joint symptoms occur first.

Inflammatory Bowel Disease

Arthritis of inflammatory bowel disease, either ulcerative colitis or Crohn disease, typically causes symptoms in patients younger than 21 years, but only 15% of patients are diagnosed before age 15 years. Arthralgia without joint effusion is twice as common as arthritis with joint effusion.

Tests

Physical Examination

A purplish discoloration around the joint is one of the distinguishing features of a juvenile spondyloarthropathy.

A child with ankylosing spondylitis may have an enthesitis, such as patellar tendinitis, Achilles tendinitis, or plantar fasciitis. Although children with ankylosing spondylitis may not have back pain, limited mobility of the spine can be present.

Mild conjunctivitis or an acute anterior uveitis causing painful red eyes and photophobia also are associated with Reiter syndrome.

In psoriatic arthritis, monoarticular involvement of the knee is the most common presentation. Progression to other joints proceeds in an asymmetric fashion. Upper extremity involvement and tenosynovitis involving the digits and nail pitting is more common in psoriatic arthritis than in other spondyloarthropathies.

Pauciarticular arthritis of the lower extremity in inflammatory bowel disease typically is of short duration and either resolves spontaneously or with treatment of the bowel lesion. Progressive ankylosing spondylitis, however, may develop in some patients.

Diagnostic Tests

The presence of HLA-B27 and a positive family history for spondyloarthropathy support the diagnosis of ankylosing spondylitis. Sterile pyuria supports the diagnosis of Reiter syndrome.

Differential Diagnosis

- Juvenile rheumatoid arthritis (often younger age at onset, upper extremity joint commonly affected, synovitis more impressive)
- Overuse syndromes (localized and more often unilateral)

Adverse Outcomes of the Disease

Many lower extremity problems associated with childhood spondyloarthropathies resolve spontaneously, but persistent erosive arthritis may develop. Ultimately, changes in the sacroiliac joint develop in children with ankylosing spondylitis.

SECTION 9 PEDIATRIC ORTHOPAEDICS

Treatment

NSAIDs, muscle strengthening, orthoses for the painful joint, and counseling about activity modifications are indicated.

Adverse Outcomes of Treatment

NSAIDs can cause gastric, renal, or hepatic complications.

Referral Decisions/Red Flags

Loss of function or inability to control pain indicates the need for further evaluation.

SECTION 9   PEDIATRIC ORTHOPAEDICS

Shoes for Children

During the past several decades, clinical studies have clarified the role shoes play in a child's life. The accumulated body of data is now sufficiently large to establish recommendations for children's footwear.

Normal Foot Development

Clinical studies have consistently shown that in societies where going barefoot is common, the human foot has the following attributes: (1) excellent mobility; (2) thickening of the plantar skin to as much as 1 cm; (3) alignment of the phalanges with the metatarsals, causing the toes to spread; (4) variable arch height; and (5) an absence of most common foot deformities. These findings show that satisfactory foot development occurs in the barefoot environment.

Arch development has been documented in several studies. The arch develops spontaneously during a child's first 6 to 8 years, and the range considered as normal is very broad. About 15% to 25% of adults have flexible flatfeet, which are considered a variation of normal and typically are not associated with disability. The military no longer disqualifies individuals with flatfeet, as long as the flatfoot was not corrected and is asymptomatic.

Choosing Appropriate Shoes

The primary role of shoes is to provide protection for the foot. If shoes are not fitted properly, toe deformities are likely to develop.

Wearing shoes does not affect how soon a child will begin to walk. Infants do not require shoes, and socks or booties are just fine; soft shoes may be used for appearance or to protect the foot when outside. Soft, flexible shoes are best for the toddler. Nonslip soles help to provide traction on hardwood and tile floors. The shoes also should have breathable uppers to avoid excessive sweating. A wide toe box also is suggested to avoid constriction across the foot. If the toddler's foot is chubby, a high-top shoe can be helpful to keep the shoe on the foot, but this type of shoe does not affect the growth or development of the foot. High-top shoes also may be beneficial in children with ligamentous hyperlaxity or hypotonia.

Characteristics of a Good Shoe

For children, the features of a good shoe include the following five Fs:

- *Flexible*. The shoe should allow as much free motion as possible. As a test, make certain that the shoe can be easily flexed in your hand.
- *Flat*. Avoid high heels that force the foot forward, cramping the toes.
- *Foot-shaped*. Avoid pointed toes or other shapes that are different from the normal foot. A straight last shoe best approximates the child's foot.
- *Fitted generously*. Better too large than too short. Allow about a fingerbreadth of room for growth.
- *Friction like skin*. The sole should have about the same friction as skin. Soles that are slippery or adherent can cause the child to fall.

The "Corrective" Shoe

Controlled prospective studies on the effect of shoe modifications on arch development showed no difference between treated and untreated feet. In essence, shoe inserts do not modify or alter intoeing, outtoeing, or flexible flatfeet. In fact, shoe inserts can be harmful. Adults who wore shoe modifications as children often remember the experience as negative and, in one study, were shown to have lower self-esteem than control subjects.

Shoe modifications that are not corrective but produce some immediately desirable effect are useful. For example, shoe lifts for the short leg equalize limb length and improve walking. Shoe inserts for older children or adolescents with rigid foot deformities can redistribute weight-bearing forces and reduce discomfort or skin breakdown if sensation is impaired. Shock-absorbing footwear with cushioned soles can help in the management of overuse syndromes.

Current Problems

The design of shoes has improved over the past decade. The major problems continue to be the prevalence of constrictive and deforming shoes, including elevated heels, pointed toes, and tight fit, which may cause deformity (bunions) and instability, both of which can increase the risk of ankle injuries.

Recommendations

Shoes should be regarded as a form of clothing and should be designed to simulate the barefoot state.

- Walking and play in the barefoot condition in a safe environment is acceptable for infants and children.
- For most children, shoes should be flexible, flat, shaped like the foot, and have soles that provide friction similar to skin.
- Cushioning of the sole can reduce the risk of overuse conditions around the foot.
- Shoe modifications are not "corrective." Inserts are useful only for load redistribution and do not change the shape of the foot.
- Prescribing unnecessary shoe inserts and modifications is expensive for the family and society. More importantly, these can be uncomfortable and embarrassing for the child.

SECTION 9 PEDIATRIC ORTHOPAEDICS

Slipped Capital Femoral Epiphysis

Synonym

Slipped epiphysis

Definition

Slipped capital femoral epiphysis (SCFE) occurs when progressive displacement of the upper portion of the femur occurs in relation to the capital femoral epiphysis. The slip occurs through the physis, typically during the adolescent growth spurt. The etiology is unknown and is likely multifactorial, involving an increase in shear stresses across a weakened physis. Anatomic variables that may predispose to SCFE include femoral retroversion, a greater inclination of the proximal femoral physis, and weakening of the perichondrial ring. Mechanical factors also are important: Most patients are above the 95th percentile for weight. African Americans are more commonly affected than Caucasians or Hispanic Americans. SCFE is most common in boys from 13 to 15 years of age and in girls from 11 to 13 years of age. Patients who are outside the typical age ranges (younger than 11 years, older than 16 years) are likely to have an underlying endocrinologic or metabolic disorder (hypothyroidism or hyperthyroidism, panhypopituitarism, growth hormone deficiency, renal disease). Bilateral involvement is seen in 40% to 50% of patients who are followed to closure of the growth plate. SCFE may be classified according to time or duration of symptoms (acute is less than 3 weeks, chronic is more than 3 weeks; acute-on-chronic has exacerbation after several months of symptoms) or stability (stable can bear weight, unstable cannot).

Clinical Symptoms

Pain is the most common presenting symptom. It is usually localized to the groin or anterior thigh, but it also may occur in the distal thigh or knee. The pain is made worse by activity, and a limp is common. The slipped epiphysis develops gradually in most patients, although some may have acute onset of symptoms following an injury.

Figure 1 Radiographs of the pelvis show mild slipped capital femoral epiphysis (SCFE) of the left hip. **A,** Posterior displacement of the femoral head (arrows) is profiled on the frog-lateral radiograph. **B,** On the AP radiograph, mild degrees of medial displacement can be recognized by drawing a Klein line on the lateral aspect of the femoral neck. When SCFE is present, the line on the involved hip will either miss the femoral head or transect less of it than on the uninvolved hip.

Tests

Physical Examination

Patients are typically in the upper ranges of weight and body mass index for age, and they ambulate with both lower extremities externally rotated. When SCFE is unilateral, external rotation is greater on the affected side. Patients with unstable SCFE are unable to ambulate even with crutches. Loss of hip internal rotation is the most sensitive and specific finding on bench examination. Hip flexion also should be tested, as progressive flexion is usually accompanied by progressive external rotation of the hip. The affected extremity is shortened, often from 1 to 3 cm, depending on the severity of the slip.

Diagnostic Tests

AP and frog-lateral radiographs of the pelvis confirm the diagnosis (**Figure 1**). On rare occasions, in the "preslip" phase, the radiographs are normal or demonstrate irregularity or subtle widening of the physis. MRI may help to confirm the diagnosis when radiographs are inconclusive. On the AP radiograph, SCFE is suspected if a line drawn along the superior femoral neck (the Klein line) does not intersect the lateral capital femoral epiphysis. The degree of displacement is best appreciated on the lateral view, and usually a prominence is seen along the anterior

SECTION 9 PEDIATRIC ORTHOPAEDICS

femoral neck. The severity of displacement is classified as mild, moderate, or severe as measured by the degree of angulation (mild, <30°; moderate, 30° to 50°; severe, >50°).

Differential Diagnosis

- Acute fracture through the physis (Salter Harris I) (history of acute trauma)
- Endocrinopathy (atypical age)
- Legg-Calvé-Perthes disease (in younger age range)
- Meralgia paresthetica (lateral femoral cutaneous nerve entrapment)
- Neoplasm (night pain, no restriction of hip internal rotation in flexion)

Adverse Outcomes of the Disease

Progressive slip may be accompanied by gait disturbance, and SCFE may predispose the hip to symptomatic degenerative changes. The prominence along the anterior femoral neck may impinge against the acetabulum, resulting in labral tears or other intra-articular pathology. The prognosis has been linked to stability of the physis: stable SCFE has a low likelihood (approximately 5%) of developing osteonecrosis, but unstable SCFE may be associated with osteonecrosis in up to 50% of patients.

Figure 2 Radiograph demonstrates SCFE treated with surgical fixation in situ with a single cannulated screw.

Treatment

The goals of treatment for adolescents with SCFE are to stabilize the physis (promote closure of the physis), avoid complications such as osteonecrosis and chondrolysis, and maximize function. Most patients are treated by in situ stabilization with a single screw (**Figure 2**), although some surgeons prefer to treat unstable SCFE with two screws. This strategy has been shown to be effective and associated with few complications. Patients are typically allowed to be touch-down weight bearing (non–weight-bearing for unstable SCFE) for the first 6 weeks, and activities are restricted until the physis has closed, typically for 6 to 9 months. Patients with greater degrees of deformity may require a realignment osteotomy, but this is only considered after the physis has been stabilized and the patient has reached a plateau in function.

Several areas of controversy and continuing study remain, especially with regard to the treatment of unstable SCFE and whether to prophylactically pin the other hip in patients with unilateral involvement. An unstable slip may be likened to a Salter Harris I fracture of the physis, and a subset of patients do present with a history of an acute event. These unstable SCFEs are often stabilized as an emergency, and many surgeons decompress the hip joint to reduce intra-articular pressure. The role of manipulative reduction before pinning remains to be determined.

Up to 60% of patients will develop bilateral disease, and the need for routine prophylactic pinning of the contralateral hip remains a subject of debate. Families of patients with routine SCFE within the typical age range are counseled regarding the pros and cons of prophylactic pining before making the final decision. Prophylactic pinning is indicated in patients with an underlying endocrinologic or metabolic diagnosis, and it is generally recommended in patients younger than 10 years.

Recently, there has been interest in the technique of open surgical dislocation of the hip to address a variety of problems, including SCFE. This technique facilitates not only realignment of the proximal femur at the site of deformity, but also the treatment of any coexisting labral problems or intra-articular pathology. These strategies are currently under investigation in selected centers, and longer-term follow-up studies are required to define any role for these procedures.

Adverse Outcomes of Treatment

Patients are at risk for recurrent slippage until the physis closes. Chondrolysis and osteonecrosis also may occur.

Referral Decisions/Red Flags

Further evaluation for surgical treatment should occur immediately upon diagnosis. Patients should be non–weight bearing once the diagnosis is made.

SECTION 9 PEDIATRIC ORTHOPAEDICS

Spondylolysis/ Spondylolisthesis

Definition

Spondylolysis refers to a unilateral or bilateral defect in the pars interarticularis, the region of bone lying between the superior and inferior articular facets. This condition is acquired. The process may start with a stress reaction, which leads to a stress fracture and often to an established pseudarthrosis (nonunion with fibrous tissue interposition). The most common level is L5, although spondylolysis may occur at higher levels in the lumbar spine and may be observed at more than one level. Up to 25% of patients with spondylolysis will develop a spondylolisthesis.

Spondylolisthesis is anterior translation, or slippage, of one vertebra in relation to the vertebral body below. The most common slip is L5 on S1, which represents more than 85% of cases (**Figure 1**). The vast majority of cases in children and adolescents are acquired (due to a stress fracture or spondylolysis); a small number of cases are congenital (or dysplastic) spondylolisthesis. Acquired spondylolisthesis, in which the amount of slip occurs through the defect in the pars interarticularis (which becomes filled with fibrocartilaginous material), is in contrast to congenital spondylolisthesis, in which elongation of the posterior elements often is associated with a dome-shaped sacrum. Higher grades of slip are often associated with kyphosis at the lumbosacral junction.

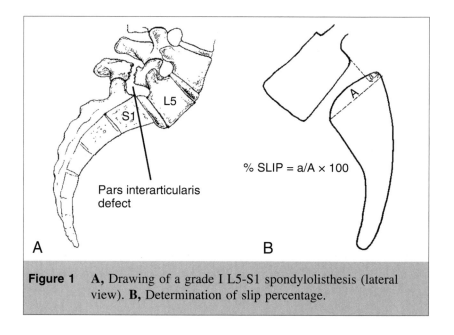

% SLIP = a/A × 100

Pars interarticularis defect

Figure 1   **A,** Drawing of a grade I L5-S1 spondylolisthesis (lateral view). **B,** Determination of slip percentage.

Clinical Symptoms

Activity-related low back pain that often radiates distally to the buttock and/or thigh is the most common symptom. Radiation to below the knee is uncommon and suggests lower lumbar radiculopathy, which may occur with high-grade spondylolisthesis (**Figure 2**). Symptoms are more common with slips greater than 50%. Hamstring spasm/contracture is common and may result in a limitation in forward bending. With higher grade lesions, neurologic abnormalities may be seen, such as nerve root symptoms (radiculopathy) from traction on the lower lumbar nerve roots, or bowel or bladder dysfunction (or symptoms of cauda equina syndrome) from compression (or traction) of the neural elements.

Tests

Physical Examination

Patients with significant spondylolisthesis have a characteristic standing alignment, including mild flexion at the hips and knees, which compensates for backward tilting of the pelvis, and flattening of the normal lumbar lordosis (often a kyphosis at the lumbosacral junction). With marked levels of slip, a step-off can be palpated, and the spinous process of the vertebra below is more prominent than the one above. Patients often experience discomfort with hyperextension of the spine (loading the posterior elements in compression); the examiner should hold the spine in this position for 10 to 20 seconds to see if discomfort can be reproduced. This may be the first sign of a stress reaction or of spondylolysis. Manual pressure on the spinous processes may produce discomfort at the involved level. The popliteal angle should be tested to evaluate for a hamstring contracture: With the patient supine and with one hip flexed to 90° and the other leg fully extended, the knee is extended and the angle between the tibia and the vertical plane is measured. (The average is 6° in toddlers, 25° in adolescents.) A neurologic examination is essential, and other regions in which back pain may be referred (abdomen, pelvis, hips) must be evaluated as well.

Diagnostic Tests

AP and weight-bearing lateral radiographs of the lumbar spine are obtained, often supplemented by oblique radiographs. Established spondylolysis will exhibit the "Scotty dog sign" on oblique views (**Figure 3**). When clinical suspicion of spondylolysis exists and plain radiographs are normal, a bone scan with single-photon emission computed tomography (SPECT) images will help establish the diagnosis. CT with thin cuts through the pars region may be required to determine if a pars fracture has healed or progressed to a nonunion. With spondylolisthesis, the lateral radiograph will demonstrate

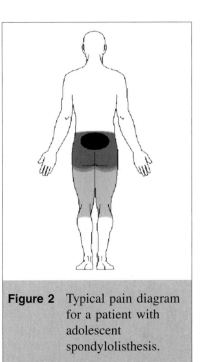

Figure 2 Typical pain diagram for a patient with adolescent spondylolisthesis.

Figure 3 Oblique radiograph shows a normal "Scotty dog" appearance in the outlined area. In the vertebra below, the Scotty dog has a "collar" (arrow), indicating the pars interarticularis defect of spondylolisthesis.

SECTION 9 PEDIATRIC ORTHOPAEDICS

Figure 4 Lateral radiograph demonstrates a grade I L5-S1 spondylolisthesis. The black arrow indicates the direction of the slip; the white arrow indicates the defect.

Figure 5 Lateral radiograph shows a high-grade spondylolisthesis for which surgical stabilization was required.

forward translation of L5 relative to S1 for an L5-S1 slip (expressed as a percentage of the anteroposterior width of the vertebral body) (**Figure 4**). The degree of lumbosacral kyphosis, or flexion of the lumbar spine relative to the sacrum (the slip angle), also is measured. Lateral lumbar radiographs are occasionally obtained in flexion and extension to determine if excessive motion or instability between the involved segments occurs.

Differential Diagnosis

- Ankylosing spondylitis (human leukocyte antigen B27 [HLA-B27] positive, sacroiliac joint changes)
- Intervertebral disk injury or herniation (no step-off or slip and no defect seen on plain radiographs, radiculopathy occasionally present)
- Intervertebral diskitis (elevated erythrocyte sedimentation rate and fever, disk space narrowing on radiographs)
- Osteoid osteoma (night pain, abnormal bone scan, pain relieved by aspirin)
- Spinal cord tumor (sensory findings, upper motor neuron signs)

Adverse Outcomes of the Disease

The natural history of spondylolysis and spondylolisthesis is variable, and many patients will be asymptomatic and able to participate in activities as tolerated. A subset will develop chronic back pain, however, with or without radiculopathy, and some patients with high-grade spondylolisthesis will develop bowel and bladder involvement or cauda equina syndrome (**Figure 5**). Spondylolisthesis may progress in children and adolescents, so clinical and radiographic monitoring is required. The frequency of evaluation, typically every 6 to 12 months, depends on the amount of growth remaining, the degree of slip, and whether a patient is symptomatic. A weight-bearing spot lateral radiograph is usually adequate for periodic monitoring.

Treatment

Patients with a stress reaction or an early case of spondylolysis are treated with activity restriction, short-term analgesics or anti-inflammatory agents, and a thoracolumbosacral orthosis (TLSO) for 3 to 4 months, often supplemented by rehabilitation. Healing may be achieved using this approach in a subset of patients (especially those with unilateral pars defects), but in many patients the spondylolysis ultimately progresses to a chronic pseudarthrosis or nonunion, which may or may not be symptomatic.

Asymptomatic spondylolysis requires no active treatment, and patients may participate in activities as tolerated. In patients with a symptomatic pseudarthrosis (limited or no healing potential), the goal of treatment is symptomatic relief rather than healing. Rehabilitation also is helpful, and involves strengthening of the abdominal and paraspinal muscles, stretching the hamstring muscles, and postural adaptations. A TLSO also may be recommended for symptomatic relief in patients with chronic pain and an established pseudarthrosis, although the goal is symptomatic relief rather than healing of the stress fracture. For patients who have chronic symptoms despite an adequate trial of nonsurgical treatment, surgical options include repair of the pars defect (with instrumentation and bone grafting) or fusion of the involved segments. Fusion is typically recommended for the less mobile L5-S1 articulation; repair is an option when higher levels of the spine are involved.

The treatment of spondylolisthesis depends on the age, degree of deformity, and whether symptoms are present. Asymptomatic children with minimal amounts of slippage may continue with activities as tolerated, although follow-up at regular intervals will be required. Skeletally immature patients with a greater than 50% slip are candidates for spinal fusion (with or without instrumentation) with the goal of stabilizing the segment, as are those chronically symptomatic patients with a lower grade spondylolisthesis (less common). Patients with high-grade spondylolisthesis, especially with neurologic symptoms or findings, will require a neural decompression in addition to the spinal fusion, and either postural or instrumented reduction of the amount of slip is considered depending upon the circumstances.

Adverse Outcomes of Treatment

In addition to the general complications of spine surgery such as bleeding and infection, surgical complications of spondylolysis repair include pseudarthrosis (nonunion); for spondylolisthesis, they include nerve root or cauda equina injury, pseudarthrosis, implant failure, and chronic pain.

Referral Decisions/Red Flags

Patients with significant or chronic back pain and/or a confirmed spondylolysis or spondylolisthesis require further evaluation.

SECTION 9 PEDIATRIC ORTHOPAEDICS

Tarsal Coalition

Synonyms

Calcaneonavicular bar
Peroneal spastic flatfoot
Rigid flatfoot
Talocalcaneal bar

Definition

Tarsal coalition is an abnormal connection (fibrous, cartilaginous, or osseous) between two tarsal bones, most commonly the calcaneus and the navicular (calcaneonavicular coalition) or the talus and the calcaneus (talocalcaneal coalition). Rarely, more than one coalition is present. The condition is bilateral in approximately 50% of patients and may be found in other family members who are asymptomatic but have no hindfoot motion.

Clinical Symptoms

If symptoms develop, they usually occur during late childhood or adolescence. In some cases, the bar is initially cartilaginous and ossifies later, during early adolescence. Symptoms are the result of a restriction in hindfoot eversion and inversion. Calcaneonavicular coalitions generally become symptomatic in children between 9 and 13 years of age; symptoms from a talocalcaneal coalition generally develop later, between 13 and 16 years of age.

The onset of pain usually is insidious but can be associated with an injury or change in activity. Ankle sprains are frequent, and a limp is common. Pain from a talocalcaneal coalition usually is vague and located deep within the hindfoot. Pain from a calcaneonavicular coalition usually occurs laterally, over the area of the coalition.

Tests

Physical Examination

Patients with tarsal coalition typically have rigid flatfoot (hindfoot valgus, forefoot abduction); that is, the longitudinal arch is absent whether in a weight-bearing position or not. Hindfoot motion (inversion and eversion) is markedly restricted. Spasm of the peroneal muscles holds the foot in a stiff, everted position and may be demonstrated by attempting rapid passive inversion of the foot.

Figure 1 Oblique radiograph of a foot with a cartilaginous calcaneonavicular coalition (arrow).

Diagnostic Tests

AP, lateral, and oblique radiographs of the foot may delineate a calcaneonavicular coalition (**Figure 1**). Talocalcaneal bars are difficult to see on these views, but they may be visualized on a Harris heel view. In most cases, CT is used to establish the diagnosis and better characterize the coalition.

Differential Diagnosis

- Accessory navicular (medial prominence and pain over the navicular)
- Congenital vertical talus (rigid flatfoot deformity noted in the infant or toddler)
- Flexible flatfoot (no restriction of subtalar motion, usually without pain)
- Juvenile idiopathic arthritis or other inflammatory disease (negative radiographs and CT, synovitis on MRI)

Adverse Outcomes of the Disease

Pain, restricted inversion and eversion of the foot, and limited walking and running are possible consequences.

Treatment

Treatment options include observation, short leg cast immobilization, resection of the coalition, and arthrodesis. Observation or activity modifications are appropriate for children who are asymptomatic or who have minimal symptoms. For more severe symptoms or for milder symptoms that persist, a 4- to 6-week trial in a short leg walking cast may be of benefit.

SECTION 9 PEDIATRIC ORTHOPAEDICS

For patients with persistent symptoms that do not respond to nonsurgical treatment, resection of the coalition with interposition of fat or muscle is the preferred treatment. Resection reduces pain in most patients, and this procedure is more reliable for calcaneonavicular coalitions. An osteotomy of the calcaneus also may be performed at the same time as resection of a coalition, when realignment of the hindfoot is needed. Hindfoot arthrodesis (joint fusion) is reserved for patients who have not responded to resection procedures or patients who are not candidates for coalition resection because the coalition is too large or arthritic changes are already present.

Adverse Outcomes of Treatment

Complications include cast sores, postoperative infection, failure of fusion, recurrence of the coalition, inadequate pain relief or persistent symptoms, and arthritic changes.

Referral Decisions/Red Flags

Significant pain following nonsurgical treatment indicates the need for further evaluation.

SECTION 9 PEDIATRIC ORTHOPAEDICS

Toe Walking

Synonym

Habitual toe walking

Idiopathic toe walking

ICD-9 Code

781.2
Abnormality of gait

Definition

Idiopathic toe walking (or habitual toe walking) is toe walking in children who are otherwise normal and have no underlying neurologic abnormalities. Toe walking can be a normal variation in children when they begin to walk. Toe walking that persists or develops after a child has been walking with the feet flat may indicate an underlying disease process. Symptoms are uncommon, and most patients respond to nonsurgical measures.

Clinical Symptoms

Parental concern is usually the reason for referral. Children with idiopathic toe walking generally are active and asymptomatic and have no functional difficulties or other medical problems. The patient may have occasional forefoot discomfort in the region of the metatarsal heads after prolonged activities. Discomfort in the hindfoot or posterior calcaneus also may occur if the child has an associated Achilles tendon contracture.

Tests

Physical Examination

The diagnosis of idiopathic toe walking is one of exclusion, and pathologic causes must be ruled out. A thorough history is critical, particularly a detailed birth history, developmental history, and family history. Cerebral palsy is suggested by a delay in reaching motor milestones and a history of prematurity, low birth weight, hypoxia, or perinatal infection. Muscular dystrophy is suspected when a positive family history and proximal muscle weakness exists. The time of onset also is important. Patients with muscular dystrophy may be slightly delayed in achieving independent ambulation, and they typically walk with feet flat for a period of time before they begin to walk up on their toes. Children with idiopathic toe walking begin ambulation at the appropriate age and are up on their toes when they begin walking. Toe walking is common in children with speech and language delays, including autism spectrum disorders.

Figure 1 Idiopathic toe walking.

Ankle range of motion should be tested to quantify the degree of dorsiflexion. When assessing range of motion, the hindfoot should be inverted to lock the subtalar joint. Patients with less than 10° of passive dorsiflexion have an Achilles tendon contracture. Toe walking varies in severity (**Figure 1**), but children with idiopathic toe walking generally can stand with their feet flat on the floor and can walk heel-toe if reminded. A subset of patients with idiopathic toe walking will also have an Achilles tendon contracture. These patients may still be able to walk with the feet flat, but they will appear to have flatfoot when standing, as dorsiflexion through the hindfoot joints compensates for a loss of dorsiflexion at the ankle. A thorough neurologic examination is essential, including evaluation for cutaneous lesions over the spine that may suggest occult spinal dysraphism

Diagnostic Tests

Diagnostic tests should be ordered only if the history is unclear or if the examination reveals some abnormality suggestive of another disorder.

Differential Diagnosis

- Autism spectrum disorder (other developmental/behavioral concerns)
- Cerebral palsy (delayed developmental milestones, spasticity of gastrocnemius-soleus complex)
- Intraspinal abnormality (cavus feet, unilateral or asymmetric involvement)
- Muscular dystrophy (proximal muscular weakness, positive family history)
- Occult hydrocephalus (upper motor neuron signs)

Adverse Outcomes of the Disease

The prevalence of long-term sequelae has not been documented; however, in some patients, persistent calluses and pain in the forefoot develop during late adolescence.

Treatment

Treatment depends on the age of the child and the severity of the problem. In the toddler who has just begun to walk, the condition often resolves spontaneously after 3 to 6 months. Observation is appropriate for older toddlers who walk on their toes only occasionally. Stretching exercises may be tried for young children with mild contractures. Children with autism spectrum disorders may benefit from physical therapy, occupational therapy, or other comprehensive interventional strategies.

Serial casting involving two to three short leg casts over a period of 6 weeks often is successful, especially if a coexisting Achilles tendon contracture exists. The degree of dorsiflexion is increased with each cast. Casting for several weeks will result in atrophy of the Achilles tendon, which theoretically can help treat any habitual component, as the child may find it difficult to stay up on the toes after the casts are removed, at least until the muscle regains its strength. Rehabilitation, possibly supplemented by nighttime splinting in dorsiflexion, may help to prevent recurrent contracture. Some clinicians recommend use of an ankle-foot orthosis to prevent recurrence. After casting, many of these children will walk heel-to-toe, but some will revert to their previous gait pattern.

Adverse Outcomes of Treatment

Observation and stretching exercises are complicated only by failure or recurrence. Recurrence and skin problems can occur with casting or with heel cord lengthening.

Referral Decisions/Red Flags

Any child with persistent toe walking despite stretching and rehabilitation or with evidence of a neuromuscular impairment requires further evaluation. Surgical treatment typically is indicated for an older child with a fixed heel cord contracture when nonsurgical treatment is ineffective or poorly tolerated. Heel cord lengthening is considered after all nonsurgical measures have failed. Postoperatively, approximately 6 weeks of cast immobilization is required. Unilateral toe walking is never normal. In these instances, thorough examination is required to identify the underlying pathologic process. The most common causes of unilateral toe walking are limb-length discrepancy, cerebral palsy, and tethering of the spinal cord (intraspinal anomaly). Consideration should be given to developmental evaluation of children with other developmental or behavioral concerns.

SECTION 9 PEDIATRIC ORTHOPAEDICS

Torticollis

Synonym

Acquired torticollis
Congenital muscular torticollis
Wryneck

Definition

Torticollis describes a head position characterized by tilting (lateral bending) of the head to one side, often with rotation. It is a finding and not a specific diagnosis. Most cases that present at or shortly after birth represent congenital muscular torticollis (CMT). CMT is a unilateral contracture of the sternocleidomastoid (SCM) muscle and is diagnosed shortly after birth. The etiology remains unknown, but fibrosis and subsequent contracture may be due to a localized compartment syndrome within the muscle caused by abnormal positioning in utero. Acquired torticollis, which presents later in infancy or in childhood and may be associated with a variety of conditions, requires a detailed workup, including advanced imaging studies and, often, subspecialty consultations. The differential diagnosis includes injuries, congenital anomalies, inflammatory or infectious disorders, neurologic abnormalities, ophthalmologic problems (nystagmus, superior oblique palsy), atlantoaxial rotatory displacement (AARD), and others. Torticollis in infants also may result from congenital anomalies within the cervical spine, either from a progressive congenital scoliosis at the cervicothoracic junction (**Figure 1**) or an anomaly at the occipitocervical junction. These deformities may present as a progressive tilt with or without significant rotational deformity. The Klippel-Feil syndrome involves a congenital fusion of two or more cervical segments, which commonly manifests as a restriction in cervical motion associated with a short neck, and is occasionally associated with head tilt.

Clinical Symptoms

Parental concern about head posture is the usual reason for the visit. Children with acquired torticollis may present with neck pain, fevers, or, rarely, neurologic abnormalities, depending on the underlying diagnosis. The contracture causes the head to tilt toward the affected side and rotate toward the unaffected side (**Figure 2**). CMT is commonly associated with plagiocephaly and facial asymmetry. A lump may be palpable within the midsubstance of the muscle during the first weeks of life, but

Figure 1 AP radiograph of an infant with torticollis caused by progressive congenital vertebral anomaly at the cervicothoracic junction.

this typically disappears within weeks to months. Associated findings may include positional foot deformities (metatarsus adductus, calcaneovalgus) and developmental dysplasia of the hip (5% to 8%).

Tests

Physical Examination

Infants with CMT hold the head in a "cock robin" position. Contracture of the left SCM muscle results in tilting to the left side with rotation of the head to the right side, with associated facial/mandibular flattening on the left side and occipital flattening on the right side. In patients with CMT, a lump or swelling in the SCM muscle that disappears over the first few weeks to months may be noted. Patients with AARD hold the head in a similar position to those with CMT; however, spasm of the SCM usually occurs on the opposite side to the tilt, in contrast to CMT. Range of motion should be evaluated, as it may be limited as a result of contracture (CMT) or because of discomfort or muscle spasm. A complete neurologic examination is essential, as well as an opthalmologic evaluation, to assess for ocular or neurologic disorders. A complete musculoskeletal examination also is required, as CMT can be associated with developmental hip dysplasia and intrauterine deformations.

Acquired torticollis requires a comprehensive evaluation. An ophthalmologic examination often is helpful, as "ocular" torticollis may be due to nystagmus or a superior oblique palsy. In such cases the findings may resolve when the eyes are closed or vision is blocked. Neurologic causes of torticollis include tumors of the posterior fossa and cervical spine, as well as developmental conditions such as syringomyelia, and neurologic consultation (and MRI) is indicated in many patients. Infections such as diskitis or vertebral osteomyelitis usually present with significant pain and systemic signs or symptoms. Benign paroxysmal torticollis of infancy involves episodes of torticollis that may last from minutes to days; the side of involvement may alternate, and the condition usually resolves spontaneously.

AARD represents a spectrum of abnormalities in the alignment and arc of motion between C1 and C2. Either subluxation or dislocation may be present, and the displacement is initially reducible but becomes fixed or irreducible over time. AARD may develop following minor trauma; in association with inflammatory disorders of the upper airway, neck, or pharynx (Grisel syndrome); or following surgical procedures on the ears, nose, or oropharynx.

Figure 2 Child with congenital muscular torticollis. The chin is rotated to the patient's right and the head is inclined to the left.

Diagnostic Tests

The indications for screening radiographs of the cervical spine in patients with CMT are controversial; some authors advise obtaining radiographs when the typical clinical features of CMT are absent or the deformity does not respond appropriately to stretching. AP and lateral radiographs of the cervical spine should be obtained in all patients with acquired torticollis to rule out underlying congenital bony anomalies, and most patients diagnosed with a cervical anomaly will require lateral radiographs in flexion and extension as well, to rule out instability. Patients with neurologic symptoms or findings also may require MRI of the cervical spine in flexion and extension to rule out neurologic encroachment. Patients with a history of trauma should be imaged with more than two views of the cervical spine; an open-mouth odontoid view, and, occasionally, oblique views. Specialized imaging studies such as CT or MRI may be indicated as well. MRI of the brain and cervical spine often is required to rule out a brainstem tumor or other pathology. Open-mouth odontoid views should be obtained when AARD is suspected; however, this diagnosis is very difficult to secure on plain radiographs. CT scans of the cervical spine with the head in neutral and in maximal rotation (right and left) characterize the rotational alignment between C1 and C2 throughout the available range of motion and will clearly show any fixed subluxation or dislocation between C1 and C2. The study may be difficult to obtain if the patient has significant pain or spasm.

Other imaging studies also may be considered, depending on the specific diagnosis. For example, screening hip ultrasonography is considered even when the physical examination is normal in patients with CMT. All patients with congenital vertebral anomalies should have coexisting visceral anomalies ruled out, typically by a renal ultrasound, a cardiac evaluation with or without an electrocardiogram, and, often, MRI of the neural axis.

Differential Diagnosis for Acquired Torticollis

Present at or Shortly After Birth

- CMT (identified during first 2 months of life)
- Congenital vertebral anomalies or instabilities
- Klippel-Feil syndrome (short neck, low hairline, may have
  Sprengel deformity)
- Pterygium colli (skin webbing)
- Unilateral absence of SCM muscle

Acquired

- **AARD** (older patient, history of minor trauma, ear/nose/throat procedure, pharyngitis, late onset)
- **Benign paroxysmal torticollis** (infants, repeated episodes)
- **Infectious or inflammatory**
  Cervical lymphadenitis (lymphadenopathy)
  Diskitis or vertebral osteomyelitis (pain with flexion)
  Juvenile idiopathic arthritis (multiple joint involvement, gradual onset)
  Soft-tissue infection in the neck/pharynx (localized tenderness in soft tissues)
- **Neurogenic**
  Cervical dystonia (increased muscle tone that fluctuates, history of developmental delay or cerebral palsy)
  Chiari malformation and/or syringomyelia (headaches, neurologic abnormalities)
  Ocular (nystagmus, superior oblique palsy) (ophthalmologic findings)
  Posterior fossa tumor (headaches, constant and increasing pain, more gradual onset, neurologic findings)
- **Posttraumatic**
  Muscle sprain, fractures (history of trauma)
- **Other**
  Hysteria (rare, diagnosis of exclusion)
  Sandifer syndrome (gastroesophageal reflux)

Adverse Outcomes of the Disease

The natural history of CMT includes persistent torticollis, facial asymmetry, and plagiocephaly. Untreated AARD will result in fixed malalignment at the atlantoaxial joint, which may be associated with chronic pain and a risk of neurologic dysfunction. The natural history in other acquired cases of torticollis depends on the underlying diagnosis. Klippel-Feil patients are at risk of cervical spinal cord injury and should be restricted from participation in contact activities or those that involve sudden acceleration/deceleration.

Treatment

Congenital Muscular Torticollis

Nonsurgical treatment of CMT consists of frequent stretching exercises that tilt and rotate the head. Supervision by a rehabilitation specialist is helpful, but the parents themselves must actually perform the stretching exercises several times a day. In addition, the infant's bed and changing table can be positioned to encourage the infant to look away from the limited side. Nonsurgical treatment is successful in more than 90% of patients. If the problem persists after 12 to 18 months, surgical release/lengthening of the SCM should be considered.

Acquired Torticollis

The treatment for acquired torticollis depends on the underlying etiology. Initial management of AARD is immobilization in a soft cervical collar and administration of analgesics for pain. If restoration of motion and alignment does not occur in approximately 1 week, cervical traction with a head halter, coupled with analgesics and muscle relaxants, should be tried. Most cases will resolve with this program, and patients are typically splinted in a collar or other device such as a pinless halo for several additional weeks. If this treatment fails, consideration is given to a period of halo traction in an attempt to reduce the malalignment. AARD that persists for more than 1 month is less likely to respond to these treatment strategies, and some patients will ultimately require an upper cervical fusion for relief of symptoms and restoration of alignment.

Referral Decisions/Red Flags

Most infants with CMT are referred for rehabilitation and for specialty evaluation, recognizing that the vast majority of cases will respond to nonsurgical measures. Referral should be considered for all patients with acquired torticollis, as well as those with head tilt and rotation to the same side.

Transient Synovitis of the Hip

Synonyms

Coxalgia fugax

Toxic synovitis

ICD-9 Code	
719.05	
Effusion of joint, pelvic region and thigh	

Definition

Transient synovitis of the hip is a sterile effusion of the joint that resolves without therapy or sequelae, typically over 4 to 6 weeks, and is a common source of limping in children from 2 to 7 years of age. Boys are affected two to three times more often than girls. The etiology is unknown. Mild trauma may explain some cases, and many patients have a history of viral illness (upper respiratory or gastrointestinal) in the days to weeks preceding the onset of limping.

Clinical Symptoms

The child presents with a limp, which may be painless or associated with discomfort that is localized in the groin, proximal thigh, or knee. Some patients with more significant symptoms will refuse to walk. The limp may be intermittent; typically, it worsens toward the end of the day and usually resolves over 1 to 2 weeks.

Tests

Physical Examination

Examination reveals a limp (typically an abductor lurch/ Trendelenburg gait) and mild restriction of hip motion, particularly in abduction and internal rotation. There may be guarding at the extremes of hip rotation. Most children are afebrile.

Diagnostic Tests

Because transient synovitis is a diagnosis of exclusion, the extent of the evaluation process depends on the degree and duration of symptoms and the findings on physical examination. A short period of observation may be appropriate if the child has minimal symptoms, no systemic signs or symptoms, and no significant pain with motion. In most patients with a limp and findings localized to the hip region, it is appropriate to order AP and frog-lateral radiographs of the pelvis and blood tests that include a complete blood count with a differential, an erythrocyte sedimentation rate (ESR), a C-reactive protein (CRP) level, and an antistreptolysin-O (ASO) test. Other blood tests may be appropriate depending on the findings, such as a Lyme titer or rheumatologic tests. If any suspicion of septic arthritis exists or if the patient has significant pain, any systemic signs or symptoms, or pain with short arc motion (mid range of motion rather than the extremes of motion), referral to the emergency department or hospital admission for further evaluation may be most appropriate.

Radiographs in patients with transient synovitis are usually normal, but they may show widening of the joint space due to effusion. If septic arthritis is suspected, hip ultrasonography is ordered urgently, and aspiration of the hip may be performed at the same time. MRI may be useful in selected cases to rule out other infections (osteomyelitis of the femur or pelvis, psoas abscess) or early Legg-Calvé-Perthes disease.

Differential Diagnosis

■ Infections

Lyme disease (similar presentation, may have swelling in other joints)

Pelvic osteomyelitis (pain that is dull, constant, and increasing; fever)

Proximal femoral osteomyelitis (pain that is dull, constant, and increasing; fever)

Septic arthritis (pain that is dull, constant, and increasing; fever)

■ Inflammatory diseases (juvenile idiopathic arthritis or other) (history of joint swelling)

■ Injuries (sprain, strain, rarely occult fracture)

■ Legg-Calvé-Perthes disease (boys 4 to 8 years old, similar presentation)

Adverse Outcomes of the Disease

No sequelae are associated with transient synovitis, and recurrence is uncommon. Legg-Calvé-Perthes disease subsequently develops in 1% to 3% of patients, but whether this disorder has any association with transient synovitis is unclear. A delay in diagnosing septic arthritis or another disease process is possible.

Treatment

Most children can be treated with activity restriction (bed rest acutely) and anti-inflammatory agents or mild analgesics. The limp typically improves within 3 to 14 days, but it may take 4 to 6 weeks for complete resolution. When the diagnosis is equivocal or the patient has significant discomfort, hospitalization for observation and further investigation is indicated.

Referral Decisions/Red Flags

Patients with significant pain and limping, with or without systemic signs or symptoms, require further evaluation. Consultation with a specialist is frequently obtained during the evaluation. Specialty follow-up is indicated if radiographs suggest Legg-Calvé-Perthes disease.

Glossary

Abduction The movement of a body part away from the midline

Acupuncture The insertion of needles into precisely defined points on the body; thought to realign imbalances of yin-yang and qi and thereby bring harmony to the "climate" of an individual

Adduction The movement of a body part toward the midline

Adhesive capsulitis Self-limiting condition resulting from any inflammatory process about the shoulder in which capsular scar tissue is produced, resulting in pain and limited range of motion; also called frozen shoulder

Aerobic exercise Exercise that uses oxidative metabolic pathways to provide energy

Allograft Biologic tissue from a cadaver that is used to surgically replace damaged tissue

Alternative medicine A wide spectrum of treatments—many finding support from collective anecdotal evidence—that is not considered standard therapy because of the lack of a scientific rationale, clinical evidence, or a favorable historic tradition

Anabolic steroid Testosterone, or a steroid hormone resembling testosterone, that stimulates anabolism in the body

Anaerobic exercise Exercise of short duration, not requiring the body's utilization of oxygen to make fuel available

Anaerobic metabolism Oxygen debt; when the cardiovascular system is unable to meet the needs of the working muscles, the anaerobic metabolism is activated

Analgesia The relief of pain

Ankylosing spondylitis An inflammatory disorder that affects the low back and pelvis and produces stiffness and pain

Ankylosis Marked stiffness of a joint typically observed with end-stage arthritis, following a complex intra-articular fracture, delayed treatment of septic arthritis, or severe rheumatoid arthritis

Anorexia nervosa A condition, common in young females, in which the patient takes in less food and may become seriously emaciated and malnourished; a manifestation of a severe underlying psychological disorder

Anterior compartment syndrome Increased soft-tissue pressure in the anterior compartment of the lower leg, resulting in pain, decreased sensation, and muscle paralysis

Anterior cruciate ligament (ACL) Ligament that passes from the lateral intercondylar notch of the femur to attach anteriorly on the articular surface of the tibia

Anterior superior iliac spine Blunt bony projection on the anterior border of the ilium, forming the anterior end of the iliac crest. Serves as the origin of the sartorius muscle.

Anterior surface Surface at the front of the body, facing the examiner

Anterior talofibular ligament One of three lateral ligaments of the ankle; arises from the anterior border of the lateral malleolus to attach to the neck of the talus

Anterior tibial tendon Structure that arises in the anterior compartment of the leg and passes downward and medially to insert on the first cuneiform and the base of the first metatarsal

Anterior tibiofibular ligament Part of tibiofibular syndesmosis; it arises from the anterior calculi on the lateral side of the tibia and blends into the interosseous membrane above the ankle joint

Anterolateral rotatory instability Anterior internal rotational subluxation of the lateral tibial condyle on the femur, reflecting damage to the anterior cruciate ligament and lateral structures

Anteromedial rotatory instability When the medial plateau of the tibia rotates anteriorly and medial joint opening occurs, indicating disruption of the superficial tibia collateral ligament, medial and posteromedial capsular structures, and anterior cruciate ligament

Anteroposterior drawer test Test for anterior and posterior laxity in which the examiner holds the knee in 90 of flexion, stabilizes the thigh, and slowly draws the tibia forward on the fixed femur, noting the degree of displacement. The examiner then attempts to displace the tibia posteriorly on the femur. The test is positive if changes in anteroposterior displacement of the tibia are noted. The injured side should always be compared with the noninjured side. The Lachman test is done similarly but with the knee in 30° of flexion.

Anulus fibrosus The outer ring of fibrous material surrounding the nucleus of the intervertebral disks

Apophysis A cartilaginous structure at the insertion of major muscle groups into bone that may be susceptible to overuse syndromes and acute fractures in pediatric athletes

Apophysitis Inflammation of an apophysis; injury from repetitive traction to the cartilaginous growth plate near the origin or insertion of muscle

Arcuate ligament Posterior third of the lateral capsule, which, together with the popliteus attachments, provides considerable stability to the posterolateral corner of the knee

Arthrocentesis Aspiration of a joint

Arthrodesis The surgical fusion of a joint. The procedure removes any remaining articular cartilage and positions the adjacent bones to promote bone growth across a joint. A successful fusion eliminates the joint and stops motion. The usual purpose is pain relief or stabilization of an undependable joint

Arthroplasty A procedure to replace or mobilize a joint, typically performed by removing the arthritic surfaces and replacing them with an implant. Total joint arthroplasty is replacement of both sides of the joint. Hemiarthroplasty replaces only one side of a joint

Arthroscopy A form of minimally invasive surgery in which a fiberoptic camera, the arthroscope, is introduced into an area of the body through a small incision

Aspiration Removal of fluids from a body cavity; often done to obtain specimens for analysis

Autograft Biologic tissue from the patient's own body that is used to surgically replace damaged tissue

Avascular necrosis A condition in which cells die as a result of inadequate blood supply; *see also* osteonecrosis

Avulsion fracture A fracture that occurs when a ligament or tendon pulls off a sliver of the bone

Axis The second cervical vertebra (C2)

Bankart fracture A small chip fracture off the anterior and inferior rims of the glenoid that is seen after an anterior dislocation of the shoulder

Biceps brachii Muscle in the anterior arm, originating from two heads (hence biceps) from the anterior glenoid and the coracoid process of the scapula and inserting into the biceps tuberosity of the radius. It is a powerful flexor of the elbow and supinator of the forearm.

Biceps muscle Large muscle that covers the front of the humerus; functions include forearm flexion and hand supination

Biceps tendinitis Inflammation of the biceps tendon in its subacromial location

Bisphosphonates Potent inhibitors of osteoclasts and bone resorption. May be used to treat osteoporosis and Paget disease.

Bone infarction Bone death that occurs as the result of ischemia

Bone remodeling A process that couples bone resorption by osteoclasts with deposition of osteoblasts (new bone cells)

Bone scan A study used to identify lesions in bone such as fracture, infections, or tumor. A radioisotope is injected into a vein and allowed to circulate through the body. The distribution of radioactivity in the skeleton is measured by a special camera that can detect the emission of gamma rays. Lesions in bone with increased metabolic activity (eg, fracture, tumor, or infection) will show increased uptake of the radioisotope and appear as a dark area in the bone. Also called bone scintigraphy

Brachial muscle Originates on the humerus, extends anteriorly across the elbow joint, and attaches into the ulna; functions in forearm flexion

Brachial plexus Network of nerves that pass from the lower part of the cervical spine and upper part of the thoracic spine down the arm

Bucket-handle tear Complete longitudinal tear of the central segment of the meniscus with the torn fragment "flipped" into the joint like the handle of a bucket

Bunion Prominence of the first metatarsal head often associated with lateral shift of the great toe (hallux valgus deformity)

Bursa A sac formed by two layers of synovial tissue that is located where there is friction between tendon and bone or skin and bone

Bursitis Inflammation of a bursa

Burst fracture A compression-type fracture of a vertebra that involves posterior displacement of the fragments, often into the spinal canal

Calcaneofibular ligament The longest of the three lateral ligaments of the ankle; inserts on the lateral surface of the calcaneus

Calcaneus Heel bone

Capsule A collagenous structure that surrounds a joint like a sleeve. The capsule allows motion of joints and protects the articular cartilage. The capsule, along with ligaments, tendons, and bony structure, provides stability of the joint

Carpal bones Bones of the wrist

Cartilage A cellular tissue that, in the adult, is specific to joints, but in children forms a template for bone formation and growth. Hyaline cartilage is a low-friction cellular tissue that coats joint surfaces. Fibrocartilage is tough with high collagen content, such as found in the meniscus of the knee, or the anulus fibrosus portion of the intervertebral disk

Cauda equina The terminal nerve roots of the spinal cord located within the vertebral canal; so named because they resemble the tail of a horse

Cavus Excessive height of the longitudinal arch of the foot

Cellulitis Inflammation of subcutaneous tissue. Can be caused by trauma or infection.

Cerebellum The brain area located posteriorly and attached to the brain stem; functions with the cerebral cortex and brain stem to regulate movement and posture

Cerebrum A mass of nerve tissue that makes up the largest part of the brain

Cervical spine The upper seven vertebrae, which extend from the base of the occiput to the first thoracic vertebra

Chondroblasts The cells that form cartilage

Chondroitin sulfate An important class of glucosaminoglycans in articular proteoglycans; the oral form is thought to prevent degradation of joint cartilage and relieve symptoms

Chondromalacia Softening of the articular surface that results from exposure of normal cartilage to excessive pressure or shear

Chondrosarcoma A primary sarcoma formed from cartilage cells or their precursors but without direct osteoid formation

Chronic rotator cuff tear Tear of the rotator cuff of the shoulder resulting from degeneration within the rotator cuff tendon

Clavicle The collarbone

Clavicular epiphyseal fracture Fracture of the growth plate of the clavicle; may appear clinically as a dislocation, especially if some displacement is present

Claw toe Deformity involving hyperextension of the MTP joint and a hyperflexion of the interphalangeal joint

Closed fracture A fracture that does not disrupt the integrity of the surrounding skin

Closed reduction A procedure to restore normal alignment of a fractured bone or dislocated joint in which the fractured bones are simply manipulated and no incision is needed

Clubfoot A complex foot disorder that includes three separate deformities: metatarsus adductus, ankle equinus, and heel varus

Coccyx The three to five fused vertebrae distal to the sacrum

Collagen A triple helix protein that is the major structural macromolecule of the extracellular matrix of articular cartilage; found also in bone, tendon, and ligament

Colles fracture Fracture of the distal radius, with dorsal displacement of the fragments; often caused by a fall on an outstretched arm with the hand extended

Comminuted fracture A fracture with more than two fragments

Common peroneal nerve Nerve lying below the head of the fibula that controls movement at the ankle and supplies sensation to the top of the foot

Compartment syndrome Ischemia of the nerves and muscles within a fascial compartment caused by elevated pressure within the compartment; frequently seen in association with tibial fractures

Compound fracture Any fracture in which the overlying skin has been penetrated

Computed tomography (CT, CAT scan) A radiographic modality that allows cross-sectional imaging from a series of x-ray beams. The x-ray tube is rotated 360° around the patient, and the computer converts these images into a two-dimensional axial image. CT is capable of imaging bone in three planes: coronal, sagittal, and oblique. This modality is particularly useful in evaluating fractures and bone tumors

Concentric contraction The shortening of a muscle during activation

Concentric exercises Exercises in which the muscle shortens while contracting against resistance

Condyle A rounded process at the end of a long bone

Connective tissue Tissue that connects and supports the structures of the body

Contusion Bruise; injury to soft tissue without a break in the skin

Copper therapy An as-yet unproven therapy in which any of a number of copper devices are applied to the body to reduce pain and inflammation associated with joint and connective tissue problems

Coracoacromial ligament Ligament lying anteromedially and superior to the glenohumeral joint; defines the subacromial space

Coracoclavicular ligaments Strong stabilizers of the acromioclavicular joint, consisting of the conoid and trapezial ligaments

Coronal plane A coronal plane is any plane of section in the anatomical position that passes vertically through the body and is perpendicular to the median plane. It divides the body into anterior and posterior sections.

Cortical bone Dense bone that is responsible for skeletal homeostasis

Corticosteroids Cortisone-like medicines that are used to provide relief for inflamed areas of the body. They lessen swelling, redness, itching, and allergic reactions. Often used for a number of other diseases such as asthma or other auto immune diseases.

Costal arch Fused costal cartilages of the sixth to tenth ribs forming the upper border of the abdomen

Costovertebral angle Angle that is formed by the spine and the tenth rib; the kidneys lie beneath the back muscles in the costovertebral angle

COX-1 Cyclooxygenase-1 enzyme; an enzyme that is present in most bodily tissues (including platelets and gastrointestinal mucosal tissues) and serves as a "housekeeping" enzyme to form prostaglandins

COX-2 Cyclooxygenase-2 enzyme; an enzyme that is thought to be present in the body only when induced in response to injury and is responsible for the formation of prostaglandins that mediate pain and inflammation

Coxa valgus A valgus or abduction deformity of the hip. The neck/shaft angle in increased.

Coxa magna A deformity of the hip in which the ball of the hip joint is enlarged. May be secondary to Legg-Perthes disease or arthritis.

Crepitus a grating or grinding sound

Cross-table lateral view Lateral view of the hip obtained by flexing the opposite hip and directing the x-ray beam "across" the table to image a true lateral of the hip. Used in imaging hip fractures, when a frog lateral view (taken with the hip abducted and rotated) would cause patient discomfort.

Crush injury An injury produced as a result of continuous pressure applied to a part of the body, usually an extremity

Cryotherapy The therapeutic use of cold

Cubital tunnel syndrome Compression of the ulnar nerve at the elbow

Cubitus (Elbow). Cubitus varus is a bowing (or adduction) deformity of the elbow. Cubitus valgus is an elbow aligned in the opposite direction.

Curettage The removal of growths from within cavity walls; in the treatment of musculoskeletal tumors, the scraping of tumor out of bone

Deep vein thrombosis (DVT) Venous clot formation caused by immobilization, hypercoagulation, obstructed venous flow, or endothelial injury, among others

Degenerative joint disease (DJD) Deterioration of the articular cartilage that lines a joint, which results in narrowing of the joint space and pain; osteoarthritis

Delayed union A delay in normal fracture healing; not necessarily a pathologic process

Deltoid The muscle that arises from the inferior surface of the lateral third of the clavicle, the acromion, and the spine of the scapula and inserts into the deltoid tuberosity of the humerus. The anterior fibers assist in flexing and medially rotating the arm, whereas the posterior fibers extend and laterally rotate the arm. Acting as a unit, the deltoid acts to abduct the arm at the glenohumeral joint.

Deltoid ligament One of the major support ligaments of the ankle; originates on the medial malleolus and spreads to attach to the medial border of the talus

Dermatome A localized area of skin that is has its sensation via a single nerve from a single nerve root of the spinal cord

Diaphysis The shaft of a long bone

Direct bone healing Method of healing of a fracture in which the approximated bone ends attach themselves to one another by laying down woven bone

Discoid meniscus A congenital deformity in which the meniscus is discoid in shape rather than semilunar

Diskectomy A surgical decompression procedure in which an intervertebral disk is removed

Dislocation Complete disruption in the normal relationship of two bones forming a joint (ie, no contact of the articular surfaces). The direction of the dislocation is described by the position of the distal bone (eg, with an anterior dislocation of the shoulder, the humerus is displaced anterior to the scapula).

Displaced fracture A fracture that produces deformity of the limb

Distal Location in an extremity nearer the free end; location on the trunk farther from the midline or from the point of reference

Dorsal Toward the posterior surface of the body

Dorsalis pedis artery The continuation of the anterior tibial artery on the anterior surface of the foot

Dual-energy x-ray absorptiometry (DEXA or DXA) A diagnostic imaging technology that uses two different x-ray voltages to assess bone density

Dynamic strength The magnitude of isotonic or isokinetic contraction

Dysplasia A broad term that describes a condition affecting growth or development in which the primary defect is intrinsic to bone or cartilage

Dystrophy A condition resulting from defective or faulty nutrition, broadly construed to include nourishment of tissue by all essential substances, including those normally manufactured by the body itself

Eccentric contraction The lengthening of a muscle during activation

Eccentric exercises Exercises in which the muscle lengthens despite resisting a force, as in slowly lowering a weight

Ecchymosis Bruising or discoloration associated with bleeding within or under the skin

Edema Condition in which fluid escapes into the tissues from vascular or lymphatic spaces and causes local or generalized swelling

Effusion The presence of fluid within a joint

Electrical muscle stimulation (EMS) Treatment in which the biphasic current delivers stimulation to muscles in a variety of ways, including pulse, surged, or tetanizing contractions

Electromyography (EMG) A test that measures the electrical response of muscle contraction

Enchondral bone healing Process in which capillaries grow among mesenchymal cells, forming a fibrovascular tissue known as callus that bridges the gap between bone ends

Endochondral ossification The formation of bone within a cartilage model

Enthesopathy A disease process occurring at the insertion of muscle, tendon, or ligament into bone or joint capsule.

Epiphysis A part of a long bone developed from a center of ossification distinct from that of the shaft and separated at first from the latter by a layer of cartilage.

Epiphyseal line The part of a long bone that produces growth

Equinus Plantar flexed position of the ankle

Ewing sarcoma A primary sarcoma of the bone that usually arises in the diaphyses of long bones, ribs, and flat bones of children and adolescents

Exercise-induced compartment syndrome A condition in which exertion leads to relative muscle swelling within a restricted fascial compartment, resulting in compression of neurovascular structures, reduced circulation, muscle ischemia, bone death, and the painful buildup of lactic acid.

Extensor A muscle, the contraction of which causes movement at a joint with the consequence that the limb or body assumes a more straight line, or so that the distance between the parts proximal and distal to the joint is increased or extended; the antagonist of a flexor

Extensor digitorum brevis Short toe extensor on the dorsum of the foot

Extensor digitorum longus Muscle in the anterior compartment of the muscles of the leg; divides and inserts on the dorsum of the small toes

Extensor hallucis longus Muscle in the anterior compartment of the leg that inserts on the dorsum of the great toe

Extensor mechanism Complex interaction of muscles, ligaments, and tendons that stabilizes the patellofemoral joint and acts to extend the knee

Extensor supinator muscle group Muscle group originating on the lateral epicondyle of the humerus and extending down the forearm dorsally into the wrist and hand that includes the extensor carpi radialis longus, the extensor carpi radialis brevis, and the supinator

External fixation Stabilization of a fracture or unstable joint by inserting pins into bone proximal and distal to the injury that are then attached to an external frame.

Fabella Sesamoid bone that is sometimes found in the lateral gastrocnemius muscle tendon

Fascia Sheet or band of tough fibrous connective tissue; lies deep under the skin and forms an outer layer for the muscles

Fascia lata Originates from the lateral crest region and continues over the lateral aspect of the knee, enveloping the lateral aspect of the thigh; iliotibial tract

Fasciculation Involuntary contractions, or twitchings, of groups (fasciculi) of muscle fibers, a coarser form of muscular contraction than fibrillation

Fast twitch muscle fibers Type II muscle fibers.

Fat embolism syndrome Respiratory distress and cerebral dysfunction caused by droplets of marrow fat released at a fracture site and deposited in the lungs or brain

Fatigue fracture Microfracture that occurs when the bone is subjected to frequent, repeated stresses, such as in running or marching long distances, and the rate of bone breakdown exceeds the rate of bone repair.

Fat pad Specialized soft tissue structure for weight bearing and absorbing impact

Fat pad sign A sign on a lateral view of the elbow with the elbow flexed 90° that indicates swelling within the joint, often from a fracture with hemorrhage

Felon Infection of the pulp of the distal phalanx of the finger

Female athlete triad The constellation of abnormal or absent menses, eating disorders, and osteoporosis/stress fractures seen in female athletes

Femoral condyles Two surfaces at the distal end of the femur that articulate with the superior surfaces of the tibia

Femoral head Proximal end of the femur, articulating with the acetabulum

Femoral neck The bone connecting the head and the shaft of the femur; fractures frequently occur in this area

Femur The thigh bone; extends from the pelvis to the knee and is the longest and largest bone in the body

Fibrochondrocytes Cells that are able to synthesize fibrous extracellular proteins and have the rounded appearance of chondrocytes

Fibula Outer and smaller of the two bones of the leg, extending from just below the knee to form the lateral portion of the ankle joint

Fibular collateral ligament Ligament that inserts from the femoral condyle to the fibular head

Flexibility The capacity of a muscle to lengthen or stretch

Flexor A muscle the action of which is to flex or bend a joint

Flexor digitorum longus muscle One of the medial stabilizers of the ankle, located in the posterior compartment of the muscles of the leg, that flexes the lateral four toes

Flexor hallucis longus muscle One of the three muscles of the deep portion of the posterior compartment that flexes the great toe

Flexor pronator muscle group A muscle group with a primary role associated with the wrist and hand and a secondary role as elbow flexors

Floating ribs The eleventh and twelfth ribs, which do not connect to the sternum

Fluoroscopy A special type of radiograph that shows continuous motion of the structure, such as wrist motion

Fracture A disruption in the integrity of a bone

Fracture callus Bone developed after a fracture; initially formed from a hematoma at the bleeding edges of bone, it eventually forms a cartilage mass that is remodeled into mature bone

Fracture-dislocation A fracture of bone associated with a dislocation of its adjacent joint.

Fracture reduction The realignment of fracture fragments to restore normal anatomy of the bone

Freiberg disease An osteochondrosis or osteonecrosis of the metatarsal head

Frequency In strength training, the number of workouts completed per unit of time; also refers to number of workouts during 1 week

Frozen shoulder A condition characterized by restricted shoulder movement resulting from acute trauma or a periarticular biceps or rotator cuff tendon injury

Fusion (arthrodesis) The joining of two bones into a single unit, thereby obliterating motion between the two. May be congenital, traumatic, or surgical.

Galeazzi fracture Dislocated ulna with a fractured radius

Gamekeeper's thumb Rupture of the ligament on the ulnar side of the thumb metacarpophalangeal joint that helps to stabilize the joint when pinching

Ganglion A mass of nerve cell bodies usually found lying outside the central nervous system

Genu (knee) Genu valgum is knock-knee deformity; genu varum is bowleg deformity

Glenohumeral dislocation Injury in which the humeral head may displace from the joint; most of these dislocations are anterior and inferior to the glenoid rim

Glenohumeral joint True shoulder joint

Glenoid labrum A soft fibrous rim surrounding the glenoid fossa that deepens the socket and provides stability for the humeral head

Glenoid labrum tear Tear of the glenoid labrum; can result from acute trauma or overuse

Glucosamine sulfate A fundamental component in the synthesis of both hyaluronic acid and chondroitin that is thought to promote cartilage repair and synthesis; the oral form is taken as a dietary supplement to treat arthritis

Glycosaminoglycans Polysaccharides consisting of long-chain, unbranched, repeating disaccharide units, such as keratin and chondroitin sulfate

Gout An inflammatory arthritis associated with deposition of urate in the joint

Gracilis muscle One of the three hamstring muscles of the knee that make up the pes anserine and help protect the knee against rotatory and valgus stress (the other ones are the sartorius and semitendinosus)

Greater trochanter Broad, flat process at the upper end of the lateral surface of the femur to which several muscles are attached

Greenstick fracture A fracture that disrupts only one side of the bone. This fracture pattern is seen in children because of the greater plasticity of their bones.

Growth factors The molecules that stimulate cell growth or activation

Guarding Refusal to use an injured part because motion causes pain; involuntary abdominal muscular contraction reflecting inflammation and pain within the peritoneal cavity

Hallux The great toe

Hammer toe Flexion deformity of the distal interphalangeal joint of the foot

Hamstring One of the large muscle groups at the back of the thigh that flex the knee

Hangman's fracture Fracture of the pedicles of C2

Head The upper or proximal portion of a structure; the head of a bone is the rounded end that allows joint rotation

Hemarthrosis The presence of blood in the joint

Hematoma A collection of blood resulting from injury

Herniated disk Rupture of the nucleus pulposus or anulus fibrosus of the intervertebral disk

Heterotopic ossification The formation of bone in any nonosseous tissue; often occurs following trauma

Hill-Sachs lesion A wedge-shaped impaction fracture of the posterolateral portion of the humeral head seen following anterior dislocations of the shoulder

Hip pointer Painful injury caused by irritation or avulsion of the attachments of the abdominal and thigh muscles at the iliac crest

Homeopathy A system of therapy developed by Samuel Hahnemann based on the "law of similia," from the aphorism, *similia similibus curantur* (likes are cured by likes), which holds that a medicinal substance that can evoke certain symptoms in healthy individuals may be effective in the treatment of illnesses having similar symptoms, if given in very small doses

ICES Ice, compression, elevation, and splinting

Iliofemoral ligament One of three extremely strong ligaments surrounding the hip joint anteriorly and posteriorly, which reinforce the capsule; the other two are the ischiofemoral and the pubofemoral ligaments

Iliopsoas bursa One of the two most important bursae (the other being the trochanteric bursa) about the hip joint; located between the capsule and the iliopsoas muscle anteriorly

Iliotibial band (ITB) Thickening of the iliotibial tract that inserts directly into the lateral tubercle of the tibia

Ilium One of the three bones (ilium, ischium, and pubis) that fuse to form the pelvic bones

Impacted fracture A fracture pattern in which the fragments are pushed together, thus imparting some stability.

Impingement syndrome Shoulder pain caused by tendinosis of the rotator cuff tendon or irritation of the subacromial bursa. *See also* Rotator cuff impingement, external, and Rotator cuff impingement, internal

Infarct An area of tissue that is cut off from its blood supply, becomes ischemic, and dies

Inflammation Heat, redness, swelling, and pain that accompany musculoskeletal injuries; occurs when tissue is crushed, stretched, or torn

Infraspinatus Muscle of the rotator cuff that arises from the dorsal surface of the scapula and inserts on the greater tuberosity

Instability Looseness; unsteadiness

Intercondylar eminence Proximal tibial process; anterior and posterior to the intercondylar eminence are attachment sites for the cruciate ligaments' menisci

Intercondylar notch Bony notch that separates posteriorly the condyles of the femur

Intercondylar tubercles A lateral spur projecting upward from the intercondylar eminence

Internal fixation Surgical insertion of a device that stops motion across a fracture or joint to encourage bony healing or fusion

Internal impingement A condition in the shoulder of throwing athletes that results in tears of the underside of the rotator cuff and the posterior labrum

Interval throwing program A program for shoulder rehabilitation that allows the athlete to get a light workout several times a day at a submaximal level without fatiguing the arm

Intervertebral disk The structure located between two moving vertebrae that stabilizes the spine, helps maintain its alignment, allows motion between vertebral levels, absorbs energy, and distributes load applied to the spine

Intramedullary nailing or rodding A procedure for the fixation of fractures in which a nail or rod is inserted into the intramedullary canal of the bone from one of its two ends

Intramembranous ossification Bone formation characterized by the aggregation of undifferentiated mesenchymal cells, which differentiate into osteoblasts

Inversion injury Ankle injury resulting from landing on the lateral aspect of the foot

Involucrum In osteomyeltis, a sheath of live bone that forms around a piece of dead bone, the sequestrum

Iontophoresis Therapeutic modality that uses galvanic electrical current to drive ionized medications through the skin to injured tissues

Ischemic Lacking oxygen, usually as the result of partial or complete blockage of blood flow

Ischial tuberosity The bony prominence felt at the base of each buttock, near the crotch; the major attachment site for the hamstrings and the major weight-bearing structure for sitting

Ischiofemoral ligament One of three extremely strong ligaments surrounding the hip joint anteriorly and posteriorly, which reinforce the capsule; the other two are the iliofemoral and the pubofemoral ligaments

Ischium One of the three bones (ilium, ischium, and pubis) that fuse to form the bony pelvis

Isokinetic Literally, "same speed"; when applied to muscle action, it implies constant velocity of shortening

Isokinetic exercise In isokinetic contractions, the muscle contracts and shortens at constant speed.

Isometric Literally, "same length"; when applied to muscle action, it implies that the muscle length is held constant even with varying loads. Accomplished by contracting the flexors and extensors of a joint at equal loads so that the joint does not move.

Isotonic When applied to muscle action, the condition when a muscle shortens against a constant load, as in lifting a weight

Isotonic exercise Contraction of muscles concentrically or eccentrically against resistance with movement of the part so that the load remains constant

Jersey finger Traumatic rupture of the deep flexor tendon of the ring finger; so named because it often occurs as a result of grabbing an opponent's jersey

Joint Articulation, place of union, or junction between two or more bones of the skeleton

Joint mobilization A manually administered treatment modality in which joints are manipulated to improve flexibility and decrease pain

Jones fracture Stress fracture of the proximal shaft of the fifth metatarsal; a fracture that frequently heals with difficulty

Jumper's knee Chronic tendinosis of the patellar tendon; frequently limited to the distal pole of the patella rather than being diffused throughout the tendon

Juvenile rheumatoid arthritis A chronic inflammatory disease in children that is characterized by pain, swelling, and tenderness in one or more joints and may result in impaired growth and development

Kohler disease Osteochondrosis of the tarsal navicular

Kyphosis Curvature of the spine that is convex posteriorly

Lamellar bone Mature, well-organized form of cortical bone

Laminectomy A surgical decompression procedure in which part of the posterior arch of a vertebra is removed; allows access to the disk

Lateral Lying away from the midline

Lateral collateral ligament Ligament on the lateral side (outside) of three joints—the knee, the elbow, and the ankle

Lateral condyle Forms the lateral border of the upper surface of a joint

Lateral epicondylitis An irritation or partial tear of the extensor tendons of the wrist near their origin at the elbow; also called tennis elbow

Lateral ligament structure The three pairs of the lateral collateral ligament of the ankle: the posterior talofibular ligament, the calcaneofibular ligament, and the anterior talofibular ligament

Lateral malleolus Bony prominence at the end of the fibula that is part of the ankle joint

Lateral meniscus The lateral C-shaped fibrocartilaginous structure of the knee

Lateral view A view that passes from side to side at 90° to an AP or PA view

Latissimus dorsi A muscle of the trunk that originates on the spinous processes and supraspinous ligaments of all lower thoracic, lumbar and sacral vertebrae, lumbar fascia, posterior third iliac crest, last four ribs (interdigitating with external oblique abdominis) and inferior angle of scapula , inserting on the floor of bicipital groove of humerus after spiraling around teres major. Extends, adducts and medially rotates arm. Costal attachment helps with deep inspiration and forced expiration.

Lavage The irrigation or thorough washing of an infected joint with high-volume saline solution

Lesser trochanter Large medial prominence distal to the neck of the femur; the site of the insertion of the iliopsoas tendon

Ligament A collagenous tissue that connects two bones to stabilize a joint

Limb salvage Surgical removal of a tumor without amputation of the affected extremity

Lisfranc fracture A fracture-dislocation of the tarsometatarsal joint

Longitudinal arch Arch along the long axis of the foot formed by the bones of the foot starting at the weight-bearing surface of the calcaneus and ending at the metatarsal heads

Lordosis Curvature of the spine that is convex anteriorly

Low-molecular-weight heparins (LMWHs) Anticoagulants that work by binding to antithrombin-III and catalyze its inactivation of factor Xa

Magnetic resonance imaging (MRI) An imaging modality that depends on the movement of protons in water molecules. When subjected to a magnetic field, protons that are normally randomly aligned become aligned. Radio waves directed at the tissue to be studied are used to change the alignment of these photons. When the radio waves are turned off, the protons emit a signal that is detected and processed by a computer into an image. In the musculoskeletal system, MRI is useful in diagnosing soft-tissue injuries, tumors, stress fractures, and infection.

Mallet finger An injury often caused by direct contact with a ball in which the finger is forced into flexion against resistance and the extensor tendons attaching to the distal phalanx may rupture

Malunion Healing of a fracture in an unacceptable position

Maximal oxygen consumption (VO2$_{max}$) Reflects the body's ability to maximally extract and use oxygen for aerobic metabolism; measures the lung's ability to extract oxygen

Mechanism of injury A representation of the patterns of energy that cause traumatic injuries

Medial Lying toward the midline

Medial capsular ligament Mid third of the true capsule of the knee joint; ligament extending from the femur to the midportion of the meniscus and then to the tibia

Medial collateral ligament Ligament on the medial aspect of the knee consisting of anterior, posterior, and oblique components and extending from the femur to the tibia

Medial condyle Forms the medial border of the upper surface of a joint

Medial malleolus The bony prominence at the end of the tibia that, together with the lateral malleolus, forms the sides of the ankle joint

Medial meniscus The medial C-shaped fibrocartilaginous structure of the knee

Medial patellar retinacula Extension of the vastus medialis that helps extend the knee joint

Medial retinaculum Structure composed of the aponeurosis of the vastus medial muscle itself; attaching along the medial border of the patella, its primary function is to hold the patella medially

Median nerve Nerve that controls sensation of the central palm, the thumb, and the first three fingers, as well as the ability to oppose the thumb to the little finger

Medullary canal The relatively hollow central core of a long bone that houses blood-forming cells

Meniscofemoral ligament With the meniscotibial ligament, it attaches the midportion of the medial meniscus peripherally to the tibia and the femur

Meniscotibial (coronary) ligament With the meniscofemoral ligament, it attaches the midportion of the medial meniscus peripherally to the tibia and femur

Meniscus A fibrocartilage structure interposed between articular cartilage. In the knee, the medial and lateral meniscus are semicircular structures on the periphery of the joint that act as protective buffers during walking and running activities

Merchant view An axial view of the patella in which the patient lies supine on the x-ray table with the knee flexed 45°. The cassette is held perpendicular to the tibia about halfway between the knee and ankle. The x-ray beam is directed caudally through the patella at an angle of 60° from vertical. This view is useful to evaluate subluxation of the patella and patellofemoral arthritis

Metacarpal bones The five bones of the hand that extend from the wrist to the fingers

Metaphysis The broad portion of a long bone adjacent to a joint. In children, the broad portion of a long bone includes the epiphysis, the physis, and the metaphysis.

Metastasis The transfer of disease from one part of the body to another; tumor metastasis usually occurs via the bloodstream or the lymphatic system

Metatarsus valgus Congenital deformity of the forefoot in which the forefoot is rotated laterally in relation to the hindfoot; also called metatarsus abductus

Metatarsus varus Congenital deformity of the forefoot in which the forefoot is rotated medially in relation to the hindfoot; also called metatarsus adductus

Microtrauma Destruction of a small number of cells caused by additive effects of repetitive forces

Midline Imaginary straight vertical line drawn from midforehead through the nose and the umbilicus to the floor

Modalities Physical agents that can create an optimum environment for injury healing, while reducing pain and discomfort

Monoarticular Affecting a single joint

Monteggia fracture Dislocation of the radial head in association with an ulnar fracture

Mortise view A view of the ankle in which the ankle is rotated internally so that the medial and lateral malleoli are parallel with the plane of the film. This view is used to assess reduction of the ankle joint as well as joint space narrowing

Morton foot Congenital abnormality characterized by a short first metatarsal, which throws weight-bearing stresses to the second metatarsal head, often resulting in pain

Myelogram X-ray study of the spine carried out after injection of a contrast material into the spinal cord sheath; helpful in diagnosing ruptured or bulging disks

Myelopathy An abnormal condition of the spinal cord, whether through disease or compression. The usual consequences are spasticity, impairment of sensation, and impairment of bowel and bladder function.

Myoblasts The embryonic cells that develop into skeletal muscle cells

Myofascial pain syndrome A painful musculoskeletal response that can follow muscle trauma

Myofibers The fibers that constitute a muscle

Myofibrils A slender thread within a muscle fiber that functions in muscle contraction

Myopathies A wide and varied group of primary muscle disorders characterized by weakness

Myositis ossificans Abnormal production of bone within muscle

Myotome

Navicular bone Bone with which the head of the talus articulates on the medial side of the foot; also a bone in the wrist that articulates with the trapezium, trapezoid, and other carpal bones

Neck The constricted portion of a structure (eg, femoral neck)

Nerve conduction studies Studies that test the speed by which motor, sensory, or mixed (combined motor and sensory) nerves transmit impulses

Neuralgia Pain along the course of a nerve

Neurapraxia A temporary loss of neural function

Neuritis Inflammation or irritation of a nerve

Neuroma A tumor composed of nerve cells

Neuropathic arthritis The chronic, progressive destruction of a joint that is caused by the loss of sensation from an underlying neurologic dysfunction; also known as Charcot arthropathy

Neuropathy An abnormal condition involving a peripheral nerve

Nocioceptive Pain-sensing

Nondisplaced fracture Fracture in which there is no deformity of the limb

Nonlamellar (woven) bone Immature bone

Nonossifying fibromas Osteolytic and sometimes painful proliferative lesions composed of spindle (fibrous) cells

Nonsteroidal anti-inflammatory drugs (NSAIDs) Inhibitors of cyclooxygenase and therefore prostaglandin synthesis

Nonunion Failure of healing of a fracture or osteotomy. With continued motion through a nonunion, a pseudarthrosis will form

Nucleus pulposus The central core of gelatinous material within intervertebral disks

Oblique fracture A fracture in which the fracture line crosses the bone diagonally

Oblique view A view in which the x-ray beam passes at an angle somewhere between an AP or PA view and a lateral view

Odontoid view An open-mouth AP view of the C2 vertebra used to identify fractures of the odontoid (dens) process of C2

Olecranon bursa Bursa in the elbow that separates the skin from the underlying ulna; allows the soft tissue to glide smoothly over the olecranon process

Olecranon process Bony process of the proximal ulna that prevents hyperextension of the elbow

Open fracture A fracture in which the skin is broken, exposing the fracture site to the environment

Open reduction An open surgical procedure in which normal or near-normal relationships are restored to a fractured bone or dislocated joint

Open reduction and internal fixation (ORIF) A procedure that involves incising the skin and soft tissue to repair a fracture under direct visualization

Origin The more fixed end or attachment of a muscle

Osteitis pubis An inflammatory condition of the pubic bones caused by repetitive stress on the symphysis pubis

Osteoblasts The cells that synthesize the organic component of bone; also thought of as the bone-forming cells

Osteochondral fractures Injuries that disrupt articular cartilage and the underlying subchondral bone

Osteochondritis dissecans (OCD) A localized abnormality of a focal portion of the subchondral bone, which can result in loss of support for the overlying articular cartilage

Osteoclasts Large cells that resorb bone matrix when activated

Osteocytes The cells of established bone

Osteogenesis imperfecta A hereditary disorder of connective tissue caused by mutations in the gene for type I collagen

Osteoid osteoma A small, benign, but painful tumor usually found in the long bones or the posterior elements of the spine

Osteolysis Dissolution of bone, particularly as resulting from excessive resorption

Osteomyelitis Infection of bone, either bacterial or mycotic

Osteonecrosis The death of bone, often as a result of obstruction of its blood supply

Osteophytes Overgrowth of bone, common in osteoarthritis and spinal stenosis

Osteosarcoma A primary sarcoma of the bone that is characterized by the direct formation of bone or osteoid tissue by the tumor cells

Osteosynthesis The process of bony union, as in fracture healing. It is a biologic welding process that is sometimes facilitated with grafts of bone from the iliac crest and insertion of fixation devices

Osteotomy Literally, cutting a bone. Used to describe surgical procedures in which bone is cut and realigned

Os trigonum A bony ossicle posterior to the talus

Overload principle States that strength, power, endurance, and hypertrophy of muscle can only increase when a muscle performs workloads greater than those previously encountered

Paget disease A condition of abnormally increased and disorganized bone remodeling

Palmar The anterior surface of the forearm, wrist, and hand

Panner disease Osteonecrosis of the capitellum seen in teenagers

Pannus A proliferation of synovium beginning at the periphery of the joint surface as seen in rheumatoid arthritis

Parasympathetic (craniosacral) nervous system A part of the autonomic nervous system that causes blood vessels to dilate, slows the heart rate, and relaxes muscle sphincters

Parathyroid hormone The major regulator of calcium homeostasis; promotes increased levels of serum calcium

Paresthesias Abnormal sensations such as tingling, burning, or prickling

Pars interarticularis Part of the vertebra posteriorly between the spinal arch and the pedicle

Patella Kneecap

Patellar ligament *see* **patellar tendon**

Patellar plicae A synovial fold that may persist into adult life and cause medial knee pain in the absence of trauma

Patellar tendon The extension of the quadriceps mechanism from the patella to the tibia; also called patellar ligament

Patellectomy Surgical excision of the patella

Patellofemoral groove Groove that runs anteriorly between the condyles of the femur; the patella lies in the trochlear groove

Pathologic fracture A fracture caused by a normal load on abnormal bone, which is often weakened by tumor, infection, or metabolic bone disease

Patient-controlled analgesia (PCA) The intravenous or epidural delivery of narcotics via a pump that is controlled by the patient

Pectoralis major A muscle of the upper chest, originating from the anterior surface of the medial half of the clavicle and the anterior surface of the sternum, the superior six costal cartilages, and the aponeurosis of the external oblique muscle and inserting on the lateral lip of the intertubercular groove of the humerus, which adducts and medially rotates the humerus; draws the scapula anteriorly and inferiorly. Acting alone, the clavicular head flexes the humerus and the sternocostal head extends it.

Pelvic cavity Space between the pelvis walls

Pelvis A bony ring, consisting of the sacrum, coccyx, and innominate bones, that connects the trunk to the lower extremities, supports the abdominal contents, and allows passage of the excretory canals

Percutaneous pinning Insertion of pins into bone through small puncture wounds in the skin for stabilization of a fracture or a dislocated joint that was realigned by closed reduction.

Periosteum A sleeve of connective tissue that surrounds the shaft of the bone and contributes to fracture healing

Peritendinitis Inflammation of the tendon sheath, marked by pain, swelling, and, occasionally, local crepitus

Permeative margin An indistinct margin visible on radiographic images that signifies the hazy transition between growing tumors and normal bone

Peroneus brevis muscle Muscle in the lateral compartment of the leg that functions to evert the ankle; it passes distal and inferior to the lateral malleolus and inserts on the base of the fifth metatarsal; acts to plantar flex and abduct the foot

Peroneus longus muscle Muscle in the lateral compartment of the leg that functions to evert the ankle; it passes under the cuboid bone and inserts on the inferior surface of the medial cuneiform and base of the first metatarsal; it acts to plantar flex, abduct, and evert the foot

Phagocytosis The process by which white blood cells ingest debris or microorganisms

Phalanges Bones making up the skeleton of the fingers or toes

Phonophoresis The transdermal introduction of a topically applied medication (usually either an anti-inflammatory or analgesic) into soft tissue using ultrasound

Physis The growth plate. Specialized cartilaginous tissue interposed between the metaphysis and epiphysis in long bones in children. Provides growth in length of the bone.

Pigmented villonodular synovitis A proliferative process of the synovial membrane of unknown etiology

Placebo effect The placebo effect is the measurable, observable, or felt improvement in health not attributable to treatment. This effect is believed by many people to be due to the placebo itself in some mysterious way. A placebo (Latin for "I shall please") is a medication or treatment believed by the administrator of the treatment to be inert or innocuous.

Plantar The sole, or flexor surface, of the foot

Plantar calcaneonavicular ligament Sling ligament supporting the longitudinal arch

Plantar fascia Fibrous tissue band that runs from the calcaneal tuberosity to the phalanges and supports the talus

Plantar fasciitis Irritation of the plantar fascia, usually from overuse; the pain is most severe at the calcaneal tuberosity

Planus Flattening of the arch of the foot

Plyometric exercises Exercises that use explosive movements to increase athletic power

Polyarticular Affecting multiple joints

Polyneuropathies Neuropathies of several peripheral nerves simultaneously

Popliteal artery Continuation of the superficial femoral artery in the popliteal space (posterior surface of the knee); supplies the knee and the calf

Popliteal fossa The hollow area on the posterior surface of the knee; popliteal space

Popliteus muscle Muscle deep to the popliteal artery with three proximal insertions on the tibia; its primary function is internal rotation of the tibia on the femur

Portable transcutaneous electrical nerve stimulation (TENS) unit A portable therapeutic modality that uses electrical stimulation to attempt to modulate pain, strengthen muscles, and enhance soft-tissue healing

Posterior cruciate ligament (PCL) Ligament extending from the tibia to the medial surface of the intercondylar notch of the femur that functions with the anterior cruciate ligament in anteroposterior and rotatory stability of the knee

Posterior glenohumeral dislocation Disruption of the glenohumeral joint in a posterior direction

Posterior interosseous nerve The major terminal branch of the radial nerve that winds around the radius to the dorsal side of the forearm to provide motor and sensory function to the dorsal forearm and wrist

Posterior process That part of each vertebra that can be palpated, as it lies just under the skin in the midline of the back

Posterior sternoclavicular dislocation Disruption of the sternoclavicular joint posteriorly

Posterior talofibular ligament one of the three lateral ligaments of the ankle; the strongest of the three, it helps to resist forward dislocation of the leg on the foot

Posterior tibial artery Artery that is just posterior to the medial malleolus; supplies blood to the foot

Posterior tibial syndrome Pain along the posterior medial border of the tibia; thought to be secondary to a tight posterior tibial muscle "pulling" on the periosteum in this area; associated with running

Posterior tibial tendon One of the structures that creates a dynamic sling supporting the longitudinal arch; attaches directly on the tuberosity of the navicular bone and indirectly on the plantar surface of the navicular and middle cuneiform bones

Posterior tibiofibular ligament Part of the talofibular syndesmosis, arises from the posterior calculi on the lateral side of the tibia; helps to hold the fibula snug in its tibial groove

Posterolateral rotatory instability The lateral tibial plateau rotates posteriorly in relationship to the femur

Posteromedial rotatory instability The medial tibial plateau rotates posteriorly on the femur, with associated medial opening

Postmenopausal osteoporosis The most prevalent form of primary osteoporosis

Postmenopausal osteoporosis The most prevalent form of primary osteoporosis

Posttraumatic arthritis A form of secondary osteoarthritis caused by a loss of joint congruence and normal joint biomechanics

Preload Reflection of cardiac muscle quality; an elastic distensible ventricle propels more blood more rapidly than a stiffer, less distensible ventricle

Primary bone healing The end-to-end repair process that occurs when the bone ends are anatomically opposed and held together rigidly; no callus forms

Primary osteoarthritis Osteoarthritis without an identified cause; characterized by progressive loss of articular cartilage and reactive changes in the bone, leading to the destruction and painful malfunction of the joint

Proprioception A sense or perception, usually at a subconscious level, of the movements and position of the body and especially its limbs, independent of vision; this sense is gained primarily from input from sensory nerve terminals in muscles and tendons (muscle spindles) and the fibrous capsule of joints combined with input from the vestibular apparatus

Proteoglycans Complex macromolecules that consist of a protein core with covalently bound polysaccharide (glycosaminoglycan) chains

Proximal describing structures that are closer to the trunk

Proximal patellar realignment Proximal soft-tissue reconstruction designed to align the muscle pull on the patella to enhance the action of the vastus medialis obliquus and to tighten the medial capsule

Pseudarthrosis A false joint produced when a fracture or arthrodesis fails to heal

Pseudofractures Lines of radiolucency that represent stress fractures with unmineralized osteoid

Pubic symphysis Firm fibrocartilaginous joint anteriorly between the two innominate bones

Pubis One of the three bones (ilium, ischium, and pubis) that fuse to form the pelvis

Pulmonary embolism Migration of a thrombus from a large vein (often in the leg) to the lung, causing obstruction of blood flow, respiratory distress, or even death

Quadriceps angle (Q angle) An angle formed by the intersection of two lines: one line is drawn from the anterosuperior iliac spine to the midpatella; the second is drawn from the midpatella to the anterior tibial tuberosity. These lines parallel the quadriceps and patellar tendons.

Quadriceps femoris Tendon located at the superior border of the patella, or kneecap

Quadriceps muscle Extensor muscle situated at the front of the thigh; composed of four components: the vastus medialis, vastus lateralis, vastus intermedius, and rectus femoris

Quadriceps tendon Convergence of the four muscles of the quadriceps—the rectus femoris, vastus intermedius, vastus medialis, and vastus lateralis; inserts in the superior pole of the patella

Radial artery One of the major arteries of the arm; it can be palpated at the base of the thumb

Radial nerve Nerve carrying sensation to the greater portion of the back of the hand and controlling extension of the hand at the wrist

Radial styloid Bony prominence felt on the lateral (thumb) side of the wrist

Radiculopathies A group of nerve root disorders often caused by nerve root compression or central or neuroforaminal stenosis

Radius Bone on the thumb side of the forearm

Range of motion (ROM) The amount of movement available at a joint

Reflex Fairly fixed pattern of response or behavior similar for any given stimulus; does not involve a conscious action

Rehabilitation Restoration, following disease, illness, or injury, of the ability to function in a normal or near-normal manner

Resection arthroplasty A procedure in which the surfaces of diseased bone are excised, allowing fibrocartilage to grow in its place

Revascularization A procedure to provide an additional blood supply to fractured bone

Rheumatoid arthritis A chronic inflammatory disease that is probably triggered by an antigen-mediated inflammatory reaction against the synovium in the joint

Rhomboid Muscle of the trunk that helps to stabilize and maneuver the shoulder girdle

RICE method A method of treatment of acute injury that is used to counteract the body's initial response to injury; RICE is an acronym for rest, ice, compression, and elevation

Rickets The childhood form of osteomalacia

Rigid splint Splint made from firm material and applied to sides, front, and/or back of an injured extremity to prevent motion at the injury site

Romberg test Used to test for deficits in the sensory systems that provide stability to the trunk. Standing with the feet together, the patient closes his or her eyes. Signs of swaying are a positive sign.

Rotator cuff The rotator cuff is made up of four muscles and their tendons. These combine to form a "cuff" over the head of the humerus. The four muscles—the supraspinatus, infraspinatus, subscapularis, and teres minor—originate from the scapula and together form a single tendon unit that inserts on the greater tuberosity of the humerus. The rotator cuff helps to lift and rotate the arm and to stabilize the ball of the shoulder within the joint.

Rotator cuff impingement, external Impingement of the rotator cuff on the acromion and the coracoacromial ligament; causes microtrauma to the cuff, resulting in local inflammation, edema, cuff softening, pain, and poor function of the cuff

Rotator cuff impingement, internal A condition in the shoulder of throwing athletes that results in tears of the underside of the rotator cuff and the posterior labrum

Sacroiliac joint The joint formed by the articulation of the sacrum and ilium

Sacrum One of the three bones (sacrum and two pelvic bones) that make up the pelvic ring

Saddle anesthesia Decreased sensation around the perineum

Saddle embolus A condition in which one or both of the major pulmonary arteries are totally occluded

Sarcolemma Muscle-cell membrane and its associated basement membrane

Sarcomeres The fundamental components of the contracting unit of the myofibril

Sarcopenia The loss of muscle mass and strength as a result of aging

Sarcoplasmic reticulum A continuous branching network of membrane, which is a specialized form of endoplasmic reticulum unique to muscle

Sartorius muscle One of the medial hamstring muscles that form the pes anserinus and help protect the knee against rotatory and valgus stress (the other pes anserinus muscles are the gracilis and semitendinosus)

Scapula The shoulder blade

Scapular Y view A lateral view of the shoulder taken so that the blade of the scapula, the coracoid process, and the spine of the scapula form a "Y." Used to evaluate anterior and posterior glenohumeral shoulder dislocations. Also called a transscapular view.

Scapulothoracic joint Articulation in which the scapula is suspended from the posterior thoracic wall through muscular attachments to the ribs and spine

Scheuermann disease Osteochondrosis of the vertebral epiphysis resulting in increased thoracic kyphosis in the preteen and early adolescent years

Schwann cell A specialized support cell that encases nerve fibers

Sclerotic border A sharp, geographic margin visible on radiographic images that signifies the transition between inactive or slow-growing tumors and normal bone

Scoliosis Lateral curvature of the spine

Secondary bone healing The repair process that is characterized by the formation of fracture callus, which then remodels to form new bone

Secondary osteoarthritis Osteoarthritis resulting from known precipitants such as bone ischemia, trauma, and neuropathy

Secondary osteoporosis Osteoporosis characterized by conditions in which bone is lost because of the presence of another disease, such as hormonal imbalances, malignancies, or gastrointestinal disorders, or because of corticosteroid use

Second-degree burns Partial-thickness burns that extend down to the dermis; characterized by painful blistering of the skin

Selective estrogen receptor modulator (SERM) A class of drugs that is thought to provide the beneficial effects of hormone replacement therapy without some of its adverse effects

Semimembranosus muscle Muscle extending from the ischial tuberosity to the tibia that acts to flex the leg and extend the thigh; important stabilizing structure to the posterior aspect of the knee

Semitendinosus muscle One of the hamstring muscles that comprise the pes anserinus and help protect the knee against rotatory and valgus stress (the other pes anserinus muscles are the gracilis and sartorius)

Senile osteoporosis Osteoporosis in which an age-related decline in renal production of active vitamin D is the probable cause of bone loss

Sensory nerve action potential (SNAP) The latency, amplitude, and conduction velocity recorded in sensory nerve conduction studies

Sensory nerves Nerves that carry sensations of touch, taste, heat, cold, pain, or other modalities to the spinal cord or brain

Septic arthritis Infection of a joint, either bacterial or mycotic

Sequestrum . In osteomyelitis, the dead portion of bone inside and walled off by the involucrum. *See also* involucrum.

Serratus anterior Muscle of the trunk that helps to stabilize and maneuver the shoulder girdle

Sesamoid bones Two small bones located beneath the first metatarsal head that function as extra weight-bearing structures and leverage points for the mechanics of the great toe

Sesamoiditis Inflammation of the sesamoid bones of the great toe

Sever disease Osteochondrosis of the calcaneal apophysis seen in children aged 6 to 10 years

Shaft The long, straight, cylindrical midportion of a bone

Sharpey's fibers The small collagen fibers that attach tendon to bone; in the spine they connect the outer edges of intervertebral disks to the vertebral bodies

Shin-splints Anterior or posterior tibial tendinitis

Short collateral ligament Ligament running parallel to the fibular collateral ligament and attaching to the fibular head posterior to the biceps tendon; also called fabellofibular ligament when it is attached to the fabella; reinforces the posterior capsule and contributes to the lateral stability of the knee

Shoulder dislocation *see* glenohumeral dislocation

Skeletal homeostasis The function of bone that supplies structural support and movement for the body

Skeletal survey Screening radiographs of the entire skeleton

Skeletal (voluntary) muscle Striated muscles that are attached to bones and usually cross at least one joint

Skeleton The skeletal system; the supporting framework of the human body, composed of 206 bones

Slocum anterolateral rotatory instability test Modification of the lateral pivot shift test in which the patient lies on his or her side with the uninvolved leg flexed at the hip and the examiner applies an internal rotation force to the proximal tibia and a valgus stress to the joint; at 20° of flexion the knee visibly, palpably, and audibly reduces

Slocum external rotation test One of the tests for anteromedial-rotatory instability conducted with the hip flexed to approximately 45° and the knee to approximately 80°; a forward motion is applied to the thigh and the degree of anterior drawer is assessed

Slow twitch muscle fibers Type I muscle fibers

Smooth muscle Nonstriated, involuntary muscle that constitutes the bulk of the gastrointestinal tract and is present in nearly every organ to regulate automatic activity

Soleus muscle Muscle, extending from the proximal fibula to the calcaneus, that acts to extend and rotate the foot

Spinal column Central supporting bony structure of the body; vertebral column

Spinal cord Extension of the brain, composed of virtually all the nerves carrying messages between the brain and the rest of the body. It lies inside of and is protected by the vertebrae and the spinal column

Spinal stenosis Narrowing of the canal housing the spinal cord; commonly caused by encroachment of bone

Spine Column of 33 vertebrae extending from the base of the skull to the tip of the coccyx

Spinous processes Palpable prominences in the vertebrae

Spiral fracture A fracture caused by a twisting force that results in a helical fracture line

Splint Device used to immobilize part of the body

Sprain Partial or complete tear of a ligament

Static stretching The passive stretching of a given antagonist muscle by placing it in a position of maximal stretch and holding it there for an extended period

Stem cells Cells with the unlimited ability of self-renewal and regeneration; serve to regenerate tissue

Stenosis A stricture of any canal or orifice. In the spine, a narrowing of the spinal canal secondary to a combination of disk narrowing, thickening of the ligamentum flavum, and osteophytes from arthritis of the facet joints.

Sternoclavicular dislocation Disruption of the articulation that lies between the clavicle and the sternum

Sternoclavicular joint Articulation between the sternum and the clavicle

Sternocleidomastoid Cervical muscle that produces rotation of the head

Sternum Breastbone

Straight lateral laxity Abnormal motion with lateral opening of the joint, or varus laxity; demonstrating injury to the fibular collateral ligament and lateral capsular structures

Straight medial laxity Abnormal motion with medial opening of the joint, or valgus laxity; reflecting damage to the tibial collateral ligament

Strain Partial tear of a muscle

Stress fracture An overuse injury in which the body cannot repair microscopic damage to the bone as quickly as it is induced, leading to painful, weakened bone

Stryker notch view A special view of the shoulder used to demonstrate a Hill-Sachs lesion (a compression fracture of the humeral head on the posterolateral aspect of the articular surface) seen after recurrent anterior dislocations of the shoulder. This view is taken with the patient supine, the hand of the affected shoulder on the top of the head, and the x-ray beam directed 10° cephalad.

Subacromial bursa Bursa that lies in the subacromial space and acts as the protective tissue between the cuff and the bony acromion

Subacute stage Time period between acute and chronic injury

Subluxation An incomplete disruption in the relationship of two bones forming a joint, ie, a partial dislocation. The joint surfaces retain partial contact.

Supraspinatus The most superior muscle that arises from the dorsal surface of the scapula and inserts on the greater tuberosity; part of the rotator cuff

Sympathetic (thoracolumbar) nervous system Part of the autonomic nervous system that causes blood vessels to constrict, stimulates sweating, increases the heart rate, causes the sphincter muscles to constrict, and prepares the body to respond to stress

Symptom Evidence of change in body functions apparent to the patient and expressed to the examiner on questioning

Synapse A specialized site at which an electrical signal is transmitted chemically across a junction to produce a similar electrical impulse on the opposite side

Syndesmosis A form of fibrous joint in which opposing surfaces that are relatively far apart are united by ligaments; eg, the fibrous union between the radius and ulna (radioulnar syndesmosis)

Synovial fluid The straw-colored fluid in the joint that is formed by filtration of capillary plasma

Synovial joints A joint formed by the articulation of two bones, the ends of which are lined with hyaline cartilage and is surrounded by a capsule which is lined with synovium.

Synoviocytes Cells that form the synovial membrane, remove debris, and secrete hyaluronic acid

Synovitis A condition characterized by inflammation of the synovial lining

Synovium The thin membrane that lines a joint capsule. There are two types of synovial cells. Type A act as macrophages and type B produce synovial fluid for joint lubrication. Marked hypertrophy of the synovium occurs with an inflammatory arthritis.

Tai chi A low-impact exercise program that is derived from the martial arts in China and was founded in accordance with the belief that chi (also called qi) is a vital life force flowing through the body

Talus One of the bones forming the ankle joint. It lies below and articulates with the distal tibia.

Tarsal bones Seven bones that make up the rear portion of the foot

Tarsal coalition Fusion of two or more of the major tarsal bones (talus, navicular, calcaneus, and cuboid)

Tarsal tunnel syndrome A neuritis of the posterior tibial nerve resulting in pain and/or numbness along the course of the nerve

Tendinitis Injury to the tendon or musculotendinous unit caused by the application of mechanical loads of high intensity or high frequency

Tendinosis lesion Asymptomatic tendon degeneration caused either by aging or by cumulative microtrauma without inflammation

Tendon A specialized type of collagenous tissue that attaches muscle to bone. Tendons transmit forces of muscular contraction to cause motion across a joint.

Tennis elbow Inflammation of muscle origins at the lateral epicondyle; *also called* lateral epicondylitis

Tenocytes The cells in tendons

Tenosynovitis Inflammation of the thin inner lining of a tendon sheath

Tenosynovium The sheath surrounding a tendon that enhances movement or gliding of the tendon as it transmits muscle forces across joints

Teres minor The most inferior muscle that arises from the dorsal surface of the scapula and inserts on the greater tuberosity; part of the rotator cuff

Therapeutic ultrasound The use of high-energy sound waves for healing purposes. Frequently used by physical therapists to reduce inflammation but increasingly used to heal enthesopathies, such as plantar fasciitis, lateral epicondylitis (tennis elbow), and impingement syndrome of the shoulder, as well as nonunions of fractures.

Thoracic outlet syndrome A constellation of symptoms arising from compression of the vascular or neural components of the brachial plexus in the thoracic outlet

Thrombus A blood clot within a vessel

Tibia Shinbone; the larger of the two leg bones

Tibial collateral ligament One of the major ligamentous support structures of the knee; extends from the medial condyle of the femur to the medial condyle of the tibia and just slightly beyond

Tibialis anterior muscle Muscle located in the anterior compartment of the lower leg; inserts on the medial cuneiform and acts to flex and elevate the foot.

Tibialis posterior muscle One of the three muscles of the deep portion of the posterior compartment of the muscles of the leg; one of the medial stabilizers of the ankle, it acts to invert the foot and extend the ankle.

Tibial nerve Provides motor and sensory function to the lower leg; courses deep to the gastrocnemius muscle.

Tibial plateaus The expanded upper ends of the tibia that articulate with the femoral condyles to form the knee joints

Tibial tubercle The bony prominence of the proximal tibia

Tibiofemoral joint Polycentric hinge joint that bears the body's weight during locomotion; joint between each tibial and femoral condyle

Tibiofibular syndesmosis One of the three groups of ankle ligaments; arrangement of dense fibrous tissues between the osseous structures just above the ankle joint that maintains the relationship of the distal tibia and fibula

Tidemark A wavy bluish line visible on histologic staining with hematoxylin and eosin that signifies the border between the deep zone and the zone of calcified cartilage

Tinel sign Percussion of the median nerve at the wrist to demonstrate the degree of nerve irritability by reproducing symptoms of carpal tunnel syndrome

Tomography A radiographic modality that allows visualization of lesions or tissues that are obscured by overlying structures. Structures in front of and behind the level of tissue to be studied are blurred, which allows the object to be studied to be brought into sharp focus. Tomography has been used to evaluate the degree of fracture healing and to evaluate tumors such as osteoid osteoma. Increasingly, CT has replaced tomography as the imaging modality of choice in these circumstances.

Tonic-clonic A generalized seizure involving rigid (tonic) muscular contractions and repetitive (clonic) muscular spasms

Tophi Chalky deposits of urate surrounded by inflammatory cells

Torus (buckle) fracture A fracture that only buckles one side of the cortex. Typically seen in children because of the greater plasticity of their bones.

Traction Action of drawing or pullng on an object

Traction splint Splint that holds a lower extremity fracture or dislocaton immobile; allows steady longitudinal pull on the extremity

Transcutaneous electrical nerve stimulation (TENS) Therapeutic modality in which electrical stimulation is applied to the body with an intact peripheral nervous system; can elicit either sensory or muscular responses by stimulating nerves when electrical current passes across the skin.

Transverse fracture A fracture in which the fracture line is perpendicular to the shaft of the bone

Transverse plane Horizontal section of the body

Transverse processes Together with the posterior processes, the transverse processes allow the attachment of strong intervertebral ligaments that support the spine and also provide anchors for muscles attached to the spinal column

Trapezius Large diamond-shaped muscle lying just beneath the skin of the shoulder girdle lying posteriorly

Traumatic spondylolysis The condition in which one vertebra slips anterior to the one below it secondary to a trauma-induced defect in the right and left pars interarticularis

Triceps The muscle in the back of the upper arm that acts to extend the arm and forearm.

Trochanter Prominence on a bone where tendons insert; specifically, two protuberances, greater and lesser, on the femur

Trochanteric bursa One of the two most important bursae about the hip joint located just behind the greater trochanter and deep to the gluteus maximus and tensor fascia lata muscle

Trochlea A groove in a bone that articulates with another bone, or serves as a channel for a tendon to track in

T-score A score used to express the results of bone density tests derived from the difference between the bone density of the patient being tested and the peak bone density of a healthy, young adult population; a T-score is equivalent to one standard deviation above or below ideal bone mass

Tuberculosis A chronic granulomatous infection caused by the bacteria *Mycobacterium tuberculosis*

Tuberosity Prominence on a bone where tendons insert

Turf toe A hyperextension injury of the first metatarsophalangeal joint associated with athletic activity on hard surfaces

Type I muscle fibers (slow twitch) Muscle fibersidentified by a slow contraction time and a high resistance to fatigue; helpful with slow movements such as marathons

Type II muscle fibers (fast twitch) Muscle fibers identified by a fast contraction times and rapid fatigue; helpful in rapid movements such as sprints. Type II fibers are further divided in Type II A and Type II B. Type II B fibers have a moderate resistance to fatigue and represent a transition between the two extremes of the slow twitch and type II A fibers.

Type B synoviocytes A type of synovial cell that secretes hyaluronic acid

Ulnar artery Artery originating from the brachial artery and supplying the forearm, wrist, and hand

Ulnar nerve Nerve originating from the brachial plexus and coursing down the ulnar side of the arm, adjacent to the medial condyle of the elbow and into the ulnar side of the forearm; controls sensation over the fifth and ulnar half of the ring fingers and controls much of the muscular function of the hand

Ulnar shaft The long cylindrical portion of the ulna between the olecranon proximally and the styloid distally

Ulnar styloid Bony prominence of the ulna felt on the medial (little finger) side of the wrist

Ultrasound (Ultrasonography) An imaging modality in which images are created from high-frequency sound waves (7.5 to 10 MHz [1 MHz = one million cycles per second]) that reflect off of different tissues. The reflected sound waves are recorded and processed by a computer and then converted into an image. Ultrasound is used to evaluate infant hip disorders and tears of the rotator cuff.

Valgus Angulation of a distal bone away from the midline in relation to its proximal partner. Genu valgum is a knock-knee deformity, with abduction of the tibia in relation to the femur. Can also be used to describe angulation of fractures or bony deformities.

Varus Angulation of a distal bone toward the midline in relation to its proximal partner. Genu varum is a bowleg deformity, with adduction of the tibia in relation to the femur. Can also be used to describe angulation of fractures or bony deformities.

Vastus intermedius A component of the quadriceps muscle that lies in the midline of the thigh and anterior to the femur

Vastus lateralis A component of the quadriceps muscle that lies lateral to the midline of the thigh and anterior and lateral to the femur

Vastus medialis A component of the quadriceps muscle that lies medial to the midline of the thigh and anterior to the femur

Vastus medialis obliquus (VMO) A smaller component of the vastus medialis muscle

Vertebral arch Part of the vertebra composed of the right and left pedicles and the right and left laminae; also called neural arch

Vertebral body compression Compression fracture of the vertebral body without damage to the ligamentous structures; the most common thoracic fracture; also called wedge fracture

Vertebral column Segmented spinal column composed of 24 movable vertebrae, 5 fixed sacral vertebrae, and 4 fixed coccygeal vertebrae

Vertebrochondral ribs Ribs that articulate directly with the sternum via their costal cartilages

Vertebrosternal ribs Ribs that connect the first 10 thoracic vertebrae to the sternum

Viscoelastic Having mechanical properties that depend on the loading rate of an applied force

Viscosupplements Intra-articular hyaluronic acid preparations commonly used to treat osteoarthritis; thought to increase joint lubrication

Volar Toward the anterior surface of the body.

Volkmann contracture Volkmann contracture is a deformity of the hand, fingers, and wrist caused by injury to the muscles of the forearm. It is most commonly secondary to compartment syndrome after fracture or other trauma to the forearm. Also sometimes caused by inadvertent injection of caustic material (drugs) into the arterial system of the forearm.

Voluntary (skeletal) muscle Muscle, under direct voluntary control of the brain, which can be contracted or relaxed at will

Warfarin An anticoagulant drug that reduces the synthesis of vitamin K–dependent clotting factors II, VII, IX, and X in the liver

West Point axillary view An axillary view of the shoulder in which the patient is prone on the x-ray table with a pillow placed under the affected shoulder, the arm abducted 90°, and the forearm hanging off the edge of the table. The cassette is placed against the top of the shoulder, and the x-ray beam is then directed at the axilla, angled 25° toward the table surface and 25° toward the patient's midline. Useful to visualize potential damage to the anterior glenoid rim and Hill-Sachs lesions after an anterior dislocation.

Wolff's law A law that states that the growth and remodeling of bone is influenced and modulated by mechanical stresses.

Woven bone Primitive, less-organized form of cortical bone

X-rays Radiant energy produced by exposing tungsten to a beam of electrons; useful in imaging many body parts

Y scapular view A view taken tangential to the scapula. Normally, the humeral head sits in the convergence of the "Y," which comprises the scapula, acromion, and coracoid. Useful view to identify anterior and posterior dislocations of the glenohumeral joint.

Yoga A variety of disciplines designed to bring practitioners into union with mankind and a higher god or life force

Z-score Compares the patient's bone mineral density (BMD) with what is expected in someone of the same age and body size. Among older adults, however, low BMD is common, so comparison with age-matched norms can be misleading and therefore the T-score is more important.

Index

Page numbers with *f* indicate figures.
Page numbers with *t* indicate tables.

diagnostic tests of, 693
differential diagnosis of, 693
exercise program for, 695–696
physical examination of, 692
rehabilitation for, 694
treatment of, 693–694
Quadriceps tendon, of rupture, 697–699
   adverse disease outcomes from, 698
   areas of, 698*f*
   clinical symptoms of, 697
   definition of, 697
   diagnostic tests of, 697
   differential diagnosis of, 698
   physical examination of, 697
   treatment of, 698–699

R

RA. *See* Rheumatoid arthritis
Rabies, 416
Radial deficiency, 1038
Radial head
   dislocation of, congenital, 1048–1049
   fracture of, 367–369
     adverse disease outcomes from, 368
     classification of, 367*f*
     clinical symptoms of, 367
     definition of, 367
     differential diagnosis of, 368, 372
     physical examination of, 368
     tests of, 368
     treatment of, 368–369
   subluxation of, 1004
Radial nerve
   capture of, 280*f*
   test of, 411
Radial tunnel syndrome
   clinical symptoms of, 385
   differential diagnosis of, 372
   exercise program for, 375–376
   treatment of, 387
Radiculopathy. *See* Cervical radiculopathy; Lumbar disk herniation
Radiography, 128–129
   advantages/disadvantages of, 128*t*
   indications for, 129
   of rheumatoid arthritis (RA), 46*f*
   of seronegative spondyloarthropathies, 56
   of shoulder arthritis, 269*f*–270*f*
   views with, common, 130*t*
Radioulnar synostosis, congenital, 1047–1048

Radius, 471*f*. *See also specific radial feature*
   distal, fracture of, adult, 474–478
     adverse disease outcomes from, 476
     clinical symptoms of, 475
     definition of, 474–475
     diagnostic tests of, 476, 477*f*
     differential diagnosis of, 476
     neurologic dysfunction with, 478
     physical examination of, 475
     progressive collapse of, 478
     treatment of, 476–477
     types of, 474*f*
   distal, fracture of, childhood, 1085–1088
     clinical symptoms of, 1085
     definition of, 1085
     diagnostic tests of, 1086
     differential diagnosis of, 1086
     physical examination of, 1086
     treatment of, 1087–1088
     types of, 1085*t*
Rand 36-Item Health Survey, 69
Range of motion
   ankle
     exercises for, 760, 760*f*, 766, 766*f*
     measurement of, 748–749
   of cervical spine, 914–915
   elbow, measurement of, 348–349
   of hand, 407
   hip, measurement of, 543–546
   of knee, measurement of, 634–635
   in musculoskeletal evaluation in, 9
   in overhead throwing shoulder, 307
   in pediatric orthopaedics, 980–981, 986
   restoration of, 176–180
   of shoulder, 246, 257–259, 986
   thigh, measurement of, 543–546
   of toe, great, 750
   of wrist, 408
Ray resection, 16
Reactive arthritis, 54
Reduction maneuver
   incomplete, 360*f*
   neurovascular injury from, 359–360
   shoulder
     adverse outcomes from, 326
     aftercare instructions for, 326–327
     gravity-assisted, 325–326, 325*f*
     longitudinal traction technique for, 326, 326*f*
     Stimson technique for, 325–326, 325*f*

Reflex
   deep tendon, 905
   Hoffmann, 918
Reflex sympathetic dystrophy, 67, 1029
Rehabilitation, 175–182
   for achilles tendon tear, 759
   for ACL tear, 642–643
   for acromioclavicular injuries, 265
   adverse outcomes from, 182
   for ankle sprain, 765
   athletic injury guidelines for, 176*t*
   canes, crutches, and walkers in, 217
   for carpal tunnel syndrome, 439
   for cervical sprain, 931
   for collateral ligament tear, 665
   for CRPS, 71
   definition of, 175
   for epicondylitis, 373
   for fibromyalgia syndrome, 107
   for frozen shoulder, 293
   for gastrocnemius tear, 681
   goals of, 175–176
   for hip strains, 593, 593*t*
   impingement syndrome treatment with, 297–298
   for knee arthritis, 653
   for LBP, acute, 942–943
   for LBP, chronic, 948
   for Legg-Calvé-Perthes disease, 1126
   for meniscal tear, 687
   for patellar/quadriceps tendinitis, 694
   for patellofemoral pain, 706–707
   for PCL tear, 722
   for plantar fasciitis, 842
   for plica syndrome, 713
   for posterior heel pain, 851
   rotator cuff tear treatment with, 314
   for SLAP lesion, 330
   for snapping hip, 587–588
   therapeutic modalities in, 180–181, 181*t*
   for thigh strains, 599
   for toe deformities, 878
   for trochanteric bursitis, 611
Reiter syndrome, 52*t*, 1174
Reproductive system, pathology of, 533
Resisted supination/external rotation test, 328–329
Retrocalcaneal bursitis, as dance injury, 787